INTRODUCTION TO HEALTH SERVICES

WILEY SERIES IN HEALTH SERVICES
Stephen J. Williams, Sc.D., Series Editor

Introduction to Health Services, second edition
Stephen J. Williams and Paul R. Torrens, Editors

Issues in Health Services
Stephen J. Williams, Editor

Health Care Economics, second edition
Paul J. Feldstein

Maternal and Child Health Practices: Problems, Resources, and Methods of Delivery, second edition
Helen M. Wallace, Edwin M. Gold, and Allan C. Oglesby, Editors

Rural Health Care
Roger A. Rosenblatt and Ira S. Moscovice

Planning Methods: For Health and Related Organizations
Paul C. Nutt

Health Care Management: A Text in Organization Theory and Behavior
Stephen M. Shortell and Arnold D. Kaluzny, Editors

Ambulatory Care Organization and Management
Austin Ross, Stephen J. Williams, and Eldon L. Schafer

Health Politics and Policy
Theodor J. Litman and Leonard S. Robins, Editors

INTRODUCTION TO HEALTH SERVICES

SECOND EDITION

Edited by

Stephen J. Williams, Sc.D.

Professor of Public Health
Head, Division of Health Services Administration
Graduate School of Public Health
San Diego State University
San Diego, California

Paul R. Torrens, M.D., M.P.H.

Professor of Health Services Administration
School of Public Health
University of California, Los Angeles
Los Angeles, California

A WILEY MEDICAL PUBLICATION
JOHN WILEY & SONS
New York • Chichester • Brisbane • Toronto • Singapore

Cover design: Wanda Lubelska
Production Supervisor: Audrey Pavey

Library of Congress Cataloging in Publication Data

Main entry under title:

Introduction to health services.

(Wiley series in health services, ISSN 0195-3907)
(Wiley medical publication)
Includes index.
1. Medical care—United States. 2. Health services
administration—United States. I. Williams, Stephen
Joseph, 1948–   II. Torrens, Paul R. III. Series.
IV. Series: Wiley medical publication. [DNLM: 1. Health
services—United States. W 84 AA1 I9]

RA395.A3I57 1984   362.'0973   83-14831
ISBN 0-471-86900-7

Printed in the United States of America

10 9 8 7

For D. and N. Williams
and C., J., C., J.C., and N. Torrens

Contributors

A. E. Benjamin, Jr., Ph.D.
Assistant Adjunct Professor and Associate Director
Aging Health Policy Center
Department of Social and Behavioral Sciences
University of California, San Francisco
San Francisco, California

Thomas W. Bice, Ph.D.
Professor and Director
Graduate Program in Health Services Administration and Planning
School of Public Health and Community Medicine
University of Washington
Seattle, Washington

Robert H. Brook, M.D., Sc.D.
Professor of Medicine and Public Health
University of California, Los Angeles
Center for the Health Sciences
Los Angeles, California
Senior Health Services Researcher
The Rand Corporation
Santa Monica, California

William L. Dowling, Ph.D.
Clinical Professor of Health Services
School of Public Health and Community Medicine
University of Washington
Vice-President, Planning and Policy Development
Sisters of Providence Corporation
Seattle, Washington

Arnold D. Kaluzny, Ph.D.
Professor
Department of Health Policy and Administration
School of Public Health
University of North Carolina
Chapel Hill, North Carolina

Robert L. Kane, M.D.
Professor
Schools of Medicine and Public Health
University of California, Los Angeles
Los Angeles, California
Senior Researcher
The Rand Corporation
Santa Monica, California

Rosalie A. Kane, D.S.W.
Social Scientist
The Rand Corporation
Santa Monica, California

Philip R. Lee, M.D.
Professor of Social Medicine
Director, Institute for Health Policy Studies
University of California, San Francisco
San Francisco, California

James P. LoGerfo, M.D.
Associate Professor of Medicine and Health Services
School of Medicine
University of Washington
Seattle, Washington

Lawrence A. May, M.D.
Assistant Clinical Professor
University of California, Los Angeles
Los Angeles, California

Ira Moscovice, Ph.D.
Associate Professor
Center for Health Services Research
University of Minnesota
Minneapolis, Minnesota

Mary Richardson, M.H.A.
Instructor, Department of Health Services
Administrator, Clinical Training Unit
Child Development and Mental Retardation Center
University of Washington
Seattle, Washington

William C. Richardson, Ph.D.
Graduate Dean and Vice Provost
Professor of Health Services
University of Washington
Seattle, Washington

Robert F. Rushmer, M.D.
Professor of Bioengineering
Center for Bioengineering
University of Washington
Seattle, Washington

William Shonick, Ph.D.
Professor
Division of Health Services
School of Public Health
University of California, Los Angeles
Los Angeles, California

Stephen M. Shortell, Ph.D.
A.C. Buehler Distinguished Professor of Hospital and Health Services
    Management
Professor of Organization Behavior
J.L. Kellogg Graduate School of Management
Professor of Sociology
Department of Sociology
Northwestern University
Evanston, Illinois

Paul R. Torrens, M.D., M.P.H.
Professor of Health Services Administration
School of Public Health
University of California, Los Angeles
Los Angeles, California

James E. Veney, Ph.D.
Professor
Department of Health Policy and Administration
School of Public Health
University of North Carolina
Chapel Hill, North Carolina

Stephen J. Williams, Sc.D.
Professor of Public Health
Head, Division of Health Services Administration
Graduate Program in Health Services Administration
Graduate School of Public Health
San Diego State University
San Diego, California

Foreword

Introduction to Health Services provides a thorough, yet succinct, description of health services in the United States and the key issues that must be addressed in the decades ahead. The book provides not only a historical perspective on the evolution of health services but also an analytic framework within which to examine policies for the future.

It is evident that the dramatic expansion of health services in the United States that characterized the post-World War II era is not likely to continue. If one examines general trends, the fiscal crisis that is squeezing the health sector, and health care developments in other Western industrial nations, the evidence is overwhelming. The coming decade will be unlike any that physicians, nurses, dentists, and other health professionals have faced in more than thirty years. The physician supply is increasing rapidly and will continue to do so. Unless current trends are altered and new policies adopted, there will be no commensurate increase in funds to finance the modernization of facilities, the acquisition of new equipment, or the expansion of third-party coverage (public or private) to assure access to adequate health care that is becoming increasingly costly. In short, resource allocation to the health sector will be increasingly constrained, not so much by planning and regulation but by changes in the economy and changing national priorities.

Although health services in the United States are often thought of as part of a single system, Torrens (Chapter 1) explains that four separate subsystems serve the middle and upper classes, the urban inner city poor, members of the armed forces and their dependents, and veterans. Rural areas are served by an additional subsystem that resembles the system serving the middle class, except that a higher proportion of family physicians and general practitioners provide services, and the hospitals are smaller with less specialized equipment than urban hospital centers. Health care professionals and policymakers must understand the nature and complexity of health care, including these various subsystems of health care, and avoid simplistic descriptions such as "mainstream" medical care when considering policy choices.

The most urgent problem facing health professionals, policymakers, and the public is the continued rapid rise in the cost of health care and the current reimbursement policies for hospitals, physicians, and nursing homes that compound the problem. The fee-for-service reimbursement method (cost-based reimbursement for hospitals and "usual, customary, and reasonable" fees for physician services) under third-party payment mechanisms have had multiple, often unintended effects on the use of services and the cost of care. Enthoven has analyzed the perverse effects of present health care reimbursement policies, including tax subsidies, and has proposed an approach based on stimulating more effective market forces and competition. Richardson (Chapter 11) cites Enthoven's arguments for an alternative approach to the current mix of public and private financing, limited regulation, and inflationary reimbursement policies. In addition, he examines the principal difficulties in implementing such an approach. Strategies for containing the rapidly rising costs of health care are considered in the chapters on health care financing, health care personnel, and medical technology.

Costs are not the only problem. In the 1960s and 1970s, equity and access were major issues. The issue of equity remains critical, while access problems have been markedly reduced in the past fifteen years. In examining issues related to equity, Richardson (Chapter 11) considers risk sharing across populations and income redistribution as a result of policies followed in the financing of health services. The tax-exempt status of health insurance premiums constitutes a major, if often unrecognized, subsidy to the employed population. Even in government programs, particularly Medicare, the bulk of expenditures subsidizes services for the middle class provided by private physicians and community hospitals. There is growing evidence that social class is a major factor in health policy, with primarily the middle and upper classes benefiting from federal policies, whereas the poor become increasingly dependent on the state discretion.

The last chapters of this book deal with formidable problems associated with organizing, planning, and regulating health services, as well as issues related to health personnel and medical technology. The most critical problems, such as those related to the rapidly rising costs of health care and the challenges posed by the shift from an acute illness burden (particularly infectious diseases) to a chronic illness burden, are discussed from a variety of perspectives. The clear and concise examination of these issues should be of value not only to the beginning student but also to teachers, health services administrators, and policymakers. The book is an important contribution to the resolution of our most perplexing health policy problems.

Philip R. Lee, M.D.
Professor of Social Medicine
Director
Institute for for Health Policy Studies
University of California, San Francisco
San Francisco, California

Preface
to the Second Edition

The success of the first edition of *Introduction to Health Services* has prompted us to maintain the philosophy and approach of the book in this edition, while at the same time expanding the coverage of material in order to make the book more inclusive and current. The preparation of a new edition has also allowed for updating of all information, especially of the quantitative data. As a result, this expanded, up-to-date version should be of value to a wider audience and will serve as a ready reference and comprehensive overview of health services. The need for such a reference source and modern textbook continues to increase with the ever-present escalation of changes in the health care industry, a rate of change that has little prospect of slowing down in the near future, and a process of change that has represented both progress and turmoil for many years in one of our most important national enterprises.

In addition to updating all chapters from the first edition, we have added a number of new chapters to expand further the scope and comprehensiveness of the book. Chapter 4, a detailed overview of public health services, has been added to Part Three, "Providers of Health Services." Long term care has been given fuller treatment in Chapter 7, which deals with nursing homes as well as other issues and aspects of the broader topic of health care and social services for the severely ill and the aged. A new chapter, Chapter 10, focuses on health care personnel, especially the physician, dentist, and nurse. The evaluation of health care services and programs, a topic which has increased in importance in recent years, is now the subject of a major new chapter (Chapter 14). Health care policy development and the politics of health care are also addressed in extensive detail in a new chapter (Chapter 15). Finally, some concluding comments have been added (Epilogue).

A number of chapters retained from the first edition include new topics or areas of focus that reflect the changing nature of health care services. Chapter 3 highlights recent trends in the use of services. Chapter 5 has increased content on Health Maintenance Organizations and other new types of ambulatory care providers. Chapter 6 discusses the increasing financial and political pressures on hospitals as well as the increasing trend toward multihospital systems.

Chapter 9 places increased emphasis on technology assessment. Chapter 11 discusses the dramatic new forms of financing and reimbursement, especially for institutional providers, such as preferred provider organizations. Chapter 12 discusses changes in the regulatory environment in this country and the challenges to historical patterns of planning and regulating health care services and providers.

We have maintained many of the philosophies that guided the development of the book originally. The book both describes and assesses the system. A multidisciplinary approach has also been retained. The use of empirical research has been emphasized, so that the knowledge presented is based on scientific evidence where possible.

Readers seeking a more extensive elaboration of topics covered in this book have a rich and extensive literature to draw upon. *Issues in Health Services,* a companion volume to *Introduction to Health Services* in the Wiley Series in Health Services, is a collection of many of the classic articles in the field and is a useful supplement to this text.

Much of the artwork in the book was drawn by Dale Leuthold of the University of Washington. We would also like to thank Cathy Somer, Andrea Stingelin, Janet Foltin, Bruce Williams, and Audrey Pavey for their assistance in the development and production of this book.

We have used the comments of persons who have reviewed the first edition, both privately and in publication, in revising the book, and we appreciate their many useful comments and suggestions. In expanding and updating the book, we have continued to present a state-of-the-art textbook applicable to advanced undergraduates and graduate students in all health profession fields, as well as to the practitioner seeking to understand better the complex environment within which he or she functions. Health care is a challenging and exciting field. We hope that our efforts will help all participants better comprehend the field and appreciate its complexities.

Stephen J. Williams
Paul R. Torrens

Preface
to the First Edition

Since the end of World War II, health services in the United States have undergone rapid and dramatic changes. New and more powerful technologies have been developed, generations of more specialized personnel have been educated, and more elaborate and expensive facilities have been constructed. At the same time, a complex network of new programs has been developed to handle the financing, planning, monitoring, and regulating of all aspects of health care.

By any measure, this country's health services system is huge and complex. It is also frequently confusing and discouraging to those who must work within its many programs. Indeed, it is sometimes so difficult to understand and so frustrating to change that the people within the system not only stop trying to understand why it is the way it is but also stop trying to improve it. They simply withdraw and concentrate their energies on their particular part of the system, trusting that someone else will make the right judgments for the system as a whole.

Unfortunately, this isolationism is a luxury we can no longer afford. It is essential, now more than ever before, that all those within the system understand its workings and concentrate their efforts towards making it work better.

This book is divided into five parts, the first of which is an introduction to the health services system of this country. It discusses the major trends that have characterized health care in the United States. This introduction is designed to set the stage for the detailed discussions of the various aspects of the system that follow.

Part Two discusses the factors associated with the utilization of health services. The bases for the needs and demands for health services are examined in two chapters. The first of these, Chapter 2, outlines the biological bases of disease, including both physiological and psychological trends. The second chapter in this part, Chapter 3, describes the primary patterns of health service utilization and presents frameworks to help us understand better why these patterns have developed.

The providers of health services are discussed in Part Three of this book. Chapter 4 covers ambulatory and community services, while Chapter 5 discusses inpatient services and the role of the hospital in the health services system. Chapter 6 examines some of the sweeping issues of long-term care, with a particular focus on the nursing home. Finally, Chapter 7 focuses on services to meet mental health needs.

The organizations and programs that provide health care require a variety of resources to carry out their mission, and these resources are the subject of Part Four. The technological resources for health are discussed in Chapter 8, while the subject of health personnel is taken up in Chapter 9. The finances and financial systems for health care are discussed in Chapter 10, and are considered both as a resource and as a mechanism for regulating the behavior of individuals and organizations within the health care system. As such, this chapter serves as a link to Part Five, which is devoted to assessment and regulation of the health services system.

Chapter 11 in Part Five discusses the setting of priorities for health services and the use of regulatory and planning mechanisms to achieve social goals. The assessment of the effectiveness of health care services, and particularly the evaluation of the quality of care, is discussed in Chapter 12.

Thus, this book addresses the reasons for providing health services, the organizations and programs that provide care, the resources needed to provide the services, and the systems of assessment and modification needed to alter the direction of the system in the years to come.

Throughout the various chapters, certain common concerns will repeatedly appear. Assuring easy access to health services for all who need them, maintaining a level of care that is of acceptable quality, understanding and controlling the factors causing the rapid rise in the cost of care, and establishing a more rational method of priority setting and planning—all these form a common thread that runs throughout all the chapters in the book.

This book has the dual purpose of both describing the health services system of this country and critically assessing various aspects and component parts of that system. The reader should develop an appreciation for the complexities and subtleties of health services, and understand that there are many biological, behavioral, and organizational factors affecting the use of health care resources.

Much of the existing empirical research in health services has been incorporated into this book, yet much more remains to be done before all the components of the system and all their interrelationships are completely understood. It is hoped that the reader will be challenged not only to better understand the present structure of health services in this country but also to develop an analytical framework for understanding new developments as they occur in the future. In that way, as new issues or new forces appear on the scene, they can be easily integrated into a framework that has already been worked out.

It is our feeling that everyong involved in providing health services has a duty to read about and reflect on the nature and structure of our health services system. At the same time, it is important for each of us to consider and understand our values and our biases, since they will affect our thoughts about health care. As the reader progresses through this book, it is important to keep these values and biases in mind and to look for their effects on his or her opinions and conclusions about health care.

It is also important to keep in mind the values of our society, particularly as they are expressed through politics and the political system. Although there is no separate chapter in this book on the politics of health care, the influence of politics is suggested throughout the text. The reader should be continuously aware that politics is a major force shaping the present and future health services system of this country.

Finally, the health services system is immense, and no single textbook could cover all of its aspects. As a result, many of the organizations, trends, and influences that are involved in health care in the United States are mentioned only briefly and some are omitted entirely. The objective has been to focus attention on those institutions of most significance or on those from which the most can be learned, while at the same time recognizing that a number of others have had to be omitted because of the realities of limited space.

For the reader who seeks a more extensive elaboration of this *Introduction to Health Services*, the Wiley Series in Health Services also includes a companion volume, *Issues in Health Services*, edited by Stephen J. Williams. All the chapters in this present volume, except one, were written especially for this book. The *Issues* volume, however, is a collection of articles from the health services literature, designed to complement and parallel the parts and chapters of this volume. Both of these books, *Introduction*, and the companion *Issues*, are intended for use by advanced undergraduate and graduate students in any of the health fields, including health services administration, medicine, nursing, and the allied health professions. They are also intended to be comprehensive primers on health services for clinicians, administrators, planners, policy analysts, and policymakers who seek a better understanding of the health services system and their roles in it.

This book has benefited substantially from assistance provided by Barbara Anderson, Colleen Gawle, Annette Lefcourt, Billee Lewis, Bernice Goldberg Maslan, Diane McKenzie, Cheryl Michels, Jan Peterson, and Marilyn Taber. Artwork in the book was drawn by Dale Leuthold of the University of Washington. Cathy Somer of John Wiley & Sons has been a most pleasant and responsive editor. Scott Klein assisted greatly in the production of this book.

Finally, in addition to the participation of our colleagues as contributors to this book, many associates and students over the years have stimulated our thinking about health services and encouraged the book's development. To all of them, we owe a significant debt of gratitude, which we hope is partially met by their satisfaction with our efforts.

Stephen J. Williams
Paul R. Torrens

Contents

PART ONE
OVERVIEW OF THE HEALTH SERVICES SYSTEM   1

1   Historical Evolution and Overview of Health Services in the United
    States   3
    Paul R. Torrens

    Historical Evolution of Health Services in America   3
    Overview of Health Services in the United States   14
    Health Services: A Summary of Perspectives   28

PART TWO
CAUSES AND CHARACTERISTICS OF HEALTH SERVICES USE
IN THE UNITED STATES   33

2   The Physiologic and Psychologic Bases of Health, Disease, and Care
    Seeking   35
    Lawrence A. May

    Defining Illness and Disease   35
    Disease Processes: The Physiologic Bases of Disease   37
    Physiologic Bases of Changing Disease Patterns   41
    Social and Cultural Influences on Disease and Behavior   43

3   Factors Associated with the Use of Health Services   49
    Stephen M. Shortell

    Analytic Categories and Conceptual Distinctions   50
    Analytic Models and Key Findings   63
    Special Issues in Health Services Utilization   80

xix

PART THREE
PROVIDERS OF HEALTH SERVICES   89

4   Public Health Services: Background and Present Status   91
William Shonick

The Period Before 1935   92
The Growing Disparity Between the Tax Base and Service Responsibilities
Among Levels of Government   101
The Period After 1935   104
Where Do We Stand?   131

5   Ambulatory Health Care Services   135
Stephen J. Williams

Historical Perspective and Types of Care   136
Office-Based Practice   139
Prepaid Group Practice and Health Maintenance Organizations   153
Institutionally Based Ambulatory Services   156
Governmental Programs   161
Noninstitutional and Public Health Services   163
Organization of Ambulatory Care Systems   165

6   The Hospital   172
William L. Dowling

Historical Development of Hospitals   173
Characteristics of the Hospital System   179
Internal Organization of Community Hospitals   189
Trends and Issues in the Hospital Industry   196

7   Long Term Care Versus Tender Loving Care   216
Robert L. Kane
Rosalie A. Kane

Why Is LTC Such an Issue?   217
Who Is at Risk?   219
What Is the Role of the Nursing Home?   222
How Did We Get Where We Are?   226
What Can be Done About It?   232
The Medical Component of LTC and Quality of Care   237
Quality of Life   239
Medical Versus Social Models   241

8   Mental Health Services: Growth and Development of a
    System   249
    Mary Richardson

    Historical Perspectives on Definitions of Mental Illness   249
    Extent of Mental Disorders   252
    Development of the Mental Health Services System in the United
    States   257
    Mental Health Personnel   260
    The Organization of Services   265
    Issues and Trends in Mental Health   268

PART FOUR
RESOURCES FOR HEALTH SERVICES   275

9   Technological Resources for Health   277
    Robert F. Rushmer

    Historical Heritage of Health Technologies   278
    Development of Diagnostic Technologies   282
    The Basis for Benevolent Extravagance   293
    Monitoring Methods   296
    Emergency Medical Services   297
    Therapeutic Technologies   297
    Technology Assessment: A New Need   302
    Future Forecasts   302

10 Health Care Personnel   305
    Ira Moscovice

    Employment Trends in the Health Care Industry   305
    The Expanding Supply of Physicians   309
    Dentistry: A Profession in Transition   323
    Nursing: Shortages and Future Role Changes   328
    New Categories of Health Care Personnel: Physician Assistants and Nurse
    Practitioners   333
    Future Issues for Health Care Personnel   336

11 Financing Health Services   340
    William C. Richardson

    Health Care Expenditures   340
    Financial Arrangements and Economic Relationships   344
    Health Insurance Coverage in the United States   355
    Public Policy Issues   367

PART FIVE
ASSESSING AND REGULATING SYSTEM PERFORMANCE   373

12   Health Services Planning and Regulation   375
Thomas W. Bice

Planning and Regulation   375
Origins and Development of Health Services Planning   378
Origins and Development of Health Services
Regulation   389
An Assessment of Planning and Regulation   396

13   The Quality of Health Care   403
James P. LoGerfo
Robert H. Brook

The Relationship Between Health and Medical Care   404
Quality Assessment in Health Care   408
Measurement Issues   410
Quality Assessment Methods   412
Illustrative Studies of the Quality of Care   420
Quality Assurance in Medical Care   423

14   Evaluating Health Care Programs and Services   433
Arnold D. Kaluzny
James E. Veney

What is Evaluation?   433
Long and Short History of Program Evaluation   440
Methods of Evaluation   443
The Future of Evaluation   454

PART SIX
HEALTH CARE POLICIES AND POLITICS   459

15   Health Policy and the Politics of Health Care   461
Philip R. Lee
A. E. Benjamin

Dimensions of Policymaking in Health   462
A Historical Framework: The Development of Health Policy From 1798 to
1982   467

EPILOGUE   ISSUES FOR THE FUTURE   481

INDEX   487

INTRODUCTION TO HEALTH SERVICES

PART ONE

Overview of the Health Services System

CHAPTER 1

Historical Evolution
and Overview
of Health Services
in the United States

Paul R. Torrens

This chapter introduces the development, background, concepts, and issues of health care in the United States. The first section presents the historical evolution and development of health services in this country; the second section describes the current organization of services. Combined, these sections set the stage for the detailed analyses of the latter chapters in the book.

HISTORICAL EVOLUTION
OF HEALTH SERVICES IN AMERICA

In *The Tempest*, a Shakespearean character is portrayed as saying, "What's past is prologue," suggesting that the events of the past merely set the stage for the future. In a more pertinent sense, George Santayana has written, "Those who cannot remember the past are condemned to repeat it." This is particularly true of the American health care system, since many of the issues and forces that have shaped and formed it in the past continue to influence us today. If we are to understand the future better, it seems appropriate to look at the past first.

The modern American health care system has had three important periods of development and now seems to be entering a fourth. The first period began in the mid-nineteenth century (1850) when the first large hospitals, such as Bellevue Hospital in New York City and Massachusetts General Hospital in Boston, began to flourish. The development of hospitals symbolized the *institutionalization of*

This chapter is adapted from material previously presented in *The American Health Care System: Issues and Problems*, Paul R. Torrens, St. Louis, The C.V. Mosby Company, 1978.

health care for the first time in this country. Before this time, health care in the United States was a loose collection of individual services functioning independently and without much relation to each other or to anything else. By today's standards, the first hospitals were not very remarkable, but they did provide the first visible institution around which health care services could be organized.

The second important historical period began around the turn of the century (1900) with the *introduction of the scientific method into medicine* in this country. Before this time, medicine was not an exact science, but was instead a rather informal collection of unproved generalities and good intentions. After 1900, stimulated by the opening of the new medical school at the Johns Hopkins University in Baltimore, medicine acquired a solid scientific base that eventually transformed it from a conscientious but poorly equipped art into a detailed and clearly defined science.

With the coming of World War II, the United States underwent a major social, political, and technological upheaval whose effect was so marked that it ended the second and signaled the beginning of the third period of health care development. The scientific advances continued unabated, but now they were paralleled by a *growing interest in the social and organizational structure of health care.* During this time, attention was first directed toward the financing of health care, with the resultant formation of health insurance plans such as Blue Cross and Blue Shield. This was also the time of increasing concentration of power in the federal government, as witnessed by the Hill-Burton Act (Hospital Survey and Construction Act), by the huge research budgets of the National Institutes of Health (NIH), and, more recently, by the passage of Medicare. Finally, during this period the principle of health care as a right, not a privilege, was widely discussed and generally accepted.

Since the early 1980s, the health care system of this country has appeared to be moving into the fourth phase of its development, an era of *limited resources, restriction of growth, and reorganization of the methods of financing and delivering care.* Before this period, it had been presumed that the health care system would always be encouraged to grow and expand, both in size and in complexity, and that there would always be sufficient resources to support that expansion. Now it seems that the limits of our resources are being approached and that the health care system is being forced to consider options or alternatives to unrestricted growth and expansion.

Predominant Health Problems of the American People

Since the dawn of recorded history, human beings have repeatedly suffered the sudden and devastating appearance of epidemics of infectious disease. Plague, cholera, typhoid, smallpox, influenza, yellow fever, and a host of other diseases raged almost at will, creating havoc wherever they struck.

During the period 1850–1900 in this country, these epidemics of acute infectious diseases were the most critical health problem for the majority of Americans. Of particular importance were those diseases related to impure food, contaminated water supply, inadequate sewage disposal, and the generally poor condition of urban housing. During this time, for example, a cholera epidemic occurred throughout the country, resulting in an official death toll of 5,071 in New York City alone and an unofficial toll several times higher. During this same period, yellow fever killed 9,000 in New Orleans in 1853, 2,500 in 1854 and 1855, and another 5,000 in 1858. Abraham Lincoln regularly sent his family away from the White House during the summer months to escape the "fevers," probably malaria, that swept through Washington.

By 1900, the epidemics of acute infectious disease had been brought under control due to improving environmental conditions. In the latter years of the nineteenth century, cities had begun to develop systems for water purification, for sanitary disposal of sewage, for safeguarding the quality of milk and food, and for monitoring the quality of urban housing. Health departments had begun to grow in numbers and in strength, and had begun to apply the methods of case finding and quarantine with satisfying results. Indeed, by 1900, as Table 1-1 shows, those epidemics that had plagued humanity for centuries were now eliminated as major causes of death in the United States.

After 1900 the predominant health problems that attracted the attention of the health services system were those acute events, either infectious or traumatic, that affected individuals one by one. The pendulum had swung away from epidemics of acute infections that affected large numbers of people toward conditions of a personal nature that require individualized treatment. As Table 1-1 shows, pneumonia and tuberculosis were the primary causes of death in 1900, with heart disease, nephritis, and accidents close behind.

Relieved from the burden of epidemic illnesses, the newly developed medical sciences turned their attention to better surgical techniques, the discovery of new

TABLE 1-1. Death Rates for Leading Causes of Death, 1900 and 1978, United States

1900		1978	
Causes of Death	_Crude Death Rate per 100,000 Population Per Year_	_Causes of Death_	_Crude Death Rate per 100,000 Population Per Year_
All Causes	1,719.0	All Causes	883.4
Pneumonia and influenza	202.2	Diseases of the heart	334.3
Tuberculosis	194.4	Malignancies	181.9
Diarrhea, enteritis, and ulceration of the intestine	142.7	Cerebrovascular disease	80.5
Diseases of the heart	137.4	Accidents	48.4
		Influenza and pneumonia	26.7
Senility, ill-defined or unknown	117.5	Suicide and homicide	21.9
Intracranial lesions of vascular origin	106.9	Diabetes mellitus	15.5
Nephritis	88.6	Cirrhosis of the liver	13.8
All accidents	72.3	Arteriosclerosis	13.3
Cancer and other malignant tumors	64.0	Certain diseases of early infancy	10.1
Diphtheria	40.3	Bronchitis, emphysema and asthma	10.0

SOURCES: _Vital Statistics of the United States_, Washington, DC: U.S. National Center for Health Statistics, August 1973; _Statistical Abstracts of the United States, 1981_, Washington, DC, Bureau of the Census, U.S. Department of Commerce, December 1981.

sera for the treatment of pneumonia, and the development of new tests for more accurate and rapid diagnoses. Hospitals began to grow rapidly, medical schools flourished, and there was a general air of excitement that suggested the world was on the brink of significant advances in the treatment of individual illnesses.

Significant advances *were* being made. In Baltimore and Boston, the students of William Halsted, the pioneer surgeon at Johns Hopkins Hospital, began to operate on patients whose disease had previously been beyond the ability of surgeons. Advances in obstetrics now made it safer for women to have babies, and for the first time women did not approach childbirth with the fear of dying in delivery. Research work by two physicians, Banting and Best, in the laboratories of the University of Toronto led to the discovery of insulin in 1922, and for the first time diabetes could be effectively treated. Other research by Whipple, Minot, and Murphy on the causes of pernicious anemia led to successful medical treatment for that condition and further spurred the rush to find new treatments for other age-old conditions.

There were new discoveries on all fronts, each of which contributed some new advances in medical treatment. In 1928, however, in a cluttered laboratory at St. Mary's Hospital in London, a Scottish researcher, Alexander Fleming, produced the first of several discoveries that were to lead to the treatment of patients with penicillin for the first time in 1941. This discovery absolutely revolutionized medical care and totally changed the patterns of disease that threatened humanity. Within a few years after the treatment of the first patients with penicillin, antibiotics became readily available, and acute illnesses that had previously caused serious illness and possible death now meant nothing more than the discomfort of an injection and a few days of disability. Many older people experienced the incredible effects of the antibiotic era. When they had contracted pneumonia as children, their families had admitted them to hospitals and despaired for their lives; now, as older adults, they were told they had "a little pneumonia," given an injection of penicillin, and treated at home.

With the arrival of the antibiotic era in the 1940s and the subsequent conquest of acute infectious disease, the predominant health problems of Americans became chronic illnesses. Since acute infections were no longer snuffing out the lives of children, people were living longer and beginning to manifest long-term chronic diseases such as heart disease, cancer, and stroke. As shown in Table 1-1, these three conditions alone now account for two-thirds of all deaths. A similar review of the causes of disability would show arthritis, blindness, arteriosclerosis, and other chronic diseases to be the predominant causes of morbidity and limitation of function.

For the future, chronic illnesses will probably continue to be the predominant health problems of the American people. Increasingly important will be chronic illnesses related to personal life styles and the environment. Evidence is rapidly accumulating to suggest that many of the more important chronic illnesses are either self-inflicted (albeit without that intent) or the result of hazards introduced inadvertently into the environment.

The predominance of chronic illness as the major threat to health in the future raises a number of relevant issues of health professionals. First, as May points out in Chapter 2, the entire method of defining a chronic illness and determining its prevalence must be reexamined to obtain a more accurate picture of the situation. At the present time, a chronic disease is identified or documented on the basis of the first appearance of symptoms or on positive laboratory test results. In most cases, however, it is known that the disease process started long before the appearance of symptoms. In a practical sense, this forces one to ask: when should a chronic disease be considered to be present? The implications of the answer to this question for the planning and financing of health services could be enormous.

Chronic illnesses also have two important characteristics that directly affect both prevention and treatment. First, as was just pointed out, they often begin early in life, long before overt symptoms appear; the exact starting date for a chronic disease is never known. For example, a study of apparently healthy young soldiers who were suddenly killed in combat in the Korean War showed that almost one-fourth had already started to develop early microscopic evidence of coronary artery disease before age 20. Second, once a chronic illness is present, it remains with the patient forever. The *disease* is not cured by medical treatment; rather, its more prominent *symptoms* or external manifestations are treated.

Unfortunately, although the pattern of predominant illnesses has changed from epidemics of acute infections in the 1850s, to individual acute conditions in the 1900s, and finally to chronic illnesses in the 1950s, thinking about prevention and treatment has been slow to catch up. Acute infections very conveniently have a clear-cut beginning, middle, and end; as a result, they are amenable to one-shot solutions. If there is an epidemic caused by contamination of the water supply, the construction of a sewage treatment facility will eliminate it completely. If there is a threat of poliomyelitis infection, the ingestion of polio vaccine once or twice will permanently protect a population.

With chronic illnesses, however, prevention and treatment cannot be a one-shot affair, even though this is still how our health care system approaches them. Arteriosclerotic heart disease, for example, begins early in life and is probably affected by diet, cigarette smoking, stress, obesity, and several other factors that are directly related to personal habits and life style. Prevention of these conditions cannot be accomplished by giving a person a single lecture on the evils of high cholesterol food or the dangers of heavy cigarette consumption. Rather, prevention must be long term, continuous, and aimed at bringing about major changes in an individual's knowledge of disease, personal values, and behavior patterns. Unfortunately, that understanding has been slow in coming, and most of our preventive efforts are focused on one-time activities or are aimed at very limited aspects of life style.

Optimal treatment for long term, continuous illness requires a system of health care that is, in itself, long term and continuous. Unfortunately, the organization of our health services is still modeled on the disease patterns that were predominant in the 1900–1945 period and concentrates on individual episodes of illness as if they were separate and distinct entities. As a result, the health care system is primarily short term and discontinuous in nature, and it treats chronic illness as if it were merely a series of separate acute episodes. This trend is further reinforced by the current method of financing of health services, with its great emphasis on paying for individual services rendered rather than on the long term, continuous nature of the underlying disease process.

It should be noted that a few efforts to develop longer term and more continuous systems of financing and patient care have begun to appear in the last few years, particularly in the area of care for the elderly (Chap. 7). Two examples of this trend are the new demonstration projects aimed at developing "social HMOs" (Health Maintenance Organizations) for the elderly and the creation of state and local government agencies to improve the coordination of health and welfare services for the elderly.

It is entirely possible (and, indeed, probable) that the predominant disease patterns will be changing again in the future, creating an entirely different set of conditions that may require an entirely different array of services and interventions. It will be important for future generations of health professionals to watch for changes in predominant disease patterns to ensure a health care system that is genuinely pertinent and responsive to the problems of the day.

Technology Available to the American People

During the three developmental periods of the American health care system, what technology was available to handle the diseases that affected the American people? What tools were available to health workers to conquer these conditions?

In the period 1850–1900, only a very rudimentary technology was available for the treatment of disease. The scientific base of medicine was still very narrow, and the number of effective medical treatments was very limited. Indeed, a great deal of energy and effort was expended on treatment, but whether a patient recovered from an illness or not usually depended more upon the patient and the disease rather than the treatment.

Physicians during this period of time were poorly trained. They usually obtained their skills by serving apprenticeships with physicians already in practice and then taking short courses at unsophisticated medical colleges. What physicians had to offer was usually contained in their black bags, which they took with them wherever they went. They spent a good deal of time in patients' homes and almost no time at all in hospitals. In general, their practice was little different from that of their predecessors for centuries before them.

Nurses during the period 1850–1900 were not much better trained. Generally they were members of religious groups who volunteered to work in the few hospitals that existed, or they were poor, desperate, discarded women who frequented these institutions anyway and were pressed into service. Their work was nonscientific in the extreme and consisted simply of assisting patients with their usual bodily functions in any way possible. Not until the first training program for nurses was organized at Bellevue Hospital in the 1860s was there any formal preparation for this important role anywhere in the country.

As for the hospitals themselves, they were merely places of shelter and repose for the sick poor who could not be cared for at home. Anyone who could stay at home usually did so, since hospitals had little to offer that would not be obtained at home if one had the money. Indeed, the hospitals of those days were often a direct threat to the lives of patients, since they were dirty, crowded, and disease-ridden. Infectious diseases frequently spread rapidly among hospitalized patients, and during the typhus epidemics of 1852 in New York City, for example, the highest mortality for the disease was among the patients and staff of the hospitals themselves.

After 1900 conditions began to change, spurred on by the new discoveries that were emerging from the research laboratories in this country and in Europe. In 1912, for example, a Polish chemist, Casimir Funk, published a paper, "The Etiology of Deficiency Diseases," in which he described "vitamines" and opened a whole new field of disease conditions to treatment. In 1908, James MacKenzie, in London, published his famous book *Diseases of the Heart*, and patients throughout the world were the beneficiaries. In countless medical schools and hospitals throughout this country and Europe, major scientific advances were achieved, each of which contributed to easier and safer diagnosis and treatment of acutely ill patients.

The medical schools led the way in many of these advances as a result of some basic reforms that took place in the early 1900s. Before this time, a large number of small, poorly staffed, free-standing medical colleges existed throughout the country, 14 in Chicago alone in 1910 and 10 each in Missouri and Tennessee. In 1910, Abraham Flexner undertook a study of medical education for the Carnegie Foundation and in his report, *Medical Education in the United States and Canada*, recommended that medical education in this country undergo radical reform. In particular, he strongly urged that the training of physicians be made a university function and that it be based on a firm scientific foundation. On the basis of his recommendations and the support of the Rockefeller Foundation, many of the small unaffiliated schools began to close and many of the remaining ones became part of universities, with the important result that physicians began to be trained as scientists as well as practitioners.

Gradually, physicians began to have more effective tools with which to work, and the range of their capabilities expanded rapidly. They still continued to spend the majority of their time in their offices or in patients' homes, but they now also began to look toward the hospital for the care of their more severely ill patients. A small but gradually increasing number of physicians began to specialize in a particular area of medicine; however, by 1940, more than 80% were still in general practice.

Hospitals in the 1900s began to play an increasingly important role in health care. As more technology developed, it tended to be concentrated in hospitals, with the result that patients and physicians began going to hospitals for the technology to be found there. St. Luke's Hospital in New York City, for example, was 50 years old in 1906 when it opened its first private patient pavilion. Before that time, there had been no reason for private patients to go to a hospital, because they could usually get the same type of care in their homes. Now, however, hospitals began to offer services and skills that were not available anywhere else.

Although the period 1900–1940 was one of rapid growth in scientific technology, it was nothing compared to what happened with the advent of World War II. With the start of the war, this country mounted a massive effort to organize the best talents available for the care of the wounded and for the solution of the health care problems generated by the war. For the first time, relatively large efforts in research were begun under the direction of the federal government, and the results were impressive. The development of antibiotics accelerated rapidly, new surgical techniques for the treatment of trauma and burns were discovered, and new approaches to the transportation of the sick and wounded were developed. The range and breadth of problems that were subjected to organized investigation were remarkable, opening the way for an even more greatly expanded research effort after the war ended. In 1950, the size of the research commitment begun during World War II had risen to $73 million per year, $35 million of which was distributed through the NIH. By 1974, this had risen to an annual research budget of $2.5 billion, with $1.6 billion coming from a now greatly expanded NIH (see Chap. 9).

After World War II, hospitals were no longer the same. Previously, they had been places for the care of patients, with great emphasis being placed on the caring function. Now they became extensions of research laboratories, places where medical science was practiced and where curing was the order of the day. New procedures, new equipment, and new techniques all flourished to such a degree that the hospitals were now captured by their technology. The technology itself was the motivating force for hospitals, and most major decisions were based on that technology.

The operation of these newly complex institutions called for waves of new workers, each more specialized and more highly skilled than the last. Before the war there had been approximately 20 major categories of health workers; by the 1970s there were hundreds. With the increasing specialization of services and skills, there was also an increasing interdependence of health workers on each other and an increasing reliance on the health care system to integrate the work of so many separate groups.

Physicians were severely affected by these trends. With the explosive growth of scientific knowledge after World War II, it was impossible for one physician to know everything, and so the trend toward specialization in a particular subarea of medicine had a strong impetus. Before the war, approximately 80% of physicians had been general practitioners and 20% specialists. In the years after the war, these percentages were reversed. In their training and practice, physicians focused more and more on the scientific aspects of diagnosis and treatment, and as a result spent more time in hospitals and less time in patients' homes. The hospital became the emotional center of the physician's life, since it was here that the most important, most challenging, and most interesting aspects of training or treatment occurred.

These trends affected nursing and the other health professionals to only a slightly lesser degree. The training of nurses and other health professionals became increasingly more scientific, more specialized, and more lengthy during the years after World War II. The desire to be recognized as competent in a particular area led to the proliferation of professional groups and to formal accreditation on the basis of scientific training and ability. It also led to university-based training programs in all of the health professions.

Today the technology available to the American health care system has advanced to an incredible degree. Intrauterine diagnosis of fetal malformations, nuclear-powered cardiac pacemakers that operate for years, and sonarlike sensing devices that let blind people "see" what is in front of them are all accepted as merely the expected developments of a technological age. The merging of technologies from other fields with those of the health field, such as in the development of computerized axial tomographic scanners, has further added to the immense range of technology available to the health care system. As Robert Rushmer points out in Chapter 9, however, this explosion of technology in recent years has not been without its problems. Indeed, the technology itself has *caused* a rather serious set of problems with which future generations of health care professionals must grapple.

One interesting problem raised by technology is evaluation of the various new discoveries and techniques. Much new (and even some old) technology is adopted without appropriate evaluation of how effective it really is and, even more important, how much *more* effective it might be than already existing technology. For a short time, a National Center for Health Care Technology existed within the federal government and was charged with carrying out these need evaluations; unfortunately, the center has recently fallen victim to budget reductions. However, it will certainly return, since the need for this type of evaluation is so apparent to everyone.

One of the most obvious problems raised by the new technology is its cost and the effect that it has on the entire financial structure of the health services system. The costs of providing this vast new technology increase each year, as do the costs of staffing that technology with the increasingly specialized and highly trained personnel that are needed. These increased costs are passed along to the public, to health insurance plans, and to the government, all of whom now ask, "Can we continue to spend our money in this way? Are we getting enough back for our money? Is there a better way in which we can use our resources for the people under our care?"

For several years, the Office of Technology Assessment of the U.S. Congress has had a unit specializing in the evaluation of the costs and benefits of technology. It has provided some extremely useful analyses of the economic impact of technology and has served as a great resource in the health policy debates in this country.

Possibly a more important problem of medical technology is its impact on the form and configuration of the health care system and on the values and patterns of practice of the professionals in that system. In many ways, the American health services system has been captured by its technology and has been subtly and seductively shaped by its demands. Decisions regarding the design of programs and institutions, the training of personnel, and the distribution of services have been governed by technological considerations that loom larger every year.

A still more profound effect of technology is its ability to insinuate itself into the values of not just the system but also of the people who work in the system. The student entering a health profession rapidly learns that academic success and, later, professional success, comes from mastery of the scientific technology. Increasingly, the student views excellence as being reached through technical achievements and gives decreasing importance to the more personal, nontechnical aspects of disease. By the time the student becomes a fully accepted member of the profession, a value system has been established that views illness as a series of technical problems to be solved by the application of specific technical solutions. This value system is then reinforced in practice by the expectations of the public and by the requirements of the regulators, both of whom have come to view quality in terms of technical excellence. The result frequently is a professional performance that is excellent in technical terms and rather poor in human terms.

A quite different problem of technology arises not from its excessiveness but rather from its inefficient distribution to society. If there is indeed more technology available than can be provided equitably to all people due to limits on funding, then large portions of society do not benefit as much as they should from technologic knowledge. Marked differences exist, for example, in mortality and morbidity measures for white and nonwhite segments of society, possibly indicating an unequal access to modern health care technology. The answer obviously is to improve the health services system to ensure adequate distribution of available resources.

In summary, virtually no technology was available to treat disease before the 1900s. Technology began to appear and grow rapidly after the turn of the century. World War II fostered an incredible surge of research endeavors, with the result that the health care system began to be overwhelmed by the range and diversity of available technology. By the 1970s, the American health care system had been captured by its technology, and the challenge was to regain mastery over the giant that had been created.

Social Organization for the Use of Technology

How has our society organized to use the technology available to it? What has been the predominant view of the role of society in health care? During the period 1850 to 1900, no organized program was available for the use of whatever technology existed. Public services were rudimentary and were concentrated upon a very narrow range of problems. There were hospitals in a few areas, but they were generally started by religious or charitable groups for the care of those who were obviously and publicly impoverished. The predominant ethic of the time was that people should care for themselves and be self-sufficient. If they become dependent, they should take advantage of and be grateful for the various charities established for these purposes.

This philosophy of rugged individualism and relative lack of large scale social organization for health care predominated in this country until the 1930s, when the Great Depression struck with full force. At that time, economic forces beyond the comprehension of most Americans struck down many people, destroying their lives and leaving them destitute. The traditional belief in being totally and personally responsible for all aspects of one's life was badly shaken by the events of the Depression.

With the arrival of Franklin Roosevelt in the White House, the New Deal was launched and a wide array of social programs appeared, all aimed at repairing the damage of the Depression. The importance of the New Deal in terms of American social thought cannot be underestimated since, for the first time, American society created large scale national programs to assist those who could not assist themselves.

In health care, governmental activity was still minimal, limited to a few specific areas of grant-in-aid programs to states to improve certain public health services such as infectious disease control and maternal and child health. Although the services were limited and aimed primarily at the poor, this small start did signify an assumption of responsibility by the national government for health care, at least for those who could not care for themselves.

The next major change in social organization and social thinking came with the arrival of World War II. As part of the mobilization effort, millions of men and women entered military service and in return received a wide array of health services simply by virtue of that service. The significance was twofold: First, the services themselves were provided without charge by salaried physicians working for the government; second, they were provided as a right of those in the service and were clearly not charity for people who could no longer take care of themselves, as previous governmental efforts had been.

Not only did World War II accustom the country to large scale health care programs provided by the society to its members, it also encouraged the growth of the health insurance industry. During the war, a freeze was imposed on wages and salaries so that very little collective bargaining for increases in salary could occur. However, considerable activity did occur in the development of pensions, disability programs, and health insurance plans, with the result that the health insurance industry began to flourish. This industry provided the American public with a new form of social organization—the "third party," or fiscal intermediary. Before the development of health insurance, the public had no form of social organization to protect it from a sudden onslaught of medical bills. With the arrival of this new phenomenon, health insurance, the American public began to gain experience in the cooperative effort of pooling many individual contributions for a common group objective—protection from financial disaster.

The period immediately after World Warr II witnessed the slow, tentative growth of the "Blue" plans, Blue Cross and Blue Shield, nonprofit community-based health care plans that insured against hospital and medical costs. With the success and growth of Blue Cross and Blue Shield, commercial insurance companies also entered the field, offering health insurance plans to employers and industry as part of their life/health/retirement/disability packages. With the rapid advances made by Blue Cross/Blue Shield and the commercial insurance carriers, the percentage of Americans covered by some form of health insurance rose from less than 20% before World War II to more than 70% by the early 1960s.

In the early 1960s, a major battle was fought and won by those advocating a greater societal role in the organization of health services. The battle involved the creation of governmental-sponsored health insurance plans for people over the age of 65 and resulted in the passage of legislation that created Medicare. Although Medicare itself was directed primarily to the needs of the country's elderly, its impact was soon felt throughout the entire health care system. The creation of the Medicare program had two immediate major social implications. First, Medicare provided financing for health care for all persons over the age of 65 simply on the basis of age; need was not a factor. The American society, in effect, determined that there were certain things the society should do for all of its members, regardless of individual need, since society could ensure equity. The second major effect of Medicare was the assumption by the federal government of the responsibility for planning, financing, and monitoring a significant portion of the health care services in this country. The society not only wanted social insurance programs for health care, but also wanted the federal government to assume a central role in operating these programs.

A further significant change in the social organization of health care in this country occurred in the mid-1960s with the development of the Neighborhood Health Centers program of the U.S. Office of Economic Opportunity. In the War on Poverty, a number of health programs were funded for underserved areas of the country, each of which was required to have significant participation of consumers, often through governing boards and committees. This involvement of consumers was a substantial change from the past and soon became standard policy in new governmental programs. This philosophy was vigorously put forward in the National Health Planning and Resources Development Act of 1974, which required a majority of consumers on all local health planning boards. Although the health planning effort in this country has recently been dismantled to a large degree, the involvement of consumer advocates in health policy matters continues and will clearly be an increasingly important aspect of the U.S. health care system in the future.

It is interesting to note that, although consumer participation in local, state, and national health policy has decreased as a result of the demise of the health planning network, its decrease has been more than compensated for by the growth of employer and industrial involvement in health affairs. The growth of employer health care coalitions, and the more active involvement of various large employer purchasers of health insurance in matters of health policy, have created a new consumer advocacy force that promises to become an important part of the U.S. health care system in the future.

In the late 1970s and early 1980s, the health care system of this country, as noted previously, entered the fourth phase of its development, an era of *resource limitation, restriction of growth, and reorganization of systems of financing and providing health care*. With the federal Medicare program experiencing annual increases in expenditures of 20% or more per year, interest has shifted toward a reduction of benefits, greater cost sharing by the elderly themselves, and a limitation on reimbursements to providers of service. Energies have now become focused less on the development of new services or the expansion of coverage and more on the control of costs through limitations and reductions.

These developments, to be discussed in detail in later chapters that deal with health care financing, planning, policy, and regulation, have also served to reinforce the increasingly powerful central role played by the federal government in the direction of health services. The federal government now not only controls a significant amount of the financial support for health care (approximately one-third of the total health care expenditures from all sources) but also, by using these massive resources in a unified and centralized manner, is able to set many of the rules by which health care, governmentally funded or not, is provided. The health care system of this country, although by no means federally operated, certainly is federally dominated.

This country entered the twentieth century with the social philosophy that people should care for themselves or be satisfied with charity. In mid-century, it adopted the philosophy that society should care for those who, through no fault of their own, could no longer take care of themselves. Finally, toward the end of the century, it had moved to a philosophy that society, operating through the national government, should assume responsibility for solving certain large-scale problems of life for all of its members, even if some individual members can solve these problems for themselves.

As for the future, society apparently has determined that government, particularly the federal government, will organize and coordinate large-scale programs of health care for the people of this country. The society has decided, to some extent, that health care is a right, not a privilege, and will increasingly expect government to make that belief a reality.

Summary of Historical Trends

The past 125 years of history have witnessed major changes in the American health care scene (Table 1-2). The predominant health problems of our people have changed from epidemics of acute infections to a different kind of "epidemic," chronic illness. The range of technology available has mushroomed from almost none in 1850 to a condition of such abundance now that the health care system has been virtually overwhelmed and captured by the technology it has created. Society's social values have changed from a *laissez-faire* approach in the 1850s that depended upon individual initiative or organized private charity to one now that assumes that health care is a right that the federal government must assure everyone enjoys to the fullest extent possible.

OVERVIEW OF HEALTH SERVICES IN THE UNITED STATES

When visitors from abroad, particularly those engaged in health services in their own country, come to the United States, they frequently want to know about the American health care system and how it works. They are usually puzzled by the answer they get:

> There isn't any *single* "American health care system." There are many separate subsystems serving different populations in different ways. Sometimes they overlap; sometimes they are entirely separate from one another. Sometimes they are sup-

TABLE 1-2. Major Trends in the Development of Health Care in the United States, 1850–Present

Trends	1850–1900	1900 to World War II	World War II to Present	Future
Predominant health problems of the American people	Epidemics of acute infections	Acute events, trauma, or infections affecting individuals, not groups	Chronic diseases such as heart disease, cancer, stroke	Chronic diseases, particularly emotional and behaviorally related conditions
Technology available to handle predominant health problems	Virtually none	Beginning and rapid growth of basic medical sciences and technology	Explosive growth of medical science; technology captures the health care system	Continued growth and expansion of technology, with attempts to repersonalize the technology
Social organization for the use of technology	None; individuals left to their own resources or charity	Beginning societal and governmental efforts to care for those who could not care for themselves	Health care as a right; governmental responsibility to organize and monitor health care for everyone	Greater centralization of responsibility and control in federal government

SOURCE: Paul R. Torrens, *The American Health Care System: Issues and Problems*. St Louis, the CV Mosby Co, 1978.

ported with public funds, and at other times they depend solely on private funds. Sometimes several different subsystems use the same facilities and personnel; at other times, they use facilities and personnel that are entirely separate and distinct.

It should not be surprising that there is a multiplicity of health care systems (or subsystems) in the United States, given the historical development of health services in this country. In the earliest days, health care was entirely a private matter, and people were expected to take care of themselves by obtaining services of private physicians and nurses when needed, purchasing medications from drugstores and chemist shops, and paying for all these services personally. For those persons who could not take care of themselves, charitable institutions were established as voluntary, nonprofit corporations to provide charity health care. These groups usually centered their efforts on hospitals and were usually located in the larger towns and cities of this country.

In the early twentieth century, a new element was added with the development of the city/county hospitals. These hospitals were established by local governments to care for the poor in their area who could not get care either by their own efforts or from the voluntary nonprofit charity hospitals. These public facilities were generally large, acute care, general hospitals, with busy clinics and emergency rooms and with close connections to local government ambulance services, police departments, and other community services. At the same time, state governments were developing mental hospitals. The cities had previously been responsible for the care of lunatics and the insane, but after the turn of the century, state governments began to assume this burden. Every state soon had at least one mental hospital where the emotionally disturbed were offered what little care was available.

With the explosive growth in the size of the federal government and in the numbers of persons in the armed forces during World War II, a separate system of care developed for active duty military personnel and their dependents, retired military personnel, and veterans. These were almost entirely self-contained systems, employing salaried physicians and nurses, working entirely in military or veterans hospitals directly operated by the federal government.

As the cost of health care began to increase rapidly after World War II, the United States experienced a rather sudden and somewhat bewildering development of a wide variety of health insurance plans. The first to be operated were community-based nonprofit Blue Cross and Blue Shield plans, developed by hospital and physician associations to spread the cost of health care more widely among the population. These were followed by labor union health and welfare trust funds, established as a consequence of benefit negotiations for union members. At the same time, the private, for-profit commercial insurance companies expanded their efforts on behalf of both individuals and large groups of employees. Finally, several large government-sponsored and publicly supervised health insurance plans evolved, such as Medicare and Medicaid, the latter to aid the medically indigent.

Private medical practitioners, voluntary nonprofit hospitals, city and state government hospitals, military and veterans hospitals, and health insurance plans with a variety of forms and origins all developed in the United States at the same time, separately, and for specific purposes. The resulting picture has been described as having a rich diversity of opportunities and approaches for meeting the health care needs of a population that has in itself a rich diversity of people and situations. It has also been described as chaotic, uncoordinated, overlapping, unplanned, and wasteful of precious personal and financial resources. The reality probably lies somewhere in between.

If there is no single, easily described American health care system, at least some of the subsystems that compose the larger entity can be identified. Although an endless set of variations is possible, it seems appropriate to examine four models or subsystems of health care in the United States, each of which serves a different group. By looking at the components, the system as a whole may be better understood. These systems serve 1) middle class, middle income families and individuals; 2) poor, inner city, minority people; 3) active duty military personnel and their dependents; and 4) veterans of U.S. military service. For each of these systems, the manner in which basic elements of health care are provided is reviewed.

Middle Class, Middle Income America (Private Practice, Fee-for-Service System)

It is appropriate for two reasons to consider first the system of health care used by a typical middle class, middle income individual or family. First, this system is frequently described as *the* American health care system (all others, therefore, immediately becoming somehow secondary to it); second, this system is frequently said to include the best medical care available in the United States and perhaps anywhere in the world.

The most striking feature of the middle class, middle income system of care is the absence of any *formal* system. Each family puts together an *informal* set of services and facilities to meet its own needs. The system, therefore, has no formal structure or organization and is different for each individual or family. Indeed, each family's system may vary widely according to the particular situation in which it is used. The only constant feature of this system is the family itself, all other aspects are transient, changeable, and widely varied.

Two other characteristics are also immediately noteworthy. First, the service aspects of the system focus on and are coordinated by physicians in private practice. Second, the system is financed by personal, nongovernmental funds, whether paid directly by consumers or through private health insurance plans. As the system is described, it will become readily apparent that these two features are not only important descriptively; they have been important in shaping the system into its present form.

Public health and preventive medicine services for the middle class, middle income system are provided by two different sources. Those services designed to protect large numbers of people, such as water purification, sewage disposal, and air pollution control, are provided by local or state governmental agencies. Frequently, these agencies are called *public health departments*. They usually provide their services to the entire population of a region, with no distinction between rich and poor, simple or sophisticated, interested or disinterested. Indeed, these mass public health services are common to all the systems of health care to be discussed. Those public health and preventive medicine services that are aimed at individuals, such as well-baby examinations, cervical cancer smears, vaccinations, and family planning, are provided by individual physicians in private practice. If a middle income family desires a vaccination in preparation for a foreign trip or wants the blood cholesterol level of its members checked, the family physician is consulted and provides the service. If it is time for the new baby to have its first series of vaccinations, the family pediatrician is usually the one who provides them.

Ambulatory patient services, both simple and complex, are also obtained from private physicians. Many families use a physician who specializes in family practice, while others use an array of specialist physicians such as pediatricians, internists, obstetrician/gynecologists, and psychiatrists who provide both primary care and specialty services. When special laboratory tests are ordered, x-ray films required, or drugs and medications prescribed, private commercial for-profit laboratories or community pharmacies are used. Many of these services, from individual preventive medicine services to complex specialist treatments, are financed by individuals through out-of-pocket payment, since most health insurance plans do not provide complete coverage for these needs. When the middle income family begins to use institutional services, such as hospital care, the source of payment shifts almost completely from the individual to third-party health insurance plans.

Inpatient hospital services are usually provided to the middle class, middle income family by a local community hospital that is usually voluntary and nonprofit. The specific hospital to be used is determined by the institution in which the family physician has medical staff privileges. Generally, the smaller, less specialized, more local hospitals will be used for simpler problems, whereas the larger, more specialized, perhaps more distant hospitals will be used for more complicated problems. Many of these larger hospitals have active physician training programs, conduct research, and may have significant charity or teaching wards.

The middle class, middle income family obtains its long term care from a variety of sources, depending upon the service required. Some long term care is provided in hospitals and, as such, is merely an extension of the complex inpatient care the patient has already received. This practice was more common in the past, but utilization review procedures have increased the pressure on hospitals to reduce the length of time people are hospitalized. More commonly, long term care is obtained at home through the assistance of a visiting nurse or voluntary nonprofit community-based nursing service. If institutional long term care is needed, it is probably obtained in a nursing home or a skilled nursing facility, usually a small (50–100 patients) institution, operated privately, for profit, by a single proprietor or small group of investors. Recently, there has been a general increase in size (100 + patients per facility) and a trend toward absorption of individual facilities into larger multifacility proprietary chains. The middle class, middle income family usually pays for its long term care with its own funds, since most health insurance plans provide relatively limited coverage for long term care.

When middle class families require care for emotional problems, they will again use a variety of mostly private services. However, as the illness becomes more serious, families may, for the first time, rely on governmentally sponsored service. When emotional problems first begin to appear in the middle class family, the patient will probably turn to the family physician, who may provide simple supportive services such as tranquilizers, informal counseling, and perhaps referral for psychological testing. The physician may even arrange for the patient to be hospitalized in a general hospital for a rest, for "nervous exhaustion," or for some other nonpsychiatric diagnosis. As the emotional problems become more severe, the family physician may refer the patient to a private psychiatrist, or to a community mental health center that most likely will be a voluntary nonprofit agency or under the sponsorship of one (such as a voluntary nonprofit hospital). If hospitalization is required, the psychiatrist or the community mental health center is likely to use the psychiatric section of the local voluntary nonprofit hospital if it seems that the stay in a hospital will be a short one. If the hospitalization promises to be a long one, the psychiatrist may use a psychiatric hospital, usually a private, nongovernmental community facility.

In those cases in which very extended institutional care is required for an emotional problem and the patient's financial resources are relatively limited, the middle class family may request hospitalization in the state mental hospital. This event usually represents the first use of governmental health programs by the middle income family, and as such it frequently comes as a considerable shock to patient and family alike.

In summary, the middle class family's system of health care is an informal, unstructured collection of individual services put together by the patient and the private physician to meet the needs of the moment. The individual services themselves have little formalized interrelationship, and the only thread of continuity is provided by the family's physician or by the family itself. In general, all the services are provided by nongovernmental sources and are paid for by private funds, either directly out-of-pocket or by privately financed health insurance plans.

For all of its apparent looseness and lack of structure, the middle class family's system of health care allows for a considerable amount of decision and control by the patient, more than that of the other systems to be discussed. The patient is free to choose the physician, the health insurance plan, and frequently even the hospital. If additional care is required, the patient can seek out and use (sometimes overuse) that care to the limit of the financial resources available. If the patient does not like the particular care being provided, dissatisfaction can be expressed in a more effective manner: The patient can seek care elsewhere from another provider. Even with the newer Preferred Provider Organization approach to health insurance, which attempts to influence people to obtain care from lower cost physicians and hospitals, the influences are indirect and economic in nature (i.e., a discount for using the lower cost providers) and certainly not coercive or directive (i.e., mandating that a person can use only certain providers in order to be insured at all).

On the other hand, the middle class family's system of care is a poorly coordinated, unplanned collection of services that frequently have little formal integration with one another. It can be very wasteful of resources and usually has no central control or monitor to determine whether it is accomplishing what it should. Each individual service may be of very high quality, but there may be little evidence of any "linking" taking place to ensure that each service complements the others as effectively as possible.

One special subset of the middle class, middle income model now involves millions of patients in this country. When people reach age 65, they are automatically eligible for Medicare, the federally sponsored and supervised health insurance plan for the elderly. A patient covered by Medicare benefits can utilize the same system of care as the middle income family, including private practice physicians and voluntary nongovernmental hospitals. The main difference now is that the bills are paid by a federal government health insurance plan, rather than the usual private plan in which the typical middle class family is enrolled. The physicians are the same and the hospitals are the same; only the health insurance plan is different.

Poor, Inner City, Minority America (Local Government Health Care)

A second major system of health care in the United States serves the poor, inner city, and generally minority population. While the specific details may vary from city to city, the general outline is well known in all major cities of the country. If it was important to study the middle class, middle income system of care because if represented the *best* health care possible in this country, it is equally important to study the poor, inner city system of care, since it frequently represents the *worst*.

The most striking feature of the health care system of the poor, inner city resident is exactly the same as that characterizing the middle class system: There is no *formal* system. Instead, just as in the middle class system, each individual or family must put together an *informal* set of services, from whatever source possible, to meet the health care needs of the moment. There is one significant difference, however: The poor do not have the resources to choose where and how they will obtain their health services. Instead, they must take what is offered to them, and try to put together a system from whatever they are told they can have.

There are two important characteristics of the system. First, the great majority of services are provided by local government agencies such as the city or county hospital and the local health department. Second, the patients have no real continuity of service with any single provider, such as a middle class family might have with a family physician. The poor family is faced with an endless stream of health care professionals who treat one specific episode of an illness and then are replaced by someone else for the next episode. While the middle class system of health care can establish at least some thread of continuity by the ongoing presence of a family physician, the poor family cannot.

The poor obtain their mass public health and preventive medicine services, including a pure water supply, sanitary sewage disposal, and protection of milk and food from the same local government health departments and health agencies that serve the middle class system. In contrast to the middle class system, however, the poor also get their individual public health and preventive medicine services from the local health department. When a poor family's newborn baby needs its vaccinations, that family goes to the district health center of the health department, not to a private physician. When a low income woman needs a Papanicolau smear for cervical cancer testing or when a teenager from a low income family needs a blood test for syphilis, it is most likely that the local government health department will give the test.

To obtain ambulatory patient services, the poor family cannot rely on the constant presence of a family doctor for advice and routine treatment. Instead, they must turn to neighbors, the local pharmacist, the health department's public health nurse, or the emergency room of the city or county hospital. It has often been said that the city or county hospital's emergency room is the family doctor for the poor, and the facts generally support this contention: When the poor need ambulatory patient care, it is quite likely that the first place they will turn is the city or county hospital emergency room.

The emergency room also serves the poor as the point of entry to the rest of the health care system. The poor obtain much of their ambulatory services in the outpatient clinics of the city/county hospitals. To gain admission to these clinics, they must frequently first go to the emergency room and be referred to the appropriate clinic. Once out of the emergency room, they may be cared for in two or three specialty clinics, each of which may handle one particular set of problems but none of which will take responsibility for coordinating all the care the patient is receiving.

When the poor need inpatient hospital services, whether simple or complicated, they again usually turn to the city or county hospital to obtain them.

Admission to the inpatient services of these hospitals is usually obtained through the emergency room or the outpatient clinics, thereby forcing the poor family to use these ambulatory patient services if they wish later admission to the inpatient services. The poor may also turn to the emergency room, the outpatient clinics, and the inpatient ward or teaching services of the larger voluntary nonprofit community hospitals. Since these hospitals are frequently teaching hospitals for the training of physicians, they often maintain special free or lower-priced wards. It is to these wards that the poor are usually admitted. Since the care in the teaching hospitals is generally as good as or better than any that might be obtained at the local city or county hospitals, many poor are willing to become teaching cases in the voluntary nonprofit hospitals in exchange for better care in better surroundings. By and large, however, city and county hospitals carry the largest burden of inpatient care for the poor.

If the long term care situation of middle income people is generally inadequate, the long term care of the poor can only be described as terrible. In contrast to the middle-class, much of the long term care of the poor is provided on the wards of the city and county hospitals, although not by intent or plan. The poor simply remain in hospitals longer because their social and physical conditions are more complicated and because the hospital staffs are reluctant to discharge them until they have some assurance that continuing care will be available after discharge. Since this status is often uncertain, poor patients are likely to be kept longer in the hospital so that they can complete as much of their convalescence as possible before discharge.

Most of the long term care of the poor is provided in the same types of nursing homes or skilled nursing facilities that are used by the middle class—either the smaller (50–100 patients) facilities, operated for profit by a single proprietor or the larger (100 + patients) facilities operated by a proprietary chain. One major difference between the systems used by the poor and the middle class is the quality of the facility used. The middle class generally has access to better-equipped and better-staffed nursing homes, while the poor are admitted to less expensive, less well-equipped facilities. Another important difference between the middle class and the poor is that middle class, middle income patients are more likely to pay for their own care in these institutions, while the poor have their care paid by welfare, Medicaid, or other public funds.

It is interesting to note that the system of health care for the middle class utilizes entirely private, nongovernmental facilities until long term care for mental illness is required; at that point, a governmental facility, the state mental hospital, is used. By contrast, the system of health care for the poor is composed almost entirely of public, government-sponsored services until long term care is required. This care is usually provided in private, profit-making facilities, the first such use of private facilities by the poor.

The convergence of poor and middle class systems of care in the private profit making nursing homes is important, since it represents an important feature of our multiple subsystems of health care. In many cases, several systems of health care that are otherwise separate and distinct will merge in their common use of personnel, equipment, and facilities. The emergency rooms of the city or county and voluntary nonprofit teaching hospitals, for example, will serve as the source of emergency medical care for the middle class family that cannot reach its own family physician. It will also serve as the family physician for the poor family that has none of its own. The private, for-profit nursing home will serve as the source of long term care for the middle class family, and may provide the same function for the poor. The radiology department of the voluntary nonprofit teaching hospital will provide x-ray tests for the middle class patient whose care is supervised by the private family physician, as well as for the poor patient whose care is supervised by a hospital staff physician in training. This does not mean that there is any real, functional integration of the separate systems of care because of their common use of the same facility or personnel. Rather, the model is more like that of a busy harbor in which a variety of ships will berth side by side for a short period of time before going their separate ways for separate purposes.

In their use of services for emotional illnesses, the poor return once again to an almost totally public, local governmental system. Initial signs of emotional difficulties are haphazardly treated in the emergency rooms and outpatient clinics of the city or county hospital. From here, patients may be referred to the crowded inpatient psychiatric wards of these same hospitals, but are just as likely to be referred to community mental health centers operated by local governmental or voluntary nonprofit community agencies. When long term care in an institution is required, the poor are sent to the psychiatric wards of the city or county hospital, and from there to the large state government mental hospitals, frequently many miles away.

In the past, health services for the poor were usually free, at least to the patients. Neither the local health department, the city or county hospital, nor the state mental hospital generally charged for its services, regardless of the patient's ability to pay. In the last few years, both local health departments and city and county hospitals have been forced to initiate a system of charges for services that were previously free. They have done this to recapture third-party payments to which the poor patient might be eligible, and patients who are unable to pay are still ordinarily provided the services they need. The imposition of these charges for previously free health services has probably changed the perception of these programs by the poor, but it is still too early to determine the implications of these changes.

As with the middle class, middle income system, there is a subset of the health care system of the poor that requires special comment. Certain persons who are poor enough by virtue of extremely low income or resources may qualify for Medicaid, the federal-state cooperative health insurance plan for the indigent, frequently termed Title 19 in reference to the section of the federal legislation by which it was created (Medicare, an entirely different program, is termed Title 18.) Under Medicaid people whose income and resources are below a level established by the individual states can use a state government-sponsored health insurance program to purchase health care in the private, middle class marketplace. The purpose of this program is to move the poor out of their usual local government health care system and into the supposedly better private practice health care system of the middle class. Unfortunately, the ability of Medicaid to move the poor into a better system of care had been limited by the reluctance of private physicians and private hospitals to assume responsibility for many Medicaid patients. This reluctance is based on Medicaid's low rate of reimbursement for service, its incredible amount of paperwork and red tape, and its frequently appalling system of retroactive denial of payment for services already provided.

Medicaid has succeeded to a degree in moving poor patients from local government hospitals into voluntary nonprofit teaching hospitals, but its greatest effect has probably been in moving poor patients into private, profit making nursing homes and skilled nursing facilities. In some states, for example, more than 60% of all patient bills in private nursing homes are now paid by the Medicaid program, providing some indication of the importance of this program to the provision of long term care. And for all its problems, the Medicaid program has allowed certain aspects of the middle class, middle income system of health care to be shared with the poor, inner city minority system of health care—a blending, merging, or sharing of resources and services that is characteristic of the American health care system and that makes it so difficult to evaluate any one subsystem cleanly and separately.

Unfortunately, with the recent tendency to cut back on the Medicaid program, at both the national and state levels, this movement of poor patients into the middle class system may abate considerably and may even be reversed. As less and less Medicaid money becomes available to purchase care in the middle class system for poorer patients, they may increasingly have to fall back once again on the resources of the city and county public hospital, as in the past.

In summary, the system of health care for the poor is as unstructured and informal as that for the middle class, but the poor have to depend upon whatever services the local government offers them. The services are usually provided free of charge or at low cost, but the patient has relatively little opportunity to express a choice and exercise options. Poor patients often cannot move to another set of services if they dislike the one first offered, since those first offered are usually the only services available.

Like the system of health care for the middle class, the system for the poor is poorly coordinated internally and almost completely unplanned and unmonitored. It is certainly as wasteful of resources as the middle class system, but because it is a low cost, poorly financed system, the exact amount of waste is difficult to document. At the same time, the great virtue of the health care system for the poor—its openness and accessibility to all people at all times for all conditions (albeit with considerable delays)—is difficult to evaluate adequately as well.

Certainly, the most important issue for the system of care that presently serves the poor is whether or not it will be able to survive much longer without a new source of financial support. As more and more city and county governments find themselves in deep financial difficulties, as more and more states and local areas pass laws limiting the amount of tax revenue a local (or even a state) government can raise, the financial situation of local government units becomes increasingly shaky; so too does the financial situation of the public health and hospital services they provide. The key issue in the survival of the system that provides care for the poor is financial, and the prospects are increasingly bleak.

Military Medical Care System

A person joining one of the uniformed branches of the American military sacrifices many aspects of civilian life that nonmilitary personnel take for granted. At the same time, however, this person receives a variety of fringe benefits that those outside the military do not enjoy. One of the most important of these fringe benefits is a well-organized system of high quality health care provided at no direct cost to the recipient. Certain features of this military medical care system (the general term used to include the separate systems of the U.S. Army, Navy, and Air Force) deserve comment. First, the system is all inclusive and omnipresent. The military medical system has the responsibility of protecting the health of all active duty military personnel everywhere and of providing them with all the services they may eventually need for any service-connected problem. The military medical system goes wherever active duty military personnel go, and assumes a responsibility for total care that is unique among American health care systems.

The second important characteristic of the military medical care system is that it goes into effect immediately whether the active duty soldier or sailor wants it or not. No initiative or action is required by the individual to start the system; indeed, the system frequently provides certain types of health services, such as routine vaccinations or shots, that the soldier or sailor would really wish not to have. The individual has little choice regarding who will provide the treatment or where, but at the same time, the services are always there if needed, without the need to search them out. If a physician's services are needed, they are obtained; if hospitalization is required, it is arranged; if emergency transportation is necessary, it is carried out. There is little that the individual can do to influence how medical care is provided, but at the same time, there is never any worry about its availability.

The third important characteristic of the military health care system is its great emphasis on keeping personnel well, on preventing illness or injury, and on finding health problems early while they are still amenable to treatment. Great stress is placed on preventive measures such as vaccination, regular physical examinations and testing, and educational efforts toward prevention of accidents and contagious diseases. In an approach that is unique among the health care systems of this country, the military medical system provides health care and not just sickness care.

In the military medical system, the same mass public health and preventive medicine services that are provided to a locality or a community by a local government health department or health agency may also be provided to the active duty military personnel. However, whenever the personnel are actually within the boundaries of a military reservation or post, an additional set of mass public health and preventive medicine services may be provided by the military itself. Sanitary disposal of sewage, protection of food and milk, purification of the water supply, and prevention of vehicular or job-related accidents may be provided for by a local government agency, but each military installation will usually have a second separate system of its own, staffed by its own public health and safety officers. Individual public health and preventive medicine services are also provided by the military medical system according to a well-organized, regularly scheduled routine of yearly examinations, surveys of patient records, vaccinations, and other measures. The persons providing the specific preventive service (for example, a routine tetanus shot) are usually medical corpsmen or other nonphysician personnel; however, their work is carried out according to carefully developed guidelines and will be monitored by well-trained supervisory medical personnel.

Routine ambulatory care is usually provided to most active duty military personnel by the same medics who provide the individual preventive services. These services are usually provided at the dispensary, sick bay, first aid station, or similar unit that is very close to the military personnel's actual place of work. These ambulatory services may also be provided by physicians or nurses at the same locations, but this is less likely. More complicated ambulatory patient care services are usually provided by physicians, frequently specialists, working at the same dispensary or medical station as the medics or, more likely, in a clinic or outpatient department of a larger facility such as a military hospital. Patients are usually referred by medics or physicians who have first cared for the patients for more simple problems; laboratory tests, x-ray examinations, and medications are obtained at the same military facility to which the patient is referred.

The most simple hospital services are provided using short-stay beds at base dispensaries, in sick bays aboard ship, or at small base hospitals on various military installations around the world. Usually the range of services that can be offered at these installations is limited, and referral to larger institutions is routinely carried out if a more complex problem is suspected. More complicated hospital services are provided to active duty military personnel in regional hospitals that possess a wide variety of specialized services and facilities. Frequently, these hospitals also have large teaching and training programs, where the atmosphere and the quality of care are similar to what might be expected at a university hospital or a large community teaching hospital.

The military medical system does not pretend to offer the same extensive range of long term care services that it provides for more acute short term problems. The military medical system does provide care for potentially long range problems in military hospitals, as long as there is some reasonable expectation that the patient will some day be able to return to full active duty. Whenever it is determined, however, that the problem is genuinely long term in nature and that complete return to active duty is not possible, the patient is given a medical discharge from the service and long term care will be provided through the Veterans Administration (VA) facilities.

If military personnel develop emotional difficulties, care is most likely to be provided initially by the medical corpsman and then by a physician assigned to that military unit. These personnel will provide short term nonpsychiatric support and counseling, and possibly prescribe certain medications, such as tranquilizers. For more severe problems, the patient is referred to the psychiatric services of larger military hospitals where the severity of the problem will be determined. If the problem is short term and is not believed to affect the patient's work seriously, an attempt may be made to provide the short term treatment at the military hospital itself, first on an inpatient and later on an outpatient basis. More likely, if there is a significant psychiatric diagnosis, the patient will be given a medical discharge, with follow-up care to be provided through the psychiatric services of the VA hospitals.

In general, the military medical system is closely organized and highly integrated. A single patient record is used, and the complete record moves from one health care service to another with the patient. Once the need for health care is identified, the system itself arranges for the patient to receive the required care and usually even provides transportation to the services. The patient does not have to search out the necessary service or determine how to use it. This service is provided at no cost to the patient, requires little effort by the patient to initiate it, and generally involves a high quality product. The system is centrally planned, use nonmedical and nonnursing personnel to the utmost, and is entirely self-sufficient and self-contained. The services are provided by salaried employees in facilities that are wholly owned and operated by the system itself. The system is not generally available to persons who are not active duty military personnel or their dependents, although in cases of emergency or pressing local need, they can be. Generally, the patient has little choice regarding the manner in which services will be delivered, but this drawback is counterbalanced by the assurance that high quality services will be available when needed.

In recent years, the military medical system has been affected by the termination of the physician draft that previously kept it well supplied with high quality young physicians who had just completed their specialty training. With the end of the physician draft, the military medical systems have had to compete with all other health care systems for physicians, and their choice of physicians has been narrowed considerably.

Dependents and families of active duty military personnel are served by a special subsystem of military medicine that combines the services of the middle class, middle income system and the active duty military system. The dependents and families of active duty military personnel are covered by an extensive health insurance plan, the Civilian Health and Medical Program of the Uniformed Services (CHAMPUS), provided, financed, and supervised by the military. This health insurance plan allows dependents and families of active duty military personnel to purchase medical care from private medical practitioners and from local community nonmilitary hospitals when similar services cannot be provided at a military installation within reasonable distance. The dependents and families of active duty military personnel can also use the same military services that the active duty personnel use, provided space and resources are available and military authorities determine that this procedure is appropriate. The resulting subsystem of care for military dependents and families generally allows them to participate to some degree in two separate systems of care: the middle class, middle income private practice system and the military medical system. Their participation in either is generally not as clearly focused or as active as it would be for someone firmly planted in either system exclusively, but it still provides them with two viable options for obtaining care.

Veterans Administration Health Care System

Parallel to the system of care for active duty military personnel is another system operated within the continental United States for retired, disabled, and otherwise deserving veterans of previous U.S. military service. Although the VA system is in many respects larger than the system of care for active duty military personnel, it is not nearly as complete, well integrated, or extensive. At the present time, the VA system of care is primarily hospital oriented and not really a health care system. The VA operates 171 hospitals throughout the country that provide most VA care. In recent years, the VA has increasingly provided outpatient services and now maintains more than 200 outpatient clinics; however, the majority of VA health care is still focused on the hospitals.

A second important characteristic of the VA system is the great preponderance of male patients with long term care problems. By and large, the patients using the VA health care system are older, inactive men in whom the occurrence of multiple and chronic physical and emotional illnesses is much higher than in the general population.

A third important feature of the VA system is its existence as only one part of a much larger system of social services and benefits for veterans. Many of the people eligible to utilize the VA health care system are also receiving other kinds of financial benefits as well; indeed, access to the VA health care system is sometimes directly dependent upon eligibility for financial benefits. The dollars represented in Table 1-3 paid for health care for over 1 million veterans annually during the period 1975–1980. During this same time period, 2.5 million veterans also received educational assistance, more than 3 million veterans received VA disability compensation, and more than 3.5 million veterans had VA home loans outstanding

TABLE 1-3. VA Medical Care Expenditures and Percent Distribution According to Type of Expenditure, 1965–1980

Type of Expenditure		1965	1970	1975	1980
				Year	
	Total	$1,150.1	$1,688.6	$3,328.2	$5,981.3
		Amount of millions			
		Percent distribution			
All expenditures		100.0	100.0	100.0	100.0
Inpatient hospital		81.9	71.3	66.4	64.3
Outpatient care		12.0	14.0	17.8	19.1
Va nursing homes and domiciles		2.9	4.3	4.8	5.1
Community nursing homes		0.0	1.2	1.4	2.0
All others		3.2	9.1	9.6	9.6

SOURCE: *Health-United States, 1981*, DHHS publication (PHS) 82-1232. US Department of Health and Human Services, December 1981.

annually. Since health care is only one of many VA programs, a great variety of social services interact with and compete for all available resources.

A further feature of the VA health care system is its unique relationship with organized consumer groups. Since the VA is organized to provide care exclusively for veterans, and since many of those veterans are members of local and national veterans clubs and associations, the VA health care system is constantly in direct communication with groups representing the interests of veterans. In a manner that is unparalleled in any other health care system in this country, the interests of the veterans are constantly conveyed to individual VA hospitals, to the VA administration in Washington, and to the U.S. Congress. In no other health care system in this country does organized consumer interest play such a constant, important, and influential role.

Since the VA system is primarily a hospital system, there are few attempts to provide general public health services or routine ambulatory care services. Veterans usually obtain these services from some other system of care, either the middle class, middle income system or the local government system that serves the urban poor. The VA does provide the more complicated ambulatory care services, usually through its hospital outpatient clinics. This care is in preparation for possible hospital admission or as follow-up after hospitalization. Many veterans who require these services obtain them from other systems of care and come to the VA system only after a condition is apparent and hospitalization is required. Admission to VA hospitals can be gained either through the ambulatory patient care services operated by the VA itself, by direct referrals from physicians in private practice, or by referrals from hospitals in the community. The services in VA hospitals are provided by salaried, full-time medical and nursing personnel; as in the military medical system, most of the VA hospitals are self-contained, relatively self-sufficient units that require little outside support or staff.

The VA health care system provides a tremendous quantity of long term care for both physical and emotional illnesses. Indeed, the VA is probably the largest single provider of long term care in the country, if not the world. In addition to providing considerable long term care in the acute, short term care hospitals, the

VA also operates a number of domiciliaries and nursing homes, and also pays for care in local community nursing homes and skilled nursing facilities. As of early 1982, 18 VA hospitals also offered hospice or hospicelike care to their patients who were dying of cancer.

The VA system of care is difficult to describe fully for two important reasons. First, it is a system that does not attempt to provide a complete range of services, but instead concentrates on acute hospital services and on long term care for physical and emotional problems. Second, eligibility for entry into the system is somewhat unclear and sometimes open to variable local interpretation. The system is designed to serve veterans with service-connected disabilities, but offers services to other veterans if they cannot obtain adequate care elsewhere and if adequate VA resources are available. In practice, the actual eligibility requirements and patient mix vary substantially from one VA hospital to the next.

If the system of health care for active duty military personnel focuses on preventive, ambulatory, and acute inpatient care, the VA system of care stresses long term, chronic inpatient care for both physical and emotional problems. Whereas the military medical system offers a complete, well integrated, well coordinated package of health care services, the services that the VA offers are primarily hospital related. In contrast to the military medical system, which actively seeks out and offers services to patients as part of their work environment, the VA provides its services to patients only when they come forward to seek them. If they do not seek out the care, the VA system does not actively pursue them. Despite these reservations about the VA as a complete system of health care, it should be stressed that the VA serves as the primary source of inpatient hospital care for 1 million veterans a year and is a potential source of inpatient care for many millions more. As such, it is the largest single provider of health care services in this country and must be considered an integral, important component of the American health care scene, both now and in the future.

HEALTH SERVICES: A SUMMARY OF PERSPECTIVES

In reviewing each of these four major systems of health care for Americans, the middle class, private practice system, the local government system for the urban poor, the military medical system for active duty military and their dependents, and the VA health care system, it becomes apparent that there are a number of additional systems that could have been included as well. Other systems of health care include the one used by rural farming families and the Indian Health Service operated for native Americans by the federal government. There are also many possible variations within the four systems discussed here. The purpose, however, is not to be exhaustive in describing the systems themselves but rather to point out that there are multiple systems providing services to different populations with different needs. No one system predominates in terms of persons served or benefits provided. Indeed, the purpose here is to point out that there is no one single American health care system but rather a mosaic of subsystems, each with its own characteristics and moving in its own direction.

Is it bad to have so many separate subsystems? Why is it even worth pointing out the obvious fact that many such systems exist? Several pressing reasons exist for reviewing this country's compartmentalized organization of health care. The first and most important is quite simple: To improve health services to everyone in this country, an understanding of the entire situation is essential; otherwise, piecemeal solutions will be proposed to specific problems without recognizing the possible long-range potentials for the entire system. In a system that could be compared to a jigsaw puzzle, it would be foolish and perhaps even dangerous to consider individual pieces of the puzzle without first viewing the puzzle as a whole.

The second reason for considering the various separate systems of health care in this country is the vigorous competition for scarce resources of money, people, and facilities. Although the four systems described are separate from one another, they all compete for the same resources since they are all dependent upon the same economy and the same supplies of health personnel and skills.

Whenever there is vigorous competition for resources, two things frequently happen. First, the stronger, more vigorous, more aggressive, or better connected competitors obtain the larger portion of the resources, whether or not this outcome is justified by their needs. In practice, this has meant that the middle class, private practice system, the military medical system, and the VA system have all done relatively well, while the local government health care system has not. Indeed, as has already been pointed out, the local government health care system for the poor has always been severely underfinanced and understaffed, a situation that seems to be getting progressively worse.

Second, intense competition for resources frequently results in wasteful duplication and ineffective use of resources. For example, in the same region, a city or county hospital, a private teaching hospital, a military hospital, and a VA hospital may all be operating exactly the same kind of expensive service, although only one facility might be needed and where undoubtedly one large integrated service would provide more efficient use of resources than four smaller ones. Because each institution is part of a separate system, serves a different population, and approaches the resource pool through a different channel, no really purposeful planning or controlled allocation of resources is possible. In the past, this situation might have been acceptable because the resources seemed endless, but in these days of very limited resources, this is no longer acceptable.

In addition to this economic inefficiency, there are other reasons for looking with a critical eye at multiple systems of care, reasons that are related to quality and accessibility of services. Unfortunately, not all of these subsystems of care serve people in the same way with the same results. There is great inequality among the various systems of health care, with the result that different people receive different levels of care simply by accident of birth or membership in a special group. Since all the separate systems of health care in this country ultimately depend on public funds for their continued existence, it is imperative that the inequalities among them be removed as rapidly as possible. This does not necessarily mean eliminating the various separate subsystems of care, but rather requires that all the systems rise to a common high level and equitably share responsibilities and resources.

In recent years, there have been various approaches to the problem of reorganizing these separate subsystems of care so that they function together in a more integrated and effective fashion. Although these proposals have often been limited to specific aspects, such as financing or quality of care, their overall purpose has generally been to move the various pieces of the American health care system into a better and more efficient relationship with each other. These approaches are interesting not in themselves but in how they will shape health care in the future. The specific scenarios for particular issues will undoubtedly change, but the overall effort to develop a more rationally integrated system will certainly continue unabated and will, indeed, expand as resources are stretched to the limit.

Two proposals can be mentioned briefly, not because they are unimportant but rather because the possibility of their implementation is so slight that they have relatively little practical impact. The first of these might be described as a *laissez-faire*, free-market approach that implies in effect, "Leave everyone alone, stop meddling, stop regulating, and let the workings of the marketplace with its active competition eventually force the health care system to reorganize." The second approach, at the other political and social extreme, implies, "What this country needs is a single, governmentally controlled health care system, such as the British National Health Service, which would allow for greater centralized control and planning for all aspects of the system." For different reasons, both of these approaches have been viewed as so politically impractical for this country at this time that they have not been seriously considered.

Another approach that has been considered has been the "health planning" approach. With the passage of the original Comprehensive Health Planning legislation and, more important, with the passage of the National Health Planning and Resources Development Act of 1975, it had been thought that providers, consumers, and public officials might come together and develop plans for all states and localities that would then become blueprints for a more rationally organized system of care. This hope did not turn into reality, and with the demise of the health planning system, this approach toward more rational coordination of health care services has been virtually abandoned for the time being, as discussed further in Chapters 12 and 15.

A somewhat different approach to rationalizing the American health care system focuses on the use of financing mechanisms to encourage or force increased coordination of effort throughout the system. The proponents of this approach suggest that the power to withhold financial reimbursement to providers who do not comply with efforts to improve the system would be so strong as to be irresistible. Although the argument is used most visibly by many of the proponents of a national health insurance plan, this approach has become more apparent in the way the Health Care Financing Administration (HCFA) uses Medicare funds to encourage compliance with its long range objectives. It is also becoming increasingly obvious in the way certain employer health care coalitions are using their influence over the industrial concerns' health insurance dollars as a means of making their wishes known.

Another possible solution, which has yet to receive considerable attention, is the "public utility" approach. In this approach toward a more rational health care system, all the components of the health care system, or at least the large institutional ones, would be placed under the regulatory supervision of public bodies that would have total control over licensing, financing, mode of function, packages of services to be offered, personnel development, and so forth. Both public and private components could continue to exist as they do at present under their own auspices (just as individual utilities do now, for example), but what they would be able to do and how much they would be allowed to charge would be controlled by a single regulatory agency. A strong argument for this approach is that all of these regulatory efforts are now conducted in a poorly coordinated and often conflicting fashion by multiple regulatory agencies. Having one single body would remove much of the present jungle of regulatory efforts. A strong argument *against* such a body is that immense power over the system would be given to a single superagency. Practically speaking, in the present antiregulatory political climate in this country, there is little enthusiasm for this approach.

A final approach toward rationalization of the present system might be called "incremental tinkering" and it is one that tacitly assumes that no major, sweeping, overall reorganization is possible. The proponents of this approach try instead to do whatever they can to increase rationality whenever an opportunity occurs anywhere in the system. A new piece of state legislation here, a new form of federal health insurance there, a new form of local cooperative planning are all added in piecemeal fashion, with no great effort to relate them to each other or to some underlying master plan. The hope in this approach is that all the individual accretions to the system will provide for a more efficient and integrated end product.

These six approaches are obviously not mutually exclusive, so it is entirely possible that someone might support several of them because they work well together. Someone interested in reorganizing the health care system through health planning might also want to institute a national health insurance program because it would provide the centralized financial leverage for mandatory health planning. In the same fashion, someone might propose a mostly *laissez-faire* approach to any intentional reorganization and also support a national health insurance plan that would allow all people to make their own choices in an open market.

In the future, all six approaches (and possibly more) will probably continue to be fostered and most likely no single approach will predominate. What certainly will continue, however, will be efforts to bring the various pieces of the subsystems and the various subsystems themselves into a more efficient and effective new relationship with one another and with the consumers who must use them. Indeed, this issue is so important and so central to all our other interests that the future of health care in this country will be shaped by the direction our society decides to follow.

The remaining chapters of this book describe, dissect, and analyze the health services system of the United States. Trends, issues, interrelationships, and problems are revealed and assessed. Only by thoroughly understanding the evolution, structure, attributes, and deficiencies of the system, or systems, can the fundamental decisions facing the nation be addressed.

PART TWO

Causes and Characteristics of Health Services Use in the United States

CHAPTER 2

The Physiologic and Psychologic Bases of Health, Disease, and Care Seeking

Lawrence A. May

In this chapter, the physiologic bases of disease and the psychologic characteristics of care-seeking behavior are explored. The concepts of illness and disease and the complexities surrounding the exact definitions of diseases are discussed. The orderly relationship between pathologic abnormality, physiologic alteration, and clinical manifestations of disease are presented, especially as they relate to care-seeking behavior. The influence of biologic, pharmacologic, and environmental factors on changing disease patterns is reviewed, and some of the effects of these changing disease patterns on the health services system are demonstrated as a prelude to the remaining chapters of the book.

DEFINING ILLNESS AND DISEASE

The distinction between illness and disease is essential for the understanding of care-seeking behavior. Illness is a lay experience that connotes both a physical and a social state (1). It is an individual's reaction to a biologic alteration, and is defined differently by different people according to their state of mind and cultural beliefs. The term *illness*, therefore, is imprecise and represents a highly individual response to a set of physiologic and psychologic stimuli.

By contrast, *disease* is a professional construct. It is perceived as being precise and reflecting the highest state of professional knowledge, particularly that of the physician. The definition of disease is used as the vehicle for informing the patient of the presence of pathology, as a means for deciding on a course of treatment, and as a basis for comparing the results of therapy. It becomes an essential element in the planning and organization of the health care system and in the allocation of resources within that system.

The accurate definition of disease is so important that it is crucial to recognize that considerable imprecision exists in the process of medical diagnosis. An individual physician using the best professional judgment available may diagnose a disease in a particular patient, but this definition may not be shared by other physicians. Even when the definition of a particular disease is similar in different patients, the impact of the diagnosis on those patients may vary widely depending upon how the definition is applied and on the unique social and biologic characteristics of individual patients.

Attempts to link illness (the individual's perception of loss of functional capacity) with disease (the professional's definition of a pathologic process) is even more complicated. Illness may occur in the absence of real disease, and disease may be present in the absence of perceived illness. It is illness, the individual's perception of impaired function, and not disease that stimulates care-seeking behavior, making the relationship between these two concepts important to understand.

The complexity of defining disease and its interaction with care-seeking behavior are well illustrated by the condition diabetes mellitus. Both the general public and the health care professional understand that diabetes results in an elevated blood sugar level, but the physiologic bases of this metabolic alteration can vary widely (2). In one person, the disease may result from impaired secretion of insulin by the pancreas, or it may be caused by a resistance to sufficient amounts of insulin in a patient who is obese. Diabetes mellitus may result from the imposition of a normal physiologic condition such as pregnancy, or it may be due to the use of exogenous drugs such as diuretics or steroids.

Aside from the varying causes of an elevated blood sugar level (referred to as *hyperglycemia*), an important issue is the amount of hyperglycemia that defines a patient as diabetic. Various criteria have been suggested to define who is diabetic, using different numerical measures of elevated blood sugar level, but these criteria do not necessarily separate those who feel healthy, nor do they define a level at which treatment is indicated (3). The myriad criteria that have been applied to diabetes at one time or another would define anywhere between 4% and 40% of the population over age 60 as having diabetes. In recognition of the fact that even objective measures of disease or health such as a blood sugar determination are variable, great effort was expended to reach a consensus on what level of blood sugar elevation defines diabetes. The criteria state that the level must be consistently elevated in the fasting and postprandial states and that this level must be found on two occasions. The current criteria for diagnosing diabetes are a fasting blood sugar level of 140 and a blood sugar level or more than 200, measured two hours after eating on two separate occasions. The previously widely used glucose tolerance test is expensive, unnecessary, and results in an excessive number of false-positive readings sacrificing specificity in a way that is unacceptable (4).

The problem illustrated by diabetes extends to many other disease conditions that are defined by an abnormal laboratory measurement or blood test result. Hypertension is a common medical problem resulting from a variety of physiologic bases, including abnormalities in hormone production and use, improper resetting of neurologic control centers, or acquired loss of blood vessel elasticity secondary to atherosclerosis.

In view of the variety of causes of hypertension, the selection of an arbitrary number to define individuals or members of a population as having an abnormal condition is a difficult and possibly futile effort. The blood pressure reading of 140/90 has been offered as the boundary of normality, but the meaning of this reading in different persons may vary markedly. A blood pressure of 150/100 in a 72-year-old woman has quite different implications from the same reading in a 26-year-old man. An elevated blood pressure after a half hour of bed rest means something quite different from an elevated blood pressure in a person waiting anxiously for half an hour in a physician's office.

To complicate matters further, as with diabetes, there is no direct relationship between the presence of elevated blood pressure and the development of either perceived symptoms or actual pathologic damage to body organs, at least at the lower ranges of hypertension. Some people with only slight hypertension will attribute a variety of functional complaints to their "blood presure," whereas others with dangerously elevated levels may not have any symptoms and perceive themselves as being well (5).

The definition of diabetes or of hypertension is relatively straighforward when compared to diseases that cannot be numerically defined, such as rheumatoid arthritis. The definition of this disease is clinical rather than numerical and is based on the presence of four or more diagnostic characteristics determined by the American Rheumatism Association to be valid criteria for the disease. Even with the use of this symptom aggregation approach, there are still many professionals who confuse rheumatoid arthritis with degenerative joint disease and with other forms of arthritis. Further, even with this more orderly approach to the definition of this disease, the ability to measure its impact on a population is comparatively limited.

In summary, the definition of disease is a more imprecise and inexact process than is usually thought. Although it is frequently associated with apparently solid, objective measurements such as blood sugar levels or blood pressure, the implications of these values may vary widely. Finally, the relationship between illness, which is a personal observation by patients, and disease, which is a scientific judgment by professionals, needs to be understood and constantly remembered.

THE PHYSIOLOGIC BASES OF DISEASE

The major pathophysiologic processes involved in disease production are vascular, inflammatory, neoplastic, toxic, metabolic, and degenerative. These processes give rise to disease conditions, but their expression is modified by factors in the host such as age, immunologic status, medication ingestion, concurrent disease, or psychologic perceptions. The combination of the pathophysiologic processes and the different host factors creates the various disease patterns.

Vascular abnormalities may produce disease in a variety of ways in multiple organ systems. The gradual narrowing and eventual blockage of blood vessels by the deposit of fatty materials in the walls and lumina of the vessels is a characteristic of arteriosclerotic cardiovascular disease. Vascular disease may also be produced by the more rapid occlusion of a blood vessel by an embolus, material from a distant site floating in the bloodstream. Other disease pictures may be produced by bleeding from a ruptured blood vessel in the brain or elsewhere. In some disease conditions, such as stroke, the same clinical picture may result from any one of these three causes. Whatever the initial cause, gradual occlusion, embolus, or rupture, the result is damage to brain tissue and resultant paralysis. It is usually easy to determine that a cerebrovascular accident (stroke) has occurred, but it is frequently impossible to determine whether it was caused by gradual occlusion, embolus, or rupture of a blood vessel.

Inflammation is the basis of disease in many organ systems, but the physiologic basis of that inflammation may be infectious, autoimmune, traumatic, or something else. A single inflamed joint may be due to autoimmune inflammation, the presence of uric acid crystals, or degeneration of cartilage as a consequence of age and use, or it may be due to infection with bacteria or viruses. The failure to identify the specific etiologic factor can be highly destructive to the patient or at least fail to resolve the problem in the appropriate amount of time. Therefore, having defined both the type of disorder and the mechanism of inflammation, physicians must seek to identify the underlying agent in the process of inflammation.

Neoplastic disease is caused by an abnormal new growth of tissue. Benign neoplasms are abnormal growths that remain localized and do not spread to distant locations in the body. Malignant neoplasms, generally called *cancer*, by contrast, not only grow locally and invade surrounding tissues but also spread to distant sites in the body, producing metastases. Benign neoplasms may cause considerable damage by continued local growth and pressure on surrounding tissues, such as pressure on the brain from a benign growth on its surface. Malignant neoplasms, by contrast, invade the organs directly and disrupt their normal functioning by replacing normal tissue with diseased tissue. Neoplasms may occur spontaneously or may be caused by environmental, toxic, or host factors (6–11).

Toxic bases for disease involve the presentation to individual organs of chemical materials that are inherently damaging. These materials may originate from environmental pollutants, from the use of potentially damaging materials such as alcohol or cigarettes, or from the ingestion of medications. Alcohol, for example, is toxic to the liver under appropriate conditions, causing hepatitis, fibrosis, and eventual cirrhosis. Cobalt in beer can be toxic to heart muscle cells, bee stings may damage the glomerulus of the kidney, and asbestos may contribute to the development of lung cancer. Cigarette smoking may destroy, inflame, or alter the cells of the lung, producing emphysema, chronic bronchitis, or cancer. Digitalis, an ordinarily useful drug in the treatment of various heart conditions, in excess doses may produce toxicity and life-threatening arrhythmias. In a society with an increasing amount of environmental pollution, drug use, and industrial exposure, toxins are unfortunately becoming a more common cause of disease.

Metabolic diseases are caused by chemical disorders within body cells, usually secondary to some excess or deficiency of a hormone or important nutrient. The excess or deficiency of a thyroid, parathyroid, or adrenal cortical hormone causes clinical disease pictures that are easily recognized by well-trained physicians. A deficiency of insulin, secreted by glands in the pancreas, gives rise to diabetes, as mentioned earlier. Deficiency of important nutrients, caused either by a scarcity of the elements in the diet or by an inability to absorb and use them, results in a wide variety of clinical pictures ranging from anemia to pellagra.

Degeneration is the final pathophysiologic cause of disease, and may occur as a primary idiopathic disorder or secondary to another process such as aging. Physicians generally resist accepting degeneration as an explanation for disease, but there are many diseases that currently cannot be otherwise explained. For example, many people with senile dementia have a pathologic process of unexplained primary degeneration of brain cells. Degenerative joint disease is usually related to age and may be accelerated by unusual use or trauma, but it remains primarily a degenerative process with no specific vascular, metabolic, or inflammatory explanation.

It should also be clear that a particular disease may be caused or affected by a variety of pathophysiologic mechanisms. Peptic ulcer, for example, is a common disease with a multifactorial physiologic basis. The ulceration of the mucosal lining of the duodenum is caused by gastric acid, may occur in genetically predisposed people, and may be abetted by the toxic effect of drugs such as aspirin or corticosteroids that impair the protective barrier of the mucosa. There may be a secondary inflammation producing pain or obstruction, and the ulcer may erode a blood vessel, producing bleeding. To say that any single pathophysiologic process "causes" ulcers would be misleading.

Once the initial pathophysiologic process has given rise to a particular disease entity, its clinical manifestations are modified by a variety of host factors such as age, immunologic status, medication ingestion, concurrent disease, or psychologic makeup. For example, in a healthy person with high tolerance for pain, a case of herpes zoster (shingles) may be perceived as a minor discomfort, whereas in a person with a low threshold for pain, it may become a disabling illness for which professional attention and potent analgesics are required. Under the influence of a concurrent disease or the ingestion of drugs such as steroids that suppress the immunologic response, a usually nonpathogenic fungal infection may produce serious illness. A minor inflammation of the connective tissue such as cellulitis, for example, may become a serious, life-threatening problem in a diabetic with an impaired vascular, sensory, or immunologic status. In a genetically susceptible host, an infectious agent may precipitate an inflammatory response and antibody production leading to systemic lupus erythematosus, whereas in a genetically nonsusceptible host it may not produce any effect.

Thus, there are a variety of pathophysiologic processes that can initiate disease, but the expression of the disease itself may be modified by a variety of factors in the host. Any review of a particular disease entity, therefore, should include consideration of both aspects, so that a complete understanding of the disease can be developed.

Symptom Production and the Pathologic Process

A pathologic process may begin and exist silently for some time without producing any evidence of physiologic alteration. Although the disease is present and active, it may be undiscovered. In many chronic disease situations, it is now well known that the disease condition may be present for a considerable length of time before becoming detectable by current diagnostic procedures. Atherosclerosis, for example, has been detected at autopsy in healthy young 18-year-olds dying from accidental causes (12–14); many prostatic cancers are discovered at autopsy that were never recognized during life.

After a pathologic process has been present for a time, it may not only begin to produce physiologic alterations that can be discovered by appropriate diagnostic tests but may also begin to produce clinical symtoms that are, for the first time, recognized by the patient or the physician. There can be a significant time lag, however, between the onset of physiologic alteration and the production of symptoms, just as there was between the onset of the pathologic process and the physiologic alteration. A pathologic process may be present and discoverable by diagnostic tests long before it produces sufficient symptoms for a patient to feel its presence. Atherosclerosis and atherosclerotic vascular disease illustrate this continuum of pathologic process, physiologic alteration, and symptom production and are reviewed to provide further insight into the disease process.

Atherosclerosis is a pathologic process characterized by focal accumulation of lipids and complex carbohydrates, producing a secondary narrowing of the arteries. The process affects arterial vessels of the body in the cerebral, coronary, peripheral, and abdominal circulations and is now the leading cause of death in the United States.

As mentioned previously, atherosclerosis without physiologic alteration has been documented in 18-year-olds. At this stage, it is a subclinical or presymptomatic process and can be identified only by direct examination of the blood vessels.

Coronary artery disease is a specific manifestation of atherosclerosis in the arteries that provide blood to the heart muscle. As it becomes progressively more serious, it interferes with arterial capability for providing sufficient oxygen to meet the heart muscle's metabolic demands. As the reduction in oxygen supply worsens, ischemia of the heart muscle may occur. With still further progression, any increased demand on the cardiac muscle, as in any kind of exertion, may produce angina pectoris, or chest pain, the cardinal symptom of coronary artery disease.

Long before the angina is present, coronary artery disease may be identified by an abnormal electrocardiogram (EKG). If an EKG with the patient at rest does not produce evidence of disease, frequently an EKG during controlled exercise will yield the necessary evidence. In these cases, the coronary artery disease may not be sufficiently serious to produce EKG changes during normal demands on the heart, but the increased cardiac demands associated with exercise will provide the necessary diagnostic evidence.

These clinical changes may not evoke any symptoms, but eventually the patient may experience intermittent chest pain on exertion and seek medical care. At this time, the chances of obtaining an abnormal EKG and confirming the presence of coronary artery disease become much greater, but even at this stage a patient may have typical angina pain with an apparently normal EKG. The difficulty of defining the specific relationship between pathology and symptoms may be even greater. Both resting and exercise EKGs produce a number of false-positive and false-negative results. The absolute criterion for the definition of coronary artery disease becomes arteriography, the injection of dye to outline the coronary artery and the areas of narrowing. However, it should be understood that many people with no symptoms have demonstrable coronary artery disease, and that many others with classic anginal symptoms and characteristic EKG abnormalities have coronary arteries free of atherosclerosis. It has been well established in the literature that the same objective alterations in the EKG and classic symptoms may be produced by spasm rather than occlusion of the coronary arteries (15).

In patients with occlusive coronary artery disease, atherosclerosis may eventually occlude a coronary artery completely, causing the heart muscles supplied by the artery to die. This clinical event is known as *myocardial infarction,* commonly called a "heart attack," and is accompanied by prolonged chest pain, nausea, sweating, shortness of breath, and weakness. However, the arterial occlusion and subsequent tissue death may occur silently and without symptoms, to be discovered by EKG at some later date.

Following the pathologic process a step further, loss of heart muscle function secondary to coronary artery disease may affect the heart's ability to maintain adequate circulation to the rest of the body and may produce a range of secondary signs and symptoms in other organs. As the heart becomes weaker, there may be progressive difficulty in breathing, swelling of the legs and feet, inability to maintain blood supply to the brain and subsequent faintness, and impairment of kidney function with reduction of urinary output. These events are sometimes labeled by the single clinical description of *heart failure*.

Atherosclerosis is a generalized disease and is usually not limited to the coronary arteries; similar events occur in the blood vessels of other organs. This process may produce primary effects in organs that are not related to the secondary effects of heart failure described above. Abdominal pain, bowel necrosis, neurologic deficits, strokes, renal failure, calf pain, and aortic aneurysms may all be produced by atherosclerotic damage to the arteries of various organs. The combination of this primary damage to the organs themselves and the secondary effects of heart failure is complicated and serious, dramatically illustrating why atherosclerosis is such a major cause of morbidity and mortality.

PHYSIOLOGIC BASES
OF CHANGING DISEASE PATTERNS

Over the years, the pattern of diseases affecting the U.S. population has changed profoundly, generally as a result of changes in the environment, in the population's demographic composition, and in medical practice. Infectious diseases as the major cause of mortality have been replaced by chronic diseases associated with aging. At the turn of the century, infectious diseases struck the young and healthy and spread rapidly, often resulting in death. The confluence of improved sanitation, a higher standard of living, antibiotics, and vaccines reduced death and disability from infectious diseases so markedly that they are now a comparatively minor cause of death (see Chap. 1).

The treatability of syphilis, for example, has reduced its incidence and impact markedly, and cases with the secondary or tertiary manifestations of this potentially devastating disorder are now increasingly rare. Smallpox, polio, mumps, diphtheria, measles, pertussis, rubella, tetanus, typhoid, and cholera, all once highly prevalent, have now all but disappeared. Bacterial infections of childhood and infantile diarrheas of all kinds are now effectively treated with antibiotics and intravenous feedings; as a result, they do not present the threat they did at the turn of the century.

While these disease entities have been diminishing or disappearing, new disease patterns have been emerging to take their place as the most important threat to life and health. Some of these patterns have resulted from the removal of diseases in early life (e.g., childhood infections), which has allowed time for diseases of later life (e.g., atherosclerosis) to appear. Other disease patterns, however, are comparatively new, are far more prevalent than they once were, and are the result of new forces in modern life and environment.

Changes in the incidence and prevalence of some cancers, for example, provide dramatic evidence of these patterns (16). In the early part of the century, cancer of the lung was not a major cause of death, but it began to increase in men as the rate of cigarette smoking in men increased. The incidence of lung cancer in women lagged behind that of men until recently, when it began to rise to a comparable level, probably secondary to the increase in cigarette smoking among women.

In the same vein, there has been a rise in endometrial carcinoma in women, attributed at least in part to the increased use of estrogens by postmenopausal women (17). Pancreatic cancer has increased in recent years and is occurring at a younger age than previously, but no clear explanation of this changed disease pattern has been proposed. The etiologic factors contributing to the increased risk of pancreatic cancer have been subject to vigorous epidemiologic debate. Coffee in its caffeinated and decaffeinated forms has been implicated, with considerable refutation of these arguments (18). Again, recent years have seen a marked rise in mesothelioma, a previously rare type of lung cancer, probably secondary to the markedly increased use of asbestos in manufacturing and construction.

In the same fashion, improvement in our medical technology has changed the patterns of disease, not just by wiping out previously existing scourges but also by creating new ones (see Chapter 9). The morbidity and mortality of common diseases such as pneumonia and wound infections have been replaced by serious infections with once nonpathogenic bacteria that are now resistant to antibiotics. Patients whose own defense mechanisms have been compromised by corticosteroids, immunosuppressive agents, and cancer chemotherapy are now susceptible to serious infections with fungi, yeast, protozoa, or bacteria that are not normally harmful (19).

A dramatic recent expression of changing disease patterns illustrating basic scientific mechanisms and a fascinating interaction between social behavioral issues has occurred in the homosexual population. Kaposi's sarcoma, a previously rare disease of elderly people of Mediterranean origin, has been diagnosed in a large number of young homosexuals (20). Other viral infections including herpes simplex and cytomegalovirus have been detected with frightening frequency, as well as infections with previously rare diseases such as *Pneumocystis carinii* pneumonia (21). In part because of sexual practices and immunosuppression, an entire spectrum of intestinal infections with parasites, viruses, and bacteria has been described and referred to as the "gay bowel" syndrome (22). There is much speculation on the implications of this devastating epidemic, but it illustrates an interaction between a behavior and the biologic basis of disease that has given rise to a spectrum of diseases previously unknown or at least vanishingly rare (23). The Council on Scientific Affairs of the American Medical Association has published a report on the specific health care needs of the homosexual population (24). This report illustrates the complex interaction and the need for involvement by planners and administrators in defining health services based on often rapidly changing disease patterns. Another example of new diseases is the often described toxic shock syndrome and its relationship to tampons. This disease illustrates a public health and political decision that one often has to make (25).

A substantial percentage of hospitalizations are now attributable to drug toxicity and the secondary effects of new surgical procedures such as ileojejunal bypass for morbid obesity or the complications of kidney dialysis for chronic renal disease. Cardiac pacemakers prolong life but also produce a new spectrum of morbidity, as do other new prosthetic devices such as cardiac valves, artificial joints, or silicone implants. Organ transplantation has created an entirely new spectrum of biologic diseases based on intentional destruction of the body's immunologic system, its own basic protection from disease. Patients with bone marrow or renal transplants require considerable care and present diseases that are rare if they occur at all in normal, nonimmunosuppressed populations. The potential for transplanting other organs creates considerable flux in the biologic nature of disease and has frightening implications for the ability of persons to provide and pay for these services. The most dramatic example is the artificial heart, developed and implanted in a patient in December 1982 by a team at the University of Utah.

The increased effectiveness of medical intervention is also having a considerable effect on the patterns of disease by changing the gene pool controlling the incidence of certain diseases. Improvements in prenatal and high-risk obstetric care allow completion of pregnancies in diabetic women who otherwise may not have reproduced. This development may increase the prevalence of an already common disease such as diabetes. The successful introduction of vigorous physical therapy and prophylactic antibiotic use have increased the survival of patients with cystic fibrosis, and a few have successfully reproduced. The impact of the longer term survival on the gene pool for this disease remains to be seen, but it is a good example of some of the potential hazards caused by new technology.

An additional powerful influence affecting our patterns of disease is environmental change. Vehicle accidents are an increasingly important cause of morbidity and mortality, and directly reflect our increasing use of the automobile for transportation. Pollution of air and water has already been suggested as at least partially causative in a number of conditions, and toxic aspects of industrial work environments have been suggested as the cause of many more. Indeed, it has been argued that as many as three-fourths of all cancers may be in part environmentally determined.

Dietary habits have also been suggested as contributing to changes in disease patterns in recent years. The most obvious result of dietary change is obesity, which is associated with hypertension, heart disease, and diabetes. Burkitt and associates have suggested that diverticulosis, hemorrhoids, appendicitis, and even cancer of the colon may be a consequence of changes in the amount of fiber in the Western diet. Epidemiologists have implicated certain foods as possible causes of atherosclerosis (26). Increased salt intake has already been indicted in certain aspects of hypertension, and increased ingestion of refined sugars has definitely been associated with increased incidence of dental caries and possibly with several other conditions.

In summary, in addition to a wide variety of causes of disease and a wide variety of responses in individual hosts, the overall pattern of disease in a society can change markedly over time. In this country, the pattern of disease has moved from one of acute infectious disease several generations ago to one of chronic disease today. Further, the pattern of disease has been influenced by our ability to wipe out certain diseases, thereby allowing others to be expressed. Finally, many aspects of modern life, such as improved medical technology and environmental pollution, have caused disease patterns that have never existed before.

SOCIAL AND CULTURAL INFLUENCES ON DISEASE AND BEHAVIOR

It has been estimated that 70% to 90% of all self-recognized illness is not generally treated in the conventional medical care delivery system (27). Conversely, it is reported that more than half of the visits to physicians are related to patient-identified problems for which no ascertainable biologic basis can be determined. It is clear, from this finding, that seeking medical care may or may not be associated with actual pathologic processes, and that social and cultural values greatly influence the individual's decision to visit a physician (28,29).

A large number of physician visits are for complaints in which the physiologic function is well within normal limits, but for which the patient feels that some abnormality exists. Many people seek medical attention for constipation, for example, when bowel function is basically normal and no serious pathology can be documented. For some reason, either internally generated or imposed by the prevailing culture, these patients believe that the situation is not quite right and seek medical attention. They have somehow been led to expect bowel function that is different from what they are experiencing, and a medical remedy is sought.

Symptoms of fatigue may be attributed by the patient to a nondisease such as hypoglycemia (30). Conversely, a disease with a well-defined physiologic basis may not produce care seeking, since it may not be interpreted as a disease. The teenager with acne, for example, has a problem with a well-understood physiologic basis and an obvious clinical manifestation. The potential patient, however, may interpret it as a normal consequence of adolescence that will eventually resolve and for which treatment is either ineffective or unavailable (31). Seeking care for serious conditions is often delayed because of fear or uncertainty (32).

Disease and the perception of illness are not the only reasons people seek medical care. Normal physiologic processes frequently are the occasion for seeking care. Pregnancy or contraception are certainly not pathologic or disease processes, but they usually require professional attention. Heavy menstrual flow, missed or irregular periods, and menopause are usually the result of basically normal physiologic processes, and yet medical attention is frequently sought concerning them. An event of modern times illustrates how medicalized normal physiologic processes can become and the interaction of social factors in creating the need for medical care. The increasing rates of infertility and the frighteningly high incidence of cesarean sections are modern medical problems. Many have attributed the current rates of infertility to the frequent delay in childbearing (33). This decrease in fertility has been well documented and has created substantial medical and psychologic problems and a tremendous base for care seeking. The rate of cesarean section is sometimes linked to this phenomenon and to the complex interaction of physician fear of litigation, the presence of monitoring equipment that allows detection of abnormalities that might not have affected the outcome, and the technologic advances that allow cesarean section to be performed with less morbidity than formerly existed. It is not only the perception of illness or the presence of disease, but also the alterations in normal physiologic functions and changes in medical practice influenced by social and technologic interventions, that create some of the reasons for care-seeking behavior.

Indeed, in many cases, medical care is sought because the patient is healthy and wants to remain that way. Parents bring infants and small children to the pediatrician for routine evaluations in order to ensure that the child is developing normally. Adults visit their physician periodically for an examination, a chest x-ray film, a Papanicolaou smear, and possibly other tests because they have been told it is important to do so. Indeed, all care seeking behavior is carried out in a framework that is intensely affected by current social, cultural, and political values, regardless of the type or severity of the pathologic process. Cultural influences frequently determine what society considers to be a medical problem, whereas economic or political realities determine whether or not medical care is sought. The complex interactions of people and doctors, the personal and cultural influence on disease, and the perception of symptoms have been well reviewed in the literature (29).

Zbrorowski (34) studied the differences in attribution between Italian and Jewish patients. Italians were generally satisfied and ceased demanding medical care once pain relief was obtained. Jews were reluctant to take medication and continued to be concerned with the underlying cause of their discomfort rather than simply relief of pain. It can be anticipated that they would continue to seek care until they were reassured that there was no serious underlying pathology.

The deep psychologic meaning of disease was explored by Cassel (35) in an article on suffering. He argued that suffering was experienced by people. It was not a physical construct and it was often underappreciated by practicing physicians. He illustrated his point by suggesting that pain in circumstances such as childbirth, in which it is expected, rarely produces suffering and does not call for much care-seeking because of discomfort. In contrast, situations in which pain is unexplained may give rise to considerable suffering and continued care seeking. He again argues that the physician's failure to appreciate and deal with the bases of suffering may lead to a failure to reassure the patient.

The complex psychologic underpinnings of care seeking are indicated by the remarkable ability of patients to respond to placebos. Placebos, which have been effective in reducing not only subjective symptoms but also objective test results, are a testament to the importance of symbolic intervention. They argue for a complex interaction between physician and patient on both verbal and nonverbal levels and demonstrate that the encounter itself and the therapeutic relationship have meaning to the individual who weeks medical services (36). Many authors have recently argued that physicians do not fully recognize the social and cultural determinants of care seeking. An illuminating article on the Couvade syndrome demonstrated failure by physicians in a prepaid practice to recognize the influence of a woman's pregnancy on the husband's medical complaints (37). In the Couvade syndrome, husbands of pregnant women have symptoms such as nausea, vomiting, anorexia, pain, and bloating—feelings often experienced by their wives—while having no objective organic abnormalities. In this study, husbands of pregnant women had two times the number of doctor visits, four times the number of symptoms, and two times the number of prescriptions without any increase in actual pathology during the period of their wives' pregnancy as compared to other periods. The study illustrates the myriad influences on the production of symptoms and the need to seek medical care. It has increasingly been argued that consumerism and a critical analysis of health care needs and physician limitations can give rise to a more productive doctor-patient relationship (38). Health care administrators must understand the complex influences on care seeking and design systems that identify both the physical abnormalities and the cultural determinants that provide the impetus for seeking medical services.

As social and cultural values change, the understanding of what constitutes disease and the subsequent care-seeking patterns may change as well (39,40). The transference of marital adjustment and childrearing problems from the category of family problems best handled by a member of the clergy to psychologic problems best handled by a physician or psychologist is one example of this trend. The recent shift toward the description of alcoholism as a disease requiring medical treatment is another. A further example is the court decision changing abortion from a criminal act to a recognized medical service. The numerous manifestations of psychologic problems, discussed further in Chapter 8, represent many examples of difficult to define illness with a substantial political and value-laden component.

In all of these examples, it should be noted that the underlying pathologic process has not changed; rather, it is the perception of these processes as disease or not that has been altered. In other circumstances, even our perception of certain conditions as illnesses does not change; instead, external social values change the way we react to them.

For example, the increased mobility and weakened family structure of modern

American life have made it more difficult to care for elderly and infirm family members at home. Smaller housing units, increased numbers of families in which both adults are employed, and a variety of other social pressures have altered the ability to handle the health problems of the elderly in the fashion of the past. Instead, society has created a new network of health institutions—nursing homes— to provide professional care for pathologic processes that previously were handled at home. The underlying pathologic processes have remained the same. It is the societal response to them that has changed (41).

The Influence of Supply

Within the total spectrum of pathologic processes that affect the health of people in this country, it is important to note that some processes receive much more interest and attention from the health care system than others. It is also important to speculate about why this occurs.

The structure and availability of health services contribute significantly to the amount and nature of the care that will be sought. Once the patient makes the initial decision to seek professional attention, much of the additional medical care results directly from the decisions of the physician (40). The physician usually decides what laboratory tests, x-ray films, treatment procedures, and hospitalizations are necessary, and in so doing shapes a particular pattern of care for each patient. In some ways, these decisions by the physician also shape the health care system itself by creating a demand for certain services. As long as the demand exists, the institutions, programs, and services will expand to fill the need.

But does the process work this way, or is the reverse true? Do pathologic processes stimulate patients to visit physicians, who in turn demand certain services as a result of their decisions? Or do the specialized services become available to physicians, thereby influencing the manner in which they approach disease, and do physicians then shape patients' perceptions and demands on the basis of what they know is available (42)? There is some evidence to suggest that the latter is true, at least in part, and is becoming progressively more important.

Physicians generally do most of their training in hospitals and are introduced early to the use and benefits of sophisticated procedures and tests. The availability of these tests and treatments then influences the physicians' view of disease, since they now make possible the treatment of conditions that were previously beyond consideration. The surgical treatment of degenerative processes such as hip replacement for osteoarthritis, laser treatment for diabetic retinopathy, and replacement of diseased heart valves with prosthetic devices have all created many new options for the physician. They have also created new reasons for patients to seek care.

Unfortunately, the development of these new approaches is not always in keeping with the real need for care among patients, as determined by the pathologic processes that threaten them. The mere fact that a particular process, such as arthritis or alcoholism, has a major impact on public health does not necessarily mean that sophisticated technology will be developed to deal with it. Instead, the more sophisticated technologies are frequently developed in areas of lesser importance, leaving more serious problems relatively less well attended. Patients' perceptions of illness and its importance are then shaped more by areas where major technology is available than by areas of perhaps greater need.

It is unclear whether the development of pathologic processes or the availability of services to treat them creates the demand for health care. It is clear, however, that the use of medical services is the result of a unique interaction involving the pathologic process themselves, the patient's and the physician's perceptions of them, and the availability of services to deal with them (43). Each of these elements must be considered if the use of health services is to be better understood by all concerned.

REFERENCES

1. Apple D: How laymen define illness. *J Health Hum Behav* 1960; 1:219–225.

2. Siperstein MD: The glucose tolerance test: A pitfall in the diagnosis of diabetes mellitus. *Adv Intern Med* 1976; 20:297–323.

3. O'Sullivan JB, Mahan CM: Prospective study of 352 young patients with chemical diabetes. *N Engl J Med* 1968; 278:1038–1041.

4. National Diabetes Data Group: Classification and diagnosis of diabetes mellitus and other categories of glucose intolerance. *Diabetes* 1979; 28:1039–1057.

5. Mabry J: Lay concepts of etiology. *J Chronic Dis* 1964; 17:371–386.

6. Lowenfels AB: Alcoholism and the risk of cancer. *Ann NY Acad Sci* 1975; 252:366–373.

7. Merliss RR: Talc-treated rice and Japanese stomach cancer. *Science* 1971; 173:1141–1142.

8. Selikoff IJ, Churg J, Hammond EC: Asbestos exposure and neoplasia. *JAMA* 1964; 188:22–26.

9. Poskanzer DC, Herbst AL: Epidemiology of vaginal adenosis and adenocarcinoma associated with exposure to stilbestrol in utero. *Cancer* 1977; 39(suppl):1892–1895.

10. Dungal N: The special problem of stomach cancer in Iceland with particular reference to dietary factors. *JAMA* 1961; 178:789–798.

11. Lowenfels AB, Anderson ME: Diet and cancer. *Cancer* 1977; 39(suppl):1809–1814.

12. Enos WF, Beyer JC, Holmes RH: Pathogenesis of coronary disease in American soldiers killed in Korea. *JAMA* 1958; 158:912–914.

13. Enos WF, Holmes RH, Beyer JC: Coronary disease among United States soldiers killed in action in Korea. *JAMA* 1953; 152:1090–1093.

14. McNamara JJ, Molot MA, Stremple JF, et al: Coronary artery disease in combat casualties in Vietnam. *JAMA* 1971; 216:1185–1187.

15. Meller J, Pichard A, Dack S: Coronary arterial spasm in Prinzmetal's angina: A proven hypothesis. *Am J Cardiol* 1976; 37:938.

16. Kritchevsky D: Metabolic effects of dietary fiber. *West J Med* 1979; 130:123–127.

17. Schwarz BE: Does estrogen cause adenocarcinoma of the endometrium? *Clin Obstet Gynecol* 1981; 24:243–251.

18. McMahon B, Yen S, Trichopoulos D, et al: Coffee and cancer of the pancreas. *N Engl J Med* 1981; 304:630–633.

19. Stamm WE: Nosocomial infections: Etiologic changes, therapeutic challenges. *Hosp Pract* 1981; 16:75–88.

20. Hymes KB, Chung T, Greene JD, et al: Kaposi's sarcoma in homosexual men—a report of eight cases. *Lancet* 1981; 2:598–600.

21. Mildvan D, Mathus U, Enlow RW, et al: Opportunistic infections and immuno-deficiency in homosexuals. *Med Ann Intern Med* 1982; 96:700–704.

22. Philips SC, Mildvan D, William DC, et al: Sexual transmission of entire protozoa and helminths in venereal-disease-clinic population. *N Engl J Med* 1981; 305:603–606.

23. Amman AJ: Acquired immune dysfunction in homosexual men. *West J Med* 1982; 137:419–421.

24. Health care needs of a homosexual population. *JAMA* 1982; 248:736–739.

25. Wanamaker LW: Toxic shock problems in definition and diagnosis of a new syndrome. *Ann Intern Med* 1982; 96:775–777.

26. Turpeinen O: Effect of cholesterol-lowering diet on mortality from coronary heart disease and other causes. *Circulation* 1979; 59:1–7.

27. Dingle JH, Badger GF, Jordan WS: Illness in the home: A study of 25,000 illnesses in a group of Cleveland families. Western Reserve University, 1964.

28. Zola IK: Culture and symptoms: An analysis of patients' presenting complaints. *Am Sociol Rev* 1966; 31:615–630.

29. Stocker JD, Barsky AJ: Attributions: Uses of social science knowledge in the "doctoring" of primary care, in Eisenberg L, Kleinman A (eds): *The Relevance of Social Science for Medicine.* Hingham, Mass: D Reidel Publishing Co, 1980, pp 223–240.

30. Meador CK: Art and science of nondisease. *N Engl J Med* 1965; 272:92–95.

31. Ludwig EG, Gibson G: Self perception of sickness and the seeking of medical care. *J Health Soc Behav* 1969; 10:125–133.

32. Battistella RM: Factors associated with delay in the initiation of physicians' care among late adulthood persons. *Am J Public Health* 1971; 61:1348–1361.

33. DeCherney AH, Berkowitz GS: Female fecundity and age. *N Engl J Med* 1982; 306:424–426.

34. Zborowsky M: Cultural components in responses to pain. *J Social Issues* 1952; 8:16–30.

35. Cassell EJ: The nature of suffering and the goals of medicine, *N Engl J Med* 1982; 306:639–644.

36. Brody H: The lie that heals: The ethics of giving placebos. *Ann Intern Med* 1982; 97:112–118.

37. Lyokinji M, Lamb GS: The Couvade syndrome: An epidemiologic study. *Ann Intern Med* 1982; 96:509–511.

38. Jensen PS: The doctor-patient relationship: Headed for impasse or improvement? *Ann Intern Med* 1981; 95:769–771.

39. Parsons T: Definitions of health and illness in the light of American values and social structure, in Jaco EG (ed): *Patients, Physicians and Illness.* Glencoe, Ill, Free Press of Glencoe, 1958, pp 165–187.

40. Fuch V: *Who Shall Live? Health, Economics and Social Choice.* New York, Basic Books, 1974.

41. Somers AR: Long term care for the elderly and disabled: A new health priority. *New Engl J Med* 1982; 307:221–226.

42. Stoeckle JD, Zola IK, Davidson GE: On going to see the doctor, the contributions of the patient to the decision to seek medical aid: A selective review. *J Chronic Dis* 1963; 16:975–989.

43. Rosenstock IM: Why people use health services. *Milbank Mem Fund Q* 1966; 44 (pt 2):94–127.

CHAPTER 3

Factors Associated with the Use of Health Services

Stephen M. Shortell

The biologic and medical bases for health care needs were presented in Chapter 2. This chapter examines the translation of these needs into actual use of services. Overall trends and explanations of differences in use among various population groups are presented. Some of the implications of these trends and differences for health care professionals are discussed. In addition, selected issues related to long term care, self-care, primary and rural health care, and child health are described. Many of these issues are elaborated further in subsequent chapters.

The ability to provide accessible and cost-effective health services to patients depends on a thorough understanding of factors associated with the use of health services, especially those factors that can be manipulated to improve the provision of care. The analysis of utilization patterns aids the understanding of such issues as the analysis of the distribution of health resources across the population to determine which groups have limited access to care, the relationship between use of services and health status, and the relationship between volume and patterns of use and strategies for controlling health care costs.

All health professionals needs to understand health services utilization patterns. For health administrators, such information is essential for forecasting demand for care, for developing strategic organizational plans, and for the marketing of services. Physicians, nurses, and other providers of care benefit from a knowledge of those utilization patterns that offer insight into such issues as delays in seeking or receiving care, comprehensiveness of services, continuity of care, and compliance with the provider's advice. Health planners use the data for many of the reasons identified above and are especially interested in the relationships among different types of use at an aggregate level (for example, in a county or geographic region). Health policy analysts require use data to examine the cost effectiveness of alternative means of providing care. For example, for some individuals home care may be less expensive and just as effective as nursing home care. Policy analysts and researchers also require utilization data to analyze the potential impact of changes in national health policies related to such issues as cost containment, financing, and personnel. Finally, it is increasingly important for all health professionals to plan, provide, analyze, and evaluate services from an epidemiologic perspective based on defined populations. Increased regulatory pressures and demands for greater public accountability underscore the importance of analyzing users and nonusers of services.

The next section presents analytic categories and descriptive trends pertaining to the use of personal health services. Subsequent sections discuss differences in use, important findings and practical implications of research studies, and the need for broader frameworks for analyzing utilization. The concluding sections highlight specific topics in health services utilization that are especially relevant to public policy.

ANALYTIC CATEGORIES
AND CONCEPTUAL DISTINCTIONS

There are many approaches to describing utilization of personal health services, but the three principal categories are the type and purpose of utilization, and the organizational setting in which care is provided. Principal types of utilization include hospital admissions, total hospital inpatient days, physician and dental visits, admissions to long term care facilities, and total inpatient days in these facilities. Utilization can also include visits to nurses, nurse practitioners, physician assistants, social workers, physical therapists, optometrists, and other types of health care professionals. Still other types of use include admissions to mental hospitals, outpatient visits to community mental health centers, drug prescriptions, and use of medical appliances. Each type of utilization can also be categorized by the purpose of the visit. Examples include preventive examinations, diagnosis, treatment, and rehabilitation.

Utilization can also be differentiated by the organizational setting in which it occurs. Examples include hospital inpatient units, outpatient departments and emergency rooms, Health Maintenance Organizations (HMOs), physicians' offices, neighborhood health centers, nursing homes, and the patient's home.

For each of the above categories of use (type, purpose, and organizational setting), measures of contact and volume of services can be examined. Contact measures might include the percentage of a population hospitalized in a specified year or the percentage seeing a physician in a year. Volume measures might include the total number of hospital inpatient days in a specified time interval or the total number of physician visits in a year. Patterns of utilization can be described from the sequential flow of providers seen and resources used during an episode of illness. Continuity of care and other system characteristics can be determined from these patterns using various summary indexes (1–3). The different categories for describing and analyzing health services utilization are summarized in Figure 3-1.

In analyzing utilization patterns, it is important to distinguish between the concepts of health needs and wants and the demand for health services (4). A population's *need* for services may be determined by either normative medical judgments or individual perceived needs. *Wants* refer to the quantity of health services that individuals feel they ought to consume, based on their own perceptions of their health needs. *Demand* is the quantity of health services that individuals wish to consume at specified prices, using available financial resources, and

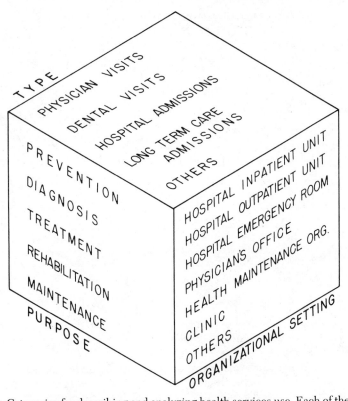

Figure 3-1. Categories for describing and analyzing health services use. Each of these categories can be further characterized by measures of *contact* with the system, *volume* of services received, and the *pattern* or sequential flow of services received.

considering preferences for all other goods and services. *Utilization* is the actual quanity of services that is consumed when demand is translated into care-seeking behavior. Individuals' wants may be more or less than their needs or demands for care.

These distinctions are important because they underlie notions of equity in, and relative shortages of, health services. Equity assumes that services are provided to meet everyone's needs for care, as determined by either professional medical judgment or the self-perceptions of patients. However, this is a value judgment that does not conform to the economist's notion of *market shortage*, which is defined as the excess of demand over supply at existing prices. Failure to achieve equity may be the result of shortages in personnel, facilities, and other resources, or it may be due to problems associated with their distribution across the population. Analysis of utilization and related data can reveal trends that influence public policy related to access, equity, and cost issues.

Descriptive Trends

Using the framework in Figure 3-1, the tables and figures in this chapter indicate the major trends in health service use in the United States in recent decades. This information is based on the most recently available data from a variety of sources,

TABLE 3-1. Use of Health Care Resources: United States, 1979

Resource	Unit of Measure	Estimated Number/1,000 Population
Practioners' offices	Visits	3,175.4
Hospital outpatient facilities, including emergency room	Visits	618.8
All other ambulatory sources	Visits	905.6
Short-stay general hospitals	Discharges	162.8
	Days of care	1,158.2
Nursing homes	Residents	6.1
	Days of care	1,888.7[a]
Mental health facilities other than hospitals	Residents	1.67[a]

SOURCES: *Excerpts of Health Resources and Utilization Statistics, 1976,* DHEW publication (PHS) 79-1245. Hyattsville, Md, Public Health Service, October 1978; *Health: United States, 1981,* DHEW publication (PHS) 82-1232. Hyattsville, Md, Public Health Service, Office of Health Research, Statistics, and Technology, December 1981.

[a] 1976 data.

especially those from national data collection efforts. The detailed comparisons are also presented for race, income, residence type, and other sociodemographic differences in the population.

Table 3-1 provides an overview of the use of selected health care resources in the United States during 1979. Heavily used facilities include practitioners' offices, short-stay general hospitals, and nursing homes. These settings reflect the major organizational settings in which care is provided in this country, and each is discussed in detail in a separate chapter.

Physician Use.   Currently, approximately 75% of the population visits a physician at least once a year. This figure is in contrast to 66% in 1958 (5). As shown in Figures 3-2 and 3-3, the gap between whites and nonwhites has closed, and the differences by income group have narrowed. Despite these changes, however, black children are more likely than white children to have had no physician visits. The difference is particularly pronounced in rural areas, where 21% of black children and 14% of white children had no visits, compared with only 10% and 9%, respectively, in metropolitan areas (6).

There have also been substantial changes in the location of care over the years. During the period 1928–1931, 40% of all physician visits occurred in the home. By 1971, this proportion was less than 2%. During the same time period, office visits increased from 50% to 70% of all visits (7). Approximately 43% of these visits were to general and family practitioners, although this proportion increased to 65% in nonmetropolitan areas and decreased to 35% in metropolitan areas (8). The majority of visits represent return or repeat visits; only 16% are first visits (9). In 1970, 14% of visits by the poor and 19% of visits by nonwhites were to hospital outpatient departments compared with 7% for the total population (10). In 1976, 16% of the low income population reported using a hospital outpatient department clinic as their regular source of care versus only 5% of the high income group (11). Further issues in ambulatory care use are discussed in Chapter 5.

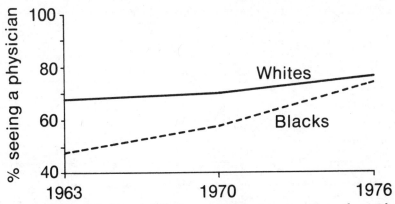

Figure 3-2. Percentage of whites and blacks seeing a physician in a 12-month period.
SOURCE: *America's Health System: A Portrait*, special report. The Robert Wood Johnson Foundation, no 1, 1978, p 7.

In 1979, Americans averaged 4.7 physician visits per person per year. The number of visits increased with age and was higher for women than men (5.2 versus 4.1). This difference was due, in part, to women's need for obstetric care (12). There have been significant shifts in the volume of physician visits per person per year by income group and race. In 1964, the number of visits for the nonpoor was 4.7 per person per year compared to 3.8 for the poor. In 1978, the poor averaged more physician visits per person per year than the nonpoor (6.2 versus 5.0). Similarly, differences by race have also changed markedly. In 1964, whites had 4.7 physician visits per person per year versus 3.3 for nonwhites; in 1978 the figures were virtually identical: 4.9 versus 4.8. Differences beween urban and rural areas have also narrowed somewhat. In 1964, urban residents had 4.8 physician visits per person per year versus 3.8 for rural residents; in 1978 the respective figures were 4.9 and 4.4 (13). Rural blacks, however, experienced only 3.7 physician visits per person per year in 1978 compared with 4.4 visits per person per year for rural whites. The differences were particularly pronounced for children under 17 years of age: Rural blacks had only 2.0 physician visits per person per year compared to 3.9 for rural

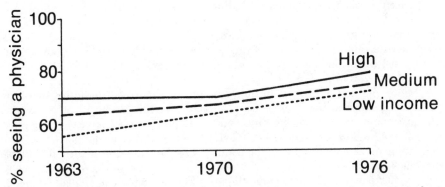

Figure 3-3. Estimated percentage of high, medium, and low income groups seeing a physician in a 12-month period.
SOURCE: *America's Health System: A Portrait*, special report. The Robert Wood Johnson Foundation, no 1, 1978, p 8.

TABLE 3-2. Physician Visits, Adjusted and Unadjusted for Health Status

	Unadjusted[a]	Adjusted for Health Status[a]	Unadjusted[b]	Adjusted for Health Status[b]
Low income[c]	4.6	44	5.1	37
Medium income	4.0	44	4.9	46
High income	3.8	45	4.9	64
Ratio of high to low income	0.83	1.02	0.92	1.73

SOURCES: Aday LA, Andersen R, Fleming GV: *Health Care in the U.S.: Equitable for Whom?* Beverly Hills, Calif., Sage Publications, 1980; Kleinman JL: *NHIS Results by Income and Insurance*, Hyattsville, Md, National Center for Health Statistics, 1980.

[a] Visits: data from Aday et al. (1980).

[b] Visits: data from Kleinman (1980).

[c] Aday et al. define low income as income below $8,000, medium income as income between $8,000 and $14,999, and high income as income above $15,000. Kleinman defines low income as below the poverty level adjusted for family size, medium income as between the poverty level and twice the poverty level, and high income as more than twice the poverty level.

whites. Overall, blacks under 17 had only 3.0 visits per person per year compared with 4.3 for whites (14).

Although overall the volume of physician visits per person per year has increased markedly for the poor and for nonwhites, these data ignore the greater medical needs of these groups, as indicated by a variety of health status measures. Two studies have attempted to adjust for differences in the volume of physician visits per person per year by taking into account differences in health status as measured by the volume of physician visits per 100 disability days. Aday et al. (15) adjusted their data by considering all reported disability days, and Kleinman (16) adjusted his data by using bed disability days only, a somewhat more stringent measure in terms of likely need for medical care. Although these adjustments are not without problems, the results, as shown in Table 3-2, indicate that the poor have fewer physician visits than the middle and upper income groups. This pattern is particularly marked in Kleinman's findings. Thus, when the data are adjusted for differences in health status, the poor continue to have fewer physician visits than higher income groups. Further analyses suggest that when age and sex are also taken into account, those whose income is more than twice that of the poverty line receive 5.2 physician visits per person per year versus only 3.5 to 4.0 for those below the poverty line (16).

Figure 3-4 and 3-5 reveal further differences. Figure 3-4 indicates that those without chronic conditions who do not qualify for the Medicaid program (non-Medicaid poor) have only two physician visits per person per year compared to those in the Medicaid program, who receive four to seven visits per person per year, depending on race and region of the country. For the latter group, the data indicate that blacks have fewer visits than whites and that persons residing in the South have fewer visits than those living in other regions. Figure 3-5 indicates a marked income effect among those who perceive their health to be fair or poor; the differences are particularly strong among children under age 17.

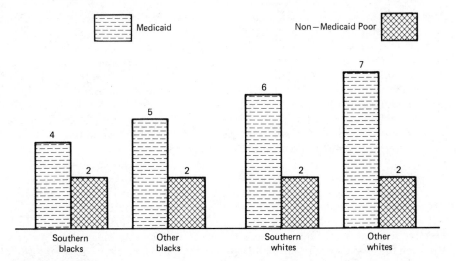

Figure 3-4. Number of annual physician visits for low income persons with no chronic conditions, 1976.
SOURCE: Link CR, Long SH, Settle RF: *The Impact of Medicaid on the Utilization of Medical Services by the Poor: Some New Evidence,* working paper. Syracuse, NY, Maxwell School, Syracuse University, April 1980.

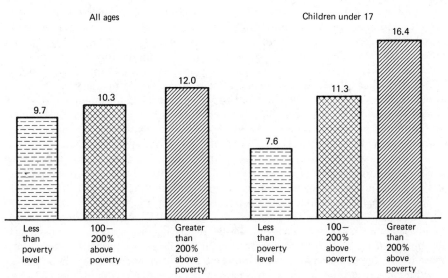

Figure 3-5. Average number of annual physician visits for persons with fair or poor health, 1976–1978.
SOURCE: Kleinman J: National Health Interview Survey results. Hyattsville, Md, Department of Health and Human Services, National Center for Health Statistics, 1980.

Other Ambulatory Care Visits.   The most recently available data for the period 1973–1974 indicate wide variations in the number of visits to outpatient facilities other than physicians' offices. For example, the number of visits per 1,000 population was 228.8 for health department clinics, schools, and insurance offices; 97.6 for family planning clinics; 41.8 for company or industrial health units; and 25.0 for community mental health centers. In addition, there was a total of 694,100 visits to public health service clinics (17). Further, outpatient care episodes involving community mental health centers ranged from a low of 88.8 per 100,000 population for persons aged 65 and over to a high of 463.9 per 100,000 or those in the 25–44 age group. There are virtually no differences by sex (18).

Use of Selected Preventive Services.   With increased concern over the rising cost of health care, more attention has been focused on preventive care. The assumption is that early prevention measures will not only help people maintain their health but will result in early detection of disease, which may be treated in a more cost-effective manner than if left undetected or detected at a later, more severe stage. Although the evidence supporting this assumption is mixed, and must await further research to indicate specific areas where prevention may be cost effective, the issue is of growing importance to health care professionals.

Overall, use of preventive services is most consistently associated with higher levels of education. For example in 1976, 56% of persons living in households headed by an individual who had 13 years or more of education received a general physical examination versus only 45% of those whose household head had 8 or fewer years of education (15). In 1970, 81% of women having live births, residing in a household whose head had 13 years or more of education, saw a physician by the end of the first trimester versus only 71% of those whose household head had 8 or fewer years of education (19).

Tables 3-3, 3-4, and 3-5 summarize data pertaining to Pap smears, breast examinations, and blood pressure tests. Table 3-3 indicates that the overall percentage of women having a pap smear increased from approximately 54% in 1973 to nearly 60% in 1979. As shown, the increase was greatest among the low income group; it was particularly significant for low income blacks, increasing from 47.1% in 1973 to 66.9% in 1979. Differences by income remain, however, particularly for those between the ages of 45 and 64; in 1979 only 42.9% of low income women received Pap smears versus 56.0% of high income women. Interestingly, all of this difference is accounted for by white women; only 38.3% of low income white women received a Pap smear in 1979 compared with 56.0% of high income white women.

Table 3-4 shows an overall increase in the percentage of women having a breast examination, from 55.6% in 1973 to nearly 63.0% in 1979. The increase was particularly significant among black women, increasing from 54.3% in 1973 to 71.4% in 1979. The most substantial increase occurred among the 45–64 age group, from 44.5% in 1973 to 58.2% in 1979. As shown, between 1973 and 1979, the percentage of low income black women aged 45–64 receiving breast examinations nearly doubled. Still, overall, higher income women in this age group in 1979 were much more likely to receive breast examinations (63.3%) than low income women (50.9%). As with Pap smears, the difference was particularly marked for white women; 63.2% of the high income group received a breast examination versus only 47.6% of the low income group.

Table 3-5 indicates a significant increase for both men and women in the percentage having a blood pressure test, rising from approximately 62% in 1974 to 75%

TABLE 3-3. Women with a Pap Test during the Past Year, According to Race, Age, and Family Income: United States, 1973 and 1979.

	Race					
	All Races		White		Black	
Age and Family Income	1973	1979	1973	1979	1973	1979
20–64 years	Percent of women					
All incomes	54.2	59.6	54.4	58.5	52.7	70.6
Low income	44.4	55.4	43.6	51.9	47.1	66.9
High income	57.2	62.5	57.2	61.9	58.5	71.5
45–64 years						
All incomes	40.9	51.0	41.5	50.0	35.5	60.6
Low income	29.8	42.9	29.7	38.3	30.1	62.1
High income	44.8	56.0	44.9	56.0	41.7	*59.5

SOURCES: National Center for Health Statistics: Data from the 1973 National Health Interview Survey and from the 1979 National Survey of Personal Health Practices and Consequences. Hyattsville, Md, US Dept of Health and Human Services, various years.

Note: Definitions of low and high income groupings in Tables 3-3 through 3-5 are based on family income for each year as follows:

Year	Low income	High income
1973	Less than $ 6,000	$ 6,000 or more
1979	Less than $10,000	$10,000 or more

in 1979 for men and from 75% in 1974 to 83.5% in 1979 for women. The increase was particularly significant for black women, increasing from 80% in 1974 to 96% in 1979. Much of this increase was accounted for by the substantial growth for low income black women. Low income black men also made significant strides, increasing from 61.2% in 1974 to 82.7% in 1979. Although not shown in the table, there was a particularly significant increase in the percentage of lower income men aged 45–64 who received a blood pressure test, increasing from 62.7% in 1974 to 81.6% in 1979.

TABLE 3-4. Women with a Breast Examination during the Past Year, According to Race, Age, and Family Income: United States, 1973 and 1979

	Race					
	All Races		White		Black	
Age and Family Income	1973	1979	1973	1979	1973	1979
20–64 years	Percent of women					
All incomes	55.6	62.8	55.7	61.8	54.3	71.4
Low income	45.5	57.5	44.8	53.5	47.9	69.0
High income	58.7	66.4	58.6	66.0	60.6	70.9
45–64 years						
All incomes	44.5	58.2	45.0	57.2	39.6	67.0
Low income	32.9	50.9	32.8	47.6	33.4	65.0
High income	48.5	63.3	48.7	63.2	46.5	*67.6

SOURCES: National Center for Health Statistics: Data from the 1973 National Health Interview Survey and from the 1979 National Survey of Personal Health Practices and Consequences. Hyattsville, Md, US Dept of Health and Human Services, various years.

TABLE 3-5. Persons with a Blood Pressure Test during the Past Year, According to Race, Age, Sex, and Family Income: United States, 1974 and 1979

	All Races		White		Black	
Age, Sex, and Family Income	1974	1979	1974	1979	1974	1979
20–64 years						
Male			Percent of population			
All incomes	61.8	75.2	61.5	74.9	66.1	79.3
Low income	58.8	69.3	58.3	67.6	61.2	82.7
High income	62.5	76.2	62.2	76.0	68.1	78.3
Female						
All incomes	75.5	83.5	75.0	82.0	80.1	96.1
Low income	74.9	86.4	74.3	83.5	77.2	96.0
High income	76.0	83.6	75.5	83.1	82.8	95.3

SOURCES: National Center for Health Statistics: Data from the 1974 National Health Interview Survey and from the 1979 National Survey of Personal Health Practices and Consequences. Hyattsville, Md, US Dept of Health and Human Services, various years.

Other data indicate that the percentage of women seeing a physician in the first 3 months of pregnancy continues to vary by income, increasing from a low of 65% for low income women to 85% for middle income women and 96% for high income women (15). But there is relatively little difference among adults 17 years of age and older in the percentage receiving chest x-ray films: 36% for high income persons versus 31% for low income persons. For the percentage receiving a flu shot, low income people were more likely to choose it than those of high income: 15% versus 9% (15).

It is also interesting to note the ratio of preventive care visits to visits for diagnosis and treatment. As shown in Figure 3-6, the ratio is higher for higher income groups. Finally, it is important to note that the earlier mentioned differences in overall physician visits between farm residents and other residents also persist for preventive care use. For example, only 42% of farm residents had a physical examination in 1976 versus 50% or more for residents of other areas; only 67% of farm residents had a blood pressure test versus 77% of residents in Standard Metropolitan Statistical Area (SMSA) central city areas; only 35% of farm women over age 17 had a Pap smear versus 58% in SMSA central city areas; and only 43% of farm women over age 17 had a breast examination versus 58% in SMSA central city areas (15).

Overall, the data indicate increased use of preventive services by high risk subgroups, especially the poor and nonwhites. In particular, significant strides have been made by black women in regard to Pap tests, breast examinations, and blood pressure tests. These increases may be due to a number of events occurring during the 1970s, including increased health education efforts such as the National High Blood Pressure Education Program, begun in 1971 and involving 150 national organizations and state health departments (20), and the Community Hypertension Evaluation Clinic Program, which served more than 1 million people during the period 1973–1975 (21). Medicaid funding, community health centers, and federally subsidized family planning services may have also played key roles. Nonetheless, some important differences in the use of preventive services continue to exist

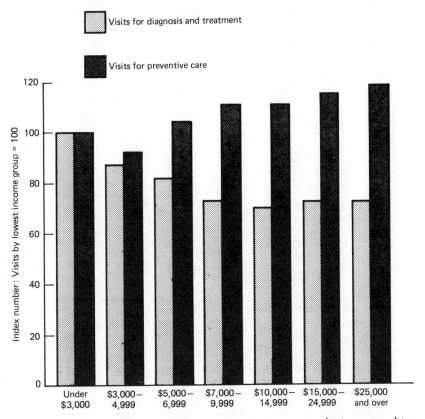

Figure 3-6. Relative number of physician visits per person per year, by income and type of visits, United States, civilian Noninstitutionalized population, 1975. Note: Preventive care visits consists of the following: a) pre- and postnatal care; b) routine checkups and checkups for specific purposes such as employment or insurance, in which no diagnosis is made; c) immunizations provided by a physician or under a physician's supervision; and d) visits for eye refractions, for preventive services not included in the preceding categories, and visits for which the type of service provided is unknown.
SOURCE: Donabedian A, Axelrod S, Wyszewianski L: *Medical Care Chartbook,* ed 7. Ann Arbor, Mich, Health Administration Press, 1980.

among the poor, nonwhite, and farm populations. Further, there is increased concern that present and possibly future cutbacks in Medicaid and federal programs may erode some of the gains made over the past decade.

Dental Examinations. Table 3-6 indicates the percentage of people with at least one dental visit during the 2-year period 1976–1978. As shown, whites are more likely to visit a dentist than blacks in every age group. National data not shown also indicate marked differences by income and residence (22). For example, in the age group 6–16, 91% of those in the highest income category saw a dentist during 1976–1978 versus only 65.3% in the lowest income category. These income-related differences were even more pronounced in the 45–64 and 65 and over age groups. For all age groups, those living in metropolitan areas were consistently 7% to 10% more

TABLE 3-6. Persons with at Least One Dental Visit during the Past 2 Years, According to Race and Age: United States, 1976–1978

Age	Race		
	All Races	White	Black
	Percent of population		
All ages	63.8	65.6	51.5
Under 6 years	25.0	26.1	18.9
6–16 years	79.0	81.8	64.3
17–44 years	72.3	74.1	60.1
45–64 years	61.4	62.9	46.1
65 years and over	39.9	41.2	26.4

SOURCE: Division of Health Interview Statistics, National Center for Health Statistics: Data from the National Health Interview Survey. Hyattsville, Md, US Dept of Health and Human Services, various years.

Note: Data from 1976, 1977, and 1978 were combined.

likely to have seen a dentist during 1976–1978 than those living in nonmetropolitan areas. Differences between blacks and whites were least in the lowest income groups but increased markedly to a difference of 23% in the highest income group. Other data indicate that in 1976 only 14% of poor rural blacks living in the South saw a dentist and only 23% of poor whites of Spanish heritage living in the Southwest (23). The probability of seeing a dentist also increases with increased education.

Data indicate that once a dentist is seen, there are few differences in the number of visits per person per year by sex, age, race, income, or education. Once again, though, farm residents tend to have fewer visits than those residing in other areas (5).

The above data indicate that dental care is particularly sensitive to differences in income, suggesting that an increase in income might improve use. One study has shown increased dental use after expansion of Medicaid coverage, with services provided through community health centers (24). But there is evidence to suggest that the poor are less likely than the nonpoor to seek preventive dental care (25).

Hospital Use. In 1978, about 10% of the population was hospitalized at least once, a decline from 13% in 1971–1972. As shown in Figure 3-7, hospital admissions per 1,000 persons per year have begun to level off after sharp and consistent growth over the past 50 years. Patient days per 1,000 persons per year have likewise leveled off. Using data on discharges per 1,000 persons per year, Figure 3-8 indicates interesting differences by geographic region. Rates are highest in the North Central region and lowest in the West, and the length of stay is highest in the Northeast and lowest in the West. These regional differences in hospital use have not been adequately explained but are believed to be due to a complex web of factors including the evolution of different styles of medical practice in different parts of the country. Other data, not shown, indicate that hospital use is higher for persons over 65, blacks, and lower income groups, all reflecting an increased need for care.

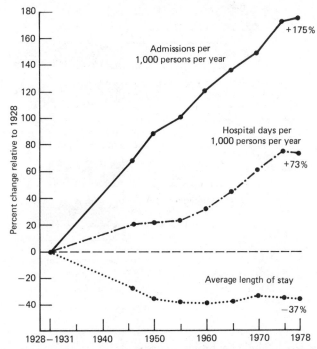

Figure 3-7. Use of general hospitals, United States, selected years, 1928–1978. For 1928, this definition includes all hospitals except tuberculosis and psychiatric hospitals; for 1946–1978, it includes all nonfederal, short term general and other specific hospitals listed by the American Hospital Association. Figures for average length of stay before 1970 include short term psychiatric and tuberculosis hospitals. After 1970, those hospitals are excluded from those figures. In 1978, short term tuberculosis hospitals had 1,895 admissions and short term psychiatric hospitals had 20,834 admissions. The 1928 data are from a sample study in 17 states and the District of Columbia conducted from February 1928 to May 1931. Data for 1946–1978 are nationwide data.
Source: Donabedian A, Axelrod S, Wyszewianski L: *Medical Care Chartbook,* ed 7. Ann Arbor, Mich, Health Administration Press, 1980.

Other aspects of hospital use include the volume of surgical operations and the volume of outpatient visits. Between 1974 and 1979, the number of surgical operations increased from 91.2 to 93.7 per 1,000 population (26). Most of this increase is accounted for by the 65 and over age group, in which the number of operations per 1,000 population increased from 165.4 in 1974 to 207.6 in 1979. Outpatient visits per 1,000 days increased from 568 in 1970 to 749 in 1979. Practically all of this increase occurred during the 1970–1975 period, with almost no increase having occurred between 1975 and 1979.

Finally, the volume of patient care episodes in state and county mental hospitals increases linearly with age, from a low of 56.4 per 100,000 population for those under 18 to a high of 652.6 per 100,000 population for those 65 and over. Rates are higher for men (418.1 per 100,000) than for women (315.3 per 100,000). The most prevalent diagnosis is schizophrenia (138.8 per 100,000), followed by alcohol disorders (61.2 per 100,000) (18). Other issues related to the use of mental health facilities are discussed in Chapter 8.

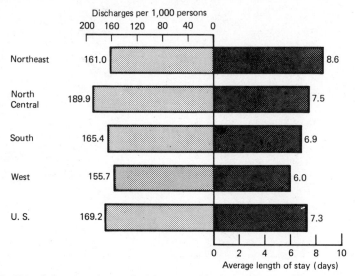

Figure 3-8. Use of short-stay hospitals, by geographic area, United States, 1977.
SOURCE: Donabedian A, Axelrod S, Wyszewianski L: *Medical Care Chartbook*, ed 7. Ann Arbor, Mich, Health Administration Press, 1980.

Nursing Home Use. The most prominent provider of long term care services is the nursing home. In 1976, more than 1.1 million people were discharged from nursing homes; 70% of these were discharged alive. The median length of stay in nursing homes is 1.6 years (27). Admission rates increase with age, are higher for women than for men, and are higher for whites than for nonwhites. The primary diagnoses include hardening of the arteries, stroke, mental disorders, senility, and old age, as discussed in further detail in Chapter 7.

Prescription Use. There are no available reliable national data on prescription use. Smaller studies suggest that approximately one-third of the population report taking prescribed drugs in a 1- or 2-day period (28–30), and more than one-third report taking a nonprescribed medicine, usually analgesic, cold remedy, or vitamin.

Summary of Descriptive Trends. These descriptive data provide an overview of the use of health services in the United States. Over the years, a larger percentage of the population has gained increased financial access to medical care, which is associated with a significant narrowing of differences by income and race in the percentage seeing a physician annually. Significant improvements have also been made in a number of preventive measures such as Pap smears, breast examinations, and blood pressure tests, although some differences between the poor and nonpoor remain. Differences in number of physician visits have also narrowed or disappeared; however, after taking into account differences in health status, the poor still receive fewer services than the nonpoor.

There is considerable variation in the annual percentage of Americans visiting a dentist, and this percentage is positively associated with income and education. But for those who see a dentist, there is little difference in the mean number of annual visits, except for farm residents.

TABLE 3-7. Gaps in Access to Care: Coverage of the Poor by Federal Programs

	Total Population	Living in Medically Underserved Areas		
		Served by Community Health Centers	Not Served by Community Health Centers	Nonmedical Underserved Areas
Total	100%	8%	29%	63%
Medicaid	34	3	8	23
Non-Medicaid	66	5	21	40

SOURCE: Assistant Secretary for Planning and Education: National Health Plan Lost Estimating Tables. US Dept of Health and Human Services, 1980.

The data also indicate several groups in the population for whom use of and access to health services remains an issue. These include children living in central cities and rural areas, and the farm population regardless of age. In addition, Davis et al. (31), as shown in Table 3-7, have identified a subgroup of the population who appear to be in "triple jeopardy" regarding the use of services. These are the 21% of the population living in medically underserved areas without Medicaid coverage *and* without being served by a community health center.

It is clear from the data that Medicare, Medicaid, and a variety of federally and foundation-funded primary care programs have improved Americans' access to health services, as reflected in the narrowing of differences in use. However, it is equally important to note that nearly two-thirds of the poor remain uncovered by Medicaid and that different primary care programs reach less than one-third of the medically underserved (32). Further, many of the gains that have been achieved may be in jeopardy, as changes in health policy suggest cutbacks in Medicare, Medicaid, and other federally and state-sponsored programs. The situation calls for creativity in generating more cost-effective approaches to the use of scarce resources. This represents a major challenge to administrators, providers, planners, and policymakers alike. In order to identify points of intervention and develop effective strategies, it is necessary to understand a number of analytical approaches to the study of health services utilization and to know the findings based upon current research.

ANALYTIC MODELS AND KEY FINDINGS

The descriptive trends presented above provide necessary background information. But from policy, planning, and administrative perspectives, factors associated with the differences in use must be examined to facilitate the design of effective intervention strategies for improving the health services system. A number of models have been developed for this purpose.

Description of Models

Six types of models have been developed to explain differences in health services utilization (33). These models are typically described as 1) demographic; 2) social structural; 3) social psychologic; 4) economic; 5) organizational; and 6) the systems model.

Demographic models of health services utilization primarily emphasize variables such as age, sex, marital status, and family size. The rationale of the demographic approach is that such variables represent physiologic states of individuals and stages of the family life cycle, which might be associated with differences in health status and the use of health services. There has been relatively little research that relies solely on demographic variables to explain differences in health services utilization, although these variables have been used extensively in more comprehensive models.

The social structural approach primarily emphasizes variables such as education, occupation, social class, and ethnicity. These factors reflect not only an individual's life style, which may predispose to the use of certain types of health services, but also reflect the general physical and social environment in which people live. For example, economists have suggested that education may affect the ability of individuals to combine their financial knowledge and other resources to use health services more intelligently and thus maximize their health status (34).

The social psychologic approach emphasizes the influence of values, attitudes, norms, and culture in explaining the utilization of health services. An example of the social psychologic approach is the Health Belief Model developed by Irving Rosenstock (35). This model suggests that four concepts influence the decision to seek preventive health care services: perceived susceptibility to the disease, perceived severity of the disease, the expected benefits of seeking care weighed against the costs involved, and a "cue," such as a media campaign, to trigger action. A number of small studies have indicated support for some components of this model, and the model is discussed further in a later section of this chapter.

The economic approach considers the factors influencing an individual's demand for services as well as the supply of services. Demand factors include an individual's income and health insurance coverage. Supply factors include the number of health facilities, such as hospital beds, and providers, such as physicians or nurses, per population in a community. The economic approach argues that the interaction of the demand and supply factors determines the volume of services consumed.

The organizational approach is primarily based on factors that influence use once patients have entered a health care system. Variables include the organization of physicians' practices, such as group practice versus solo practice, use of ancillary personnel, and professional referral patterns.

The systems approach argues that factors in all of the above models must be considered in explaining differences in health services utilization. The approach considers the nature of the inputs providing medical care services, the transformation of these inputs into services to patients, and the resulting outputs, or outcomes, or the transformation process. While this approach is probably the most realistic, since it considers many of the complex interrelationships that shape health services utilization, systems models also present difficult measurement problems. However, a number of studies (36–38) are beginning to indicate the potential utility of the systems approach.

In each of these models, it is important to identify those variables that can be directly affected by planners, providers, and administrators through health policy or direct intervention (Table 3-8). Variables in the demographic and social structural models cannot be directly influenced. Rather, these factors represent target group

TABLE 3-8. Classification of Health Services Utilization Models by Degree to Which They Can Be Influenced by Changes in Public Policy or Administrative Intervention

Model	Variables	Subject to Direct Policy or Administrative Intervention	Useful in Identifying Groups in Need	Health Professionals Who Can Exert the Most Influence
Demographic	Age, sex, marital status, family size, residence	No	Yes	Not relevant
Social structural	Social class, ethnicity, education, occupation	No	Yes	Not relevant
Social psychologic	Health beliefs, values, attitudes, norms, culture	No—short run Possibly—long run	No	Health educators, providers, administrators
Economic	Family income, insurance coverage, price of services, provider/population ratios, regular source of care	Yes	Yes	Planners, policymakers
Organizational	Organization of practice, referral patterns, etc.	Yes	No	Providers, administrators
Systems	Most of above considered as complex set of interrelationships	Yes	Yes	At the level of the overall system, planners and policymakers; at the level of individual organizations, providers and administrators

variables that aid the identification of subgroups in the population that have limitations in access to health services. In contrast, variables in the economic and organizational approaches are more susceptible to changes in health policy and direct administrative intervention. Examples include changes in third-party insurance coverage, changes in provider and facility ratios, and changes in the organization of services. Planners and policy analysts can influence economic variables, whereas providers and administrators are more likely to influence organizational factors. The variables in the social psychologic approach represent an intermediate degree of intervention potential. Such factors as values, attitudes, norms, and culture are difficult to change in the short term but may be influenced eventually through health education and related efforts. The advantage of the systems approach is its consideration of the relationships among the many variables contained in the other approaches. It suggests the need for a more coordinated effort among policymakers, planners, providers, and administrators in the attempt to initiate change.

The distinction between variables that are potentially susceptible to intervention and those that comprise target group variables is not intended to suggest that the latter are unimportant. Realistically, both types of variables must be considered in any interventions in a health services system and in local planning. It is the interaction of the target group variables and the other variables that will ultimately determine the success of specific programmatic efforts. For example, having a regular source of care may be more important for some age groups than for others. The distinction between manipulable variables and target group factors, as well as the relationship between them, needs to be considered in reviewing the empirical findings from the literature.

The Behavioral Model: Research Findings

One model that incorporates a number of the variables contained in the demographic, social structural, economic, and social psychologic approaches was developed by Ronald Andersen and is known as the behavioral model of health services utilization (39). The model (Table 3-9) proposes three sets of factors that influence differences in initial contact with the health services system and in volume of utilization by those who achieve access: predisposing, enabling, and and medical need variables. Predisposing variables include age, sex, marital status, family size, education, ethnicity, personal beliefs about the value of health services, and attitudes toward physicians. Enabling variables include family income, insurance coverage, the availability of a regular source of care, and facility and provider per capita ratios. Medical need variables include disability days, symptoms, perceived health status, and physician-evaluated severity of the diagnosis and symptoms.

Some of the variation in utilization may be explained by such predisposing characteristics as age, sex, education levels, ethnicity, and personal beliefs about medical care. For example, age is highly correlated with levels of illness in the population. Variables such as ethnicity, education, and occupation suggest the possible importance of life styles and the physical and social environments of individuals in relation to the use of health services. Personal beliefs about medical care, physicians, and disease can also influence care-seeking behavior. For example, people who believe strongly in the efficacy of health care treatment might be more likely to seek services sooner than those without such beliefs.

The predisposing variables alone are inadequate to explain differences in utilization. Individuals must also have the necessary means to seek and receive care.

TABLE 3-9. Overview of the Behavioral Model of Health Services Utilization

Predisposing Component	Enabling Component	Medical Need Component	Types of Utilization to be Explained
A. Demographic	A. Family resources and related factors	A. Perceived illness	
Age	Family income	Disability days	A. Hospital
Sex	Insurance	Symptoms	contact
Marital status	Coverage	Perceived health	volume
Family size	Group enrollment	Worry about	B. Physician
Birth order	Physician office	health	contact
Past hospitalization	Coverage	Pain frequency	volume
Neighborhood tenure	Dental coverage	Dental symptoms	C. Dentist
	Regular source of care		contact
	Group practice		volume
	Appointment time		
	Travel time		
	Waiting time		
B. Social structure	B. Community resources	B. Physician evaluated	
Education	B. Residence	Diagnosis	
Social class	Region	Symptoms	
Occupation	Physician/popula-tion ratio		
Ethnicity	Hospital bed/population ratio		
Religion			
C. Beliefs			
Value of health services			
Value of physicians			
Knowledge of disease			
Response threshold			

SOURCE: Adapted from Andersen R, Kravits J, Anderson OW: *Equity in Health Services: Empirical Analysis in Social Policy,* Cambridge, Mass, Ballinger Publishing Co, 1975, pp 14, 15.

Thus, such demand factors as family income, level of health insurance coverage, and the availability of a regular source of care, and supply factors such as the number of health facilities and professionals in the community, can be expected to influence utilization. Region of residence, particularly rural versus urban, may influence utilization as a result of the geographic distance to a source of care, as well as local attitudes toward medical care.

The level of illness in the population, as perceived by consumers or as evaluated by physicians, is also an important correlate of utilization. Illness levels can be measured by the number of disability days or symptoms experienced by individuals, self-perceived health status, and ratings by physicians or other providers of the severity of reported conditions and symptoms in terms of the relative need for care.

In an equitable system of health care, the primary determinants of access, measured by initial contact and volume of services used, should be need for care and not factors such as income, health insurance coverage, education, and occupation. Thus, to the extent that differences in use are explained primarily by medical need variables and demographic correlates of need, the distribution of services would be relatively equitable. However, to the extent that enabling or predisposing variables explain differences in use, there would be some inequity in the use of health services.

Effect of Predisposing Variables.   Among the empirical tests of this model is a 1970 nationwide survey of 3,880 families comprising 11,882 individuals (40). Information was collected from household interviews, health providers and insurers, and employers. Age was significantly and positively related to length of hospital stay and to initial contact with, and number of visits to, a dentist, even adjusting for the other factors that were correlated with age. Age was not related to number of physician visits after adjusting for other age-related factors such as medical need. Sex had no impact on the rate of physician visits, hospital admissions, or dental visits. Individuals, especially children, in larger families had fewer physician visits than those in smaller families.

Race (white versus nonwhite) was significantly and positively related to number of physician and dental visits; nonwhites had significantly lower utilization than whites even when all other variables in the model were considered. High income blacks were less likely to seek physician care for discretionary services (elective and preventive care) than high income whites. Furthermore, low income whites were even more likely than high income blacks to have seen a dentist during the survey year.

Personal beliefs about physicians and the efficacy of medical care were generally not related to health services utilization. However, beliefs explained more of the differences in use of dentists than any other variable, probably because dental care is highly discretionary. Among high income blacks, a favorable attitude toward health care was associated with increased discretionary dental care use. None of the other predisposing variables was consistently related to differences in utilization.

Effect of Enabling Variables.   A regular source of health care was positively related to having some contact with a physician, and, for individuals with major illness episodes (five or more annual visits or $100 or more in annual expenditures), a regular source of care was an important predictor of differences in the number of visits. Income, even independent of education, was an important variable in explaining differences in the rate of dental visits, but was not related to the frequency of physician visits or of hospital admissions. Although previous analyses in a 1963 study had indicated that income was an important determinant of the physician visit rate, the introduction of Medicare and Medicaid in 1966 and the expansion of major medical insurance coverage essentially eliminated these effects. Insurance coverage in 1971 was important only as a predictor of the number of physician visits for individuals with major illness episodes. As might be expected, people with comprehensive insurance coverage tended to be higher users of physician and hospital services. Finally, the physician/population ratio in the community showed a positive correlation with the number of physician visits.

Effect of Medical Need Variables.   The number of disability days and individual concern about health status were the best predictors of hospital care; severity of diagnosis was the best predictor of the physician visit rate. The number of dental symptoms was the best predictor of whether or not dental care was sought.

The results of all aspects of the model indicate that measures of illness and demographic factors, such as age, are the primary predictors of hospital use, suggesting that these services are approximately equitably distributed among population groups. To an extent, physician services also appear to be somewhat equitably distributed since diagnostic severity is the principal predictor of differences in physician visits. However, other factors are also important, including the availability of a regular source of care, insurance coverage, and the number of providers in the community. In addition, some population groups, such a nonwhites, used fewer services than other groups, controlling for the other variables in the model.

Dental care was more highly related to predisposing and enabling variables than hospital and physician services and was less related to need. Dental care is poorly distributed among population groups. Whites who have a higher education, live in a higher social class, and enjoy a better than average income are more likely to obtain dental services than people in other social, economic, or racial groups.

These results can be evaluated in terms of their potential for public policy or administrative intervention (Table 3-10). Of the 19 most important relationships, 7 are related to predisposing variables that cannot be manipulated, 5 are related to enabling factors that can be manipulated, and the remaining 7 concern medical need. The predisposing variables suggest target groups for which public policies might be developed. Among the enabling variable relationships, family income, insurance coverage, and physician/population ratios are of relevance to policymakers. The availability of a regular source of care can be affected by federal health personnel policies and by the actions of administrators and providers. It is also of interest to note that most of the significant relationships are related to the volume of services, rather than to contact with providers, suggesting that somewhat more is known about total volume of use than about those factors associated with initial contact.

The findings outlined above are also supported by other studies. For example, a study of 2,168 households in five New York and Pennsylvania counties indicated that need for care, insurance coverage, age, and average cost of a visit strongly affected the volume of physician visits (41). Analysis of national data by Berki and Kobashigawa suggests that medical need variables such as chronic disability days and education were positively, and family size was negatively, related to the number of ambulatory visits (42). Chronic disability also had indirect effects through its association with increased incidence of acute conditions. An evaluation of a Health to Underserved Rural Areas (HURA) project in Washington State revealed that poor health status and a regular source of care were positively associated with the number of visits, although no relationship was found between increased access to care and use (43).

Strong relationships between use and number of disability days, usual source of care, insurance coverage, and price for services have also been demonstrated by Bice and associates in their study of a low income population (44). In a 1970 national study of 839 children between the ages of 1 and 5 years, Colle and Grossman (45) found that family income was associated with likelihood of a child's visiting a physician, having a physical examination for preventive services, and annual num-

TABLE 3-10. Summary of Strongest Predictors of Health Services Utilization Using the Behavioral Model

Variable	Directly Manipulable	Hospital Utilization		Physician Utilization		Dental Utilization	
		Contact	Volume	Contact	Volume	Contact	Volume
Predisposing							
Age	No		X[a]			X	X
Race	No						X
Beliefs	No (short run)						X
Family size	No				X		
Enabling							
Regular source of care	Yes			X	X		
Family income	Yes						X
Insurance coverage	Yes				X		
Physician to population ratio						X	
Medical need							
Disability days	No		X		X		
Worry about health	No (short run)		X		X		
Diagnostic severity	No					X	
Symptoms	No				X		X

[a]X = strongest predictors.

ber of physician visits. Having Medicaid coverage also increased the likelihood of physician contact and the probability of a preventive care examination.

The importance of insurance is especially evident from the effect of coinsurance or copayment by the patient, as discussed further in Chapter 11. For example, Scitovsky and Snyder found that a 25% coinsurance rate resulted in a 24% decrease in the per capita volume of physician visits (46). In a Canadian study of 40,000 families conducted between 1963 and 1973, Beck and Horne (47) found that the introduction of copayment resulted in a statistically significant decline in the use of ambulatory services, but no relationship was found in regard to the use of hospital services. Further, in a true experiment designed to assess the effect of various health insurance plan and organizational features on use, cost, and quality of care, Newhouse et al. (48) found that persons fully covered for medical services spent about 50% more than similar persons with an income-related catastrophic insurance plan. In this study, both ambulatory services and hospital admissions increased. Other reviews of the literature generally support these research results (27).

The Health Belief Model: Research Findings

The research described above does not deal in a central way with the role of health beliefs in explaining use of services. This section examines a widely used model that incorporates health belief concepts. First, however, it is important to differentiate health behavior, illness behavior, and sick role behavior.

Health behavior has been defined as "any activity undertaken by a person who believes himself (herself) to be healthy, for the purpose of preventing disease or detecting disease in an asymptomatic stage" (49 p. 246). *Illness behavior* is "any activity undertaken by a person who feels ill, for the purpose of defining the state of his (her) health and of discovering a suitable remedy." In contrast, *sick role behavior* is "the activity undertaken by those who consider themselves ill, for the purpose of getting well." Examples of health behavior include visits to health care providers when individuals do not perceive symptoms but are seeking to prevent or detect disease in the absence of symptoms (e.g., general physical examinations). The concept could also be extended to include such health-promoting activities as exercise, proper nutrition, and attention to hygiene. Illness behavior includes visits to health care providers for the purpose of defining the state of one's health in the presence of symptoms. Sick role behavior includes actions in response to the care-seeking process, such as compliance with medical regimens.

The health belief model was originally developed to explain differences in health and illness behavior (50), but it has also been used to explain differences in sick role behavior, particularly in regard to patient compliance with medical advice. In addition to the previously noted concepts of perceived susceptibility, perceived severity, benefit versus cost of action, and a cue, various demographic, social psychologic, and structural variables have been incorporated into the model (Figure 3-9) (51). Studies have also included the variable "behavioral intent to act" (52).

Empirical investigations over the past 20 years have indicated consistent support for several of the variables contained in the model, but the associations with health services use have generally indicated that perceived susceptibility and perceived benefits are related to preventive health behavior, whereas the role of perceived severity has been less strongly supported (51). For example, in a study of swine flu vaccination, Rundall and Wheeler (53) found that perceived susceptibility to the disease was positively associated with immunization, whereas perceived danger from immunization was negatively associated with use. The more highly educated and those with more physician visits in the previous year were also more likely to receive the vaccination. The results were further elaborated in a Michigan study of 374 households in which past flu shot experience, behavioral intention to act, social influence, and physician's recommendations directly affected use of vaccinations (54). Measures of behavioral intention to act had the strongest direct influence on the probability of receiving immunization.

Other studies have examined the relationship between the health belief model and different kinds of preventive health behavior, while at the same time testing such "social network" variables as socioeconomic status and frequency of interaction with friends. Results indicate that individuals who belong to a high socioeconomic group and interact frequently with friends are more likely than other groups to manifest preventive health behaviors such as seat belt use, exercise, and immunizations (55). Social network variables, however, have little effect on other behaviors, such as safe driving and avoidance of smoking.

In regard to illness behavior, such as physician visits, most of the studies indicate some relationship between perceived benefits and use (55). The evidence is somewhat less clear concerning the impact of perceived susceptibility. None of the results indicate that the combination of variables in the model have an additional effect on explaining differences in use.

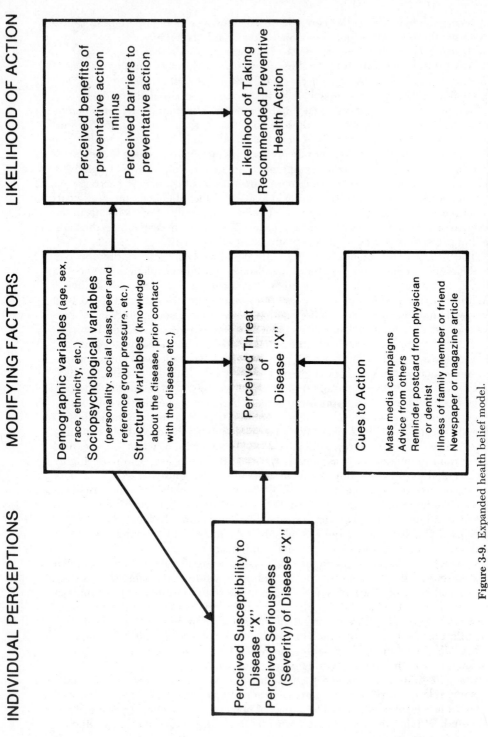

INDIVIDUAL PERCEPTIONS   MODIFYING FACTORS   LIKELIHOOD OF ACTION

Demographic variables (age, sex, race, ethnicity, etc.)
Sociopsychological variables (personality, social class, peer and reference group pressure, etc.)
Structural variables (knowledge about the disease, prior contact with the disease, etc.)

Perceived benefits of preventative action minus Perceived barriers to preventative action

Likelihood of Taking Recommended Preventive Health Action

Perceived Threat of Disease "X"

Cues to Action

Mass media campaigns
Advice from others
Reminder postcard from physician or dentist
Illness of family member or friend
Newspaper or magazine article

Perceived Susceptibility to Disease "X"
Perceived Seriousness (Severity) of Disease "X"

Figure 3-9. Expanded health belief model.

SOURCE: Rosenstock IM: Historical origins of the health belief model. *Health Educ Monogr* 1974; 2:344. Adapted from Becker MH, Drachman, RH, Kirscht, JP, et al: A new approach to explaining sick role behavior in low income populations. *Am J Public Health* 1974; 64:205–216. Reprinted by permission.

In regard to sick role behavior, specifically the use of medication, a number of studies have indicated positive relationships between perceived susceptibility, perceived severity, and perceived benefits and costs (57). Most of these associations are relatively weak, but they tend to be consistent across studies.

Other factors that have been found to be related to compliance or adherence with medical advice include the patterns of communication between providers and patients (58), continuity of physician care (59), and age (60). In general, existing evidence indicates no relationship between compliance and sex, intelligence, education, or marital status.

Since experimental studies using the health belief model variables are only beginning to be conducted, it is not possible to draw any inferences concerning the possible causal relationships involving these factors and actual health services use. Thus, although the current findings have little predictive value for health professionals, the relationships found thus far suggest approaches to influencing health care-seeking behavior. Particularly relevant is the importance of demonstrating the possible benefits and costs of certain health behaviors, factors that are more easily affected by health professionals than are perceived susceptibility and perceived seriousness.

The Impact of Organizationally Related Variables

A number of studies have examined the effect on use of different organizational forms such as prepaid group practices. These results are important because many of these organizational factors can be influenced by managers, planners, policymakers, and providers.

A number of studies have indicated that enrollees in prepaid plans have significantly lower hospital use than people receiving care under fee-for-service arrangements (60–63), as discussed further in Chapters 5 and 11. However, differences in benefit packages, consumer characteristics, and financial arrangements for paying for care have limited many analyses. For example, most studies of ambulatory care use have not simultaneously considered differences in enrollee characteristics, benefit packages, and financing mechanisms. Results have not conclusively demonstrated that any one organized arrangement, such as prepaid practice, is associated with consistently lower use of ambulatory care services (64–69).

The Seattle Prepaid Health Care Project offered an unusual opportunity to examine differences in use between two systems for providing services for patients with comprehensive care at no cost to the enrollee and with geographic access to care (70). In this 4-year experiment involving more than 8,500 people, low income residents of the Seattle Model City area had the choice of receiving care from a well established, consumer operated, prepaid group practice or from a plan comprising most independent office based private practitioners in the community. Approximately one-third of the residents chose the group practice plan. The findings indicated that hospitalization was significantly lower among the group practice enrollees compared to those enrolled in the private practice plan (110 versus 140 admissions per 1,000 enrollees annually). These results confirm other research findings that utilization patterns can be affected by different organizational systems even when enrollee characteristics, benefit packages, financing arrangements, and geographic access are not factors.

In the Seattle study, there were also no significant differences in ambulatory care use, as measured by overall visit rates in the two systems of care. However, the number of visits per user was greater in the private practice plan, whereas the percentage of people having any contact with a provider was significantly higher in the group plan. Despite the absence of financial barriers, whites had more physician visits than blacks in both plans, especially among younger enrollees. Among enrollees in poorer health, those in the private practice plan had significantly more provider visits than those in the group plan, suggesting that in prepaid group practices economic barriers may be replaced by other barriers, such as long waiting times for an appointment. Interestingly, there was no relationship between enrollee perceived access to care and the volume of services used, although significant relationships did exist between perceived access and patient satisfaction, particularly in the group plan (38).

A study by Riedel and associates of the Federal Employees Health Benefits Program compared hospital and ambulatory care use for employees under a Blue Cross/Blue Shield insurance plan and a prepaid group practice plan (71). Substantial differences in hospital admission rates (121 versus 69 admissions annually per 1,000 memberships) remained even after correcting for demographic differences between the two groups. The Blue Cross/Blue Shield admission rate was also significantly higher in 39 of 46 diagnostic categories examined in detail.

Controlling for race, there was virtually no difference in ambulatory visits between the two plans (72). However, as in the Seattle study, the volume of visits for whites was higher under both plans than for blacks. Nearly all younger people in smaller families with high incomes had at least one annual visit. In large, low income families, only 14% of Blue Cross/Blue Shield and 44% of the group plan enrollees had at least one visit. Interestingly, in families with four or more persons, children and young teenagers used significantly more health services if only one parent was working full time. As in previous studies, the need for care explained most of the difference in physician visits. There was no evidence for any substitution of ambulatory care for inpatient services.

Studies have also been conducted of network model independent practice associations (IPAs); arrangements whereby an insurance plan enrolls a defined group of individuals on a prepaid basis and, in turn, contracts with private practice physicians in the community to deliver services. Results from an evaluation of one such plan, United Health Care, in comparison with a fee-for-service system and a large prepaid group practice, revealed the following: 1) 88% of United Health Care enrollees used at least one service compared with 90% for the prepaid group practice and 70% for the fee-for-service system; 2) overall use and total outpatient use were higher in both United Health Care and the fee-for-service system than in the prepaid group practice plan; 3) total ambulatory visits were higher in the prepaid group practice plan and United Health Care than in the fee-for-service plan; and 4) ambulatory care visits, specifically to primary care physicians, were highest among United Health Care enrollees (2.76 per person per year) versus 1.78 for the prepaid plan and 0.95 for the fee-for-service plan (73). Interestingly, there was no evidence to suggest adverse selection by sicker individuals of United Health Care despite its comprehensive benefits.

Another study, by Gaus and associates, compared use in ten Health Maintenance Organizations (HMOs) and a fee-for-service plan for a Medicaid population (74). The only important difference between the plans was significantly lower hospital use in the HMOs that were organized as group practices; however, foundation model HMOs similar to United Health Care did not have lower use than the fee-for-service plans. These findings suggest that capitation payments to HMOs alone do not appear to be associated with changes in use. Rather, the organized, multi-specialty group practice arrangement with largely salaried group physicians may be a more significant factor.

An important question, from a federal and state cost containment policy perspective, is whether prepaid group practices ca.. reduce the hospital use of Medicaid recipients. Existing evidence, although preliminary, suggests that they can. For example, a study of Medicaid members of the Kaiser Foundation health plan in Multnomah County, Oregon, revealed significantly lower hospital use for Kaiser Medicaid and non-Medicaid low income enrollees in comparison with sex- and age-matched groups of non-Kaiser Medicaid recipients (75).

A similar question may be posed in terms of Medicare enrollees. One study of Medicare enrollees in several prepaid group practices and fee-for-service plans indicated that prepaid enrollees incurred higher physician services costs, including care provided by practitioners outside the plans, and lower costs for provider-initiated services such as in-hospital care and extended care but excluding home health care. Inpatient hospital services did not reduce the use of extended care or home care services. Group practices that were relatively small and hospital based appeared to provide care at the least cost in the plans studied (76).

In general, more studies indicate that HMO enrollees receive more preventive services than studies that show no differences or that show greater preventive use by non-HMO enrollees. This finding was true for the HMO enrollees in the Seattle Prepaid Health Care Project, noted earlier, and is also supported by findings of Berki and Ashcraft in a study of 626 families in Rochester, New York (77). To some extent, the higher preventive services use of HMO enrollees may be due to the comprehensive coverage provided rather than to an explicit intention of HMOs to promote preventive care (78).

All of these studies suggest that enrollees in prepaid group practices have significantly lower hospital admission rates than people who receive care in fee-for-service and other settings. The rates are lowest for those receiving care in group and staff model HMOs and somewhat higher for IPAs; the latter, however, have lower rates than fee-for-service patients (79). There is little evidence of the direct substitution of ambulatory care for inpatient care, although this issue has not been fully examined. Beyond the organizational factors, medical need is the most important factor in explaining differences in use of services, although sociodemographic characteristics such as race and family size also explain some percentage of the variation.

More research is needed on the relative performance of different organizational forms for providing care. The existing results raise some interesting questions regarding what forms should be encouraged. What are the comparative advantages of independent fee-for-service practice plans, freestanding groups, hospital-sponsored groups, HMOs, and other organizational forms? Of particular interest is the extent to which HMOs can provide cost-effective care to Medicare and Medicaid populations while remaining financially viable as organizations. Also of interest is the extent to which HMOs and other new forms of delivery can encourage more competition in the delivery of care, which might be associated with more cost-effective services. Some of the answers to these and related questions will be forthcoming from research currently in progress, but others will become apparent only as further innovations are undertaken and evaluated.

Critique of Existing Models of Health Services

Existing models of utilization have been helpful for thinking about health services and have suggested possible avenues for intervention in the health services system. But these models explain relatively little of the variation in use (generally 15–25%). The inability of the models to explain a greater amount of variation may be due to measurement error, specification effort, and dependent variables that are too aggregate and too heterogeneous. For example, the variable race and ethnicity may not allow for heterogeneity within ethnic subgroups (80); income may not represent social structure or purchasing power; poor health may lead to low income, as well as low income leading to poor health; and insurance variables may not adequately reflect the comprehensiveness of coverage. Traditional measures of utilization such as hospital admissions and number of physician visits, may also be too heterogeneous or aggregate (81). For example, physician visits include prevention, diagnosis, treatment, and rehabilitation, may be initiated by the patient or another family member, and may be a first visit or a return visit. Further, the large-scale aggregate studies of utilization seldom include detailed psychosocial variables involving the processes that lead people to seek health care services (82).

Models of utilization need to be developed that include more refined variables and are specific to the different types of situations that people experience in using health services. Further, the issue of what constitutes appropriate use must be addressed if health care professionals are serious about providing cost-effective care. One approach to addressing these concerns is to analyze episodes of illness from symptom perception to subsequent care and outcomes. This approach builds on the use/disability ratio (number of physician visits per 100 disability days) and the symptoms/response ratio (actual number of persons who contacted a physician at least once for symptoms minus physician estimates of the number of persons who should contact a physician for symptoms, divided by physician estimates). These ratios have been developed by Aday and Andersen (83). As suggested by Yergen et al. (84), the episode of illness approach links use and disability to a specific series of medical encounters that includes seeking care because of worry, in addition to perceived symptoms. Physician judgments about the need for care for particular episodes, not symptoms, can then be developed. It thus becomes possible to combine professional judgments about the need for care with degree of patient worry using the classification scheme developed by Aday et al. (15) and presented in Table 3-11.

An example of the above typology might be used to derive an index of appropriate use or expected use, as shown in Figure 3-10. In this figure, all episodes categorized as a cure and for which care was elective (cells $1+$, $1-$, $5+$, and $5-$) would be classified as adequate care. In contrast, all episodes not cured and of illness type III or IV should have an associated visit (cells $10+$, $11+$, $12+$, $14+$, $15+$, and $16+$); otherwise, the use pattern would be classified as inadequate (cells $10-$, $11-$, $12-$, $14-$, $15-$, and $16-$). Illnesses of type III that are not cured and yet are associated with a physician visit would be classified as adequate (cell $9+$), whereas type IV visits not cured and with no physician visit would reflect inadequate access (cell $13-$). All other episodes with physician visits would be considered adequate. Yergen et al. suggest that type II illnesses without care might be considered inadequate if they are not improved (cells $7-$ and $8-$). Such a summary index, although not without limitations, provides a beginning approach to the issue of assessing appropriate use (84).

TABLE 3-11. Physician's Judgment and Respondent's Worry Level: Classification Scheme

Type	Physician's Judgment	Respondent's Worry Level
I	Care is elective	Not a lot
II	Care is elective	Cares a lot
III	Care is mandatory	Not a lot
IV	Care is mandatory	Cares a lot

SOURCE: Aday LA, Andersen R, Fleming GV: *Health Care in the United States. Equitable for Whom?* Beverly Hills, Calif., Sage Publications, 1981.

Broader Frameworks for the Study of Health Services

Health services utilization is of interest primarily in relation to issues of equity and access to care, and the relationships between utilization costs of care, and health status. As a result, utilization must be analyzed within a broader context that includes not only patient and provider characteristics but also the issues of access, costs, continuity, quality, and outcomes of care. There have been few efforts thus far to develop models of the health services system that examine the interrelationships among these factors. This process would involve examining relationships among sociopsychologic (patient's beliefs, perceptions, and attitudes toward care), structural (type of providers and organizational characteristics), and behavioral (use of services and technical quality of care) variables.

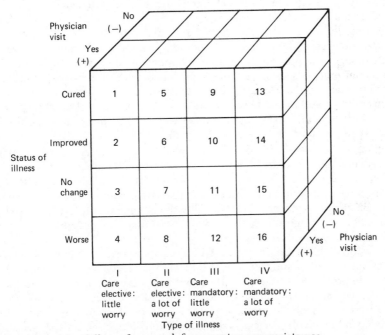

Figure 3-10. Episode of illness framework for assessing appropriate use.
SOURCE: Yergen J, LoGerfo J, Shortell SM, et al: Health status as a measure of need for medical care, a critique. *Med Care* 1981; 19(suppl):65.

An example of a more complete model of use is presented in Figure 3-11 (37). In this model, patient and provider characteristics are considered as exogenous (predetermined by external factors not included in the model), and the remaining variables are considered endogenous (determined by the other variables in the model). The model includes structural variables (patient and provider characteristics), process variables (access to care, utilization of services, continuity of care, and physician performance), and outcome variables (costs, technical quality of care, and patient satisfaction). Arrows indicate those variables hypothesized to affect other variables. For example, costs are directly affected by patient characteristics, provider characteristics, utilization of services, and continuity of care, but there is no assumed direct effect of perceived access on costs because this relationship is predicted to be indirect through the utilization of services. Access to care is determined by patient and provider characteristics, and all three, in turn, determine utilization of services. For example, older patients should have more visits because they are sicker, regardless of the degree of access to care. In this model, perceived access refers to the patient's perception of the ease with which services can be obtained when needed, whereas actual access refers to organizational, financial, and geographic realities facing the patient in seeking care.

Continuity of care is an intermediate outcome of use and is affected by patient and provider characteristics. Costs depend on continuity (poor continuity contributes to higher costs), use, and patient and provider characteristics. Technical quality (provider skill) is determined by the provider's characteristics, whereas technical outcome of care depends on technical quality, provider characteristics, and, in some instances, the patient's initial health status. Finally, patient satisfaction is determined by provider and patient characteristics, access to care, and the quality, costs, and continuity of care.

This model is intended only as an example of possible relationships among structural, process, and outcome variables and is not the only model that might be constructed. For example, an alternative model would be to suggest direct effects of use and continuity of care on the technical outcome of care, assuming that greater use of physician services corresponds to closer monitoring of the patient's condition and thus might result in an improved outcome. A single contact point for care might lead to improvement in coordination of services, adherence to a medical regimen and, thus, better outcomes of care (59, 85, 86).

Although the model in Figure 3-11 appears complex, it is actually oversimplified; feedback loops should be drawn between some variables, reflecting the dynamic nature of human behavior. For example, patient satisfaction might change over time and would affect subsequent use and compliance behavior, which might, in turn, affect future outcomes of care. The development and testing of such nonrecursive two-way causation models involving feedback loops represents an important avenue for future research.

A version of the model in Figure 3-11 has been tested on hypertension (37) and diabetes patients (38), and the results indicated modest support for several of the hypothesized relationships, especially between patient characteristics and satisfaction, perceived access and satisfaction, and provider characteristics and use of services. Alternative models need to be further tested to provide more systematic knowledge of the health services system. Such knowledge can provide a foundation for more realistic changes in public policy and administrative and provider practices.

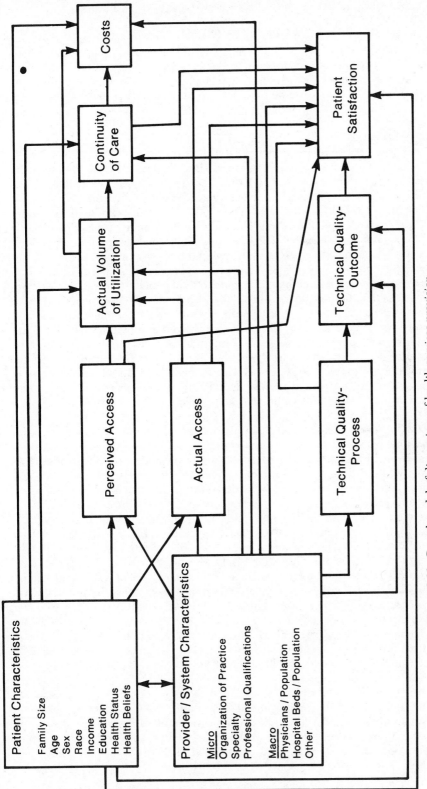

Figure 3-11. Causal model of dimensions of health services provision.
SOURCE: Expanded from Shortell SM, Richardson WC, LoGerfo JP, et al: The relationships among dimensions of health services in two provider systems: A causal model approach. *J Health Soc Behav* 1977; 18:139–159. Reprinted by permission.

SPECIAL ISSUES IN HEALTH SERVICES UTILIZATION

A number of special issues concerning the use of health services require further discussion. These are use by the elderly and by children, primary care services and self-care, and rural health care. Many of these topics are further elaborated in later chapters, as is mental health services.

Long Term Care. Use of health services among the elderly will continue to expand over the next 25 years as people live longer and as the number of older Americans increases. For example, life expectancy increased from 68.2 years to more than 74 years between 1950 and 1979. By the year 2000, it is estimated that 20% of the population will be over 65 years of age (87), and individuals 75 years old and older (the "old-old," while those aged 65–75 are "young-old") will represent 45% of the elderly population (88). The elderly, particularly those 75 and over, suffer from more diseases, have higher rates of hospital admission and longer lengths of stay, and have per capita health expenditures that are three times higher than those of adults under age 65. Perhaps 15% of the elderly over age 65 and 30% of those over age 80 need treatment for some form of mental illness (89). Medicare now pays less than half of the total health care costs for those over age 65.

As discussed in Chapter 7, a complex web of genetic, biomedical, mental, social, organizational, and financial issues are involved in providing services to the increasing number of elderly people. This interplay of forces requires that administrators, planners, policymakers and providers think across organizational and institutional lines, using a systems perspective. Those individuals who can play effective brokerage and coordinative roles will likely assume increased power and influence, as opposed to those who manage or plan for single institutions.

Child Health Care. Young children in low income families are less likely to have contact with a physician than those in higher income families; they also use fewer services. Nonwhite children, regardless of family income, have fewer physician visits than white children. These use data suggest target groups in particular need of services and illustrate the value of health services utilization data for assessing patterns of care.

There are other potentially alarming data. In 1976 an estimated 14.4% of the population under age 18 had an excessively long interval since their last contact with a physician. (90). The figure was nearly 24% for children in families with low education (8 years or less), 19.5% for blacks, and 21.4% for children from large families. Children in families with incomes of less than $6,000 were nearly eight times as likely to be without a regular source of care as those in families with incomes above $11,000 (91). Furthermore, only 44% of children in these lower income families reported a physician as a regular source of care compared to 75% in higher income families; 15% of all child care and 33% in poor urban areas is obtained from hospital emergency rooms and outpatient departments. When the use/disability ratio is considered, the differences by race, income, and education become even more pronounced.

As of 1976, 38% of children aged 4–17 had not seen a dentist the previous year (92). The figure was 53% for low income children, 58% for children from low education families, and 57% for blacks. When children reach school age, they have an average of three decayed teeth, and about 50% of all school age children suffer from periodontal disease (93). In 1975, one-third of all children were not adequately immunized against polio, and nearly 40% were not vaccinated against rubella (94). Preventive medical care is also more likely to occur among white children, those from wealthier families, and those from better educated families (95, 96).

The substantial variation in child health indicators in different areas of the country (97) suggests a need for more preventive and health-promoting services, such as prenatal care and immunizations, particularly for the poor and for nonwhites. Given past experience, however, it is unlikely that extending financial coverage alone will have much of an impact unless effective health services systems are also designed.

There are also other related problems in health care for children that have received relatively little attention. These have been labeled the "new morbidity" (98) and include learning difficulties, behavioral disturbances, allergies, speech difficulties, child abuse, and societal adjustment problems. Although these problems may not constitute traditional illnesses, and labeling them as such may increase the medicalization of social deviance, many parents and teachers seek solutions and help from the health services system. Since these problems encompass social and health services, the ability to manage and plan across institutional and organizational boundaries is essential.

Expansion of Primary Care.   Primary care includes the first contact and continuous care for meeting most of a person's health care needs. There has been renewed interest in primary care as a substitute for more expensive inpatient care, and as the most appropriate approach to meeting many health needs, especially in underserved areas where resources are scarce (99–102). However, there is little evidence that the provision of a higher volume of ambulatory services substitutes for hospital inpatient care. Primary care also raises issues related to composition of providers, new role relationships involving nurse practitioners and physician assistants, inadequate third-party coverage for ambulatory care, the need for different management and medical information systems from those that presently exist in hospitals, and the need to develop quality assurance systems.

Hospitals are also concerned with the role of primary care as a means of capturing more patient referrals. Various primary care initiatives have been incorporated into hospital marketing and long term strategic plans (103).

Self-Care.   Increasing costs, barriers to access, attention to consumer participation, increased interest in the nursing field to new approaches to patient care, interest in behavior modification, and other factors have resulted in a new "self-care" movement. Self-care is a "process whereby a lay person can function effectively on his (her) own behalf in health promotion and prevention, and in disease detection and treatment at the level of the primary health resource in the health care system" (104). The impact of self-care on health services use, costs, quality, and related issues is largely unknown. However, it is important for health professionals to anticipate the potential impact of this trend. For example, research on health beliefs suggests that interest in self-care may be highest among young educated whites and low among blacks, suggesting that health programs serving minority groups would find it difficult to promote a self-care program (105).

Increased emphasis on self-care may result in decreased health services use and costs. However, there is no evidence yet to support this possibility. Further, any decreased use would likely be in routine visits and not in expensive, high technology inpatient care.

Available evidence indicates that that there is a definite trend, of unknown magnitude, in consumer health education toward self-diagnosis and self-care, with consumers increasingly assuming responsibility for tasks previously performed by health providers, including diagnosis, screening, and treatment (106). Although it is difficult to predict the exact implications of this trend, a number of general issues can be suggested. First, to what degree can consumers be trained to diagnose and treat themselves, versus acquiring enough knowledge and judgment to recognize when they need to contact health care providers? Second, what is the utility of consumer algorithms (diagrams that aid consumer decision making)? Third, if higher income, better educated groups are more likely to adopt self-care, what is the potential for generalizing health education and self-care education strategies to other population groups that could also benefit from such knowledge? Fourth, to what degree can self-care be integrated into the existing health care delivery system? Finally, and perhaps most significantly, what impact will self-care have on the self-image and professional identity of health care professionals themselves; that is, how will they adjust to a change in their role from healer to educator?

Rural Health Care.   A consistent finding throughout this chapter is that rural residents, particularly those in farm areas, receive fewer health care services than urban Americans. The deficiency of health resources in rural areas is widely known. For example, 25% of the nation's population resides in rural areas, but only 13% of the nation's physicians practice there. Rural areas also include a higher proportion of people living in poverty (21%—twice that in urban areas), a higher concentration of children and elderly people (9 dependents for every 10 working-age adults, compared to 7 in urban areas), and notable environmental and social health hazards, such as impure water supplies, inadequate sewage treatment, and considerable substandard housing (107).

Rural health care is complicated by Medicare reimbursement rates that are 30% lower than those in urban areas; lack of payment for nonphysician services provided without the presence of a physician, which discourages the use of other types of practitioners; and noncoverage for preventive care, nutrition, and transportation services. As a result of these and other constraints, the average Medicaid expenditure in 1973 per poor child was $76 in metropolitan areas and only $5 in nonmetropolitan areas. The availability of services is further limited by restrictive income eligibility requirements in such rural states as Alabama, Arkansas, Louisiana, Mississippi, and South Carolina, where only 1 of every 10 poor children is covered by Medicaid. In most states, Medicaid also fails to cover two-parent families and families with an employed head of household. As a result, less than one-half of the rural poor are eligible for Medicaid. A number of programs, such as the National Health Service Corps, Health to Underserved Rural Areas, and Rural Health Initiative, as well as a number of foundation programs, were established in the 1970s to address some of these issues. Overall, they have had relatively little impact thus far and are threatened by funding cutbacks in the 1980s.

An Assessment of Utilization

This chapter has taken a descriptive and analytical approach to the determinants of health services utilization. The existing data suggests that there have been improvements in access to care that have resulted in increased use of services and higher total health care costs. Many of the improvements have been among low income and minority groups. However, evidence suggests that when medical need is considered, the number of visits is less among lower income groups than among higher income groups. There are also differences in use among population groups such that children aged 0–5 in low income families, rural residents, and blacks experience comparatively less use of medical and dental services than other groups. Maurana and associates (27) provide a useful summary of these and other findings from numerous studies in the literature.

Models that explain some of the differences in use and selected results from these models were presented. Generally, need for care is the best predictor of differences in use, although the availability of a regular source of care, insurance coverage, and sociodemographic characteristics such as age are also associated with various patterns of use. Some variables in the health belief model, such as perceived suceptibility, concern about one's health, and behavioral intent to act, have been associated with certain forms of preventive health care use, such as compliance with medical regimens. Studies of organizational influences on utilization indicate that enrollees in prepaid group practices consistently experience lower hospitalization rates than those in fee-for-service plans, possibly as a result of employing salaried physicians in the groups. In general, prepaid group practice enrollees appear to receive somewhat more preventive services. The evidence regarding the volume of ambulatory care services is mixed, as discussed in this chapter and in Chapter 5. An episode of illness approach to addressing the issue of appropriate use was also discussed. Broader models that incorporate continuity of care, costs, quality, and patient satisfaction in an integrative and more comprehensive framework are needed.

Finally, a number of special issues related to use of services were discussed. These issues are of increasing concern to providers, planners, policymakers, and managers, and suggest the need for health professionals to think about systems of care and to provide linkage among primary, secondary, and tertiary levels of care, not only in the health care system but in the larger human services system as well. A number of the issues and challenges raised in this chapter are discussed further in the chapters that follow.

REFERENCES

1. Shortell SM: Continuity of medical care: Conceptualization and measurement. *Med Care* 1976; 14:377–391.

2. Bice TW, Boxerman SB: A quantitative measure of continuity of care. *Med Care* 1977; 15:347–349.

3. Steinwachs DM: Measuring provider continuity in ambulatory care: An assessment of alternative approaches. *Med Care* 1979; 17:551–565.

4. Jeffers JR, Bognanno MF, Bartlett JC: On the demand versus need for medical services and the concept of "shortage." *Am J Public Health* 1971; 61:46–63.

5. Andersen R, Lion J, Anderson O: *Two Decades of Health Services.* Cambridge, Mass, Ballinger Publishing Co, 1976, p 44.

6. Kleinman JC: Medical care use in non-metropolitan areas, in *Health, United States, 1981.* Hyattsville, Md, US Dept of Health and Human Services, Public Health Service, December 1981, p 55.

7. Donabedian A, Axelrod S, Wyszewianski L: *Medical Care Chartbook*, ed 7. Ann Arbor, Mich, AUPHA Press/Health Administration Press, 1980.

8. US Dept of Health, Education, and Welfare: Provisional data from the national ambulatory medical care survey. Hyattsville, Md, Division of Health Resources Utilization Statistics, National Center For Health Statistics, 1976.

9. *Health, United States, 1981*. Hyattsville, Md, US Dept of Health and Human Services, Public Health Services, December 1981, p 160.

10. Andersen R, Lion J, Andersen O: *Two Decades of Health Services*, Cambridge, Mass, Ballinger Publishing Co, 1976, p 47.

11. Davis K, Gold M, Makuc D: Access to health care for the poor: Does the gap remain? *Ann Rev Public Health* 1981; 2:169.

12. *Health, United States, 1981*. Hyattsville, Md, US Dept of Health and Human Services, Public Health Service, December 1981, p 156.

13. *Health, United States, 1981*. Hyattsville, Md, US Dept of Health and Human Services, Public Health Service, December 1981, p 157.

14. Kleinman JC: Medical care use in non-metropolitan areas in *Health, United States, 1981*. Hyattsville, Md, US Dept of Health and Human Services, December 1981, p 60.

15. Aday LA, Andersen R, Fleming GV: *Health Care in the United States. Equitable for Whom?* Beverly Hills, Calif, Sage Publications, 1981.

16. Kleinman JC: *NHIS Results By Income and Insurance*. Hyattsville, Md, US Dept of Health and Human Services, Public Health Service, National Center for Health Statistics, 1980.

17. Division of Health Interview Statistics, National Center for Health Statistics: Number and rate of visits to selected free-standing outpatient facilities: U.S. 1973–74. Dept of Health, Education, and Welfare, 1976.

18. National Institute of Mental Health: Utilization of mental health facilities, 1971. *Analytical and Special Study Reports*, Series B, No 5, Publication No NIH (74-657). US Govt Printing Office, 1973.

19. Andersen R, Lion J, Andersen O: *Two Decades of Health Services*, Cambridge, Mass, Ballinger Publishing Co, 1976, p 57.

20. Ward GW, Johnson R: Recent trends in hypertension control. *Urban Health*, June 1976, pp 38–39.

21. Stamler J, Stamler R, Riedlinger WF, et al.: Hypertension screening of one million Americans. *JAMA* 1976; 235:2299–2306.

22. Foster JE, Machlin SR, Kleinman JC: *Use of Dental Services*, in *Health: United States, 1981*. Hyattsville, Md, US Dept of Health and Human Services, Public Health Service, December 1981, p 64.

23. Davis K, Gold M, Makuc D: Access to health care for the poor: Does the gap remain? *Ann Rev Public Health* 1981; 2:172.

24. Okada L, Wan T: Factors associated with increased dental care utilization in five urban, low-income areas. *Am J Public Health* 1976; 69:1001–1009.

25. Nikias MK, Fink R, Shapiro S: Comparisons of poverty and non-poverty groups on dental status, need, and practices. *J of Public Health Dent* 1975; 35:237–259.

26. *Health, United States, 1981*. Hyattsville, Md, US Department of Health and Human Services, Public Health Service, December 1981, p 169.

27. Maurana CA, Eichhorn RL, Lonnquist LE: *The Use of Health Services: Indices and Correlates for a Research Bibliography, 1981*. West Lafayette, Ind, Health Services Research and Training Program, Purdue University, November 1981.

28. Bush PG, Osterweis M: Pathways to medicine use. *J Health Soc Behav* 1978; 19:179–189.

29. Osterweis M, Bush PJ, Zuckerman AE: Family context as a predictor of individual medicine use. *Soc Sci Med* 1979; 13:287–291.

30. Rabin DL, Bush PJ: Who is using medicine? *J Community Health* 1975; 1:106–117.

31. Davis K, Gold M, Makuc D: Access to health care for the poor: Does the gap remain? *Ann Rev Public Health* 1981; 2:178.

32. Davis K, Gold M, Makuc D: Access to health for the poor: Does the gap remain? *Ann Rev Public Health* 1981; 2:181.

33. Andersen R, Anderson OW: Trends in the use of health services, in Freeman HE, Levine S, Reeder LG (eds): *Handbook of Medical Sociology,* ed 3. Englewood Cliffs, NJ, Prentice-Hall, Inc, 1979, p 385.

34. Grossman M: *The Demand for Health: A Theoretical and Empirical Investigation.* National University Press, 1972.

35. Rosenstock I.: Prevention of illness and maintenance of health, in Kosa J, Antonovsky A, Zola I (eds): *Poverty and Health: A Sociological Analysis.* Cambridge, Mass, Harvard University Press, 1969, pp 168–190.

36. Anderson JG: Causal model of a health service system. *Health Serv Res* 1972; 7:23–42.

37. Shortell SM, Richardson WC, LoGerfo JP, et al.: The relationships among dimensions of health services in two provider systems: A causal model approach. *J Health Soc Behav* 1977; 18:139–159.

38. Williams S, Shortell SM, LoGerfo J, et al.: A causal model of health services for diabetic patients. *Med Care* 1978; 16:313–326.

39. Andersen R: *Behavioral Model of Families' Use of Health Services,* research series 25. Chicago, Center for Health Administration Studies, University of Chicago, 1968.

40. Andersen R, Kravits J, Anderson OW: *Equity in Health Services: Empirical Analysis in Social Policy.* Cambridge, Mass, Ballinger Publishing Co, 1975.

41. Wan TH, Soifer SJ: Determinants of physician utilization: A causal analysis. *J Health Soc Behav* 1974; 15:100–108.

42. Berki SE, Kobashigawa B: Socioeconomic need determinants of ambulatory care use: Path analysis of the 1970 health interview survey data. *Med Care* 1976; 14:405–421.

43. Moscovice IS: *An Evaluation of the Eastern Grays Harbour HURA Project.* Final Report Submitted to Washington State Department of Health and Social Services, December 1981.

44. Bice TW, Eichhorn RL, Fox PD: Socio-economic status and use of physician services: A reconsideration. *Med Care* 1972; 10:261–271.

45. Colle AD, Grossman M: Determinants of pediatric care utilization. *J Hum Resour* 1978; 13 (suppl): 115–153.

46. Scitovsky AA, Snyder NM: Effect of co-insurance on use of physician services. *Soc Secur Bull* 1972; 35(6):3–19.

47. Beck RG, Horne JM: Utilization of publicly insured health services in Saskatchewan before, during and after co-payment. *Med Care* 1980; 19:787–806.

48. Newhouse JP, Manning WG, Morris CN, et al: Some interim results from a controlled trial of cost-sharing in health insurance. *N Engl J Med* 1981; 305:1501–1507.

49. Kasl SV, Cobb S: Health behavior, illness behavior, and sick role behavior. *Arch Environ Health* 1966; (part I) 12:246–266; 1966; (part II) 12:534–541.

50. Rosenstock IM: Why people use health services. *Milbank Mem Fund Q* 1966; 44:94–127.

51. Rosenstock IM: The health belief model and preventive health behavior. *Health Educ Monogr* 1974; 2:354–386.

52. Fishbein M, Ajzen I: *Belief, Attitude, Intention and Behavior: An Introduction to Theory and Research.* Reading, Mass, Addison-Wesley, 1975.

53. Rundall TG, Wheeler JRC: Factors associated with utilization of the swine flu vaccination program among senior citizens in Tompkins County. *Med Care* 1979; 17:191–200.

54. Rundall TG, Wheeler JRC: The effect of income on use of preventive care: An evaluation of alternative explanations. *J Health Soc Behav* 1979; 20:397–406.

55. Langlie JK: Social networks, health beliefs, and preventive health behavior. *J Health Soc Behav* 1977; 18:244–260.

56. Kirscht JP: The health belief model and illness behavior. *Health Educ Monogr* 1974; 2:387–408.

57. Becker MH: The health belief model and sick role behavior. *Health Educ Monogr* 1974; 2:409–432.

58. Svarstad B: Physician-patient communication and patient conformity with medical advice, in Mechanic D (ed): *The Growth of Bureaucratic Medicine.* New York, John Wiley & Sons, Inc, 1976, pp 220–238.

59. Becker MH, Drachman RH, Kirscht JP: A field experiment to evaluate various outcomes of continuity of physician care. *Am J Public Health* 1974; 64:1062–1070.

60. Blackwell B: Drug therapy: Patient compliance. *N Engl J Med* 1973; 289:249–252.

61. Donabedian A: An evaluation of prepaid group practice. *Inquiry* 1979; 6:3–27.

62. Klarman H: Economic research in group practice, in *New Horizons in Health Care.* Proceedings of the First International Congress on Group Medicine, Winnipeg, 1970, pp 178–193.

63. Roemer M, Shonick W: HMO performance: The recent evidence. *Milbank Mem Fund Q* 1973; 51:271–317.

64. Anderson OW, Sheatsley P: *Comprehensive Medical Insurance—A Study of Cost, Use, and Attitudes Under Two Plans.* New York, Health Information Foundation, Research Series No. 9, 1959.

65. Hastings J, Mott FD, Barclay A, et al: Prepaid group practice in Sault Ste Marie, Ontario: Part I: Analysis of utilization records. *Med Care* 1973; 11:91–103.

66. Hetherington RW, Hopkins C, Roemer M, et al: *Health Insurance Plans: Promise and Performance.* New York, John Wiley & Sons, Inc, 1975.

67. Robertson RL: Comparative medical care use under prepaid group practice and free choice plans: A case study. *Inquiry* 1972; 9(3):70–76.

68. Shapiro S, Williams JJ, Yerby AS, et al: Patterns of medical use by the indigent aged under two systems of medical care. *Am J Public Health* 1967; 57:784–790.

69. Williams J: *Family Medical Care under Three Types of Health Insurance.* New York, Foundation on Employee Health, Medical Care, and Welfare, 1962.

70. Richardson WC, Boscha M, Diehr P, et al: *Comparison of Health Services Delivery in a Competitive Market.* Hyattsville, Md, National Center for Health Services Research, Department of Health and Human Services, Research Summary Series, August 1980.

71. Riedel DC, Walden DC, Singsen AG, et al: *Federal Employees Health Benefits Program. Utilization Study.* Rockville, Md, National Center for Health Services Research, Health Resources Administration, US Public Health Service, 1975.

72. Meyers SM, Hirshfeld SB, Walden DC, et al: Ambulatory and medical use by federal employees: Experience of members in a service benefit plan and in a prepaid group practice plan. Paper presented at the 105th annual meeting of the American Public Health Association, Washington, DC, November 1, 1977.

73. Richardson WC, Martin, DP, Diehr, PD, et al: Comparison of a primary care network model with traditional plans in a competitive market. Baltimore, Office of Research and Demonstrations, Health Care Financing Administration, US Dept of Health and Human Services, forthcoming 1983.

74. Gaus CR, Cooper BS, Hirschman CG: Contract in HMO and fee-for-service performance. *Soc Secur Bull* 1976; 3(5):3–14.

75. Johnson RE, Azevedo DG: Comparing the medical utilization and expenditures of low-income health plan enrollees with Medicaid recipients and with low-income enrollees having Medicaid eligibility. *Med Care* 1979; 17:953–956.

76. Weil PA: Comparative costs to the Medicare program of seven prepaid group practices and controls. *Milbank Mem Fund Q* 1976; 54:339–365.

77. Berki SE, Ashcraft ML: On the analysis of ambulatory utilization. An investigation of the roles of need, access and price as predictors of illness and preventive visits. *Med Care* 1979; 17:1163–1181.

78. Luft H: *Health Maintenance Organizations: Dimensions of Performance*. New York, John Wiley & Sons, Inc, 1981, p 205.

79. Luft H: *Health Maintenance Organizations: Dimensions of Performance*. New York, John Wiley & Sons, Inc, 1981, p 176.

80. Geertsen R, Kane RL, Klauber MR, et al: A re-examination of Suchman's view on social factors in health care utilization. *J Health Soc Behav* 1975; 16:225–237.

81. Ware J: *A Cross-Sectional Study of Patient Perceptions in Use of Health Care Services*, Rand Paper P-5691. Santa Monica, Calif, Rand Corporation, 1977.

82. Mechanic D: Correlates of physician utilization: Why do major multi-variate studies of physician utilization find trivial psycho-social and organizational effects? *J Health Soc Behav* 1979; 20:387–396.

83. Aday L, Andersen RM: Equity of access to medical care; a conceptual and empirical overview, *Med Care* 1981; 19(suppl):4–27.

84. Yergen J, LoGerfo J, Shortell SM, et al: Health status as a measure of need for medical care, a critique. *Med Care* 1981; 19(suppl): 57–68.

85. Becker MH, Drachman RH, Kirscht JP: Continuity of pediatrician: New support for an old shibboleth. *J Pediatr* 1974; 84:599–605.

86. Starfield B, Simborg DW, Horn SD, et al: Continuity and coordination in primary care: Their achievement and utility. *Med Care* 1976; 14:625–636.

87. Cambridge Research Institute: *Trends Affecting the U.S. Health Care System*, DHEW Publication No. (HRA) 76-14503. US Dept of Health, Education, and Welfare, July 1976.

88. Neugarten B: Age groups in American society and the rise of the young-old. *Annals of the American Academy of Political and Social Science* 1970; 415:187–198.

89. Butler RN: Questions on health care for the aged. *Conditions for Change in the Health Care System*, DHEW Publication No. (HRA) 78-642. Health Resources Administration, September 1977, pp 98–106.

90. Kovar MG: Health status of US children and use of medical care. *Pub Health Rep* 1982; 97:12.

91. Butler JA, Baxter ED: Current structure of the health care delivery system for children, in *Developing a Better Health Care System for Children*, Harvard Child Health Care Project, vol III. Cambridge, Mass, Ballinger Publishing Co, 1977, p 42.

92. Unpublished data from health interview survey. Hyattsville, Md, US Dept of Health, Education, and Welfare, National Center for Health Statistics, 1974.

93. *Dentistry and National Health Programs*. Chicago, American Dental Association, 1971.

94. *Immunization Surveillance Report*. Atlanta, Center for Disease Control, 1977.

95. Richardson WC: Poverty, illness, and use of health services in the United States. *Hospitals* 1979; 43(13):34–40.

96. Richardson WC: Measuring the urban poor's use of physician services in response to illness episodes. *Med Care* 1970; 8:132–142.

97. Conditions of health and health care, in *Baselines for Setting Health Goals and Standards*, DHEW Publication No. (HRA) 77-640. US Government Printing Office, 1977.

98. Haggerty R, Roghmann K, Pless J: *Child Health and the Community*. New York, John Wiley & Sons, Inc, 1975.

99. Ullman R, Kotok D, Tobin JR: Hospital-based group practice and comprehensive care for children of indigent families. *Pediatrics* 1977; 60:873–880.

100. Blendon RJ: The reform of ambulatory care: A financial paradox. *Med Care* 1976; 14:526–534.

101. Kane RL: Primary care: Contradictions and questions. *N Engl J Med* 1977; 296:1410–1411.

102. Lewis CR, Fein R, Mechanic D: *A Right to Health: The Problem of Access to Primary Medical Care.* New York, John Wiley & Sons, Inc, 1976.

103. Shortell SM, Wickizer TM, Wheeler J, et al: *Hospital Sponsored Primary Care: A Study of Organizational Change and Program Implementation.* Ann Arbor, Mich, Health Administration Press, forthcoming, 1984.

104. Levin L: The lay person as the primary health care practitioner. Paper adapted from an address to the *Patient Education Symposium*, sponsored by the Department of Social Perspectives in Medicine, University of Arizona, 1975.

105. Fleming GB, Andersen R: *Health Beliefs of the U.S. Population: Implications for Self-Care*, Perspectives Series A-11. Chicago, Center for Health Administration Studies, University of Chicago, 1975.

106. Green LW, Werlin SH, Schauffler HH, et al: Research and demonstration issues in self-care: Measuring the decline of mediocentrism. *Health Educ Monogr* 1977; 5(2):161–189.

107. Davis K: Health care financing: A rural perspective. Paper presented at the American Public Health Association Meeting, New York, fall 1977.

PART THREE

Providers of Health Services

CHAPTER 4

Public Health Services: Background and Present Status

William Shonick

Public health services have traditionally focused on the prevention of disease. As a new capitalist society, seeking a more comfortable life for more people with its dynamism and mobility, evolved out of the decline of the relatively stable and immobile feudalism in Europe, new ways of living and traveling brought with them the side effects of new threats to health. Disease threatened whole communities and regions with severe illness and death. Early efforts in Europe, and later in America, were directed at preventing or mitigating epidemics of acute infectious diseases such as smallpox, bubonic plague, cholera, typhoid fever, malaria, yellow fever, venereal disease, tuberculosis, and the childhood diseases of measles, mumps, scarlet fever, diphtheria, and whooping cough. (The biologic nature of these and other diseases is discussed in Chapter 2, and the current status of the battles against infectious disease is described in Reference 1, this chapter.)

The change in living conditions created by capitalism—rapid growth of city life, worldwide exploration and trade, and formidable technology—was accompanied by an ever-changing set of diseases as people struggled to adapt to their new environment (2). These threats to health changed over time. During the earlier stages of capitalism, the greatest scourges were epidemics of acute, infectious, and highly lethal disease. With the advent of better public health measures and other factors, such as the development of genetic immunity in large portions of the population, these threats were replaced by chronic and debilitative diseases such as emphysema, asbesteosis and other pulmonary diseases, cancer, stroke, heart disease, arthritis, and mental and emotional dysfunction associated with modern life. Throughout these changes, public health practitioners, policymakers, and researchers have attempted to learn the nature of the new threats and to organize public measures to combat them. To be fully effective, these measures had to be based on a correct assessment of what caused the disease and how it spread, and methods to control its spread had to be developed. In most cases, some form of organization was necessary to combat the spread of disease. Since this organization usually involved governmental authority, the term *public health* arose. Thus, the development of public health services had four aspects: a) identifying the diseases that were the leading causes of death and debility; b) learning their cause and method of transmission; c) finding methods to prevent or control them; and d) learning how to organize society to apply the controls effectively.

As each new threat to public health arose, it drew a response from lay people and professionals, who tried to organize preventive services for mitigating or eliminating it, with varying degrees of success. In describing the organization and development of public health services in the United States, this chapter will follow the pattern suggested by the actual evolution of public health programs described above. First, we will identify the major threats to health existing during a particular period, the social conditions that led to prevailing patterns of disease, and the scientific discoveries that revealed what caused the disease, how it was transmitted, and how it could be combatted. Subsequently, we will show how the understanding of the disease patterns, the state of scientific knowledge, and the current status of the society shaped the organization of public health services in response to the prevailing threats to health.

The organization of American public health agencies has involved an interplay of federal, state, and local governments and authorities. Although the form and functions of public health organizations were largely determined by the nature of the diseases and the knowledge of their causes, as well as the relationships among medical professionals, the structure of the public health system was also strongly affected by the roles played by these three levels of government. Great changes in these roles have occurred over time, but the most significant one for the development of U.S. public health services was the passage of the Social Security Act in 1935. For the first time, the federal government began to play a major role in the development of state and local public health services. The following discussion of the development of public health services is therefore arranged in two major sections: the period before 1935 and the period after 1935.

THE PERIOD BEFORE 1935

Local Public Health Services

During the colonial period, 1620–1781, small agricultural communities generally existed. In addition to farming, they engaged in some trade, and a few port towns, such as Boston, New York, Philadelphia, and Charleston, were beginning to develop into cities. The principal health threats were epidemics of infectious diseases, probably resulting from a combination of unsanitary and unhealthy local conditions—unsafe water supplies, swamps, poor sanitation in housing—and diseases brought in by ships anchored in the harbors. The port towns were the site of some of the more serious epidemics.

Local organization to counter these epidemics consisted of voluntary boards of health set up, for the most part, on a temporary basis to meet particular threats. These ad hoc boards applied what were considered to be the appropriate sanctions, namely sanitation measures and quarantines. Quarantine was (and is) the practice of confining persons who are suspected of harboring a communicable disease to restricted quarters—a house or ship—until there was no further evidence there of such disease. All persons who had had contact with the infected person would also be confined. Only special persons such as physicians, nurses, and ministers were permitted to enter the house or board the ship as it lay in the harbor.

After the American Revolution, local public health services were carried on much as before. Community boards, meeting as the occasion required, used their powers of quarantine and summons to force compliance with a sanitary code. In time, a practicing local physician was occasionally designated as the local public health officer. For his public duties he was recompensed, always modestly and often not at all. However, the continued development of sea trade increased the frequency and severity of epidemics in the port cities. This threat was abetted by the slow but accelerating industrial development, which further increased the size and congestion of the cities, both ports and others, in which manufacturing was developing. However, the epidemics in the port cities continued to be especially severe, indicating that the most serious epidemics were imported at this time. Yellow fever attacked these port cities in a series of epidemics, of which the Philadelphia epidemic of 1793 "was in many ways the worst calamity of its kind ever suffered by an American city" (3:216). It was particularly serious because Philadelphia was then the capital and cultural center of the infant United States, and virtually the entire government deserted the city. One-tenth of the population died. The usual measures of quarantine and sanitation were followed, with emphasis on sanitation.

Before about 1850, local public health activities were largely reactive to the onset of epidemics. (This had been the pattern in much of Europe for hundreds of years.) Local elected officials, aldermen or council members, generally passed ordinances establishing house quarantine, ship quarantine, and sanitation measures during epidemics. On an ongoing basis, they passed ordinances providing for street drainage, cleanliness of public markets, and waste disposal. With the development of biologic science in Europe, methods of preventing and controlling outbreaks of contagious disease became more effective. As a consequence, professional health departments arose during the years 1850–1900, and full-time officials who came to be known as *health officers* were appointed to head them. The use of quarantine and sanitation was guided by the rapidly developing bacteriologic and pathologic sciences and the new knowledge of animal and human disease carriers. The development of vaccines and antitoxins made immunizing inoculations a public health method, and increased knowledge about the causes and method of transmission of venereal diseases and tuberculosis led local health departments to engage in case-finding and some treatment of these diseases. These practices came to be included, along with immunization, under the category of "communicable disease control."

In addition to sanitation, quarantine, and communicable disease control, the collection and analysis of vital statistics was becoming a local public health activity. Like many other measures, this was an American adaptation of European, and especially British, public health practice. Records were kept of deaths by cause and demographic composition and, in later years, physicians were required to report the incidence of communicable diseases to the local public health authority. These data were used to monitor disease rates and to alert governmental authorities to the development of epidemics. They were also used to establish causes of disease by association with environmental factors—for example, the higher prevalence of yellow fever in areas with stagnant water. The increasing sophistication of bacteriologic and pathologic science created a growing appreciation of the importance of appropriate laboratory facilities to determine what communicable disease agents were prevalent in the environment or in the population. This method, in turn, led to the addition of a fifth function for local public health departments—maintenance of a public health laboratory. Since most private physicians had no laboratories, a public health department laboratory that could test human tissue or fluid samples sent by private practitioners and water or food samples submitted by health authorities or other citizens became an important local public health facility.

By 1925, most of the leading communicable diseases that had afflicted humanity for thousands of years and produced devastating epidemics in Europe and America since about 1300 had been identified as to cause and methods of transmittal. Preventive measures had been developed for most of these: water and food sanitation; identification, treatment and perhaps isolation; immunization; and control of disease carriers (principally the mosquito, louse, and rat). The requirements for applying these controls helped to shape the structures and operations of health departments. By the 1920s, it was largely true worldwide that epidemic and even widespread endemic occurrence of acute communicable diseases was due to a failure to organize public health services for the entire population. Thus, the very presence of these diseases was considered to be a social rather than a scientific or medical problem, because methods for preventing them were known.

As mentioned previously, given these developments, localities increasingly found it necessary, or at least desirable, to employ full-time, professionally trained staff. The size of this staff grew, especially in the large cities. Toward the end of the 1800s, a medium-sized to large community with a fairly adequate public health organization had a voluntary board of health, policymaking members appointed by the executive of the local government, and a department of public health with full-time professional staff headed by a medically trained health officer. Large departments often had more than one health officer heading bureaus or divisions that specialized in various aspects of public health work such as communicable disease control. The head of the agency might then be designated the commissioner of health or chief health officer. Helping the health officer were the public health nurses, who in large departments might be organized in a bureau or division of public health nursing. They aided in administering immunization, managing clinics, and making home visits to determine the need for quarantine or to encourage immunization and perform other health education functions. Together with the local coroner, they were frequently the main collectors of vital statistics.

In a large city, sanitation functions were typically headed by civil engineers who specialized in sanitation. Working under these sanitary engineers were specially trained technicians known as *sanitarians*. Sanitary engineers framed the ordinances and planned the water works and waste disposal systems to ensure freedom from contamination. If they did not actually plan sanitary construction, they were consulted on proposals. The sanitarians inspected places of business (especially food establishments), houses, streets, and other areas for violation of the sanitary code. They often had the power to collect food and water samples and send them to the local or state public health department laboratory for analysis. They also reported violations to the health department, where the reports were routed to the appropriate health officer or sanitary engineer. The vital statistics were assembled by trained personnel known as *registrars*.

The typical bureau or division of communicable disease control ran diagnostic clinics for identifying venereal disease and tuberculosis, and also provided or arranged for treatment as well as enforced isolation or hospitalization for identified cases. In many places, attempts were made to identify and locate the persons from whom the disease had been acquired. It also offered immunization against those diseases for which vaccines and antitoxins were available, and supervised vector (disease carrier) control measures such as drainage of stagnant water to control mosquitos and rat and louse eradication.

The division of public health laboratories provided diagnostic services for physicians, public health clinics, and sanitarians. Samples sent to such laboratories would be tested for contagious disease organisms. Many laboratories also distributed vaccines to private physicians, although in some places this was done by the division of communicable disease control.

Smaller health departments rarely had a full complement of bureaus or divisions, each performing a major specialized function and headed by a highly trained specialist. They usually operated with only sanitarians and had no sanitary engineers on staff; general clerks instead of specially trained registrars handled whatever vital statistics were collected; communicable disease control might be handled by the health officer who also headed the agency; and tissue, food, and water samples would be sent to the state public health laboratory for analysis. In very small health departments, a single health officer, often a local private practitioner serving part time, handled all these functions or shared them with a single public health nurse and perhaps a clerk.

In addition to changes in local public health practice resulting largely from scientific advances, the approach of the turn of the century brought with it a marked change in local health department practice due to social developments in the U.S. population. Important demographic changes were taking place in the large cities of the East Coast and the Midwest. Immigration had been an important factor in the population growth of the United States throughout the 1800s (4), but particularly large waves of immigrants began arriving in New York City and other cities beginning about 1892. Immigration peaked during the 1901–1910 decade and then subsided slowly, reaching its low point during 1931–1940. Working in the factories and mills, these immigrants were predominantly poor and settled into many urban ghettos, especially in New York City. The resulting slum conditions produced illnesses similar to those that had arisen in Great Britain during the Industrial Revolution of 1750–1850, when the cities became very unhealthy and unsafe because of massive immigration from the countryside. Reformers and volunteer organizers worked and propagandized to alleviate the living conditions of the tightly packed slums. The health condition of the immigrants, a principal concern, focused on communicable disease and infant mortality, housing and especially sanitation, and nutrition. Volunteer agencies opened milk stations in slum areas to provide uncontaminated milk and started clinics for child care. The outpatient departments of public and some private hospitals were inundated with patients seeking primary care.

This period saw the first sign of schism in public health professional circles concerning a basic issue: the appropriateness of including personal health care in a public health department. As noted previously, until about 1900 the functions of local public health departments had generally focused on community-wide control measures—sanitation, quarantine, and immunization. Sanitation was an engineering and inspection activity; quarantine called for examination at times, but it was basically an administrative and police activity (the government's right to quarantine superseded even property rights); and much immunization was done by private physicians with vaccines obtained from the health department. Thus, most health departments were operating out of one or perhaps a few centers.

Given the overwhelming problems of slums in the big cities after 1890, many in public health were saying that the most significant new need of the immigrants was for preventive health centers in their neighborhoods; public health departments in large cities should develop chains of neighborhood public health centers. Furthermore, at these centers, additional preventive services of a personal nature—maternal and child health (well-care only) and health education, including nutrition—should be offered. The subject remained controversial until about 1910, when the New York City Health Department implemented a system of neighborhood health centers in poor areas that offered not only maternal and child health care but also examinations (and even some treatment) for venereal disease and tuberculosis detection. These latter programs, involving the part-time use of private clinicians, rapidly gained almost unanimous acceptance in professional public health circles as the sixth function considered to be basic to public health services.

By 1935, then, the local public health department in the large city was typically performing six basic functions that were later to be specifically defined by the American Public Health Association, as discussed below in the section on the Emerson Report. The typical staff consisted of health officers and public health nurses; sanitary engineers and sanitarians; pediatricians and general practitioners, who practiced privately and served part-time in the maternal and child care programs, being paid on the basis of a fixed fee per clinic session; registrars and clerks; and assorted supporting personnel. These were the basic programs in large cities. Many cities also had additional services such as mental health, and the rural and smaller cities had correspondingly fewer specialized staff. Their services rarely exceeded the basic functions, and they often could not cover even those well.

Much of the professional literature in the public health field during the active developmental period, 1900–1935 and then on to about 1945, was devoted to defining the resources required to cover populations of specified geographic areas, providing public health services of adequate depth. Services actually available were surveyed by several study groups. As minimal standards were being developed, these findings were compared with the standards, and the difference was expressed as a need. These studies assembled and published data on such matters as the number of existing local health departments, the composition of their staffs, the methods by which they were financed, the populations covered by their services, the allocation of their expenditures among various activities, and the types of activities in which they engaged. The key to obtaining good local health department coverage outside large urban centers was considered to be the expansion of the *full-time* staff.

The last study made before 1935 was that of Ferrell and associates, carried out under the direction of the Surgeon General of the United States and published by the U.S. Public Health Service in 1929 (5). The purpose of this study was to identify areas in the United States that were served by full-time health departments in 1925 and to estimate the geographic extent and population of these areas. It should be noted that the focus was on county areas *outside* large cities because the latter had their own, usually sophisticated public health departments. The number of full-time county health departments was found to have risen from 13 to 303 since 1915. The division of the funding of local health departments between state and local sources was found to vary greatly from state to state. In some states the funds emanated almost exclusively from the state governments, whereas in others the localities contributed more or less substantially.

Although the federal government did not really enter the local public health picture until 1935, the early years of the twentieth century did witness the introduction of some federal funding of local health departments, foreshadowing the complicated patchwork quilt that was later to become the predominant pattern. This topic is discussed later in terms of the federal role in public health.

Although the issue of public health departments providing general personal health (i.e., medical) services became a more serious policy issue in public health circles after 1935, the expansion of local public health departments into any aspect of curative or therapeutic general medicine, as opposed to preventive services, was watched closely and nervously by local medical societies even before 1935. The local and national medical societies jealously guarded their exclusive right to give medical care, and their resistance to perceived challenges often took on a truculent tone. Their insistence on the sole right to dispense personal medical treatment was largely responsible for the restriction of public health departments to communitywide activities such as communicable disease and sanitation control. If a patient was completely indigent and could not afford to pay for treatment, then the organized medical profession had no objection to local or other government agencies providing it in clinics or via government-reimbursed physicians. But the preference was for fee-for-service reimbursement to private physicians rather than the use of salaried physicians, and for welfare department rather than health department sponsorship. During the relatively prosperous 1920–1929 period, the operation of general medical care clinics by local health departments was occasionally tolerated by the medical profession. However, during the Depression years many of these programs were effectively discontinued, and the public health profession was sharply reminded that its scope of function did not extend to curative care.

In summary, then, the proper role of a local health department has been seen to lie in the areas of sanitation, communicable disease control (including the provision of laboratory services to practicing physicians), and the necessary collection of vital statistics appropriate to such control. Health education and other preventive areas were included, and occasionally it was considered proper for the health department to engage in restricted areas of direct medical care to populations that could not be treated privately either because the patient could not pay or because the condition was communicable. Those aspects of maternal and child care that were primarily concerned with health education and preventive measures were also permitted the local public health department, with prenatal and well-baby clinics becoming common features. Accepting, and for the most part actively and even enthusiastically acquiescing in these delimitations of its scope of function, the leaders of the public health profession turned with renewed vigor after 1935 to development of the requisite professional staffing standards for carrying these functions out.

State Public Health Agencies Before 1935

Permanent state health departments developed later than their local counterparts, as states were being pressed to exercise their police powers under the Constitution with respect to health. The power of the state to carry out functions such as protecting the health of its citizens "is generally referred to as the state's police power . . . i.e., the power 'to enact and enforce laws to protect and promote the health, safety, morals, order, peace, comfort, and general welfare of the people' . . . and local agencies, including state and local public health departments and agencies, derive their power by delegation from the state legislature" (6:5–6). The permanently organized state health department became a familiar part of state government during the years 1870–1910, when it was becoming increasingly apparent that many health problems were wider in geographic scope than the local community. As commercial and industrial development became statewide and regional rather than local, statewide public health action came to be needed. One of the principal immediate factors leading to the formation of a state public health organization often was a request "from a comparatively large number of localities which shared a common problem or when some powerful local jurisdiction such as a large city, demanded state action" (7:91).

The first permanent state board of health was organized in 1869 in Massachusetts. It is not surprising that this should have happened since the functions and structure of such a department were first formulated in that state. Lemuel Shattuck, a bookseller and a student of the work of the English public health reformer Edwin Chadwick, had been campaigning for the improvement of public health measures in Massachusetts when in 1849 he was named chairman of the Massachusetts Sanitary Commission, which had been appointed by the governor to make a "sanitary survey" of the state. The report of this commission, issued in 1850, "has become a classic in public health literature and documents" (7:93), with many of its recommendations serving as guides for the organization of subsequent state and local health departments. The recommendations were remarkably comprehensive. In fact, many of them formed the basis for the later organization of public health departments, and others are still regarded as desirable even though they remain largely unrealized to the present day.

By 1900 forty states had state health departments, and by 1909 all states had organized some form of health department. The previously cited study (5) found that in 1925 a total of seventeen states had separate bureaus of county health work with a full-time director in charge. This discovery was highlighted because of the importance attached by the authors to the promotion of local health work as a function of the state health department. The interrelationship of the state and local public health agencies remains an important aspect of the public health system to the present day. The Ferrell Study found the proportion of the funds for local full-time health departments provided by the states to vary greatly, another condition that still prevails. One state met 48% of the total expenses for full-time county health service, and in 10 states the state's share of county budgets ranged from 20% to 30% of the total. The study found that "the trend toward increasing the aid from the state is growing." Functions found to be performed or promoted most often by state health departments in 1925 were rural or district health work; development of local health units; communicable disease control, particularly tuberculosis and venereal disease; vital statistics; public health laboratories; sanitary engineering; child hygiene; public health nursing; public health education; and food and drug regulation and control. In many states, full-time divisions were organized in the state health department to direct some of these functions.

This report described the situation existing before the Social Security Act of 1935 began pumping federal monies into the states, thus expanding state and local health department facilities and functions. It was used as a benchmark to measure later progress ascribed to the availability of such funds.

Federal Role in Local and State Public Health Services Before 1935

Although the primary focus of this chapter is on public health services supervised or delivered by state and local health departments, the pattern and nature of these services have, over the years, been formed largely by federal government policy.

This discussion of federal health policy is therefore confined to those aspects that affected state and local health departments directly. This section describes the pre-1935 period, during which the foundations for a greater federal role were laid, so that after 1935 federal grants-in-aid and the regulations accompanying them increasingly determined the direction of state and local policy until the period after World War II, when federal policy became dominant. An intricate and unique federal system has been created by the fact that states supervise public health, set standards, and do only a small amount of direct service delivery; that localities deliver most of the direct services; and that the federal government has been paying for these services and, in the process, setting national policy. The intergovernmental relations involved are sometimes baffling. Under the U.S. Constitution, the protection of public health is, as a general proposition, implicitly reserved to the individual state under its police powers, since a health function is not explicitly assigned to Congress. Whenever constitutional authorization was invoked to justify early federal action in public health matters, one or both of two sections of the Constitution were cited. Under the first of these sections, Congress is specifically given the power "to regulate commerce with foreign nations, and among the several states." This proviso was used to justify the earliest federal activities centering on control of communicable diseases at ports of entry and, somewhat later, included attempts to control communicable disease in interstate commerce. Under the second proviso, that of Article I, Section VIII, Congress is empowered "to . . . provide for the . . . general welfare of the United States." This clause was the justification advanced by those who sought federal intervention in health problems in the interests of countrywide uniformity, equity, and efficiency (6).

Early federal legislation, beginning in 1796, concentrated on attempting to control the introduction into the United States of communicable diseases such as malaria, yellow fever, and cholera. To this end, various laws were passed establishing aid for quarantine procedures at the major ports of entry. The 1796 law merely provided for cooperation of the federal government with states and localities in enforcing state and local laws on ship quarantine. Quarantine power itself was still regarded by Congress as resting with the states, but opposition to this view also existed. In 1878 the Marine Hospital Service, which had been established in 1798 to provide medical care for merchant seamen, was designated as the agency that would assist any state or community that requested its services in helping to prevent the introduction of contagious or infectious diseases into this country. In 1879, a National Board of Health with a 4-year term of office was voted by Congress. Its duties included having "charge of interstate and foreign quarantine" (7:54). Because of serious dissent among its participants and various public health bodies, it became effectively defunct at the end of the mandated 4 years and officially ceased to exist in 1893. At the end of its effective life in 1883, quarantine duties were restored to the Marine Hospital Service (7:54). Under an act of 1893, ship quarantine became a federal function, and by 1921, all quarantine stations had been acquired and were being operated by the federal government.

Congress also passed laws regulating interstate quarantine measures, with enforcement powers delegated to the National Board of Health in 1879. These powers were strengthened and specifically given to the Marine Hospital Service in 1893. Thereafter the public health aspects of the work of the Marine Hospital Service were concerned primarily with control of communicable diseases with respect to both introduction of disease from abroad and its spread among the states. The agency used this internal power very cautiously, for the most part helping states with advice and personnel only when asked, despite the 1893 law entitling it to use enforcement.

Another aspect of the Marine Hospital Service's work in communicable disease control consisted of administering federal grants-in-aid to localities and lending personnel for demonstration projects in the various states, hoping thereby to encourage better practice. This was a relatively minor facet of its operations, however. Despite the change of name of the Marine Hospital Service, first to the United States Public Health and Marine Hospital Service in 1902 and finally to the United States Public Health Service in 1912, it continued to concentrate mainly on medical care for seamen and other stipulated eligible persons and on foreign quarantine. Beginning in 1913, however, a gradual broadening of perspective occurred when Congress began appropriating funds for local research in public health. During the years 1914–1916, the service conducted a series of field studies in typhoid fever control with the cooperation of about 16 states. These field investigations contained a large demonstration component and, beginning in 1917, funds were appropriated annually by Congress for rural sanitation work by the U.S. Public Health Service. The grants had to be matched in equal amount by the states receiving them. This arrangement lasted until 1934.

Between 1915 and 1935, two other types of federal stimulation of state and local public health work were also in evidence: grants for venereal disease control and for maternal and child hygiene. Grants for venereal disease control began with the Chamberlain-Kahn Act of 1918, which allocated funds to the states according to population. The appropriations for this program eventually dwindled away, disappearing in 1926, but strengthened venereal disease control laws and programs remained in effect in many states. Grants for maternal and child health began in 1921 with passage of the Sheppard-Towner Act. Administration of the act was assigned to the Children's Bureau, established in 1912 as part of the Department of Labor, which had been doing research and educational work on matters pertaining to the welfare of children and had been a leading proponent of the 1921 legislation. The act provided for allocation of the appropriated money among the states by a formula. Mustard writes that "between 1922 and 1927 the Division of Maternal and Infant Hygiene carried on an aggressive and productive program" (7:76). In 1929, the program ended after the discontinuation of federal funds.

Thus, the period up to 1935 was one of development of public health both as a profession to combat epidemics of acute communicable disease and as an organ of government. The organization was principally local, with many of the large cities having impressive departments and boards. The states were running organizations that concentrated on setting standards and monitoring local services, encouraging the formation of local health departments in areas where none existed, and providing direct local public health services via state "districts" in areas that needed the services but did not have a local department. The federal government, which was represented in the United States Public Health Service in 1912, was by 1900 performing quarantine services at major ports and providing modest amounts of aid to localities, in financial cooperation with states, for improving sanitation services in rural areas. This agency also supervised interstate quarantine when asked to do so.

However, fundamental changes, especially economic, in U.S. society were creating great fiscal strains. The responsibilities for performing local public health services (and many other social services such as education) continued to rest with the states, which delegated them to the cities and localities, but the base for tax collection was steadily moving from the localities and states to the federal level.

The disparity between service responsibility and available revenue was becoming too great to be ignored, and the question of the federal government returning some of its tax money to localities for local services came increasingly to the fore as 1935 approached.

The minimal federal aid provided by the demonstration grants for public health work was insufficient to rectify the growing disparity, and the Sheppard-Towner and Kahn-Chamberlain acts had proved temporary. During the upheaval created by the Great Depression of 1929, new legislation was passed giving the federal government more power to aid states and localities. Perhaps the most important of these laws, the Social Security Act of 1935, breathed renewed life into the federal grant-in-aid for health programs. Before turning to this legislation, it is useful to consider some general questions relating to grants-in-aid and tax sharing among levels of government.

THE GROWING DISPARITY BETWEEN THE TAX BASE AND SERVICE RESPONSIBILITIES AMONG LEVELS OF GOVERNMENT

Before discussing the fiscal interrelationships among the three levels of American government as they affect financing of health activities, it is useful to identify two aspects of such relationships: a) the service responsibilities of the respective levels and b) the tax revenue resources available to them.

The disparity between the responsibility for providing health services and the proportion of total tax revenue collected by the respective levels of government has grown ever wider since the establishment of the United States. It is common sense to suppose that if a particular level of government is assigned responsibility for a specified function, part of the total tax revenues needed to perform it would be allotted. Indeed, at the inception of our government, allocation of revenue roughly matched the responsibilities of each level of government. In time, however, although local governmental responsibility for providing services grew enormously, its share of total taxes collected by all governmental levels declined. Most of the taxes collected eventually went to the federal government, whose service responsibilities were minimal. Furthermore, the basis of most of the national wealth and income shifted from family-operated agriculture to commerce and industry operated by national corporations, including rapid growth in the service sector of the economy. With these changes, most of the tax base shifted from land and building capital to money income and money capital. Taxes on money capital, including investment securities, are not collected at all in the United States; and taxes on money income are collected primarily by the federal government and secondarily, at a far lesser rate, by the state governments. Furthermore, money income and capital can be concentrated in a few states to a greater degree than can land and property values. Despite this unequal distribution, money income can be reached by federal taxes, but not by those states whose citizens have relatively low incomes. Taxes on land and the property on it (real property) are the principal sources of taxes for local governments. Thus, whereas the proportion of the available tax base has shifted in favor of the federal government, responsibility for health services (and other social services) remains with state and local governments. The problems attendant upon this "cultural lag" will be considered in further detail.

In its early years, the federal government was assigned functions that involved mainly conducting foreign affairs, providing for national armed forces, and regulating commerce both with foreign governments and among the states. The Founding Fathers clearly seemed to believe that the basic regulatory and administrative unit of government, as far as the individual citizen was concerned, was the state, with the federal government handling only those problems that involved all or at least several of the states. It was thus entirely appropriate that the federal government's revenues came mostly from various excise taxes and tariffs. The principal function of these tariffs was to protect the development of the infant American industry; the fact that they also produced revenue was an added benefit.

As late as 1910, 54% of the population was still listed as rural and only 46% as urban. By 1970, 73% of the population was urban. Between 1910 and 1920, the majority of the population shifted from rural to urban and remained so thereafter. During this same period, there was a basic shift from a primarily agricultural population to one engaged in commerce, industry, and services.

With increasing regulatory functions after the Civil War to serve the burgeoning and ever-centralizing American capitalism, and with rising military expenditures, the federal government's need for additional revenue was growing and becoming a permanent feature of national operations. As the major source of personal income shifted markedly from real property and agricultural production to money capital and nonagricultural sources, the federal government sought to tap these new sources of wealth. After an attempt in 1894 to legislate a federal income tax was struck down as unconstitutional by a five to four decision of the Supreme Court (*Pollock v. Farmer's Loan and Trust Co.*), the Sixteenth Amendment to the Constitution was ratified in 1913, explicitly permitting the federal government to levy income taxes. Thereafter, the federal income tax rapidly became the most important single source of tax revenue for the federal government, accounting for $26 billion out of the total $35 billion, or 75% of federal receipts by 1950, and $173 billion out of $201 billion, or 86% in 1976. Customs revenues, which accounted for 84% of total revenue in 1800, 91% in 1850, and as much as 41% even as late as 1900, had shrunk to less than an insignificant 1% by 1950.

Equally illuminating is the change over time in the percentage of total government tax revenues collected by state and local units compared with that collected by the federal government. In 1902, 64% of total taxes were collected by the states and localities and 36% by the federal government. These percentages remained relatively the same until after World War II. By 1950, the picture was almost exactly the reverse of the 1900–1940 pattern, with 69% of all taxes being collected by the federal government. Thus, during the immediate post-World War II years, some 65% to 70% of all taxes were being collected by the federal government.

The shift of the major tax base from real property to money income has resulted not only in a movement in taxable resources from the states and localities to the federal level but also in a heavily unbalanced geographic distribution of these taxable money resources (tax base) among the states. States with industrial—including large scale, industrially organized agriculture (agribusiness)—commercial, and financial centers had high per capita incomes; those that were predominantly rural and had few or only secondary centers of industry, commerce, and finance suffered from low per capita incomes. The available base for local taxes became more and more unevenly distributed, not only among states but also among localities. Furthermore, the need for health services from state and local governments was often inversely related to the available tax base. Study after study of expenditures for health services of the various states in the 1920s, 1930s, and 1940s revealed two important facts: a) the amount spent per capita varied greatly from state to state; b) states with a lower per capita income were often spending more relative to their total tax resources and income than were the more affluent states.

Clearly, increasing local and state taxes could not equitably provide a uniform level of public health services to match local needs, because local taxable income was generally inversely related to such needs. Further, although the tax base now favored the federal government, the responsibility of the states for providing public health and other services remained. A solution to the problem boiled down to a choice between two alternatives or some combination of them. Either a) the responsibility for many health and other services could be directly transferred to the federal government by legislative, constitutional, or judicial action or b) the states could keep their responsibilities but receive money back from the federal treasury to discharge them. Federal revenues would thus be shared with the states and localities, but program control could continue to remain largely in state and local hands. Revenue sharing did eventually occur, but with it came a shift in responsibility and program control in the public health (and other) fields to the federal government. This change corroborated the well-established maxim that "control follows the dollar."

After 1935, the principal mechanism used to correct the disparity between tax base and service responsibilities was the grant-in-aid, under which the federal government shared its revenue with the states and localities. Different schemes for distributing these grants have been used. Some formulas are better for achieving one set of goals and other formulas for other goals. Let us now consider various mechanisms and the objectives of each in supplying grants-in-aid to various levels of government. Subsequent sections will discuss how the federal health grants actually operated with respect to state and local public health work after 1935.

Redistribution of Tax Revenues Among the Different Levels of Government

Two basic methods have been used to allocate federal money among states and localities: the formula grant and the project grant. Formula grants are distributed among the states according to a formula established by law. The basis for distribution may be equal allocation, variable allocation, or a combination of both. Under the infrequently used equal allocation, an equal fixed amount is allocated to each state. Under variable allocation, certain characteristics of each state determine the percentage of the total national appropriation it receives. This type of grant allocation was the more common one for health purposes until about 1965, and it is still widely used. Its main attribute is that it permits the appropriation to be distributed in a manner that helps equalize services and tax burdens throughout the nation.

The preceding discussion deals with formulas for *distributing* money among the states. In addition, grants to states often carry stipulations about how the money may be *spent*. Formula grants have been further identified as either general purpose (block grants) or earmarked (categorical grants), depending on the restrictions imposed. Block grants may be used without detailed, specific restrictions for broadly defined purposes such as improving and expanding local health department services. Categorical grants, on the other hand, if given to a local health department, may be spent only for a specific type of activity, such as cancer control. It is important to note that what may seem to be a block grant at one level of administration is viewed as a categorical grant at a higher level. For example, a general purpose health grant to a local health department is a block grant for that department, but it is categorically restricted from the point of view of the local government, which may prefer to use part of it for law enforcement.

Project grants, a type of grant-in-aid, are principally designed to carry out a federal program rather than to help a local health agency accomplish its own objectives. This grant transfers money directly from the federal government to a state or local government, or to any other type of governmental or nongovernmental organization, for carrying out a specific project previously approved by the federal granting agency. Often the grant award has been made to one of several competing applicants. This type of grant requires an application from a would-be recipient and is not given automatically to any governmental unit according to a preset formula.

Federal health grants that have often been used may be classified as follows:

a. General purpose health grants distributed to states by formula, with little or no restriction on expenditure categories. The states redistribute most of these grants to local public health departments.
b. Categorical formula grants distributed to states by formula, with specific program restrictions on expenditure categories. The states redistribute some of these grants to local public health departments.
c. Project grant awarded to applicants that are not necessarily government bodies. Spending is restricted by a budget that was submitted with the application. Project grants may be awarded to nongovernmental organizations. This trend has proved to be particularly important in the development of intergovernmental relations in public health.

THE PERIOD AFTER 1935

Local Health Department Growth, 1936–1945

The period from 1936 to 1945 was characterized by growth in local and state public health departments financed substantially with federal assistance. The programs appropriate to a professionally respected health department were determined by leading members of the American Public Health Association (APHA) working in special committees, and the financial aid made available by the federal government was used to expand the coverage of the U.S. population by professionally staffed health departments.

The Social Security Act of 1935 established annual grants-in-aid from the federal government to the states, part of whose purpose was to further the development of full-time local health departments. This landmark in the development of intergovernmental relations in the health field marked the first major entrance of the federal government into local and state public health operations. Although all the provisions of the act were interrelated and a number of them affected health services, two sections directly mandated federal support for state and local public health departments. Title V, Part 1, provided grants to the states for aiding state and local health departments to render maternal and child health services and was administered by the U.S. Children's Bureau, then part of the Department of Labor. These were categorical grants earmarked for maternal and child health. Title VI provided grants to the states for aiding the work of state and local public health departments. Title VI funds were administered by the U.S. Public Health Service (PHS). They were formula block or general health grants that could be spent as each public health department saw fit, within very broad limits. For both Title V and Title VI grants, the states had to match the federal money by spending a dollar of their own funds for each dollar of federal grant money.

The Mountin Report.   The development of these departments through 1946 has been described by Joseph W. Mountin, an Assistant Surgeon General of the PHS well known for his public health writing, and his associates. In a PHS monograph (8), they described a substantial expansion of local and state services.

The Mountin report indicated that the number of counties covered by full-time local health services grew from 762 in 1935 to 1,577 in 1940 to 1,851 in 1946. In addition, the proportion of the population covered *outside the cities with their own municipal health departments* grew from 37% in 1935 to 72% by 1946. The influence of these funds on the growth of local health department staffs, again exclusive of independent metropolitan centers, was equally marked. Total full-time personnel, again excluding cities, increased from 3,435 to 10,320, more rapidly in nonmedical than in medical personnel. This improvement was accomplished in spite of the fact that "a considerable proportion of established positions for medical—and others—were vacant for war-related reasons" (8:38). The data also indicated that at least 60 cities with populations of 10,000 or over were added to the list of cities with "some type of full-time official public health organization." Mountin et al. define municipal health departments as "those city health units which operate under full-time technical direction and are independent of county or district organization" (8:16).

Despite this progress, by 1946 approximately 30% of the nonmetropolitan population and almost 20% of the total population still remained without full-time local health coverage. Furthermore, some of the expanded coverage was of questionable depth; often it represented a reporting artifact resulting from a simple blanketing in of additional areas via consolidation of counties into multicounty health districts without a proportionate increase in staff and other needed resources. Public health professionals and analysts were insistently and increasingly stressing that extending coverage by full-time local health services of at least *minimally acceptable quality* to the entire population was an important and perhaps overriding goal of public health. Clearly, the extent of such coverage could not be accurately measured if standards defining minimally acceptable services were not available.

The Emerson Report.   Because of this expressed professional desire to define minimally acceptable local health service more clearly, the growth of local health departments due to federal grants was accompanied by a heightened interest in defining adequate quality or depth of service. A special committee of the APHA chaired by a well-known public health officer, Haven Emerson, worked on this question. In 1945, it prepared and issued a definitive set of standards for measuring minimally adequate public health services. The committee also estimated what resources would be needed to cover the entire population with public health services that met these standards. Standards were set for staffing, types of services to be offered, organization of both the board and the department, and other matters. Staffing standards were based on ratios of personnel (by occupational categories) to population. All needed improvements were projected as increases over the 1942 data, which were used as a baseline from which such improvement might be measured. This information was embodied in what has come to be known as the Emerson Report (9).

The Emerson committee recommended the elimination of *all* part-time employees except visiting clinical physicians and dentists. The number of part-time clinicians, especially dentists, was to be increased. This recommendation was in accordance with the previously noted belief of local public health leaders that personal medical care, provided under the "prevention" rubric of communicable disease control and maternal and child care, should be given by local private practitioners at public health department clinic sessions. All other part-time employees, in particular the 4,316 part-time health officers, were to be dismissed. An increase of approximately 60% in the number of public health nurses was recommended, and it was suggested that much of the laboratory work of small public health departments should be done by the state health department. The section of the report dealing with scope of function probably had the most lasting influence and came to be known as the "basic six." The committee defined the six basic functions of a local health department as follows:

a. Vital statistics—recording, tabulation, interpretation, and publication of the essential facts of births, deaths, and reportable diseases
b. Communicable disease control—tuberculosis, venereal disease, malaria, and hookworm
c. Sanitation—supervision of milk, water, and eating places
d. Laboratory services
e. Maternal and child hygiene—including supervision of the health of the school child
f. Health education

The application of these standards would have reduced the statistical legerdemain used in reporting populations having supposedly full-time coverage, but these standards were never achieved.

Public health goals for the future were described in these terms: "The Committee is of the opinion that a present goal should be the creation of such number and boundaries of areas of local health jurisdiction in every state in the union as will bring within the reach of every person and family the benefits of modern sanitation, personal hygiene, and the guidance and protection of trained professional and accessory personnel employed on a full-time basis at public expense, selected and retained on a merit or civil service basis, and free from disturbance by the influence of partisan politics" (9:26). The emphasis on the merit civil service system of personnel practice as a necessary reform to curb the abuses of an earlier day is worthy of note. The importance that this committee and the APHA attached to the goals stated in this report may be inferred from their efforts to obtain approval of the professional and political organizations whose cooperation would be needed to implement the recommendations. In addition to being approved by the health officers of 37 states, the principles were endorsed by the House of Delegates of the American Medical Association (AMA), the APHA, and the State and Provincial Health Authorities of North America. Thus armed and motivated, the leaders of the public health profession set forth in 1945 to bring full-time, minimally adequate public health services to all Americans.

Developments After the Emerson Report: The Period 1946–1965. The period 1936–1945 had been one of consolidating the position of local health departments. With the new federal Title V and Title VI monies and the matching state contributions, local public health departments became well established in performing the standard basic six functions. The Emerson Report provided visible evidence of the progressive nature and professional vitality characterizing many of the leaders of public health departments. In general, the leaders of the federal government's health activities accepted the role of the local public health department as delineated by leading public health executives through the APHA and worked with local and state leaders to develop public health departments with more personnel and wider geographic coverage. Here and there, dissent was raised about the inadequate scope of function of these departments. It was noted that times were changing and that the basic six functions would no longer suffice. In particular, more work was needed to prevent and control chronic and degenerative diseases and to provide general medical care in public health department clinics. These criticisms began to multiply until after World War II.

The mounting problems in the large cities, the growth of private health insurance that covered only the nonpoor, and the social reformism of some administrations and Congresses all combined to put pressure on local public health departments to deliver services that were essentially alien to the spirit of the Emerson Report. The recommendations of this report had stressed preventive services based on suppressing acute infectious disease. The nature of the new demands upon these departments and how they were met is the subject of this section. Of course, the story must include the role of the federal government, which grew rapidly. This account will be given later, and will include the changing role of the states as well.

An analysis made in 1957 by Barkev S. Sanders (10), a technical consultant for the PHS, indicated that the percentage of the population covered by full-time local health services had risen from 75% in 1946 to 86% by 1950, reaching about 90% in 1957. The number of counties included rose from about 1,850 to 2,100 in 1950 and to about 2,300 in 1957. Similarly, expenditures, when adjusted for population and price changes, increased between 1946 and 1950, and thereafter remained static or declined slightly. The same is true of the percentage of the Gross National Product spent by local health departments. A similar pattern is shown in the number of full-time public health workers employed. The analysis also indicates a sharp decline in the amount of federal funds given to local health department operations, which dropped from $15 million (19% of the total spent by local health departments) in 1947 to $9 million (5% of the total) in 1956, so that the brunt of expenditures fell increasingly upon states and especially localities. This decline in federal contributions came in spite of increased local contributions, from $54 million to $127 million, and increased state contributions, from $10 million to $40 million, during the same period. The relative decline in federal money, therefore, was even greater than the absolute reduction.

Dr. Sanders speculates upon the possible causes for this slowdown in the rate of increase of public health services: "This could mean that other agencies are taking over certain needed health services, or that American communities are not so much interested in health, or perhaps health needs that can be dealt with effectively by local health departments have diminished" (10:18). The causes of this declining federal contribution to local public health departments have not been widely investigated, but the first and third of Sanders' suppositions, and especially the third, seem to have been corroborated by subsequent events. Many of the functions of protecting the public's health have indeed become increasingly less amenable to local control, and regional, state, and federal agencies have been doing them more and more often. These functions include such matters as pollution control, safety, food and drug monitoring, and a host of others. It is also true that "other [than public health] agencies have been taking over . . . health services," but this is true more at the state than at the local level and will be discussed below in the context of the state health department after 1935.

By 1960, some 94% of the population was judged to have access to the services of full-time health departments (11). Such departments numbered 1,557 and included 2,425 of the 3,072 counties in the United States. Clearly, widespread coverage had been achieved, but the depth or quality of coverage recommended by the Emerson Report was lacking. Other data of this 1960 study clearly indicate that the per capita personnel implied in the Emerson Report recommendations was not achieved by 1960. In the all-important categories of public health nurses and dental personnel, the staffing was far short of the recommendations; dental hygienists and public health nurses per population had actually declined from 1942 levels. Indeed, the overall staff/population ratio was somewhat lower in 1960 than the Emerson Report baseline 1942 figures showed, and yet the development of the standard local public health department had gone about as far as it was to go.

Thus, there is every indication that by 1960 most of nonmetropolitan America had access to full-time local health department services, and the small part that did not appear to have access perceived little need for it. "Full-time" continued to mean only having a separate public health department address (i.e., not a physician's private office) and at least one full-time employee, even if only a clerk. But public sentiment for enriching standard public health department staffs in rural and semirural areas was not strong. The political pressures for improvement in public health services were coming from another quarter—the metropolitan areas. In metropolitan areas, defined here similarly to the Census Bureau's Standard Metropolitan Statistical Area (SMSA) as consisting of a large city and its surrounding trading area, two civilizations were developing: that of the central, or inner, city and that of the more affluent suburbs. These two cultures, although distinct, interacted with each other, usually to the detriment of the former. The members of each culture had different public health needs. The inner city populations and their advocates were pressing for more and better public medical services, especially primary care. The social structure of working class and middle class areas in the large cities before World War II had changed, leaving them, among other things, almost bereft of private physicians. In many places, they were also demanding better protection against unsafe and unclean dwellings and streets, but the demand for medical care was more prominent politically.

Many urban areas had long had health departments that met or exceeded the minimum standards of the Emerson Report, but the standard health department was not set up to cope with the newer inner city needs. By long-standing tradition, providing general medical care was alien to it. Fighting for improved sanitation in housing *was* part of the tradition and function of local public health departments, but the widespread deterioration of the inner cities overwhelmed their resources. Coping with the widespread physical devastation of slum areas and the fiscal plight of the cities was simply too much for these departments. Even standard public health activities such as public health nurse home visits often could not be properly carried out given the increasingly unsafe neighborhoods and hostile clients. The two major requirements of the inner city for public health services—medical care and aggressive enforcement of sanitation (including safety)—found the local public health department unable to respond adequately.

The demands of the suburban populations were different. Their intellectual and artistic leaders demanded environmental control—air pollution, radiation emissions, solid waste—consumer product protection, automotive safety, and similar matters. The local public health departments existing in the newly built-up suburban areas were holdovers from previous rural environments and were operating on a relatively modest scale. They were ill-equipped and insufficiently empowered to handle these new demands and the rapid surge of development. Further, even the most efficient and forward-looking local public health leaders could see that most of the problems were being caused by large, powerful industries—automotive, petrochemical, nuclear power, and extractive. They could scarcely be controlled by a local health department, even a very well run one. Only the regional, state, and, in many cases, federal (and even international for many important problems) agencies could realistically be expected to deal with them.

The confluence of these two sets of problems in the metropolitan areas, neither of which proved very amenable to the work of the standard local public health department as it had developed, greatly diminished the public standing of and federal support for these departments in performing their standard roles.

Congress and the federal executive were being pressed to consider means of using governmental powers more effectively to make better medical care available to all the people, especially those in the lower income brackets, and to improve the quality of the environment. The leadership of the local public health department, finding itself faced with a changed and seemingly intractable set of problems and rapid alterations in the composition of its clientele, became disoriented as it was pushed from all sides to do different things. Various experts and commentators were counseling different courses. Writers and practicing professionals advised local public health departments to stick to prevention, basically as defined in the Emerson Report. Others called for a bold expansion into delivering primary medical care. Still others sought to define the fundamental role of the local public health department as one of areawide health planning, standard setting, and monitoring. Examples abound of the probing, questioning, and exhortation that was appearing everywhere, reflecting confusion about the "true" role of local public health departments. (Similar questions were being raised about the role of state health departments.)

Perhaps the most vivid indication of attempts within the ranks to redefine the function of public health departments is provided by the annual efforts of the APHA leadership to spell them out in official policy statements. The nature of these changing formulations is illustrated by comparing the policy statements adopted at three annual conventions: 1940 (essentially the same as those represented by the position in the Emerson Report of 1945), 1950, and 1963.

The official APHA position in 1940 (repeated in the Emerson Report of 1945) evinces no doubts or qualms about the functions of the local health department. They are encompassed in a neat six-point package and are directed at communitywide preventive services, carefully avoiding contact with the curative aspects, which, by implication, are left to private practitioners and welfare departments. Subsequent position statements, however, although reiterating the continuing importance of the basic six, stressed that these functions were minimal. The 1950 position statement adds the important new ingredients of operation of *health cen-*

ters and *coordination* of all community health services, while broadening the scope of the original six functions. Vital statistics now becomes recording *and analysis* of health data and maintaining data on *both* disease *and* health facilities. Environmental sanitation now includes inspection of health facilities. The 1963 statement again reiterates the importance of maintaining the standard functions at a high level of efficiency, but includes almost complete responsibility for community *leadership* to achieve a coordinated, nonoverlapping, and comprehensive health services system. The importance of integrating behavioral science and statistical disciplines into the activities of the local health department is stressed. Research, development, and evaluation of methods of providing widespread health care coverage efficiently are recommended.

An APHA 1970 policy statement essentially reiterated the 1963 local public health department functions but added the responsibility to cooperate in comprehensive state and regional planning. This cooperative role was to consist of providing health data, supplying details of health program activities and achievements, giving staff support including professional judgments and interpretations of problem areas, and engaging in studies and surveys that would assist the planning agency better to understand and define issues. This change from a *leadership* planning role advocated in the 1963 statement to one of *cooperation* with the state and regional health planning agencies was made necessary by the Comprehensive Health Planning Act of 1966, which provided funds for state health planning that were administered in many states by other than the health agency, as discussed further in Chapter 12. It also provided funds for local health planning agencies other than the public health department. This subject is discussed further in a later section on state and federal roles.

The official stance of the APHA on the organization of local boards of health and staffing of local health departments was also changing, although to a lesser degree. For boards of health, the principal change called for broadening the composition of the board. The changes in staffing standards involved abandoning fixed ratios of staff to population in favor of flexibility for meeting specific local needs. Thus, the laboriously worked out ratios of the 1945 Emerson Report were officially abandoned in 1970. This development was not surprising. In light of the many years of experience with local areawide health planning that followed the issuance of the Emerson Report, it became quite clear that flat staff/population ratios are not a good way of estimating *local* needs. Estimates of needs for particular health services and resources should be based on local population characteristics (12).

Public Policy Implications. As has been noted, the adaptive abilities of local public health departments were strongly criticized by the federal government. This criticism was reflected in changes in its mechanisms for giving grants to local governments. This issue will be discussed in greater detail later, but it must be mentioned here. The federal grants-in-aid to states that had been used since 1936 largely to help local health departments develop their traditional functions—the so-called formula grants for general health purposes—declined, while the formula grants for categorical purposes and the even more specially targeted project grants increased (13). The latter were aimed at promoting carefully focused demonstration projects to encourage an innovative approach to expanding public health functions in directions desired by the federal government. Many articles and speeches by public health figures and federal analysts, and the changing positions of the APHA, showed that changing social conditions were placing demands on local health departments in large metropolitan areas that were perceived in Washington as not being met. These demands centered on medical care for the poor, enforcement of local environmental health conditions in the ghettos, particularly housing conditions, and regional environmental control, demanded primarily by sections of the middle classes. None of these demands were met to any great degree despite the infusion of federal and state funds, policy statements by public health organizations, and the writings of professional public health administrators, academics, journalists, and a wide assortment of general pundits. Why were changes not being made?

Solving these problems involved tackling adversaries for which the local health department was no match politically. Eliminating the unhealthy conditions of ghetto life meant fighting slum landlords, urban redevelopers, and urban political machines to obtain adequate and meaningful inspection and to enforce compliance. This meant taking on the entire problem of the deterioration of the inner city. Providing adequate medical care for the poor in the cities involved tackling the entire system of medical care distribution, including the traditional treatment of the public medical care sector as a charity, second class "track." The problem of environmental decay that was troubling the middle class was not amenable to local solution. The large corporations and their polluting activities, as well as the attendant problems of automobile transportation and housing sprawl, could scarcely be tackled by the states, let alone the local governments. Thus, despite suggestions for policy changes appearing in APHA resolutions and goading by speeches and writings of commentators, and that of officers of the federal government and by grant mechanism manipulation, the local health department, as an institution, departed little from its well-beaten paths.

This is not to say that no attempts were made to meet some of these problems. There were a number of such efforts, nearly all in the direction of supplying medical care on a more comprehensive basis than the basic six. These are described in References 14 and 15. In other places, some metropolitan and county governments sought solutions to their health services problems in administrative reorganization. Faced with a combination of unsatisfactory service by municipal hospitals (16) and slow response from the health department, these governments sought to improve access to ambulatory care by merging local public hospitals with local public health departments. The complaints about large urban public hospitals (17) often centered on their inaccessibility and, when they were affiliated with a large teaching institution, on their lack of orientation to ordinary patient complaints. The health department, on the other hand, was often seen as lacking the medical expertise and facilities required for comprehensive health care. It was hoped that the mergers would combine the best of both worlds—the "people" orientation of the health department, with its neighborhood health centers, with the medical expertise and facilities backup of the public hospital (18,19). These merges had varying outcomes, and a comprehensive discussion of these results is beyond the scope of this book. Briefly, one merger was successful and a few others moderately so in the sense of providing a better system of ambulatory care for poor persons. Public health professionals generally complained that hospitals were using their funds, but the validity of this argument cannot be established because the merger period (1965–1975) was accompanied by the beginning of serious reductions in public funds in large cities, and unmerged public health departments in large cities suffered as much as or more retrenchment than those that had been merged. In any case, most cities whose agencies merged have either in fact or by actual legislation dissolved the mergers. It seems clear that although the mergers may have helped improve public ambulatory care in a few places, they have been so infrequent and unstable that they did not address the question of what, if anything, more than the basic six functions a local public health department should do today.

The fundamental problems of the health delivery system and the inner cities could not be solved by local public health departments, although vigorously and skillfully led ones could do more than others. The problem of medical care for low income groups was also shifting to a national focus, and the battle to preserve the environment was shifting to the state and federal arenas. Local health departments continued to perform the basic six functions and reacted to developments in medical care and environmental control in a variety of ways, depending on local conditions. In some areas, they became the local agents of new federal programs for operating neighborhood and migrant health centers, and became actively involved in fostering federally and state-financed systems of medical care for low income people. In most areas, they did not.

Because the federal government attempted to broaden the scope of local health department activities by the use of grants, the changes in this mechanism after 1950 should be considered in some detail. To obtain a better view of these changes, let us turn to the state health department and then to the role of the federal government in public health. The interactive effects on health policy among these governmental levels and the place and future of the local public health agency can be discussed more meaningfully after looking at state health departments and the federal effort.

State Public Health Agencies After 1935: 1936–1945

The Mountin study of 1946 (8), previously discussed, also analyzed the effect of 10 years of the Social Security Act on the expansion of state health department activities. Mountin found that expenditures of the 48 states for health departments went from $12.9 million in 1930 to $18.7 million in 1940 to $37.0 million in 1946. The breakdown of these expenditures by category showed that "such activities as communicable disease control (including tuberculosis and venereal disease control), sanitation, laboratory services, and maternal or child hygiene, which accounted for a majority of State expenditures in 1930, still received more than half of the funds available in 1946." According to the study, "At the same time, the growth of newer programs is illustrated by such figures as these for dental hygiene: 37,000 in 1930, 227,000 in 1941 and 708,000 in 1946."

That these data represented real expansion of services and were not all due to price increases is shown by the corresponding increase in full-time personnel from 4,672 in 1930 to 10,128 in 1940 to 12,414 in 1946. An additional indication given by Mountin that the expansion in the years 1935–1946 was real, and not merely an artifact of price increases, is the number of activities reported as an "identified project" by state health departments. Although this sort of measure taken alone does not necessarily imply an increase in total service volume, it was used by Mountin as an indicator of expanding scope of function. Of the 46 states reporting, 39 listed communicable disease control projects for 1935, 43 in 1940, and 45 in 1946. The number of states reporting tuberculosis control programs rose from 19 in 1935 to 32 in 1940 and 45 in 1946. Virtually all the traditional public health functions showed similar increases. Mental hygiene and cancer control, however, were listed by only 7 and 27 states, respectively, in 1946. (At the time of Mountin's report, the states were heavily involved in psychiatric care, maintaining large censuses in state mental hospitals. However, these functions were generally lodged in state hospital departments or special departments of mental hospitals. The separation of what is today called *mental health* from *public health* functions is still generally true.)

Planning, chronic disease work, and other more modern functions did not appear as identified projects at all. If they were in effect, they are subsumed under the catchall category "other central services." Thus, the increased scope of function was not mainly in areas new to public health, but represented expansion in standard areas by departments that had not yet been engaging in them.

A noteworthy exception was the striking increase in the number of states operating industrial hygiene programs. In 1935, this activity was listed as an identified project by only 4 states, compared with 26 states listing it in 1940 and 38 in 1946. The two states that did not respond to the question regarding identified projects did, in fact, have industrial hygiene units in both 1940 and 1946. In addition, New York and Massachusetts provided industrial hygiene units through their departments of labor. Thus, by 1946, 42 states had such units covering 96% of the country's labor force. The services most commonly supplied by such units were "general surveys or inspection of plants for occupational health hazards with recommendations for improvement" (8:25). As early as 1946, state health departments had begun to look for occupational health hazards; this was one of the relatively few new areas they had entered. (It was not until 1970 that the federal government established the Occupational Safety and Health Administration.)

Later Trends in Organization and Functions.   The state health department of recent years may be characterized as a supervising, coordinating, equalizing, and mediating agency, whereas the local health department has been the principal agency carrying the responsibility for the day-to-day operation of public health programs. There are exceptions (in some states the state health department carries on all the functions of local public health work, with no local government health departments; these cases are discussed later), but generally the state agency provides a complete set of personal public health services directly only when local organization is lacking or inadequate, and then only as an interim measure pending local organization. More often, it provides only isolated special services, if any. Many of the substantive areas covered by local health departments are among those most frequently assigned by state law to the state health department, again with the exception that the state health department's functions are supervisory rather than involved with direct delivery. Examples of such areas are sanitation and maternal and child health. In addition, because of the breadth of the state's police powers, many state health departments engage in health-related functions that are never or rarely practiced by local public health departments, such as licensing and accreditation of health professionals and health facilities, standard setting for automobile safety devices, and supervision of the quality of public medical payment programs such as Medicaid.

The functions considered appropriate for state health departments were outlined in a policy statement of the governing council of the APHA adopted at its 96th annual meeting on November 13, 1968 (20). These may be summarized as a) health surveillance, planning, and program development; b) promotion of local health coverage; c) setting and enforcement of standards; and d) providing health services. The complexity of the monitoring and supervision that results from local programs operating with both state and federal support and supervision will be treated in greater detail in a later discussion of the federal role. The quality of local public health work throughout a state is strongly influenced by the quality of the state health department leadership, as constrained by its budget and the responsibilities assigned it by the state government. This is particularly true outside the big cities and highly urbanized counties. In urban areas, the local health department often depends less on the state health department, has more direct ties with Washington, and is often lax in reporting to the state health agency.

A study of the composition of state boards of health by Gossert and Miller (21), completed in 1972, revealed that the standards of Shattuck or the APHA were far from having been met. Alaska and Rhode Island had no statutory boards. In Illinois and Delaware there was statutory provision, but no board was currently appointed in Illinois and the Delaware board consisted solely of two state officials. In 16 states, the health function was combined with at least one other agency, and four states had a conglomerate human resources agency. Of the 46 states with functioning boards, 32 had at least one-third medical doctors on them, and in 12 they comprised a majority of the board. In two states, Alabama and South Carolina, the state medical society was the board of health. Shattuck had warned in 1850 against domination of the board of health by any one profession. Only 12.5% of the 433 seats in 46 states were occupied by persons identified as consumers in 1972. Appointments to the board were almost always made by governors, with some form of legislative approval being required in half of the states. The trend was to merge state health departments with other departments. In 1969, there were eight such states, and in 1972 there were 16.

The trends in the development of attitudes regarding the functions of local health departments have also occurred at the state level. Over time, there has been a shift away from a conception of function restricted to a few communitywide preventive measures toward one of responsibility for making the total system of health care available to all citizens of the state.

Comparison of the 1968 APHA statement of policy with the actual activities of state health departments in recent years reveals that the traditional functions are still paramount, with the newer ones of community coordination for total health care, particularly medical care, being less evident.

A 1961 study (Shubick and Wright [22], summarized in Hanlon [23]) listed the principal activities of state health agencies in terms of how many of the 50 states were actually practicing them. Table 4–1 lists a few of the most frequently encountered activities and the number of states in which they were carried on. However, this list is not complete. It should be noted that these activities are usually either the traditional programs or the "programs which are categorically funded by the federal government." On the other hand, newer programs such as "program planning, development, and evaluation" appeared as activities in only 7 state health departments; "radiologic health" in 11; and heart disease control in 25. Other programs that are infrequently encountered, such as "professional registration and licensure," appearing in only three states, represent the type of program generally administered by a special licensing body of the state.

The Most Recent Picture: The NPHPRS Data.   Since 1970, annual statistics on state health departments have been assembled via questionnaire by the National Public Health Program Reporting System (NPHPRS), an arm of the Association of State and Territorial Health Officials (ASTHO). The first comprehensive NPHPRS report was published for 1974, so that with the publication of the most recent one

TABLE 4-1. 16 Most Frequently Conducted Activities of State Health Departments, 1961

Rank	Activity	Number of States
1	Environmental health	50
2	Health education	50
3	Maternal and child health	50
4	Nursing	50
5	Vital statistics	49
6	Laboratories	47
7	Dental health	46
8	Communicable diseases	45
9	Engineering	43
10	Tuberculosis control	43
11	Hospital survey, planning, and construction licensure	42
12	Local health services	42
13	Industrial health	36
14	Personnel	34
15	Cancer control	31
16	Chronic disease control	30

SOURCE: Shubick HJ, Wright EO: Composite study of fifty health department organizational charts representing forty-nine states and the District of Columbia. Unpublished report, 1961, cited in (22:224).

for fiscal year (FY) 1978, 5 consecutive years of comprehensive data were available. Most of the following remarks about the 1978 status of these departments, *State Health Agencies (SHAs)*, as they are called in the reports of this reporting system, are based on the 1980 report (24).

In FY 1978, all 57 "states" (50 states and seven territories) had SHAs. Together, they spent $3.26 billion on their public health programs, of which $2.52 billion, or 77%, was allocated to personal health services and the rest to other program categories. These other programs are classified under the categories of environmental health, health resources, and laboratory. The data indicate a substantial transfer from state and local to federal sources of financing over these years. In 1974, 25.5% of the funds were of federal origin; by 1978, this proportion had grown to 34.8%. It is worth noting that total public health expenditures by state and local public health agencies in 1978 were $5.0 billion, so that state health agencies spent 65% of this amount. Despite the widespread discussion of public health in recent years, only 2.6% of the total $192.4 billion spent for health in 1978 was for public health, and of this amount, 1.7% was spent by SHAs (25).

The principal functions being performed generally emphasize those areas that Mountin found in 1946, in terms of both the relative distribution of the dollar and the number of SHAs involved. Comparison of the state health department functions cited by Mountin for 1930, 1940, and 1946, on the one hand, with the number of states presently reporting programs and the 1961 tabulation shown in Table 4–1, on the other, indicates that the scope of activities has not been significantly enlarged. Local consumer protection and sanitation are still the leading environmental functions, and maternal and child health, communicable disease control, and their supporting services are still the mainstays of most state health departments in the area of *personal* services. This persistent emphasis on traditional functions in spite of the widespread recognition of newer health threats reflects important political developments that will be discussed later. In fact, the dominance of a single functional area, maternal and child health, is striking. Expenditures for these programs comprise almost one-fourth of the total expenses and more than 45% of personal health care expenditures. The percentages are even higher if one includes crippled children programs. The dominating position of Maternal and Child Health (MCH) program expenditures is, in turn, also largely due to a single item, Women and Infant Care (WIC) nutrition, a diet supplement program supported by the Department of Agriculture. In 1978, $286 million of the $770 million in MCH expenditures, or 37%, went for this single program. The predominance of the MCH and Crippled Children's programs, even without the WIC component, raises provocative questions about the future. If a national medical care program, with universal eligibility and comprehensive benefits, were ever put in place, it presumably would include prenatal care, mother and infant care, and care of crippled children. It would, parenthetically, also include much of the care now provided under categorical programs for venereal disease, dental health, chronic disease, and other personal health programs. The direct personal health care functions of the SHAs might then be much reduced. In that event, the environmental, planning, and monitoring functions would be likely candidates to become the most important functions. It is interesting, therefore, to look at the status of these program categories in SHAs in 1978.

Environmental protection is one area that exemplifies the widespread use of agencies other than SHAs for health protection functions. In Idaho, Pennsylvania, and the District of Columbia, all environmental services are provided by agencies other than the SHA. (As previously noted, the data for 1978 are taken from Reference 24.) The remaining 54 SHAs provided these services in varying degrees, with one-third of the $238 million in expenditures going for consumer protection and sanitation programs. Another 25% went for water quality programs. However, most of the environmental health activities were of the standard type. The ASTHO report for 1978 (22) puts it well:

> All of the SHAs reporting environmental health programs provided *consumer protection and sanitation* [emphasis in original] services, including food, or milk control, substance control and product safety, sanitation of health care facilities and other institutions, housing and recreational sanitation, or vector and zoonotic disease control. *Water quality* services, provided by 51 SHAs, were usually related to public drinking water, individual water supply, and individual sewage disposal. Public water pollution control services were more often provided by an agency other than the SHA. *Radiation control* services were offered by 45 SHAs. Fewer SHAs provided other environmental health services: *occupational health and safety and related services* (38 SHAs), *waste management* (34), and *air quality* (emphasis added).

Environmental health expenditures of state health agencies were funded predominantly (57%) by the state. A little over 25% came from federal sources, and the rest from local government and other sources. The Environmental Protection Act of 1970 called for the governor and/or the legislature of each state to designate a "lead environmental agency" to have overall responsibility for environmental activities. There are three generally recognized models for such agency selection: an SHA, a state environmental protection agency, and a state national resources agency (26). In 1978, 19 of the 54 SHAs that had environmental programs were designated as lead environmental agencies (the 19 states in which the SHA was the lead environmental protection agency in 1978 were Alabama, Arizona, Colorado, Hawaii, Indiana, Kansas, Louisiana, Maryland, Montana, New Hampshire, New Mexico, North Dakota, Oklahoma, South Carolina, Tennessee, Texas, Utah, Virginia, and West Virginia). The four services that a lead agency generally supervised were air quality, noise pollution control, solid waste management, and water pollution control. By contrast, the services most often assigned to an SHA were consumer protection and sanitation, water quality excluding water pollution control, and radiation control.

Turning to the role of SHAs in statewide health planning, the picture is similar to, but not quite the same, as that in environmental health. In many states, other agencies are mainly responsible for health planning, but more SHAs have been given this function than in environmental health. Under the Health Planning and Resource Development Act of 1974 (PL 93-641), discussed in Chapter 12, each state was to appoint a single agency as the State Health Planning and Development Agency (SHPDA). Of the 57 "states," 36 designated their SHA as the SHPDA in 1978 (similar to the number that did so under the Comprehensive Health Planning Act of 1966). An additional 15 SHAs performed planning functions for their states under PL 93-641, including one (Tennessee) that prepared the State Plan for the SHPDA. SHAs also were active in making state plans outside the requirements of PL 93-641. SHAs were also involved in making plans for categorical programs such as MCH and family planning, as well as for Emergency Medical Services (EMS), health personnel, family services, and financing.

The drive of the public health profession for full public health coverage of the entire population and its efforts to define standards of coverage have been alluded to. One of the most important activities of state health departments is the development of local public health departments, or "local health departments (LHDs)," as the NPHPRS refers to them, and the supervision and monitoring of their work. It is interesting to see, therefore, how these matters stood in 1978 according to the NPHPRS data and the interpretations of ASTHO, its sponsoring body. The definition of an LHD (and therefore of what constitutes public health coverage) has been relaxed from some previous definitions by no longer requiring medical leadership. The NPHPRS definition asserts a local health department to be:

> An official (governmental) public health agency which is in whole or in part responsible to a substate governmental entity or entities. The latter may be a city, county, city-county, federation of counties, borough, township, or any other type of substate governmental entity. In addition, a local health department must meet these criteria: (A) it has a staff of one or more full-time professional public health employees (e.g., public health nurse, sanitarian); (B) it delivers public health services; (C) it serves a definable geographic area; and (D) it has identifiable expenditures and/or budget in the political subdivision(s) which it serves.

Clearly, ASTHO is now defining an LHD even more liberally than the full-time public health departments in the older literature by Ferrell, Mountin, and Emerson. The relaxation of the previous requirement for a medically trained health officer to head the agency was not merely a compromise with reality. Some of the literature in the intervening period (19,27) had reported the belief, often including strong advocacy, that it is desirable, not just expedient, to discontinue this requirement. The health officer position was seen by some as largely administrative, requiring a grasp of overall public health knowledge and of principles of administration rather than of medicine.

Three types of LHD are identified: an LHD operated by the SHA as part of a centrally directed state system of local public health agencies; a largely autonomous LHD receiving some technical assistance and consultation from the SHA; and a partly autonomous LHD that shares control with the SHA, with the latter having direct operating authority in some areas. In 1978, there were 2,700 LHDs meeting the definition of the NPHRPS. Ten "states"—four states and six territories—had no LHDs by NPHPRS definition (Delaware, District of Columbia, Rhode Island, South Dakota, Vermont, American Samoa, Guam, Northern Mariana Islands, Trust Territory, and the Virgin Islands). In 35 of the 47 states with LHDs, 90% of the population lived in areas served by these departments (i.e., were covered by full-time public health services); in the remaining 12 states, the SHA or the Indian Health Service (in New Mexico) provided local public health services.

About 30% of SHA money spent on public health went to the LHDs in the 42 states reporting this item for 1978. Most of this money went for personal health programs (items such as public health nursing, health education, maternal and child health, chronic disease, etc.). A little more than one-half of the money originated with the state itself, and 31% was federal money transmitted to the local government via the SHA. The total of $215 million in federal funds included $62 million from Title V (MCH) funds and $23 million from 314 (section 7A) Public Health Service Act funds, the successor to the old Title VI of the original Social Security Act. The proportion of local public health services funded by the SHA (not all of it from state money, however) continued to vary greatly from state to state. Of the 47 states with LHDs, three (Virginia, Florida, and Mississippi) operated their LHDs entirely with funds from the SHA. For 44 states, the NPHPRS estimates that about 42% of LHD funds came from the SHA. This seems to be a modest increase in the proportion of LHD funds supplied by the SHA over the percentages found for 1925 by the Ferrell study (5) cited previously. At that time, 20–30% was found to be most common but only 17 states then had separate "bureaus of county health work." Because the reporting of "funds from other sources" by LHDs to the NPHPRS is fragmentary for many states, the NPHPRS also separately reports data for 25 states from which it received "reasonably accurate" estimates of total LHD expenditures (that is, good estimates of non-SHA funds). For these 25 states, the average state contribution was 40%, much higher than in 1925, but the variability was again great from state to state. For these 25 states, the total public health expenditure (total SHA expenditures including SHA-operated institutions) per capita ranged from $9.00 to $68.50, with a median of $16.43. The interquartile range was from $11.50 to $25.

Public Policy Implications.   At the beginning of this section, it was noted that the state's responsibilities for health protection are much broader than those of the local government. Consequently, there is a wider range of possible functions that could appear in the list of programs engaged in by any particular state health department. Despite this greater breadth of choice, the number of functions that SHAs actually perform is generally only a small proportion of the health functions carried on by different state governments, and the ones assigned to the health department vary markedly from state to state. Responsibility and control are shared with other agencies. The reasons that health functions are so widely distributed among the different SHAs are complex. They reflect a growing tendency to assign health problems to agencies other than health departments since 1960. Although much rhetoric ascribes the "need" to choose another agency to the alleged fact that the SHA is technically inadequate and/or managerially inefficient, some have argued that various special interest groups seek such a choice because they think it advantageous to them. Whatever factors are actually most influential, the trend away from SHAs is undeniable. This issue will be further addressed in the discussion of the federal role, but it is so important in the development of SHAs that it is worth pausing to review the evidence that establishes this trend as a fact.

One of the principal functions of the SHA, especially after the passage of the Social Security Act, has been that of liaison and administrative agent for the distribution and supervision of federal grants among local health agencies within the state. In general, use of the SHA health agency was mandated by the early post-1935 legislation. Later, beginning in the 1950s, the SHA began to be bypassed with increasing frequency as the state agency distributing federal monies to localities for health activities; project grants for local services given directly by the federal agency to the local grantee became increasingly prevalent. In addition, many subsequent health program grants distributed via the states did not specify the SHA as the mandatory administering agency. For example, the comprehensive Health Planning Act of 1966 specified only that a single state agency in each state was to administer federal grants to that state under this act; 23 states placed this function not in their SHAs but in other agencies. Under the provision of the 1975 Planning Act, in 1978, 36 states designated the SHA as their State Health Planning and Development Agencies (SHPDAs), the remaining 21 naming other agencies. Under the Medicaid Act, only nine SHAs are the designated state agency for administering Medicaid, although nearly all SHAs have their own programs of general ambulatory care; in 1978, SHAs spent $800 million for inpatient care, of which 83% went for SHA-operated institutions. Other examples could be cited, but these are sufficient to support the assertion that SHAs have been bypassed since 1950 as the chief administrator of new statewide health programs. This tendency has been widespread even in the area of health planning, despite the fact that public health professionals and others have long advocated that areawide and state health planning be *the* basic function of state and local health departments.

The tendency to use agencies largely staffed with general technical program planning personnel represents a trend that has been gaining momentum since the end of the 1960s: improved health delivery through increased application of generalized ("generic") managerial, model making, and computing technology, generally subsumed under such terms as *cost-benefit analysis* and *systems analysis*. It remains to be seen whether predominantly managerial solutions to deep-rooted social problems will succeed. Thus far, they have not been very effective in alleviating the problems in education, urban decay, transportation, or other areas. It seems justifiable to doubt that they can protect public health. From about 1950 on, the changing functions of the SHA in response to demands by the federal government and the public have been inextricably intertwined with developments in federal legislation. The role of the federal government in public health is presented next.

Federal Role in State and Local Public Health Services After 1935: 1936–1945

It was noted previously that passage of the Social Security Act in 1935 heralded the beginning of a major program of grants-in-aid to the states for health purposes, and that the portions of the act that affected public health departments were Titles V

(Section 1) and VI. Administration of these two titles comprised the major public health activities of the federal government in the 1930s. Some details of the original provisions of these titles, especially Title VI, are presented to illustrate some of the characteristics of revenue-sharing grants discussed earlier.

Under Title V, federal grants could be given to the states for "promoting the health of mothers and children" (7:77). The funds were distributed by the Children's Bureau to the state health departments, to be used for supporting these services in state and local health departments. These programs were subsequently expanded; amendments passed in 1965 as part of the Medicare Act later provided for project grants to state and local health agencies for comprehensive maternity care to high risk mothers and for the development of high quality comprehensive health services to children and youth of school or preschool age. The operating agency could be a public or an appropriate nonprofit private agency. Amounts were subsequently also appropriated for research projects "relating to maternal and child health and crippled children's services." Expanded federal support of maternal and child health activities by state and local health departments continued until 1981, when these grants were consolidated with six other programs into a Maternal and Child Health Services Block Grant. This action was part of the reduction in social programs of the Reagan Administration embodied in the Omnibus Budget Reconciliation Act of 1981, which will be further discussed below.

Title VI of the act directly addressed the buildup of state and local health departments, and the monies appropriated under it have been administered by the PHS. In the original act, federal funds were appropriated annually, under a block grant formula, for the years 1936–1940, "For the purpose of assisting States, counties, health districts and other political subdivisions of the States in establishing and maintaining adequate public health services" (7:63). In 1944 this title, with some changes, was transferred from the Social Security Act to Section 314 of the newly constituted Public Health Service Act. The original act required that funds be allocated among the states on the basis of a formula to be promulgated by the U.S. Surgeon General, taking into account three factors: a) the state's population size; b) the state's relative economic status; and c) the prevalence of special health problems in the state. Each state health department was required to file an acceptable plan with the Surgeon General indicating how the grant was to be used, and a report at the end of the year detailing how it had indeed been used.

Several important aspects of the allocation and administrative provisions of Title VI were as follows: a) all funds were to be administered nationally by a general health agency; b) the system of tax sharing was partially a per capita redistribution of federal tax revenues and partly an attempt to equalize relative local and state tax burdens among the states; c) the filing of state plans and the requirement of annual reports was a modest attempt to achieve quality control and to encourage statewide planning; and d) the funds went directly to a single state agency, which was mandated to be the state health department, to be redistributed within the state.

The Period 1946–1968

The previous discussion of local public health departments noted that public health professionals, some members of Congress, and the Democratic presidents came to believe that the state and local health departments were being inordinately slow to enter the newer fields of public health work. These fields, dealing principally with primary care in medically underserved areas, chronic disease abatement, and control of the more recent environmental threats, were being defined by students of personal health care organization and environmental control as belonging to the local health department. It has also been mentioned that attempts by the federal government to encourage local health departments to pursue these special programs led to increased use of categorical grants as opposed to general purpose formula grants (13). The categorical grants were still formula grants and required matching—usually on a one-to-one basis—but were intended to stimulate spending for specific activities that the federal government deemed desirable nationally rather than to support the budget of the health department. From about 1950 on, the federal health grant structure increasingly encouraged state and local public health agencies to move more aggressively into areas of national health priorities. The number of classes of categorical formula grants increased over the years, as did the proportion of total formula grants so earmarked. By 1965, out of about $50 million in formula grants, only $10 million, or 20%, were for general health; the rest were designated for specified categories (28). Considerable difficulties were experienced by some states and localities, which found these earmarked funds to be inappropriate for the programs needed in their areas. After 15 years of continued efforts to encourage greater activity in chronic disease control, pollution abatement, medical care services, and similar programs, the federal government attempted in 1966 to discontinue the use of earmarked grants funneled through state governments for accomplishing these goals. The Comprehensive Health Planning and Public Health Service Amendments of 1966 (PL 89-749) and the Partnership for Health Amendments of 1967 (PL 90-174) abolished all categorical earmarking of formula grants (29). These amendments are discussed in the next section.

Project Grants. Development of the programs being promoted by the federal government via categorical grants was inhibited by the conflict between large metropolitan centers and state governments (30). Many state legislatures were so structured that the influence of rural sections was out of proportion to the size of their populations. These states had been slow to assign comprehensive health care and wide ecological control responsibilities to their state health departments. The population and organization of the large municipal centers and their suburbs, on the other hand, had increasingly attempted to expand such activities; unable to prevail in the state capital, they turned increasingly to Washington for direct aid. These factors, among others, led to the emergence of project grants as an increasingly important segment of federal grants in the 1960s.

Project grants for rural sanitation projects had been made in very modest amounts before 1935. After 1935, the first project grant to be administered by the PHS was made in 1946 for venereal disease control (8), and between 1947 and 1959, the project grant program for this purpose remained unique. "The first half of the 1960s was marked by a flood of new project grant programs" (27). Although formula (including categorical) grants were 77% of the total $76 million in health grants in 1963, they were only 48% of the $105 million given in 1965. In the latter year, the proportion of total grants-in-aid for project grants exceeded that for formula grants for the first time.

Different attitudes developed among health administrators with respect to project grants. A state chief health officer might feel that project grants going directly to applicants in a state helped to undermine the state health authority in its efforts to plan for the health care of the entire state in a coordinated and efficient manner.

Opposing points of view countered that although the desire to have federal grants essentially unearmarked and given entirely to the SHA might be desirable for a state with an aggressive state health department, such a course would be quite inappropriate for other states. Another argument supporting project grants was that direct federal grants are becoming increasingly necessary to meet interstate problems such as the Ohio River Valley Sanitation Compact, which involved seven states in an effort to control pollution (30). Subsequent federal legislation attempted to reconcile these opposing points of view and satisfy each to some degree.

The overall thrust of the amendments to Section 314 of the Public Health Service Act not only removed the categorical earmarking from formula grants, as noted previously, but also attempted to establish the project grant as a permanent form of aid and, to meet the various objections to the disintegrative effects of such grants on planning, provided support for statewide comprehensive health planning. All formula grants were block grants, and no categorical formula grants were included in the 1966 act. The federal government's attempts to encourage local public health departments *and other agencies* to act on its high priority health targets were continued and intensified, but this would be done only by the use of project grants. It should be noted that project grants are, by their very nature, well suited to promoting categorical programs. The formula public health grants that were continued as block grants in subsequent years came to be known as "314d" monies after the section of the Public Health Act that provided for them.

The important changes in grant-in-aid structure under this act may be summarized as involving four basic elements: a) introduction of a heavy element of planning activity; b) abolition of categorical formula grants; c) introduction of a state comprehensive health planning authority that need not be the same as the state health department; and d) reinforcement of the practice of awarding health services grants directly to nongovernmental grantees through the increased emphasis on project grants.

Declining Prestige of the PHS.   Public demands for improvements in health services became marked in the 1960s. These demands centered on a number of areas previously mentioned: providing medical care in underserved areas; motivating existing public health agencies to take an active if not a leading part in ensuring that their constituents were being served by a good system of health care; combatting the newer threats to environmental safety; and continued maintenance of traditional preventive community services. Efforts of the PHS to encourage innovative approaches at the state and local levels via categorical and project grants were perceived as inadequate. PHS leaders were viewed by some commentators as not presenting a strong public image of working vigorously to change medical services and to protect the environment. The practice of giving health protection functions to specialized technical agencies rather than to the health agency that was observed in the states was also occurring at the federal level. The perennial battles over the introduction of national health insurance, for example, were being waged largely by medical care and social welfare professionals rather than public health professionals, so that when Medicare and Medicaid were passed, one was given to the Social Security Administration to administer and the other to Social and Rehabilitation Services—Welfare. On the other hand, the newer environmental control acts, such as the Clean Air Act of 1965, were assigned first to independent agencies and then to the Environmental Protection Agency established in 1970. The power of the PHS and its chief, the Surgeon General, was greatly curtailed within the Department of Health, Education, and Welfare (HEW). As one leading public health writer stated (31:1577):

> By the early 1960s there appeared to be substantial disenchantment and dissatisfaction on the part of the Administration toward the Commissioned Corps of the PHS. It was considered by many to be unwilling or unable to meet modern problems related to the administration and the delivery of health services. . . . The status of the Commissioned Corps was not helped during the long battle over Medicare when it was believed that many members of the corps remained aloof . . . over the past few years, the existing organization of the PHS, with its limited number of career personnel and its traditional orientation, was overwhelmed and was bypassed. Health programs were developed at the federal level outside of HEW, such as Head Start and Neighborhood Health Centers under the Office of Economic Opportunity, and Model Cities under Housing and Urban Development.

A number of subsequent reorganizations weakened the Office of the Surgeon General. The status of that office and the role of the PHS remained in flux for a number of years, with the position of Surgeon General being actually abolished for a time under the reorganization of the PHS in 1973. The position was reinstated under the Carter administration, and its incumbent attempted to strengthen the role and prestige of the PHS with emphasis on prevention. Despite the 1966 legislation, which intended formula grants to public health departments to be of the block type, Congress was apparently unable to resist the pleas of various advocates of specific programs. Categorical programs continued to proliferate, while the block 314d money continued to dwindle away.

The Period 1969–1980

Following the election of Richard M. Nixon as president in 1968, the federal executive branch began to reverse certain aspects of the relationship between the federal, state, and local governments. This attempted change was directly pertinent to public health policy because of the federal grant system of supporting public health programs. The main goal of this policy, dubbed the "New Federalism" by his administration, was summarized by President Nixon early in 1970: "after over a century and a half of power flowing from the people and from the local communities and from the States to Washington, D.C., let's get it back to the people and to the cities and to the States where it belongs" (32). The legislative and organizational changes that the administration expected to use to translate the goals of the New Federalism into action had three principal elements:

a. There was to be greater reliance on state and local governments in the operation and administration of federal grant programs. Categorical grants were to be eliminated as far as possible in favor of block grants (revenue sharing). It should be noted that the term *block* meant a lump sum for all purposes, health included. The amount of grant to be used for health would be decided solely by the local government.
b. Federal granting programs were to be streamlined, making them simple to administer. Federal programs were to be decentralized to regional offices, with increased interagency standardization of requirements and procedures for federal grant programs. Local governments and federal regional offices were to have broad decision-making power.

c. There was to be a major realignment of federal departments "to conform better to major purposes of government and to coordinate better the management of federal programs" (33:56). On October 20, 1972, general revenue sharing was enacted into law (PL 92-512) as the State and Local Fiscal Assistance Act of 1972. An amount of $30.2 billion was appropriated to states or localities, to be distributed over a 5-year period beginning January 1, 1972. About one-third of the money went to the states and two-thirds to local governments. The program was extended in 1977 for 5 years through 1981. The budget program proposed by President Ronald Reagan for 1983 envisaged a continuation of the revenue-sharing program, at least through 1986, at slightly increased levels over 1981 and 1982 (34). This revenue sharing program was of great potential importance to state and local public health programs, for the block grants it gave to states and localities increased state and local decision-making power that could be used to reduce or augment public health programs in relation to other spending areas.

Although agreeing to the president's revenue-sharing proposals, Congress opposed eliminating appropriations for many ongoing categorical programs that had been funded in past years. The president's 1974 budget had called for discontinuing many of these programs and cutting others substantially. In general, cutting federal funds for health care services was the overriding aim (35). For this reason, the more costly programs involving medical care rather than public health were the first ones slated for termination. Formula grants for state public health programs were, for the time being at least, to be maintained at the previous year's level, but the appropriation for Maternal and Child Health Title V Project Grants was to be "folded in" to the general 314d public health department grants. In addition to making program cuts for FY 1974, the budget proposed cancellations totaling about $550 million appropriated in 1973 that the administration had not spent (rescissions). An apparent truce in the administration-Congress battle over the federally funded programs was declared when the president, in June 1973, signed a law extending expiring health programs for 1 year.

The proposed 1975 budget contained greatly modified reductions of these programs. Further contests between Republican President Nixon and the Democratic Congress was ended with Mr. Nixon's resignation on August 9, 1974, and the accession of Gerald R. Ford to the presidency. President Ford generally continued Nixon's health policies. The principal thrusts continued to be overall reduction of health budgets and consolidation of existing categorical programs into block formula grants. In his last State of the Union Address, President Ford called for budgetary consolidation of 16 health programs, including a number of public health programs such as formula public health grants (314d), immunization, rat control, lead paint poisoning prevention, maternal and child health, state health grants, and family planning. Because the states were not required to match the federal funds under this budget proposal, they could have offset reductions in federal funds by reducing their own expenditures and cutting programs back. The proposal seemed clearly tied to a reduction of health services, and was opposed by Congress. In January 1977, President Jimmy Carter assumed office.

The Carter administration discontinued Ford's attempts to consolidate most public health categorical grants into a single block grant. However, the total sum allotted for health programs in the Carter budget for 1977–1978 was little higher than it had been in the Ford budget (35). Throughout the Carter administration, three major goals were emphasized in public health: expansion of preventive and some treatment services for poor children; health promotion and prevention; and mental health services, especially in the community. Mental health is discussed in Chapter 8.

The measures suggested to expand services for children were embodied in a proposal called Comprehensive Health Assessment and Treatment for Poor Children (CHAP). It was to have reached 1.8 million children in addition to the 12 million who were already eligible for such services through Medicaid. During 1977, CHAP bills were introduced in both the Senate and the House of Representatives; throughout President Carter's term of office this proposal was pushed in Congress, but it failed to pass. A leading factor in its defeat was the attached antiabortion amendment by legislators opposed to abortion, a tactic that split congressional support.

The health promotion and disease prevention program consisted of stepped-up national campaigns to inform people about the importance to health of matters such as smoking, eating, and exercise, and a reorganization of the Communicable Disease Control section of the PHS into the Centers for Disease Control. The program was the centerpiece of the agenda of Dr. Julius Richmond, the new Surgeon General of the PHS. It will be recalled that under the Nixon-Ford administration, the role of Surgeon General had been played down, and after 1968, the position had at times been unfilled. It was combined with that of Undersecretary for Health in the Carter administration, which sought to restore its prestige by appointing a prominent physician to the post. Dr. Richmond, appointed in July 1977, set out to revitalize the PHS largely by promoting the idea of prevention and health maintenance. In documents issued in 1979 and 1980 (36–38), the importance of prevention and health promotion was carefully delineated and national "achievable" goals for 1990 were laid out. An introductory section established the orientation (36:7):

> In the modern era, there have been periodic surges of interest leading to major advances in prevention. The sanitary reforms of the latter half of the 19th century and the introduction of effective vaccines in the middle of the 20th century are two examples.
>
> But during the 1950s and 1960s, concern with the treatment of chronic disease and lack of knowledge about their causes resulted in a decline in emphasis on prevention.
>
> Now, however, with the growing understanding of causes and risk factors for chronic diseases, the 1980s present new opportunities for major gains.
>
> Prevention is an idea whose time has come. We have the scientific knowledge to begin to formulate recommendations for improved health. And, although the degenerative diseases differ from their infectious disease predecessors in having more—and more complex—causes, it is now clear that many are preventable.

The 1979 report called for allocating a greater portion of the health dollar to prevention. The 1980 report set targets for the following priority areas: high blood pressure control; family planning; pregnancy and infant health; immunization; sexually transmitted diseases; toxic agent control; occupational safety and health; accident prevention and injury control; fluoridation and dental health; surveillance and control of infectious diseases; smoking and health; misuse of alcohol and drugs; physical fitness and exercise; and control of stress and violent behavior (38). Thus, the approach followed by public health leaders in the 1800s and early 1900s in solving the health problems of their day, posed by the then imperfectly understood acute infectious diseases, was now being followed with respect to the imperfectly understood chronic and degenerative diseases. First, the current leading health problems were being identified; the next step was to identify their causes. Using extant research writings, the reports concluded that of the 10 leading causes of death in 1976, 50% were due to unhealthy behavior or life style; 20% to environmental factors; 20% to human biologic factors; and 10% to inadequacies in the existing health care system. It seemed to follow clearly that changing unhealthy behavior was the most important way of preventing or controlling the diseases that were the leading causes of death. Having pinpointed the threats and their probable causes, the third step in long-standing public health methodology was to determine what methods were effective for controlling them. These methods were suggested throughout the reports. The fourth, or final, step was to determine the appropriate organizational form to use in implementing the campaign. The principal decision was to expand the Center for Disease Control. This was done in October 1980 with a reorganization that changed the Communicable Disease Center to Centers for Disease Control (CDC).

The CDC contained six bureaus: the Center for Prevention Services, the Center for Environmental Health, the National Institute for Occupational Safety and Health, the Center for Health Promotion and Education, the Center for Professional Development and Training, and the Center for Disease Investigation and Diagnosis. Thus was the campaign to restore prevention as a priority of the federal health agency organized along the lines of the previous campaign to prevent communicable disease. There was the identification of health threats, determination of probable causes, methods for combatting them, and an organizational form with which to do it. The early public health measures of sanitation and quarantine had often been successful even though they were based on imperfectly understood causes of acute disease and the method of their transmittal. As one historian of public health put it: "the program of the sanitary reformers was based to a large extent on a structure of erroneous theories, and while they hit upon the right solution, it was mostly for the wrong reasons" (4:225). It seemed reasonable to hope that a public health campaign to curb the ravages of degenerative disease could also result in partial success. Even though the precise mechanisms of these disease processes were only imperfectly understood, their association with certain risk factors was being taken as a guide to proper preventive measures.

Not all commentators on the health scene agreed fully with the strong advocacy of prevention exemplified by President Carter's Assistant Secretary for Health/ Surgeon General, especially the emphasis on changes in life style. It was seen by some as a one-sided overemphasis on personal responsibility for ill health, an attempt to blame the victim (39) for illness. Some claimed that this policy diverted attention from the lack of access to proper medical care experienced by many people and the failure of the Carter administration to grapple strongly with polluters—who, they claimed, were responsible for much, if not most, of the current burden of disease. However, the Surgeon General's approach had strong supporters among health writers, administrators, and various public figures. Crawford (39) lists many such supportive writings (e.g., References 40 and 41) and gives partial summaries of their views. Although the writers supporting the Surgeon General's approach did not agree on all particulars, two ideas characterize their writings as a whole. First, access to modern medical care in developed countries, especially the United States, is a very small determinant of a population's health status; in fact, it even causes or exacerbates some illnesses (iatrogenic effects) (40). Second, most illnesses are caused by unhealthy personal behavior; therefore, changing such behavior is the fundamental aim of health services. It should be the principal aim of public health programs in particular.

The opponents of this view did not argue that prevention was unimportant. However, they stated that at present, and for a long time to come, persons will continue to get sick, and when they do, they need medical care. Poor people get sick more often and more seriously than do the nonpoor (42), and the only reason they often do not get it is that they are socially and economically disadvantaged. Furthermore, they disagreed that most illness is now caused by individual failure to pay attention to healthful behavior. It is due, they asserted, to the effects of polluters and unhealthful working conditions (43–45), including unemployment. Therefore, they distrusted those who advocated developing healthful behavior and what they perceived to be a consequent neglect of the campaign to ensure access to good medical care for all who need it. The medical care problem must be solved, they argued, before real political support could be mustered behind prevention. Persons facing imminent financial ruin because of impending medical bills could not be expected to concentrate on preventing ill health in the future. The various repercussions of this rift prevented unified support for President Carter's health proposal in Congress. It may fairly be said that financial support for public health did not advance substantially under Carter, despite his avowed commitment to increasing public health. In fact, considering inflation, it retrogressed. Carter's own budgets for FYs 1980 and 1981 mandated cuts in public health funds. The principal contribution was the theoretical leadership provided by the Surgeon General in beginning to define more completely what a modern program of prevention might look like.

The Reagan administration took office in January, 1981, determined to slash all government social programs to the maximum, with public health one of its main targets. The new president called for a severe cutback in federal support for public health, to be accomplished by discontinuing some programs, cutting appropriations for others, and turning as many as possible back to the states. He hoped eventually to consolidate all remaining federal money for public health given to the states into one block grant. The first major legislative result of the new administration was the Omnibus Budget Reconciliation Act, PL 97-35, passed on August 13, 1981. The act included a continuing resolution funding it until March 15, 1982. Funds for the balance of the fiscal year after March 15, 1982 were later appropriated by various further continuing resolutions that treated programs on a piecemeal basis. For example, a supplemental appropriation bill increasing the funding for the community health centers and the Maternal and Child Health Block grants to carry them through the remainder of FY 1982 was passed in July of that year.

The Reagan administration did not get its request that 26 programs be combined into two block grants for public health, but it did succeed in getting 20 programs combined into four block grants. (Different people writing about the folding-in process come up with differing counts of the number of programs involved. The differences are due to the various definitions of what constitutes a program, but the resulting discrepancies among accounts do not alter the general pattern being described.) Six programs remained categorical. The block grants were set up as a new section of the Public Health Service Act, Title XIX. The folding in of programs into block grants consists of the following:

a. Preventive Health and Health Services Block Grant. The programs folded in are 1) rodent control, 2) fluoridation, 3) hypertension control, 4) health services and centers (rape crisis centers), 5) old 314d money, 6) home health services, and 7) emergency services. The grants would be distributed among the states according to a formula based on population and other factors deemed appropriate by the Secretary of Health and Human Services (HHS). Each state had to apply for these grants.

b. Alcohol Abuse, Drug Abuse, and Mental Health Block Grant. The programs folded in are 1) Community Mental Health Centers Act, 2) Mental Health Systems Act, 3) Comprehensive Alcohol Abuse and Alcoholism Prevention, Treatment, and Rehabilitation Act of 1970, and 4) Drug Abuse Prevention, Treatment, and Rehabilitation Act.

c. Primary Care Block Grant. This section consists of the Community Health Centers. States could begin to take them over beginning with FY 1983.

d. Maternal and Child Health Services Block Grant (amends Title V of the Social Security Act). The programs folded in are 1) maternal and child health and crippled children's services of Title V of the Social Security Act, 2) supplementary security income to provide rehabilitation services for blind and disabled children, 3) lead-based paint poisoning prevention, 4) genetic disease service, 5) sudden infant death syndrome, 6) hemophilia treatment, and 7) adolescent pregnancy under the Health Services and Centers Amendment of 1978. The SHA is to be the administering agency and the formula for FYs 1982 and 1983 was based on the number of low income children. Alternative bases for the formula in the future were to be submitted to Congress by the Secretary of HHS by June 1982. The states had to give $3 for every $4 of federal funds received.

Left as categorical grants were six programs: a) childhood immunization, b) tuberculosis control, c) family planning, d) migrant health centers, e) venereal disease control, and f) an amount equal to 15% of the total Maternal and Child Health Services Grant that was to be set aside for use by HHS to fund projects of "regional or national significance" in training and research, genetic disease testing, counseling, information development, and for comprehensive hemophilia diagnostic and treatment centers. In addition, the Women, Infants, and Children (WIC) nutrition program funded by the Agriculture Department was also left categorical. As has been noted, this food supplement program is an important LHD activity. Thus, six programs were left as categorical and the remaining 20 were folded into four block grants, instead of all being folded into two block grants, because of vigorous lobbying in Congress by advocates of the varying programs.

Not only were block grants being turned over to the states to administer, but their total funding for the programs in each block grant was reduced 21%. Further, when one accounts for inflation, the actual reduction in resources was expected to be even higher, perhaps 30%. When one considers the simultaneous reduction in state and local tax revenues because of the recession of the early 1980s and the tax revolt of the late 1970s and early 1980s, it is clear that local and state public health services faced and continue to face a severe financial shortfall bordering on crisis.

As of fall 1982, the FY 1983 budget was being formulated, and political jockeying between the president and his supporters and opponents in Congress was proceeding apace. For 1983, the president's present budget proposals map a further reduction in federal grants for public health, to be accomplished by further folding remaining categorical grants into blocks and reducing the total. In his State of the Union Address, the president called for turning over 43 federal programs to the states by 1984 and giving them the choice of continuing or discontinuing them. Included in these programs were the preventive health and health services block grant; alcohol drug abuse and mental health block grant; family planning; migrant health centers; and the WIC nutrition program (35). Family planning, migrant health centers, and black lung clinics would be added to the primary care block grants and WIC to the Maternal and Child Health Services Block Grant. The stampede to approve Mr. Reagan's 1982 budget has subsided considerably, and the request for further cuts has been met with considerable opposition in Congress. By the middle of 1982, Congress was attempting to write its own budget for FY 1983 instead of waiting for the president to send one.

Public Policy Implications.   The Reagan program has been termed a basic reversal in U.S. federal policy (Chap. 15):

> The administration has endorsed a special interpretation of the federal government's past relations with the state-local and nonprofit sectors. This interpretation holds that the federal government has improperly supplanted—"usurped" is the term sometimes used—the roles of both lower levels of governmental and nonprofit organizations. . . . Viewing the federal government as a competitor with other organized associations is a distinctly conservative perspective. It contrasts with the cooperative model of federal relations. The ties to the federal government that the president condemns were developed in the belief that they fostered a constructive partnership between Washington and the States and localities. . . . Eliminating this "cooperative federalism" is a fundamental and controversial element of the Reagan experiment. (34:10–11)

What essential features of the Reagan policies have important implications for public health in the United States? First, Reaganism calls for an end to federal grants to the states and localities for public health services. A transition period would give money to the states for public health and ambulatory care services on a block grant basis, with little or no categorical restrictions on how it is to be spent by programs. Regulation of operations by the federal government would be minimal. Second, direct federal activities would be limited to a few programs that are clearly national in scope, such as research. Environmental protection activities would be sharply reduced. Third, federal income taxes would be substantially reduced so that persons would have more disposable income available. Thus, citizens could vote more state or local taxes if they wanted particular public health programs. Finally, federal grants would go to the states, and direct federal-local government contact would be avoided wherever feasible. The SHA would be the administering agency for the Maternal and Child Health Services Block Grant.

Persons favoring this program argue that the federal government has become too large and its influence too pervasive on state and local health activities (and other activities, as well). Local requirements and needs are not well determined in distant Washington and should be made locally. The massive amount of federal regulation has made most programs inefficient; they are top-heavy with administrative personnel and procedures, and stifle innovative initiatives for effective operation. Many of the environmental and workplace protections have been extreme and have hurt the growth of the economy, which is basic to the national welfare. Furthermore, many programs have not achieved their purpose. The basic and almost the only lasting solution to the problem of maintaining and improving the well-being of the American populace is to give private industry unfettered liberty to expand its activities. The mechanisms of the marketplace will see to it that industry's operations in a competitive world serve the American people in the best manner. In particular, the Reagan program will revitalize industry and result in an increased tax base for states and localities. They will then be able to decide for themselves what programs they want, and can raise the taxes to pay for them.

Persons opposing the Reagan program include many who have personally lived through or studied the history of the development of the federal system of grants and environmental protections. They point to the shift of the American economy from a local to a regional and national one. Some of these features were outlined in previous sections, but recall that these developments led to a centralization of tax revenue in the federal government, while the responsibility for public health services remained with the states and localities. This divergence, in turn, led to ever-growing disparities between needs and available tax bases in states, and among localities within states. A growing consensus holds that persons, especially children and youth, should have equal or as nearly equal opportunity as possible to develop their *potential* (46), regardless of the state or locality in which they were born or reared. This belief requires either that programs be run entirely out of Washington or that federal tax money be redistributed among states and localities according to measures of need. These people also point to the fact that the American economic system is increasingly consolidating and centralizing its control. The organization needed to protect the public interest, they would argue, also needs to be increasingly centralized to correspond to this changing system. In the public health field, the emergence of chronic and degenerative diseases as the leading health threats points to nationwide causation and the need for nationwide preventive measures. Local agencies cannot act to control activities of national and international combines. Returning environmental control to the states, for example, could result in competition among the states to offer the fewest environmental controls possible in an effort to attract national industry.

This is not to say that the opponents of Reaganism uniformly advocate complete control and administration from Washington. Most of them want to have as much local administration as possible, but with goals and aims coordinated on a national basis. That was the central idea of the federal "partnership" system, as differentiated from President Nixon's approach and President Reagan's New Federalism. Finally, the federal partnership system grew in a typically American way: It developed as a series of responses to specific problems. The Reagan program, its opponents argue, is based on an abstract ultra-right ideology that has never been tried and consists merely of a set of assertions stemming from theoretical assumptions about the functioning of the market. The reply of Reagan policy supporters is that the federal partnership really became a federal dictatorship and that its programs have not worked. Something else must be tried.

A final question is, how has Reagan's New Federalism been working so far, and what are the prospects for its success? States and localities have been reporting that it has created great stress for them and that needed services have had to be cut back (34). A feature of the Reagan agenda was the assumption that sharp cuts in federal income taxes would make more disposable income available to local and state governments for raising more taxes to operate the transferred programs. Large federal tax cuts did indeed take place, but the huge military buildup that was also part of the Reagan program increased the federal deficits to all-time highs. As a result, some of the tax cuts have already been rescinded, and it is questionable if all remaining cuts will remain. In addition, as has been noted, an economic depression, stemming partly from government monetary policy, has reduced the income tax and sales tax revenues of the states, thus decreasing their ability to continue past programs, much less take on public health (and other) programs newly transferred from federal sponsorship. Finally, many states have now passed Proposition 13 type laws strongly restricting government taxes, especially local property taxes, the former mainstay of local services financing. The Reagan administration's answer is that more time is needed to let its program revitalize industry and produce the increases in income that will reduce the deficits and provide more state and local tax revenues. It argues that it cannot hope to undo the mistakes of several decades in a few years, and that its agenda deserves a fair trial.

WHERE DO WE STAND?

What does the future hold for public health? With respect to administration and financing, the directions established in 1935 for the support of state and local public health work have been labeled inappropriate for today by the Reagan administration. After almost 50 years of proceeding in one direction, a reversal of cooperative federalism was attempted by the Nixon and Ford administrations and is now being strongly pushed by the Reagan administration. The question is whether this "counterrevolution" is an aberration or a harbinger. How one answers this question depends largely on how one views the arguments for and against the Reagan program.

With respect to the organization and content of public health services, an overriding fact is the changed nature of the major threats to health—the chronic and degenerative diseases. It may be that public health now stands with respect to these diseases where it stood with respect to acute infectious diseases in the mid-1850s. We are beginning to know something about the determinants or risk factors of these diseases and, therefore, certain preventive measures that can reasonably be advocated. For these measures to be as effective as public health measures became against acute infectious diseases after 1915, considerably more epidemiologic and biologic research is needed. As the results of this research continue to be revealed, and as the smoke settles from the political battles being waged over the future structure of our federal system, decisions will have to be made about the structure of our public health system. The structure and roles of local, state, and federal public health agencies and of other agencies doing health-related work will need to be determined. If past history is any guide, these relationships and functions will be worked out in a combination of theoretical formulation, experiments in administrative accommodation, and political battle. After a period of change and turmoil, an attempt will be made to codify the existing arrangement into a comprehensive federal law. The nation will continue to need public health leaders who keep up with findings and have the political and administrative ability to incorporate the pioneering ones into public health practice, not only as experiments in individual places but also as national and state policy. The foremost leaders will need to have a good grasp of health problems and what is known about meeting them—both preventive and curative. They will also need to understand the political, social, and historical background of health services and the society as a whole.

Given the nationwide nature of the new health threats and their suspected environmental causes, it is difficult to see how anything less than strong federal coordination of a national effort can be successful in combatting them. However, whatever the answers to these questions may prove to be, one thing is certain: A challenging period lies ahead for future public health services administrators that will test the mettle of even the most talented and hardworking aspirants.

A number of developments in the federal role in public health have not been addressed here. These include the Food and Drug Administration, the Occupational Safety and Health Act, the federal Community Mental Health Act, the Alcohol Abuse and Drug Abuse Act, and the Environmental Protection Act of 1970. Although these are extremely important to a total understanding of government's public health roles, this chapter has addressed public health activities of the federal government from the viewpoint of the federal system of public health agencies— the PHS, the SHAs, and the LHDs. Descriptions of many activities not covered in this brief overview may be found in References 23, 35, and 47 and in other chapters, especially Chapters 12 and 15.

REFERENCES

1. Last JA (ed): *Maxcy-Rosenau Public Health and Preventive Medicine*, ed 11. New York, Appleton-Century-Crofts, 1980.
2. Dubos R: *The Mirage of Health*. Garden City, NY, Doubleday and Co, Inc, 1959; *Man Adapting*. New Haven, Conn, Yale University Press, 1965.
3. Shryock R: *The Development of Modern Medicine*. Madison, University of Wisconsin Press, 1979.
4. Rosen G: *A History of Public Health*. New York, MD Publications, 1958.
5. Ferrell JA, Wilson GS, Covington PW, et al: *Health Departments of States and Provinces of the United States and Canada*, Public Health Bulletin 184. US Public Health Service, Treasury Department, April 1, 1929.
6. Grad FP: *Public Health Law Manual: A Handbook on the Legal Aspects of Public Health Administration and Enforcement*. Washington, American Public Health Association, Inc, 1970.
7. Mustard HS: *Government in Public Health*. New York, Commonwealth Fund, 1945.
8. Mountin JW, Hankela EK, Druzin GB: *Ten Years of Federal Grants-in-Aid for Public Health, 1936–1946*, Public Health Bulletin 300. US Public Health Service, 1947.
9. Emerson H: *Local Health Units for the Nation*. New York, Commonwealth Fund, 1945.
10. Sanders BS: Local health departments: Growth or illusion? *Public Health Rep* 1957; 74:13–20.
11. Greve CH, Campbell JR: *Organization and Staffing for Local Health Services*, Public Health Service publication 682. Government Printing Office, 1961 revision.
12. Shonick W: *Elements of Planning for Area-Wide Personal Health Services*. St Louis, CV Mosby Co, 1976.
13. Kenadjian B: Appropriate types of federal grants for state and community health services. *Public Health Rep* 1966; 81:9.
14. Mytinger RE: *Innovation in Local Health Services*. US Dept of Health, Education and Welfare Public Health Services, Division of Medical Care Administration 1968.
15. Mytinger RE: *What Thirteen Local Health Departments Are Doing in Medical Care*. US Dept of Health, Education and Welfare Public Health Service, Division of Medical Care, 1967.

16. Cooney JP Jr, Roemer MI, Ross MB: *The Contemporary Status of the Large Urban Public Hospital—Ambulatory Services.* Summary Report. University of California, Los Angeles, School of Public Health, November 1971.

17. The plight of the public hospital. *Hospital* (special issue), 1970; 44:40–92.

18. Shonick W, Price W: Reorganizations of health agencies by local government in American urban centers: What do they portend for public health? *Milbank Mem Fund Q/Health Society* 1977; 55:233–271.

19. Shonick W: Mergers of public health departments with public hospitals in urban areas: Findings of 12 field studies. *Med Care* 1980; 18(suppl):1–50.

20. American Public Health Association: The state health department, policy statement of the governing council of the Association, November 13, 1968. A condensed version appeared in *Am J Public Health* 1969; 59(1):158–159.

21. Gossert DJ, Miller CA: State boards of health, their members and commitments. *Am J Public Health* 1973; 63:486–493.

22. Shubick HJ, Wright EO: Composite study of fifty health department organizational charts representing forty-nine states and the District of Columbia. Unpublished report, 1961, cited in [22:224].

23. Hanlon JJ: *Principles of Public Health Administration.* St Louis, CV Mosby Co, 1969. (See also the 1974 edition for additional information.)

24. Association of State and Territorial Health Officials: *Services, Expenditures and Programs of State and Territorial Health Agencies, Fiscal year 1978.* Comprehensive NPHPRS Report. Silver Spring, Md, National Public Health Reporting System of the Association of State and Territorial Health Officials, 1980.

25. *Health United States, 1981,* publication (PHS) 80-1232. US Dept of Health, Education and Welfare, Public Health Service, Office of Health Research, Statistics and Technology, National Center for Health Statistics, National Center for Health Services Research, 1981.

26. *Book of States, 1976–1977.* Washington, Council of State Governments, 1977.

27. Cameron CM, Kobylarz A: Nonphysician directors of local public health departments: Results of a national survey. *Public Health Rep* 1980; 95(4):386–397.

28. Zwick DI: Project grants for health services. *Public Health Rep* 1977; 82:131–138.

29. Cavanaugh JH: Comprehensive Health Planning and Public Health Service Act of 1966 (PL 89-749). *Health Educ Welfare Indicators* 1967; 9–18.

30. Ingraham HS: Federal grants management: A state health officer's view. *Public Health Rep* 1965; 80:670–676.

31. Snoke AW: The unsolved problem of the career professional in the establishment of national policy. *Am J Public Health* 1969; 59:1575–1588.

32. Executive Office of the President: *Restoring the Balance of Federalism,* Second annual report to the president on the federal assistance review. Office of Management and Budget, June 1971.

33. *Federal Assistance Review: A Special Report from the Department of Health, Education and Welfare,* DHEW publication (OS) 72-38. Office of the Secretary, Dept of Health, Education and Welfare, June 1972.

34. Palmer JL, Sawhill IW (eds): *The Reagan Experiment: An Examination of Economic and Social Policies under the Reagan Administration.* Washington, DC, Urban Institute Press, 1982.

35. *Washington Report on Medicine and Health,* a McGraw-Hill weekly publication. February 1973, February 1977, February 1982.

36. *Healthy People,* the Surgeon General's report on health promotion and disease prevention, DHEW (PHS) publication 70-55071. Public Health Service, Office of the Assistant Secretary for Health and Surgeon General, 1979.

37. *Healthy People,* the Surgeon General's report on health promotion and disease prevention, DHEW (PHS) publication 79-05571A, Background Papers. Public Health Service, Office of the Assistant Secretary for Health and Surgeon General, 1979.

38. *Promoting Health/Preventing Disease: Objectives for the Nation,* US Dept of Health and Human Services, Fall 1980.

39. Crawford R: You are dangerous to your health: The ideology and politics of victim blaming. *Int J Health Services* 1977; 7:663–680.

40. Illich, I: *Medical Nemesis: The Expropriation of Health.* New York, Pantheon Books, 1973.

41. McKeown T: An historical appraisal of the medical task, in McKeown T, McLuchlen G (eds): *Medical History and Medical Care: A Symposium of Perspectives.* London, Oxford University Press, 1971, pp 29–55.

42. Hurley R: The health crisis of the poor, in Dreitzel HP (ed): *The Social Organization of Health.* edited by H.P. Dreitzel, New York, Macmillan Publishing Co, 1971, pp 83–122.

43. Epstein S: The political and economic basis of cancer. *Technology Rev* 1976; 78(8):1–7.

44. Page JA, O'Brien M: *Bitter Wages.* New York, Grossman Publishers, 1973.

45. Brodeur PL: *Expendable Americans.* New York, Viking Press, 1974.

46. Tobin J: Reaganomics and economics. *The New York Review of Books,* December 3, 1981, pp. 11–14.

47. Wilson FA, Newhouser D: *Health Services in the United States,* ed 2. Cambridge, Mass, Ballinger Publishing Co, 1982.

CHAPTER 5

Ambulatory Health Care Services

Stephen J. Williams

Ambulatory health care services are the primary source of contact that most people have with the health services system. Although there are few concise definitions of *ambulatory care,* it can be defined as that care provided outside of inpatient institutional settings. Sometimes ambulatory care is termed *care for the walking patient.* It includes an array of services ranging from simple routine treatment and counseling to relatively complex specialty services. Since so many types of organizations, providers, and services are included in this category of health care, the broad designation of *ambulatory services* is used here to denote care that involves the noninstitutionalized patient. These services form the backbone of the health services system and are integral to providing effective and comprehensive care.

This chapter presents a brief overview of the scope and history of ambulatory care services, including the different types or levels of health care that are provided. Office-based practice is discussed in detail, including both solo and group practice. Institutional services are also discussed in detail, with an emphasis on recent developments in hospital-based ambulatory care. Noninstitutional and government-sponsored ambulatory care services are also reviewed. Finally, the important concepts that must be understood to build a health care system in which ambulatory care services are integrated with each other and with other types of care are outlined, leading to the theoretical concept of a cohesive health services system that meets the needs of both consumers and providers.

The huge range of ambulatory care services preclude a discussion of every provider, setting, and type of service in detail. However, the most important providers and services are discussed, and many of the other chapters of this book are concerned with aspects of ambulatory care. For example, Chapter 4 deals with public health-related ambulatory care services and Chapter 3 covers in detail the use of these services from a quantitative perspective.

HISTORICAL PERSPECTIVE AND TYPES OF CARE

Ambulatory care originated with the healing arts themselves. In primitive societies and for many years thereafter, until the advent of institutional care, all care was provided on what might be termed an ambulatory care basis. Of course, the types of care given have little resemblance to today's health care, but the history of civilization demonstrates a consistent commitment to caring for the sick, using whatever knowledge has been available at the time. Remarkable efforts to develop medicine occurred in Greece, Rome, and other relatively sophisticated societies, and many primitive societies had their own practitioners such as religious healers and medicine men.

In more recent times, ambulatory care was provided in many settings by a variety of practitioners. In Europe and later in the United States, many of these services were given to wealthy patients in their homes, and poor people were cared for in dispensaries and public clinics. As hospital care improved, more and more patients of all social classes received both inpatient and outpatient care in hospital settings. In the United States the poor have always been more likely to obtain health care from the hospital than from a private physician.

In the United States, ambulatory care services have traditionally been provided by individual medical practitioners in their offices and in patients' homes, and by public clinics operating primarily for poor and indigent patients. The limited technological armament that physicians required allowed them to travel easily, carrying with them their principal equipment and supplies. Thus, home care was common, especially among wealthier patients. Physicians' offices were frequently located in their homes or in other small buildings, as opposed to today's medical office building or large medical centers (1). The general practitioner who made house calls, provided guidance, and offered available treatments was typical of the primary care provided before World War II.

Since World War II, however, there has been an explosion of medical knowledge, leading to increasing specialization, more complex technology, and rapid changes in the setting and nature of services. Fewer physicians are able or willing to travel to the patient's home, and many can no longer carry or have with them either the equipment and supplies or the specialized personnel and other resources available in an office. The growth of specialization and other considerations have led to the rapid expansion of new settings for providing care, such as group practices and hospital clinics, both of which are discussed further below. Increased knowledge has led to the phasing out of the traditional general practitioner.

For the poor, both in Europe and in the United States, care, when available, was often limited to public or philanthropic clinics or dispensaries. Private practitioners may have given their time, but their devotion to the patient was probably limited, as was the availability of care and the atmosphere in which services were provided. These public care provisions eventually led to public hospitals, government-sponsored clinics, and other settings discussed in this chapter. At the same time, especially in the early and mid-1900s, public health services were being directed to the needs of large populations, as discussed in Chapter 4, with the recognition that everyone is affected by the spread of contagious and communicable disease.

Efforts to link ambulatory care services and to integrate them formally with inpatient care were promoted in this country and in Europe through concepts that are now termed *regionalization*. In Great Britain, these concepts were presented in the Dawson Report (2), which eventually lead to the National Health Service. In the United States, however, centralization of the health care system has not been accepted as a politically viable alternative. In its place is a diverse but somewhat fractured network of providers that is especially characteristic of ambulatory care. Even efforts by prestigious groups such as the Committee on the Costs of Medical Care have done little to organize the health care system. The result has been the development of many settings and providers of ambulatory care, each with its own advantages and limitations. These range from hospital clinics to group practices to government-sponsored health centers.

Table 5-1 demonstrates the diversity of services, providers, and facilities that are involved in ambulatory care today. Many of these services and organizations will be discussed in this chapter. Particular attention is directed toward rapidly expanding and innovative settings such as group practice.

Levels of Ambulatory Care Services

Ambulatory care services can be differentiated into a number of distinct levels or types of care. Primary prevention seeks to reduce the risks of illness or morbidity by removing disease-causing agents from our society. These activities include, for example, efforts to eliminate environmental pollutants that are suspected to cause diseases such as cancer and emphysema. Other examples of primary prevention include encouraging people to use seat belts, treatment of water and sewage, and sanitation inspections in restaurants. Preventive health services are more direct interventions to detect and prevent disease. Examples of these services include hypertension, diabetes, and cancer screening clinics and immunization programs. The combination of primary prevention and preventive services is our first line of defense against disease (3).

Medical care that is oriented toward the daily, routine needs of patients, such as initial diagnosis and continuing treatment of common illness, is termed *primary care* (4). This care is not highly complex and generally does not require sophisticated technology and personnel. The vision of the general practitioner of bygone days traveling from house to house ministering to the sick is the traditional role of primary care, replaced in today's society by more skilled practitioners in fancier facilities.

In addition to providing services directly, the primary care professional should serve the role of patient advisor and advocate. In this coordinating role, the provider refers patients to sources of specialized care, gives advice regarding various diagnoses and therapies, and provides continuing care for chronic conditions.

The evolution of technology and medicine's increasing ability to intervene in illness have led to more specialization of medical services. These more specialized services are termed *secondary* and *tertiary care* and include both ambulatory and inpatient services. The content of secondary and tertiary care practices is usually more narrowly defined than that of the primary care provider. Subspecialists also often require more complex equipment and more highly trained support personnel than do primary care providers.

There are no clear dividing lines between primary and secondary and secondary and tertiary care. Secondary services include routine hospitalization and specialized outpatient care provided by specialists. These services are more complex

TABLE 5-1. Partial List of Providers of Ambulatory Care Services

Settings	Principal Practitioners	Level or Type of Services
Private office-based solo and group practice	Physicians, dentists, nurses, MEDEX, therapists	Primary and secondary care
Hospital clinics	Physicians, dentists, nurses, MEDEX, therapists	Primary and secondary care
Hospital emergency rooms	Physicians, nurses	Primary and urgent care
Ambulatory surgery centers	Surgeons, nurses, anesthesiologists	Surgical secondary care
Communitywide emergency medical systems	Technicians, nurses, drivers	Emergency transportation, communications, and immediate care
Poison control centers, community hotlines	Physicians, technicians, nurses	Emergency advice
Neighborhood health centers, migrant health centers	Physicians, dentists, nurses	Primary and secondary care
Community mental health centers	Psychologists, social workers	Mental health services
Free clinics	Physicians, nurses	Primary care
Federal systems—Veterans Administration, Indian Health Service, Public Health Service, military	All types	All types
Home health services	Nurses	Primary care
School health services	Nurses	Primary and preventive care
Prison health services	All types	Primary and secondary care
Public health services and clinics	Physicians, nurses	Targeted programs (e.g., family planning, immunization, inspections, screening programs, health education)
Family planning and other specialized clinics (nongovernmental)	Physicians, nurses, aides	Specialized services
Industrial clinics	Physicians, nurses, environmental health specialists	Preventive, primary, and emergency care
Pharmacies	Pharmacists	Drugs and health education
Optical shops	Optometrists, opticians	Vision care
Medical laboratories	Technicians	Specialized laboratory services
Indigenous	Chiropractors, medicine men, naturopaths	Primary and supportive care

that those of primary care, including many diagnostic procedures and more complex therapies. Tertiary care includes the most complex services, such as open heart surgery, and usually is provided in inpatient hospital facilities. Most of the care discussed in this chapter involves primary care and those secondary services that can be provided in office-based practice, hospital outpatient departments, or community clinics.

The differences between the types of services provided within the ambulatory care sector are an important concern throughout this chapter since one objective of improving or rationalizing the health services system is to match the capabilities of providers, or levels of care, with the needs of consumers. As different settings for providing ambulatory care are presented, consider the advantages and disadvantages of each to patient care needs and the optimal relationships that should be developed between the different levels of care.

OFFICE-BASED PRACTICE

Most of the ambulatory care that people receive is provided in office-based practice settings. Table 5-2 deals with physician office visits in the United States for 1979. Although a significant amount of care is provided in hospitals, the predominant setting is the physician's office, including solo, group, and noninstitutional clinic practices. More detailed information on the use of ambulatory care services is presented in Chapter 3.

TABLE 5-2. Physician Visits, by Source of Care and Patient Demographic Characteristics, United States, 1979

| Characteristic | | Source of Care | | |
	All Sources	Physician's Office	Hospital	Telephone
		Visits Per 1,000 population		
Total	4,699.8	3,175.4	618.8	603.5
Age				
Under 17 years	4,140.0	2,601.5	535.6	756.4
17–44 years	4,470.3	3,069.8	588.1	496.7
45–64 years	5,230.3	3,617.6	762.7	508.9
65 years and over	6,349.1	4,589.9	709.4	693.3
Sex				
Male	4,114.6	2,723.4	654.5	454.8
Female	5,236.0	3,581.9	591.7	740.8
Race				
White	4,764.3	3,278.9	556.4	650.1
Black	4,538.0	2,641.3	1,110.5	348.5
Family income				
Less than $7,000	5,358.2	3,141.6	1,128.4	543.9
$7,000–$9,999	5,139.7	3,445.3	790.9	570.5
$10,000–$14,999	4,582.1	3,035.9	618.1	631.5
$15,000–$24,999	4,624.6	3,253.5	519.3	637.4
$25,000 or more	4,658.3	3,349.9	425.4	624.1

SOURCE: US Dept. of Health and Human Services: *Health, United States, 1981.* US Government Printing Office, 1981.

TABLE 5-3. Estimated Distribution of Ambulatory Care Visits by Type of Service

Type of Service	Estimated Number and Percentage of Total Visits (Mid-1970s)	
	Number (Thousands)	Percentage
Private solo medical practice	545,000	49.5
Hospital outpatient departments	200,000	18.2
Private group practice	185,000	16.8
School health services	55,000	5.0
Industrial health units	40,000	3.6
Public health clinics	30,000	2.7
Special governmental programs (e.g., neighborhood health centers)	25,000	2.3
Special voluntary agencies (e.g., free clinics)	20,000	1.8

SOURCE: Roemer MI: From poor beginnings, the growth of primary case. *Hospitals* 1975; 49:38–43.

The two predominant private settings or forms of practice are solo and group practice. Solo practice is usually a one-physician private practice, although dentists and other health professionals also practice in solo settings. Group practice is the combination of three or more practitioners in a medical or other office-based practice. Two practitioners, although seemingly left out of all of the formal definitions, can also be considered a group practice. Each of these forms of practice is discussed in detail in this chapter. First, however, an overview of office practice is presented.

Most ambulatory care services have traditionally been provided by physicians in solo office-based practice. Although solo practice still accounts for more ambulatory services than any other setting (Table 5-3), group practice and hospital-based services are expanding dramatically (5). Changing life styles, the cost of establishing a practice, external pressures on practitioners, and governmental programs have also adversely affected the traditional dominance of solo practice. But solo practice remains an important setting for ambulatory services and one that will continue to have a major role in the nation's health services system.

Although there is little information available on the practice patterns of solo practitioners, an ongoing national study of all private office-based physicians, the National Ambulatory Medical Care Survey (NAMCS), has been initiated by the federal government. Although many of the participants in the study are solo practitioners, the study reflects the nature of office-based practice for physicians in all settings.

The NAMCS involves a random selection of the nation's office based nonfederal physicians, who are asked to complete a data collection form for each patient treated during a 1-week interval (6). Table 5-4 lists the most common reasons and principal diagnoses for all office visits included in the study in 1981. The high ranking of routine care, follow-up or ongoing care, and relatively simple primary care problems is striking, reflecting the predominance of these types of problems in office-based practice (7). Table 5-5 presents the diagnostic and therapeutic services provided to patients, excluding drugs prescribed, which are shown separately in Table 5-6.

TABLE 5-4. Most Common Reasons and Principal Diagnoses for Office Visits, 1981

	Reasons for Visit				Principal Diagnoses		
Rank	Most Common Principal Reasons for Visit	Number of Visits in Thousands	Percent	Rank	Most Common Principal Diagnosis	Number of Visits in Thousands	Percent
1	General medical examination	30,222	5.2	1	Essential hypertension	28,765	4.9
2	Prenatal examination	23,501	4.0	2	Normal pregnancy	25,051	4.3
3	Postoperative visit	18,071	3.1	3	Health supervision of infant or child	18,583	3.2
4	Symptoms referable to the throat	15,098	2.6	4	Acute upper respiratory tract infections of multiple or unspecified sites	14,853	2.5
5	Progress visit not otherwise specified	14,864	2.5	5	General medical examination	14,132	2.4
6	Well-baby examination	12,922	2.2	6	Suppurative and unspecified otitis media	13,106	2.2
7	Cough	12,783	2.2	7	Diabetes mellitus	10,772	1.8
8	Blood pressure test	10,662	1.8	8	Special investigations and examinations	10,548	1.8
9	Back symptoms	10,318	1.8	9	Follow-up examinations	10,207	1.7
10	Head cold, upper respiratory tract infection	9,185	1.6	10	Diseases of sebaceous glands	9,661	1.7
11	Fever	9,160	1.6	11	Neurotic disorders	9,590	1.6
12	Skin rash	8,882	1.5	12	Acute pharyngitis	8,473	1.4
13	Earache or ear infection	8,745	1.5	13	Allergic rhinitis	8,441	1.4
14	Headache, pain in head	8,436	1.4	14	Disorders of refraction and accommodation	8,216	1.4
15	Chest pain and related symptoms	8,368	1.4	15	Bronchitis, not specified as acute or chronic	6,731	1.2
16	Abdominal pain, cramps, spasms	8,240	1.4	16	Other forms of chronic ischemic heart disease	6,498	1.1
17	Eye examination	7,790	1.3	17	Osteoarthrosis and allied disorders	5,691	1.0
18	Hypertension	7,531	1.3	18	Contact dermatitis and other forms of eczema	5,228	0.9
19	Knee symptoms	7,102	1.2	19	Acute tonsillitis	5,148	0.9
20	Vision dysfunctions	6,834	1.2	20	Asthma	5,024	0.9
	All other reasons	346,463	59.2		All other diagnoses	360,460	61.6

SOURCE: Lawrence L, McLemore T: 1981 summary: National ambulatory medical care survey, in *Advance Data from Vital and Health Statistics*, no 88, DHHS publication (PHS) 83-1250. Hyattsville, Md, Public Health Service, 1983.

TABLE 5-5. Diagnostic and Therapeutic Services Provided, 1981

Diagnostic Services			Therapeutic Services		
Diagnostic Service	Number of Visits in Thousands	Percent	Nonmedication Therapy	Number of Visits in Thousands	Percent
None	47,056	8.0	None	322,019	55.0
Limited history/examination	379,544	64.9	Physiotherapy	26,743	4.6
General history/examination	88,570	15.1	Office surgery	42,844	7.3
Pap test	25,154	4.3	Family planning	11,399	2.0
Clinical laboratory test	129,123	22.1	Psychotherapy/therapeutic listening	28,038	4.8
X-ray film	44,813	7.7	Diet counseling	44,692	7.6
Blood pressure check	202,159	34.6	Family/social counseling	11,068	1.9
Electrocardiogram	18,457	3.2	Medical counseling	133,648	22.8
Vision test	33,875	5.8	Other	13,444	2.3
Endoscopy	5,656	1.0			
Mental status examination	7,861	1.3			
Other	28,045	4.8			

SOURCE: Lawrence L, McLemore T: 1981 summary: National ambulatory medical care survey, in *Advance Data from Vital and Health Statistics*, no 88, DHHS publication (PHS) 83-1250. Hyattsville, Md, Public Health Service, 1983.

TABLE 5-6. Drugs Prescribed or Provided during Office Visits, 1981

Therapeutic Categories	Number of Drug Mentions in Thousands	Percent Distribution
All categories	651,153	100.0
Antihistamine drugs	43,511	6.7
Anti-infective agents	104,804	16.1
Antibiotics	89,209	13.7
Antineoplastic agents	4,019	0.6
Autonomic drugs	24,102	3.7
Blood formation and coagulation	8,020	1.2
Cardiovascular drugs	68,779	10.6
Cardiac drugs	30,184	4.6
Hypotensive agents	24,263	3.7
Vasodilating agents	13,730	2.1
Central nervous system drugs	104,391	16.0
Analgesics and antipyretics	58,841	9.0
Psychotherapeutic agents	15,140	2.3
Sedatives and hypnotics	23,012	3.5
Electrolytic, caloric, and water balance	55,277	8.5
Diuretics	45,239	6.9
Expectorants and cough preparations	17,864	2.7
Eye, ear, nose, and throat preparations	23,546	3.6
Gastrointestinal drugs	24,196	3.7
Hormones and synthetic substances	53,999	8.3
Adrenals	20,731	3.2
Serums, toxoids, and vaccines	22,068	3.4
Skin and mucous membrane preparations	49,026	7.5
Spasmolytic agents	10,654	1.6
Vitamins	20,507	3.1
Other therapeutic agents, pharmaceutic devices and aids	11,553	1.8
Therapeutic category undetermined	4,840	0.7

SOURCE: Lawrence L, McLemore T: 1981 summary: National ambulatory medical care survey, in *Advance Data from Vital and Health Statistics*, no 88, DHHS publication (PHS) 83-1250. Hyattsville, Md, Public Health Service, 1983.

Limited examinations, laboratory tests, and blood pressure checks were the most common diagnostic services, and counseling is the most common therapeutic service provided, exclusive of drug counseling. For patients receiving medication, the most common categories of drugs prescribed or provided were antibiotics, analgesics and antipyretics, cardiovascular drugs, and hormones. Finally, Table 5-7 presents information on the characteristics of the visits themselves. According to the physician's judgment or the patient's request, more than half of the visits required a follow-up visit. Nearly all of the visits lasted for less than 30 minutes, and almost half of the visits were for 10 minutes or less. Although more extensive analyses of these results will be required to expand our understanding of office-

TABLE 5-7. Characteristics of Office Visits in NAMCS, 1981

Disposition and Duration	Number of Visits in Thousands	Percent Distribution
Disposition[a]		
No follow-up planned	65,970	11.3
Return at specified time	357,694	61.1
Return if needed	131,996	22.6
Telephone follow-up planned	20,059	3.4
Referred to other physician	14,735	2.5
Returned to referring physician	4,670	0.8
Admit to hospital	13,699	2.3
Other	1,205	0.2
Duration		
0 minutes[b]	16,164	2.8
1–5 minutes	74,471	12.7
6–10 minutes	173,441	29.6
11–15 minutes	165,206	28.2
16–30 minutes	121,047	20.7
31 minutes or more	34,847	6.0

SOURCE: Lawrence L, McLemore T: 1981 summary: National ambulatory medical care survey, in *Advance Data from Vital and Health Statistics*, no 88, DHHS publication (PHS) 83-1250. Hyattsville, Md, Public Health Service, 1983.

[a]May not add up to 100.0 since more than one disposition was possible.

[b]Represents office visits in which there was no face-to-face contact between the patient and the physician.

based patient care, the NAMCS aids our understanding of the nature of physician office visits by providing useful descriptive data.

Solo Practice

Solo practitioners are difficult to characterize for a number of reasons. First, there are few data available on their practice patterns and activities. Although a few studies have been conducted, they tend to focus on specific questions, such as referral patterns or quality of care, and do not provide a comprehensive picture of what the solo practitioner does (8,9). The studies that do contribute to a more complete understanding of the activities of solo practitioners are based on physicians in one geographic area or a particular specialty, and the results of these studies, although interesting and useful, may not be generalizable to other practices or areas. The second problem in attempting to characterize solo practitioners is their heterogeneity; they include many types of health care professionals and provide an immense array of services.

The available evidence indicates that physicians in private solo practice generally work hard, although they often earn less, on average, than their counterparts in group practice. Many solo practitioners are specialists who provide secondary care only, often on referral from primary care practitioners. These practitioners include, for example, allergists, dermatologists, and surgeons. Some specialists provide both primary and secondary care since they have insufficient work in their own specialty to achieve desired income levels. Many solo practitioners, including those trained in general and family practice, internal medicine, pediatrics, and obstetrics and gynecology, provide primary care services. There is some controversy and competition among practitioners concerning which specialists should be providing primary care. The emerging specialty of family practice, in particular, represents a challenge to internal medicine in providing adult primary care and to pediatrics in child care (10).

Little detailed information exists on how the individual practitioner's time during the workday is allocated among various activities. Most solo practitioners perform a number of functions in the office, including patient care, consultations, and administration and supervision of office staff. Exactly how much time each of these activities requires is difficult to assess, but the requirements for administration and the supervision of personnel have been increasing in recent years.

Solo practice is often associated with a greater feeling that the provider cares about the welfare of the patient, possibly resulting in a stronger patient-provider relationship than occurs in other settings. There is some evidence that this situation, where it occurs, is a result of the lower level of bureaucracy or organizational complexity in solo practice (11). Since there is also some evidence that the relationship between patient and physician is related to patient compliance with medical regimens, patients who perceive that they are receiving more personalized care may respond to the care process more positively (12). Solo practitioners are also not as restricted in referrals to specialists as are providers in some other settings, such as group practice, where organizational loyalties intervene. Finally, the solo practitioner may feel a greater identification with the community served since there is a more direct relationship between patient and provider.

From the provider's perspective, solo practice offers an opportunity to avoid organizational dependence and to be self-employed; there is also no need to share resources or income. Philosophically, solo practice is most closely aligned with the traditional economic orientations that have characterized medicine. On the other hand, all of the increasingly complex problems of administering a practice must be dealt with unless a professional manager is hired. Thus, solo practice offers distinct opportunities and has philosophical and emotional appeal, but is far from devoid of problems and constraints.

Group Practice

Office-based practice includes, in addition to solo practitioners, group practice. This form of practice has been growing in popularity in recent years, especially as the increasing pressures of practice have led many providers to seek alternative settings in which to work.

Group practice is an affiliation of three or more providers, usually physicians, who share income, expenses, facilities, equipment, medical records, and support personnel in the provision of services through a formal, legally constituted organization (13). Although definitions of a group practice vary somewhat, the essential elements are formal sharing of resources and distribution of income.

Traditionally, group practice has meant participation and ownership by physicians. In the future, however, as new and more diversified models for the provision of services are developed, other practitioners will participate in group practices. In some communities, for example, group practices of nurse practitioners may be the only sources of health services. Dentists, optometrists, and other specialized personnel are also increasingly developing group practices.

History of Group Practice.   Some of the earliest group practices in the United States were started by companies that needed to provide care to employees in rural sites where medical care was unobtainable. For example, the Northern Pacific Railroad organized a practice in 1883 to provide care to employees building the transcontinental railroad. This industrial clinic was one of a number of such clinics founded in the nineteenth century. Even more significant, however, was the establishment of the Mayo Clinic in Rochester, Minnesota, the first successful nonindustrial group practice. The Mayo Clinic, originally organized as a single-specialty group practice in 1887 and later broadened into a multispecialty group, demonstrated that group practice was feasible in the private sector. Mayo Clinic also represented a reputable model for group practice in a national atmosphere of fierce independence where group practice was viewed with skepticism and distrust. By the early 1930s there were about 150 medical groups throughout the country, with many located in the Midwest. Most included or were started by someone who had practiced or trained at the Mayo Clinic.

In 1932 a national committee, the Committee on the Costs of Medical Care, was established to assess health care needs for the nation. It issued a report that suggested a major role for group practice in the provision of medical care. The committee recommended that these groups be associated with hospitals to provide comprehensive care and that there be prepayment for all services (14).

Other constituencies, including some unions, also developed group practices. After World War II especially, a number of pioneering groups were established. In New York City, the Health Insurance Plan of New York was organized to provide prepaid medical care to the employees of the city, an idea promoted by Mayor Fiorello LaGuardia. In the West, the Kaiser Foundation Health Plans were established to provide health care to employees of Kaiser Industries; Kaiser is an affiliation of plans and providers that is now serving millions of Americans. In Seattle, a revolutionary development was the establishment of Group Health Cooperative of Puget Sound, a consumer-owned cooperative prepaid group practice, which now provides comprehensive care to more than 200,000 people. It was founded by progressive individuals who were dissatisfied with the private medical care available to them in the late 1940s. It is probably a measure of how far group practice has developed that many of these early groups are now huge organizations, viewed by some as establishment medicine but by others as still radical concepts.

Developments in medical practice also spurred the group practice movement. Perhaps most notable was the increasing specialization of medicine and the rapid expansion of technology. This increasing sophistication meant that no individual practitioner could provide all the expertise that patients would require. It also meant that more complex and expensive facilities, equipment, and personnel were needed to care for patients. Group practice provided a formal structure for sharing these costs among providers. Many people believed that resources would be used more efficiently in groups. In addition, multispecialty groups, encompassing more than one specialty, could provide patients with more of their health care under one roof and thus reduce problems of physical access to care.

Group practice was also thought to promote higher quality care since most of the different specialists that a person required would be practicing together, and would thus have the opportunity to discuss patient problems among themselves, share a common medical record, and be more able to ensure the quality and continuity of care. Thus, group practice was seen by many as offering opportunities to the physician, such as easily developed referral arrangements, sharing of after-hours coverage, more flexibility in working hours, and less financial risk, while also benefiting the patient.

Opposition to group practice has occurred mostly for political and philosophical reasons. The American Medical Association and local medical societies have at times opposed group practice. Many early group practices had difficulties when physicians were denied privileges in local hospitals. There have been many legal constraints on group practice in medicine. Community-based specialists sometimes refused to treat patients referred by group physicians. Some people still believe that group practice is antithetical to capitalistic entrepreneurism. In more recent years, however, opposition to group practice has somewhat lessened and laws have been changed; where there is still strong opposition, fears of competition and socialized medicine are common. The federal government has also had a role in the development of group practice through reimbursement policy and the development of new programs in ambulatory care.

The most recent surveys of group practice were conducted in 1975 and 1980 (15,16). In 1975, there were nearly 8,500 groups employing more than 66,000 physicians. The majority of these groups had a single specialty, and most were relatively small. Detailed data from this survey are presented in Table 5-8. Figure 5-1 gives the national distribution of physicians and groups in 1975 and reflects their national popularity.

By 1980 there were more than 10,000 groups employing more than 88,000 physicians, again primarily in small groups (Table 5-9). Although as recently as the 1960s most groups were partnerships, by the 1970s and throughout the early 1980s, most were organized as professional corporations (70.6% in 1980).

Organization of Group Practices. There are many possible organizational affiliations for group practice. Some groups are independent or free-standing, whereas others may be affiliated or owned by a hospital or health plan. Many hospitals have been developing affiliated group practices that may be hospital owned or under contract to provide specific services such as emergency, radiology, and pathology services. Some group practices are fee-for-service, and others are associated with prepayment plans in which enrollees pay a predetermined monthly fee for all health care. Thus, the legal and organizational arrangements for the establishment of group practice are numerous, and depend on group philosophies and objectives and state and local regulations.

A group practice can be legally organized as a sole proprietorship, in which one individual is the owner and all other providers are employees; as a partnership, in which a group of individuals share ownership and liability; as a professional corporation, in which stock is issued and the stockholders, who are usually the providers, own the corporation; or as one of a number of other legal forms, including associations and foundations. The tax and personal liability arrangements are most advantageous for corporations, especially in moderate and larger-sized groups. In some instances, however, the group may not have a separate legal identity, but rather exist within the structure of a larger organization such as a hospital.

The governance of the group practice depends on the legal form of organization. A corporation requires a board of directors. In many larger groups, an executive committee may be elected to conduct most of the administrative business of the

TABLE 5-8. Number and Percentage Distribution of Medical Practice Groups and Group Physicians, by Type of Group and Size, 1975

Type of Group	3–7	8–15	16–25	26–59	60–99	100+
	Number of groups					
All types	6,721	1,148	326	187	66	35
Single specialty	4,079	465	43	7	3	4
General/family practice	875	41	6	2	0	0
Multispecialty	1,785	642	277	178	63	31
	Percent of groups[a]					
All types	79.2	13.5	3.8	2.2	0.8	0.4
Single specialty	88.6	10.1	0.9	0.2	0.1	0.1
General/family practice	94.6	4.5	0.7	0.2	0.0	0.0
Multispecialty	60.0	21.6	9.3	6.0	2.1	1.0
	Number of physicians					
All types	28,398	11,828	6,363	6,463	4,364	9,428
Single specialty	6,918	4,554	807	206	156	931
General/family practice	3,364	385	113	97	0	0
Multispecialty	7,306	6,889	5,443	6,160	4,208	8,495
	Percent of physicians[a]					
All types	42.4	17.7	9.5	9.7	6.5	14.1
Single specialty	71.7	19.3	3.4	0.9	0.7	3.9
General/family practice	85.0	9.7	2.9	2.5	0.0	0.0
Multispecialty	20.5	17.5	13.8	15.7	10.7	21.6

SOURCE: Goodman L, Bennett E, Odem R: Current status of group medical practice in the United States. *Public Health Rep* 1977; 92:430–433.

[a]Some horizontal lines of percentages do not add up to 100.0 because of rounding.

group without requiring that all partners or members of the board be frequently convened. In many groups, committees composed of group members with specifically designated responsibilities are appointed or elected. Examples include a building committee to oversee new construction and a credentials committee to approve new members of the group. Larger groups often evolve into highly complex organizations.

The organizational structure of groups can vary tremendously. Larger groups are divided into departments, often based on clinical specialties. Many groups have professional managers with overall responsibility for the administration of the group and its facilities. Larger groups may have administrators for each department or may divide responsibilities along functional lines such as finance and patient care. In most groups, however, the professional manager only recommends major policy to the owners and thus does not have ultimate authority for all decision making.

Larger group practices usually have a medical director. The medical director and the administrator share authority and responsibility to an extent that varies from group to group. However, unlike the dual lines of authority in community hospitals, the providers often own the group and are the ultimate authority to whom the administrator reports. The medical director is usually responsible for policies re-

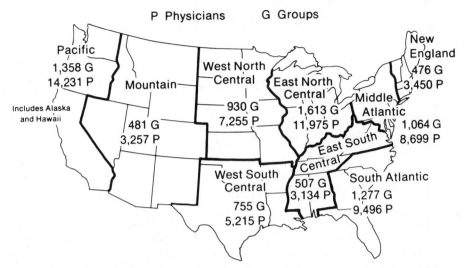

Figure 5-1. Geographic distribution of group practices and group physicians, United States, 1975.
SOURCE: Goodman L, Bennett E, Odem R: Current status of group medical practice in the United States. *Public Health Rep* 1977; 92:430–443. Reprinted by permission.

lated to clinical services including quality of care, scope of services, and productivity of practitioners. The administrator is usually responsible for personnel practices involving most nonphysician employees, patient flow and scheduling, financial management, and daily administrative matters.

Physicians in Group Practice. As discussed elsewhere in this section, there are distinct advantages and disadvantages to physicians and other practitioners in group practice. Many of the advantages involve attributes of the setting to physician time allocation between medical practice and administration. Interestingly, the quantitative information available from a national survey of physicians indicates that there is little difference in the time spent in practice as measured in hours per week or weeks per year between solo and group physicians (17). On the average,

TABLE 5-9. Results of the 1980 Survey of Group Practices, United States

Characteristics	Groups	Physicians
Type of Group		
Single specialty	6,156	29,456
Multispecialty	3,552	54,122
Family practice	1,054	4,712
Total	10,762	88,290
Size of group		
Five or fewer physicians	7,277	
More than five physicians	3,485	

SOURCE: Freshnock L, Jensen L: The changing structure of group medical practice in the United States, 1969–1980. *JAMA* 1981; 21:2173–2176.

TABLE 5-10. Average Net Income for Solo and Group Physicians, 1979

| | | Specialty of Practice | | |
Type of Practice	All	General Practice	Internal Medicine	Pediatrics
Solo	$75,800	$62,400	$74,400	$59,200
Group (number of physicians)				
8 or More	82,000	60,200	73,300	67,400
4–7	91,200	64,900	87,500	67,900
2–3	86,100	65,200	85,300	62,000

SOURCE: Goldfarb D (ed): *Profile of Medical Practice, 1981.* Chicago, Center for Health Services Research and Development, American Medical Association, 1981.

general solo practitioners worked 47.3 hours per week, internists 51.1, and pediatricians 48.5. For group practice physicians in these specialties, the averages were 48.5–52.7, 53.1–54.4, and 50.2–47.6, the range being from larger to smaller groups. Nearly all physicians in the survey worked approximately 47 weeks per year.

The net income of the practitioner, however, did vary somewhat by practice setting, as reflected in Table 5–10. Although generalization is difficult, solo practitioners did not earn the highest incomes by specialty category based on these average reported income data. Although the differences are generally not large, and may be the result of differences in the number of hours worked per year, there is also the possibility that income differences are attributable at least partly to greater efficiency or higher productivity per hour of work in group practice.

Physicians and other health care practitioners are increasingly turning to group practice, sometimes as an alternative to solo practice and all the administrative demands of that form of practice on the practitioner, but increasingly because of the very positive attributes of groups. These advantages, along with the negative aspects of group practice, are discussed next from both the consumer's and the physician's perspectives.

An Assessment of Group Practice. A critical assessment of group practice yields distinct advantages and disadvantages for both patients and providers compared to other modalities for providing ambulatory services (18). Some of these are summarized in Table 5-11. Specific advantages and disadvantages vary from group to group, and Table 5-11 lists the major considerations generally associated with group practice. Some of the topics listed under patient or provider perspectives could readily pertain to both.

The advantages of group practice from the perspective of the provider include shared operation of the practice, joint ownership of facilities and equipment, centralized administrative functions, and, in larger groups, a professional manager. The professional manager can provide expertise in areas often lacking among the providers such as billing, personnel management, patient scheduling, and ordering of supplies.

Financially, the group relieves the provider of the heavy initial investment often required to establish a practice. However, in most groups, co-ownership requires that new members buy into the group through purchase of a share of the group's capital over a long period of time.

The burden of operating costs is also lessened for any individual member of a group. Rather than having to absorb the ups and downs of a practice alone, the

TABLE 5-11. Some Advantages and Disadvantages of Group Practice[a]

Advantages	Disadvantages
From the perspective of the health services provider	
Availability of professional manager	Less individual freedom
Organizational responsibility for patient	May lead to excess use of specialists
Less physician administrative time	
Shared capital expense	Fewer outside consultants
Shared financial risk	Possible reduced identity with patient and community
Better coverage and shared on-call	
More flexible working hours	Group rather than individual decision making
More peer interaction	Share all problems
Increased access to specialists	Must work with others
Broader array of ancillary services	Less individual incentive and more security oriented
Stable income for providers	
No direct financial concerns with patient	Income limitations
Lower initial investment	Income distribution arguments
More time for continuing education	
More flexible vacation time	
Generally excellent benefits	
Possible efficiencies of scale	
Use of nonphysician practitioners	
From the perspective of the group practice patient	
Care under one roof	Less freedom of choice of provider
Availability of specialists, laboratories, etc.	
Improved coverage and emergency care	Possible lessening of provider-patient relationship
Medical and administrative records centrally located	Possible overuse of ancillary services
Referrals simplified	
Peer interaction among providers	Possible high provider turnover
Better administration of group	Heavy patient loads and waiting times may be increased
Efficiency may be promoted in patient care	
Possibly better knowledge of medical care costs	Less provider incentive for care
	More bureaucracy

[a]Some advantages and disadvantages could be included under both provider and patient categories.

sharing of income and expenses within the group allows for some fluctuations in individual practices. For example, a solo practitioner who becomes ill may have no practice income, whereas a group member's income may continue during short periods of illness since other providers are generating revenue. However, the provisions of income distribution plans vary substantially among groups.

Patient care responsibilities are also shared in group practice. This sharing results in more flexibility in working hours for the provider, as well as more time for vacation and continuing education without sacrificing the quality of care for the patient. For example, providers cover for each other during vacations and after normal working hours. And although most practitioners in solo practice arrange for patient care coverage, the continuity of care and the extent of coverage are probably greater in group practice since the patient's medical records and the full resources of the group are always available even if a specific provider is not working.

Sharing of patient care has some other potential benefits. These include more peer interaction as a result of informal discussions and referral of patients among providers. The inclusion of more providers also results in the availability, by necessity, of a wider range of specialists and ancillary services, which is a convenience for both providers and patients and a source of added revenue for the group.

Does the sharing of administrative and patient care activities within group practice produce better care at lower cost? Although many people believed that group practice, through shared facilities, equipment, and personnel, as well as more effective management, would use resources more efficiently than solo practice, the evidence is mixed. The early evidence tended to refute these beliefs, but more recent research indicates some economies of scale, or efficiencies, attributable to the grouping of resources for smaller groups but not for larger and more bureaucratic groups (19). In addition, there is some question as to whether any savings that are achieved will be returned to consumers or simply represent higher income for providers. There may be other savings in the costs of providing services in group practice through bulk purchasing of supplies, centralized administrative functions, and more efficient patient care activities such as scheduling, but there is currently little empirical evidence to support these assertions.

The use of personnel may be more advantageous in group rather than solo practice. Receptionists, medical records specialists, laboratory and radiology technicians, nurses, and other types of personnel may be used more efficiently and in the specialized areas of their training in many medium and larger-sized groups. There is some controversy over whether group practices use new health care professionals, such as nurse practitioners, more efficiently than solo practices. Empirical research has produced conflicting results, although some evidence suggests that solo practitioners and small groups use these personnel more efficiently than larger groups (20). The efficient use of such personnel depends on provider practice patterns in each situation.

The effect of grouping on patient care, especially on the quality of care, has rarely been investigated in the fee-for-service setting. Most studies examine prepaid group practices in which the incentives are substantially different since providers are paid a salary and consumers pay in advance for all care. Sharing of medical records, peer interaction, easy referrals and consultations with specialists, more sophisticated and accessible ancillary services, and more skilled and diversified support personnel are all arguments suggested in support of higher-quality care in group practice. Convincing comparative studies of quality of care in solo and group practice remain to be performed.

Group practice also offers advantages to patients and their communities. For the patient, the group offers a wide range of services under one roof so that travel between providers is reduced and access is increased. A unified medical record can contribute to continuity of care and less duplication in diagnosis and treatment. Some groups also own or operate hospitals and thus further extend the integration and scope of the services that they provide.

Group practices usually offer more accessible care after normal working hours. Some groups also offer emergency services through their own emergency room or clinic. Groups with a broader community perspective may even be involved in programs such as school health services and community immunization efforts.

The use of a professional manager should benefit the patient through more efficient scheduling and patient flow and improved overall management of the practice. Billing is simplified since all care received can be included on one statement.

Whether group practice is, overall and on balance, more efficient than solo practice remains an unanswered question at the present time. Furthermore, issues of productivity and efficiency must be related to the quality of care and the contribution, if any, to the patient's health status.

On a communitywide basis, group practice may offer a means of attracting providers to areas with inadequate numbers of medical care personnel. By offering peer interaction, support services, and other advantages, groups may increase the appeal of practicing in rural areas or inadequately served urban centers (21).

There are also distinct disadvantages to group practice for providers, patients, and communities. From the perspective of the provider, practicing in a group implies less individual freedom, with a variety of restrictions imposed through the sharing of a practice. Ideologically, the limitations of a group in this regard may be difficult for some people to accept since medicine has traditionally been an individualistic enterprise. In addition to reduced freedom, group practice means sharing responsibilities and problems with others. The interpersonal requirements for working out these responsibilities may not appeal to all practitioners. Older individuals who have been working in solo practice may be especially unlikely to adapt readily to group practice.

The financial advantages for group practice are a tradeoff against some imposed restrictions on income and the necessity of complying with the group's income distribution and practice pattern requirements. Thus, there often is more security and less risk, but also less incentive and reward for individual initiative and production.

The shift of some patient care responsibilities from the individual practitioner to the group also may adversely affect the patient-provider relationship by introducing a degree of impersonalization. If a group has high turnover, the patient may have to change providers frequently. Groups that have too few providers for the number of patients that they serve, which is common when excess capacity is being avoided, will also have waiting times for appointments and in the office that the patient may believe are excessive. The group may result in more restrictions on referral practices and limit the practitioner's willingness to use the expertise of other specialists in the community.

From a community perspective, grouping may reduce the geographic dispersion of providers and thus increase difficulties of physical access to care. In addition, groups may reduce competition in the health care marketplace by consolidating what would otherwise be competing providers.

Many of the hypothesized advantages of group practice remain to be empirically verified, and there are some distinct disadvantages to both consumers and providers. However, group practice is an increasingly popular and, on balance, attractive modality for providing health services.

PREPAID GROUP PRACTICE AND HEALTH MAINTENANCE ORGANIZATIONS

Group practice that is reimbursed on a prepaid, rather than a fee-for-service basis is an increasingly popular approach in designing health care plans. In recent years, this approach has been given government encouragement through the development of Health Maintenance Organizations (HMOs). Although group practice requires that physicians practice together in one organization and under one roof, the concept of prepayment has also been applied to community-based solo and small group practitioners through the development of Independent Practice Plans (IPPs), a form of HMO. Chapter 11 discusses both of these approaches, prepaid groups and IPPs, in more detail from a financing perspective. This chapter addresses organizational issues, with an emphasis on prepayment in group practice. The increasing importance of prepayment has led even fee-for-service group practices to participate at least partially in prepayment options through insurance companies. The rapid escalation of health care costs, increased employer interest in alternative financing methods, and encouragement of competition in health care also suggest an increasing role for prepayment, and medical group practices will seek to develop responsive packages with prepayment characteristics.

Prepayment within group practice alters the incentive system for the provider organization and for the professionals delivering care. Although most of these plans, such as the Kaiser Foundation Health Plan, incorporate many of the principles of group practice, physicians and other providers are on salary, sometimes supplemented by an incentive reimbursement program. Since the plan itself is reimbursed prospectively through a monthly fee for all health care provided, there is an incentive to avoid unnecessary use. This fact ensures that the plan's prospective budget is not exceeded and that the plan can maintain its competitiveness in the health services marketplace.

Most prepayment plans have achieved lower costs for all care through hospitalization rates that are lower than those in the fee-for-service sector. Ambulatory care use has generally been at least as high and often higher in prepaid plans as compared to fee-for-service insurance programs. Prepaid group practices attempt to ration the availability of both ambulatory and inpatient services through a number of mechanisms. Ambulatory visits initiated by the patient can be constrained by limiting the availability of care. This result is achieved through longer waiting times for appointments than patients desire, for example, although the plan must schedule in such a manner that only low priority care is discouraged, while patients with more serious or urgent problems are assured access. Other forms of use can be moderated by changing practice patterns to encourage outpatient care and by limiting the availability of inpatient beds. There is also little evidence that for any specific service, such as an office visit, prepaid groups can provide care at lower cost than fee-for-service groups or solo practitioners. Thus, their primary cost advantage is in reducing hospitalization rather than in achieving economies for individual services, as discussed further below.

Prepaid group practices can assume many organizational forms. Figure 5-2 presents a simplified organizational structure of a typical health plan. The fundamental components include the plan itself, which administers the health program, recruits enrollees, and arranges all contractual relationships. The hospitals and the medical group practices are often organizationally separate from the plan administration and are the direct providers of all care. The medical groups are composed of physicians who contract with the plan to provide care and who use facilities administered by the plan. The hospitals may be owned by the plan, but in many smaller prepaid groups, community hospitals are used through contractual arrangements.

Another type of prepaid practice is the foundation plan, in which community physicians remain in private practice using their own offices but contract individu-

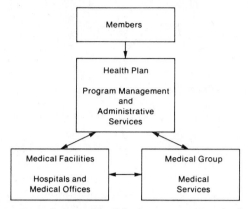

Figure 5-2. Typical prepaid health plan organizational relationships.

ally with a central plan that, in turn, contracts with prepaid enrollees (22). The physicians in this situation are reimbursed by the plan on a fee-for-service basis. This arrangement provides for prepaid services to enrollee populations without requiring that physicians either practice together or be paid on a salaried basis. Foundation type plans were started as an alternative for preserving private fee-for-service practice within a prepayment framework. One of the earliest and best known foundations is the San Joaquin Foundation in California.

The HMO program was instituted in 1973 to promote prepayment plans and incorporates both the group practice and foundation models. The concept was originally proposed by President Richard M. Nixon as a means of promoting private sector medicine through self-regulation while at the same time incorporating some incentives for containment of health care costs (23). The HMO law provides grants and loans for the planning and establishment of HMOs and requires that certain services, including those listed in Table 5-12, be provided.

The HMO program and prepaid group practices had early success in providing comprehensive and acceptable quality health services at lower total costs than the

**TABLE 5-12. Health Services Originally Required
Under the Health Maintenance Organization Act of 1973**

Physician professional services

Outpatient services

Short term mental health services

Short term rehabilitative services

Certain services for substance abuse

Laboratory and radiology services

Home health services

Family planning services

Certain social services

Immunizations and preventive health services

Health education

Arrangements for emergency care

Arrangements for out-of-area coverage

fee-for-service sector (24). However, many HMOs have had difficulties attaining financial viability. This problem may be partially the result of program requirements that include offering a full range of services and having a period of open enrollment during which anyone can join. Some provisions of the program, however, have helped developing HMOs. These provisions include the dual choice requirement under which certain employers must offer the HMO as a health care option to employees in competition with other insurance plans. The most successful prepaid groups have generally been the larger plans or those serving populations with high levels of insurance coverage. Poor management and lack of commitment on the part of organizers and providers have been identified as major reasons for the failure of some HMOs (25).

Under the competitive concepts of the Reagan administration, HMOs have had considerable appeal due to their internal incentives for cost containment and their ability to provide relatively comprehensive services for a predetermined monthly premium. However, federal support for the development of HMOs has been reduced on the assumption that the appeal of HMOs will lead to their creation without external governmental financing. The original legislation has also been amended to reduce the restrictions on HMOs in the health care marketplace—for example, decreasing open enrollment requirements and allowing premiums to be computed on a more financially sound basis (26). The number of HMOs has grown from less than 50 in the early 1970s to more than 200 today. The number of people who have received health care from HMOs has similarly grown to more than 9 million and continues to increase, as shown in Figure 5-3.

The empirical evidence, although not entirely consistent throughout all studies, has accumulated over the past few years and suggests distinct advantages for HMOs. These advantages have been reviewed in a comprehensive and analytical manner by Luft (27). The results of this review are presented in brief form in Table 5-13. It is evident that although much is now known, more remains to be discovered. But the accumulated evidence does support many of the proclaimed advantages of HMOs, although there are also distinct disadvantages. An eclectic health care system that offers many alternatives is probably likely to allow both providers and consumers the opportunity to select the type of plan that is most appealing and that meets their unique health care needs.

INSTITUTIONALLY BASED AMBULATORY SERVICES

In addition to solo and group practice in the private sector, many institutions are expanding their involvement in ambulatory care. These institutionally based settings, especially those associated with hospitals, are discussed next.

The hospital has evolved from an institution for poor people who could not be cared for at home to a provider of a full range of health services from primary to tertiary care. As technological advances have brought more services into the hospital and expanded the scope of care provided, the hospital has assumed an especially important role in the provision of highly complex health services. At the same time, more and more people have sought primary care from hospitals, sometimes due to a lack of access to other sources of care.

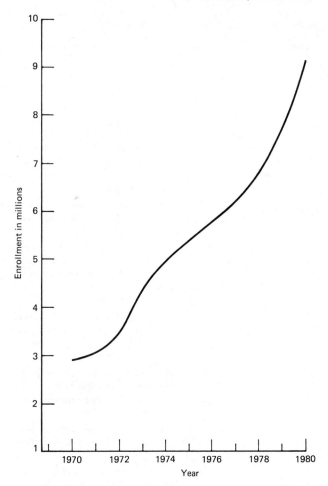

Figure 5-3. The growth in enrollment of health maintenance organizations
SOURCE: Meyers SM: Growth in health maintenance organizations, in *Health, United States, 1981*. US Government Printing Office, 1981.

Outpatient Clinics

The increased demands placed on hospitals for care have taxed the ability of many facilities to respond with appropriate and adequate resources. The result has sometimes been overcrowded facilities, the wrong mix of services, equipment, and personnel to respond to patient needs, and extremely dissatisfied consumers and providers. Some hospitals have successfully responded to these demands by expanding outpatient services and hiring full-time providers to staff-redesigned hospital ambulatory facilities (28).

Traditional hospital outpatient services have been provided in clinics and emergency rooms. In many hospitals, clinics have had second-class status compared to the complex and expensive inpatient services. However, as hospitals increasingly recognize the important role of primary care and seek to expand the base of

TABLE 5-13. Empirical Evidence Concerning HMOs

Area of Knowledge	Evidence
Consumer enrollment	Some people prefer HMOs due to broader coverage or types of benefits; other people prefer to maintain existing relationships with community physicians.
	Consumers selecting HMOs sometimes have used hospital services less and ambulatory care more than those selecting other plans. Adverse selection less likely in HMOs than in other plans.
Health care costs	Prepaid group practice (PGP) members have 10–40% lower costs than those in other plans. IPPs do not appear to have similar low costs.
	HMOs tend to offer broader coverage for the same premium as other plans. Consumer out-of-pocket costs are often lower and usually more predictable.
Health care use	HMOs deliver fewer units of service, due to lower hospitalization. PGPs have significantly lower rates of hospitalization. IPPs have somewhat lower rates than traditional insurance plans, but the evidence is less conclusive than for PPGs.
	Length of stay is similar to HMOs to other plans, but the case mix may differ. PGPs have lower admission rates for diagnoses and tests, suggesting more use of ambulatory care for these purposes.
	IPPs have a lower admission rate for surgical procedures than other plans, but PGPs do not. The use of discretionary surgical procedures does not seem to differ between PGPs and other plans.
	HMOs tend to have higher rates of ambulatory care use than other plans, in part due to broader coverage.
Use of resources	HMOs probably do not provide individual services, such as a hospital day or an office visit, at significantly lower cost than other types of providers.
	Fewer total resources per consumer probably exist in HMOs than in fee-for-service medicine.
	PGPs provide more laboratory tests and radiologic services than traditional plans.
	Productivity of specialists, especially surgeons, is much higher in HMOs due to more stringent staffing.
	Use of allied or mid-level health personnel probably does not differ between HMOs and other providers, although some HMOs rely on these personnel more heavily than do other providers.
Trends over time	There are few consistent patterns over time in HMO total costs, premiums, ambulatory care visits, or inpatient costs per day. Hospital admission and use rates and physician productivity have been falling, as has been the case for all health care providers.
Preventive care	HMOs probably provide more preventive care than other insurers.

TABLE 5-13. (Continued)

Area of Knowledge	Evidence
Quality of care	Limited evidence does not clearly favor HMOs. The quality of medical records, tests performed and appropriateness of care, and health status may be more favorable in HMOs. Use of drugs and outcome of care may not differ between HMOs and other providers.
Consumer satisfaction and access to care	Little conclusive evidence exists.
	PGP enrollees wait less time in the office when they have an appointment, and are less satisfied with scheduling delays in obtaining appointments.
	HMO enrollees tend to be more satisfied with their coverage and financial arrangements.
	Continuity of care may be lower in PGPs.
	PGP enrollees tend to be less satisfied with their interaction with physicians, and possibly with the quality of care.
	PGPs probably have a relatively low disenrollment rate. Out-of-plan use in PGPs is about 5 to 10%.
Physician perspectives	Physicians work fewer hours, earn less, have less autonomy, may be less happy with patient relationships, and are attracted by the prepayment concept in PGPs and HMOs in general. Turnover of physicians is not a problem, nor is recruitment.
HMOs and competitors	HMOs have generally been able to compete in the insurance marketplace. Restrictive laws have been eased, complex management has been improving, and relationships with other providers have been established. HMOs may select certain types of enrollees and providers. They may also force other providers to be more efficient.

SOURCE: Luft HS: *Health Maintenance Organizations: Dimensions of Performance.* New York, John Wiley & Sons, Inc, 1981.

patients that are potential users of inpatient and ancillary services, more attention is being directed toward improving clinic operations and services.

Hospital clinics include both primary care and specialty clinics. Many hospitals differentiate between clinics for walk-in patients without appointments and those for scheduled visits. Specialty clinics are usually organized by department and provide services such as ophthalmology, neurology, and allergy care. In teaching hospitals, clinics serve as important settings in which house staff members provide ongoing care to patients and follow-up after hospitalization. Increasingly, clinics also provide an opportunity to expose medical students and house staff to ambulatory care services to complement the traditionally more extensive experience with inpatient care. In teaching hospitals, there may be more than 100 different clinics reflecting the diversity of subspecialties. In nonteaching hospitals there are fewer specialty clinics and may be more emphasis on primary care.

Many hospital primary care clinics evolved from an orientation of service to the poor and were staffed by physicians who served without reimbursement in exchange for staff privileges. The level of commitment to the patient under such circumstances was, not surprisingly, less than desirable. Hospitals are now increasingly employing physicians and other practitioners as full-time clinic staff. Some hospitals are also establishing primary care group practices to complement other outpatient services and to assume the burden of providing primary care to patients who seek most of their care from the hospital. The development of a group practice has advantages for both consumers and the hospital by providing comprehensive and accessible care and removing primary care patients from facilities that are not designed to serve their needs, such as emergency rooms. The development of these group practices also has the potential of increasing use of the hospital's inpatient and ancillary services, an advantage if occupancy is low (29). However, questions have been raised concerning the ability of hospitals to compete effectively in an arena in which they have not been overly successful in the past (30). But the increasingly competitive nature of the hospital and the health care marketplace is forcing many hospitals to enter this area of practice even if they are uncertain about doing so.

Ambulatory Surgery Centers

A further innovation in hospital-based care has been the development of ambulatory surgery centers. Originated in hospitals in Washington, D.C., and Los Angeles, these organized hospital units provide 1-day surgical care. Patients are usually screened for acceptability by their personal surgeon and then report at an assigned date and time for surgery. The surgeon is supported by the unit's facilities, equipment, and personnel, and the patient is discharged 1 to 3 hours after surgery when recovery from anesthesia is sufficiently complete.

In the early 1970s free-standing ambulatory surgery centers were opened, one of the first of which was in Phoenix. These facilities are independent of hospitals and usually provide a full range of services for the types of surgery that can be performed on an outpatient basis. Community surgeons are granted operating privileges and can perform surgery in these facilities when the patient agrees and there are no medical contraindications.

Other facilities are also used for ambulatory or outpatient surgery. Many physicians traditionally performed surgery in their offices, although this practice has declined due to malpractice concerns and the increasing availability of better-equipped and staffed alternative facilities.

Free-standing emergency centers have also opened in many cities, paralleling the success of ambulatory surgery centers. These emergency centers sometimes provide a wide range of primary care in addition to responding to urgent problems. The future of specialized ambulatory centers, both in hospitals and as free-standing facilities, will probably include further expansion into other areas of health care.

Emergency Medical Services

The emergency room, like other hospital departments, has undergone transformation in recent years. The emergency room has expanded in the range of services offered and in complexity. An especially important trend has been the increasing use of the emergency room for primary care. Since the emergency room requires sophisticated facilities and highly trained personnel and must be accessible 24 hours a day, costs are high and services are not designed for nonurgent care. To reduce the burden on the emergency room and to meet patient needs more effectively, many hospitals triage patients. This is a process, often performed by a nurse, in which the patient's health care needs are determined and the patient is referred to a more appropriate source of care within the hospital. The misuse of the emergency room has received considerable attention and is compounded by third-party insurers, who have often reimbursed for primary care only if it was provided in the emergency room.

Emergency medical services have also been increasingly integrated with other community resources. Included are drug and alcohol treatment programs, mental health centers, and voluntary agencies. Many communities are developing formal emergency medical systems that incorporate all hospital emergency rooms and transportation and communication systems. In these communities, people needing emergency care either transport themselves or call an emergency number. An ambulance is dispatched by a central communications center, which also identifies and alerts the most appropriately equipped and located hospital. In many communities, regional hospital-based trauma centers have been built with extremely sophisticated capabilities. Specialized ambulance services, including mobile coronary care units and shock-trauma vans, are also increasingly prevalent. The Red Cross and other voluntary agencies have also administered programs for many years to train people to respond to accidents, drownings, and other emergencies. In Seattle a program was initiated, now expanding to other cities, to augment emergency capabilities by teaching as many people as possible to respond to heart attacks by administering cardiopulmonary resuscitation. Since accidents and heart attacks are major sources of mortality, these programs have the potential of contributing to reductions in deaths.

GOVERNMENTAL PROGRAMS

In addition to private sector and institutionally initiated efforts, governmental programs have been designed to increase the availability of health care resources in many communities. These programs have adapted some of the concepts of private institutional settings, especially those of group practice.

Neighborhood health centers have been funded since 1965. Originally intended to serve approximately 25 million people, this federal program never reached its initial objectives and now serves about 1.3 million people in more than 130 centers. The program was designed to provide primary medical care with a family orientation. It was targeted for population groups in severe need of services, as reflected by such indicators as disease prevalence and income level. At the same time, the centers were intended to employ people from the communities they serve in positions that would offer opportunities for training and advancement. Responsiveness to community needs was to be ensured by a community board or advisory panel. The centers were to recognize that the broad attributes of a community, such as housing and employment, contributed to health and illness.

Most of the neighborhood health centers are free-standing group practices, although some are affiliated with other institutions such as hospitals, medical schools, or community associations. The majority of centers are located in urban areas. There is considerable diversity in the types of services provided by the centers, but all give primary care and most offer pharmacy, laboratory, radiology, and, to a lesser extent, dental services. Some centers also provide transportation for patients and social services to address broader health needs. Although these health centers were originally intended to serve the poor, changes in federal policy that encouraged them to collect fees from patients and from third-party insurers have broadened the socioeconomic mixture of patients obtaining care. However, the centers still predominantly serve the poor and medically indigent.

Neighborhood health centers have been subjected to considerable criticism, especially from traditional medicine. Some of the criticisms include low productivity and substandard care as compared to the private sector, unwarranted federal intervention in the provision of health services, and high administrative costs. Although it is not possible to generalize across all of the centers, some probably have had high costs and low productivity. This circumstance is partially attributable to their goals of employing and training local residents, and to sometimes inexperienced management, constraints imposed by the federal government, and local politics. Neighborhood health centers have also had difficulties in finding adequate facilities, problems in physician recruitment, and high staff turnover. There have been practical problems in designing family-oriented comprehensive care for clients used to receiving few services and episodic care. Studies to measure the quality of the care provided in these centers have generally concluded that they meet acceptable standards and, in some instances, provide a higher quality of care than other community practitioners (31). The neighborhood health centers have succeeded in increasing access to care under difficult circumstances and have served as an interesting experimental model for the provision of ambulatory care.

Other community health centers that have been funded by the federal government include migrant health centers serving transient farm workers in agricultural areas and rural health centers. The National Health Service Corps supports practitioners who are placed in urban and rural areas with shortages of medical resources. Other innovations, such as mobile health vans in rural areas, have also been used to expand the scope of services.

Community Mental Health Centers and Mental Health Programs

The Community Mental Health Center program was established to provide ambulatory mental health services in underserved areas. This program has suffered from limitations in federal funding and has not been as extensive as originally envisioned. Community mental health centers were intended to provide outpatient services and emergency care and to work with other community agencies to foster action and concern for mental health. Problems of inadequate management have also troubled this program. However, the centers have succeeded in providing mental health services, primarily through nonphysician professionals, to many individuals who would otherwise not obtain such care. These centers are discussed further in Chapter 8.

Other Federal Government Programs

The federal government, in addition to supporting a variety of community-based health services organizations, directly operates many health care facilities. The Veterans Administration includes the largest health services system under a unified management structure in the United States with more than 170 hospitals and clinics. This system provides needed care to millions of veterans throughout the nation.

The military services also provide health care to millions of individuals in the armed forces and have developed extensive facilities throughout the world, as discussed in Chapter 1.

The government has a special responsibility for providing health care to a number of groups within the country. The Indian Health Service is charged with ensuring access to medical care on Indian reservations and in certain other locations. Although the difficulties of operating a largely rural system are immense, the Indian Health Service has succeeded in bringing modern medicine to many people.

The U.S Public Health Service operates eight hospitals. Although they were originally intended to serve seamen, eligibility has been expanded and the scope of care now includes a wide range of both ambulatory and inpatient services. Faced with frequent threats of closure by past presidents, the Public Health Service hospitals had difficulty obtaining sufficient financial resources to meet the demands for care of their eligible populations, and were finally phased out by the Reagan administration.

NONINSTITUTIONAL AND PUBLIC HEALTH SERVICES

As noted in the introduction to this chapter, there are many ways in which ambulatory and community health services are provided. Although only the most prevalent types of providers and services are discussed here, each helps to meet the many health care needs of a community. The list is nearly endless, and a number of services warrant further discussion.

Home health services are provided by visiting nurse associations, some hospitals, public health departments, and other agencies. These services allow people to remain in their homes and yet receive essential health services, thereby reducing costs and increasing the quality of life for many (32). These services, however, often require that the patient have special facilities or equipment and family support at home. For example, home dialysis for chronic renal failure, discussed in Chapter 9, is substantially less expensive than institutional services but requires a specially trained family member.

Rural health care has required unique and innovative solutions in many communities, especially in the absence of physicians and extensive facilities. In rural Alaska, many towns are served by physicians and other professionals who regularly fly in to treat patients. Satellites have also been used experimentally to facilitate communications with specialists in urban medical centers since even ordinary communications in remote areas may be difficult. In rural Kentucky, nurses in the Frontier Nursing Service provide much of the care to the rural mountain people. These hardy nurses have progressed from horseback to jeep in recent years but continue to provide primary health care, often by traveling from house to house through rugged and remote territory. Rural health care in many areas remains a challenging test of the ingenuity and resourcefulness of the health services system and of community residents.

In urban areas, some creative and innovative efforts to provide health care to people with limited access to services have been attempted. Among the most interesting of these has been the development of free clinics in many cities (33). These clinics provide primary medical care and referrals for specialty care, and emphasize counseling and patient education. Clients of the free clinics are often working poor who are unable to qualify for publicly assisted care but do not have the financial resources necessary to obtain services from the private sector. The clinics are usually developed by coalitions of community groups or collectives of individuals dedicated to providing care in a nonbureaucratic atmosphere through an egalitarian organizational structure. Although they employ physicians, there is often an effort to demystify the role of the physician and to rely heavily on other types of health providers, such as nurse practitioners. Free clinics have had to struggle to survive since they are funded through donations from patients, community groups, and sometimes local health departments. They have also faced opposition from traditional health care providers in some communities and have had difficulties in arranging backup support for hospitalization, specialty referrals, and other services.

Other community health services not discussed in detail here include school health services, prison health services, dental care provided by solo, group, and institutionally based practitioners, foot care from podiatrists, and drug dispensing from pharmacists, who often also extensively advise and educate consumers. Voluntary agencies also provide health care services such as cancer screening clinics and health education. Finally, many indigenous health practitioners offer their services in this country and abroad. These practitioners include chiropractors, medicine men, naturopaths, and others. The supportive and sometimes curative role of these individuals is often underestimated.

Public Health Services

Among the most important contributions to reductions in mortality and morbidity in the twentieth century have been public health measures such as the improvement of sanitation, ensurance of potable water supplies, and upgraded housing. In recent years there has also been an increased awareness of the need to control air and water pollution, to reduce exposure to carcinogens, and to improve and ensure the quality of the environment. The contribution of these efforts to health far exceeds, dollar for dollar, efforts to treat illness once it occurs. A comprehensive discussion of these services is presented in Chapter 4, and other reviews are available (34). Their importance to ambulatory care is mentioned here, however, because public health agencies have responsibility for a remarkable range of relevant services.

Public health services have addressesd serious national problems related to health and illness. Increasing numbers of unwanted births and a lack of family planning services, for example, have led many public health departments to operate family planning clinics offering contraceptive services and advice. Identification of, treatment for, and education about venereal disease have long been major activities of public health agencies.

Many health departments operate specific federally funded categorical programs. These programs range from detection of serious diseases in infants, such as phenylketonuria, to immunizations, The Women, Infants, and Children Program, for example, is a federal effort to improve the nutritional status of low income pregnant women and young children. Screening programs have been developed to detect sickle cell anemia, cervical cancer, and hypertension. Major efforts have been made to avoid and react to accidental poisoning, especially in children.

Health education is an important activity of many health departments. The avoidance of some illnesses is possible through a better-informed public. For example, use of seat belts combined with defensive driving could substantially reduce the number of deaths and injuries from automobile accidents. Avoidance of tobacco products, reduced exposure to radiation and carcinogens, and better nutrition are all examples of health education objectives that benefit society through reduced mortality and morbidity. Although few health education program efforts have been extensively evaluated, there is evidence that they have had only mixed success and that people will continue to kill or injure themselves, relying on medical services to undo the damage where possible.

Other efforts, by occupational medicine specialists in industry and government, have been directed toward reducing accidents and exposure to disease-causing agents, including chemicals, dangerous working conditions, and even noise in the workplace. Over the years these efforts, which have been controversial and often unpopular among special interest groups, have substantially improved employment conditions in the nation. However, far more remains to be done in this area, particularly in the identification and removal of potential sources of illness such as excessive radiation, chemical contamination, and unsafe facilities and equipment.

Finally, there is an increasing awareness that ambulatory and community health services are only part of the answer to the advancement of health. Self-reliance is essential if health is truly the nation's goal. Each individual has to live responsibly by avoiding unnecessary risks of injury and illness, eating adequate diets, exercising, and avoiding excessive stress. There is an increasingly popular movement toward self-reliance for prevention and treatment of disease. Protocols and instructional books have been published to assist people in evaluating their health and health care needs. This movement is a response to the reality that medicine is limited in its ability to prevent and treat disease (35).

ORGANIZATION OF AMBULATORY CARE SYSTEMS

The preceding sections of this chapter have outlined the scope and nature of ambulatory and community health care services. The remainder of the chapter discusses the organization of ambulatory care services. Within this framework, the design criteria that are desirable in ambulatory care systems are presented. Although no single unified structure currently exists in the United States for providing health services, and although ambulatory care services in particular are often poorly organized, experience and research have led to an ever-increasing understanding of the factors that are associated with the optimal design of ambulatory care systems. These factors are summarized in Table 5-14, and some are discussed in detail in the following section.

Perhaps the most important criterion that has been identified for the system is access to care. As discussed in Chapter 3, there are many complex factors that affect the use of health care services and the structure of the system itself, especially in ambulatory care systems, can be a critical factor in facilitating access to care.

Ambulatory care services are affected by several access factors. The number and distribution of providers throughout a community determine, in part, the physical access of individuals to the health care system. Decisions such as the hours of operation and the scope of services provided are important to ensure that services can actually be used. Facilities should be located so that the target patient population can reach them. The hours of operation must be consistent with employment

TABLE 5-14. Design Criteria for Ambulatory Care Systems

Criteria Topics	Criteria Requirements
Community criteria	
Availability and distribution of resources	Adequate number of facilities and practitioners Geographic dispersion Adequate transportation
Use of resources	Integration of community resources Effective referral network Appropriate mix of services Constrained excess capacity (few underused services)
Consumer criteria	
Convenience and satisfaction	Physical access assured Availability (hours of operation, after-hours coverage) ensured Efficient scheduling (appointments, follow-ups, waiting times) Financial access (insurance coverage, reasonable prices) Caring providers
Quality services	Continuity and coordination of care (medical records, follow-ups, etc.) Comprehensive services Technical quality of care ensured Multilingual staff and other special needs ensured Health education and instruction provided
Provider criteria	
Work environment	Pleasant and humane Appropriate roles for all providers Adequate income Productivity encouraged Personnel duties match skills and training
Patient care services	Efficient use of resources (personnel, capital, and technology) Use of most appropriate personnel Adequate support services available
System concerns	Technological progress readily adopted

patterns, traffic flows, and other factors. Ensurance of physical access and availability of services is further complicated by such considerations as public transportation, parking, accessibility for the handicapped, and changing population characteristics. Access to care is a highly complex topic for which researchers have attempted to construct equally complex theories and models (36). All health care professionals should assign high priority to ensuring access to care.

Comprehensive services should be available to all consumers that fulfill legitimate health care needs. Who should decide what are legitimate needs, however, is a major issue. For example, a consumer may seek care for a cold, believing that this is a high priority need due to discomfort, whereas providers may believe that little relief can be offered and services should be directed toward those who are more ill. And, who should ensure that all services are available? For example, should providers be required to offer services such as preventive care and health education, or is this a responsibility of government, insurers, or the consumer?

The scope of services is also related to controversies over who is most skilled for providing care. Numerous examples of "turf" struggles are developing in ambulatory care. For example, both general internists and family practitioners seek the central role in providing primary care services. Nurse practitioners and MEDEX are seeking an increasing role in providing services independent of physicians. Optometrists and ophthalmologists seek increasing shares of the eye care market. Pharmacists seek to expand their functions beyond dispensing drugs. Deciding who provides which service most appropriately will be among the most complex and politically charged issues to be tackled in the future.

The availability of services and access to care are often affected by special needs of consumers. For example, individuals without an adequate knowledge of the English language have difficulty in using health services unless multilingual staff or translators are able to assist them. Health education in areas such as the correct use of drugs, dietary habits and practices, and infant care is essential when the population served lacks such information. Provision of drugs may be essential when clients are unable to afford needed supplies. The health administrator, planner, or provider must consider the total environment in which services are provided and not assume that the physical presence of a facility or service alone will ensure needed care.

The organization of services requires consideration of how units of service are related to each other. Rationalization of ambulatory care requires that services not be duplicated. The absence of duplication ensures that individuals are not subjected to unnecessary and repetitive services that can be harmful, as in the case of excess radiation, and costly. However, in some instances, such as second opinions for surgery, there may be some justification for duplication.

Reductions in redundant services can be achieved through improved coordination and continuity in ambulatory care. Ambulatory services have a central role in the achievement of coordination for all health care services. Coordination and continuity imply that there is some centralization of responsibility for care on the part of both the patient and the provider. A primary care provider who directs the care of the patient with respect to specialized services can promote coordination. Common medical records in group practices also promote coordination. Returning to a previous provider for subsequent care when indicated can promote continuity. Both the patient and the provider have responsibility for ensuring the maximum degree of coordination and continuity.

In reality, of course, there are limits to the actual degree of coordination and continuity that can be achieved. Patients become dissatisfied with providers and seek care elsewhere, communications break down, referral patterns change, access to the same provider is not always possible, and numerous other problems can develop. But there is some evidence that coordination and continuity are associated with higher levels of patient compliance (37), which may in turn lead to better health outcomes. It is also likely that greater continuity and coordination will result in an overall higher degree of access and thus patient satisfaction (38), may increase the overall rationalization of the system, and finally, may reduce health care costs through reduced duplication of services.

The consumer also expects high quality services. As discussed in Chapter 13, quality of care is difficult to define and measure. However, reasonable efforts should be taken to ensure that unnecessary procedures are not performed and that individuals are treated by practitioners using an acceptable degree of skill, judgment, and current knowledge. Operationalizing these concepts is difficult, especially in ambulatory care, in which many episodes of treatment are brief and for poorly defined problems.

The quality of care provided should reflect not only adequate technical skills but also a caring attitude on the part of the provider. Consumers are capable of detecting some aspects of the technical quality of care (39), but are even more perceptive regarding the extent to which the provider and the system care about the patient. Since there are limitations to medical practice and since much health care is supportive rather than curative, consumer feelings about the treatment process are especially important and may contribute to higher levels of well-being and contentment.

The provider, as well as the consumer, must be satisfied with the structure of the system. Provider satisfaction requires acceptance of individual and organizational roles in the provision of services. From the perspective of the individual worker, whether nurse, physician, technician, or aide, the rewards and structure of the work environment must stimulate productivity and a high quality of performance.

To many, all of the arguments for designing the system to match the needs of consumers or providers center on the system's role in serving the community. Should the ambulatory care system primarily serve the consumer or the provider, or is there a happy middle ground in which both can be satisfied?

For the community, ambulatory care, first and foremost, should provide primary and specialty services in response to the needs of the community or population. Although these needs are not always easy to determine, there is at least a minimum number of services that are critical to any community. Second, the provision of ambulatory care services should be relatively efficient, however defined, so that community resources are not wasted, and should be distributed so that all members of the community have access to care. And third, the organization of ambulatory care systems should integrate providers of service and, in a sense, should orchestrate care for clients. This process extends far beyond the provision of primary medical and dental services, however, and must also include public health services, voluntary agency efforts, community health education, and all other activities that contribute to the health and well-being of a community.

Whether it is possible or even desirable to establish any single managerial entity to coordinate all of these activities has yet to be determined. This function is now performed in a fragmented way by many individuals and organizations ranging from public health departments to private practitioners. In some countries, such as England and Sweden, such activities are much more centrally organized. In the United States, the health planning agencies discussed in Chapter 12 are an early effort to move toward a somewhat more structured system for health care. The extent to which the nation moves further in this direction will be determined in a highly charged political arena.

There are many other forces affecting the design of community systems for ambulatory care. The changing technology of health care directly affects the types of services provided on an ambulatory basis. For example, the rapid expansion of testing and monitoring of the body, discussed in Chapter 9, which can be performed relatively easily on an outpatient basis, has resulted in more ambulatory care services. New screening techniques have resulted in community programs to detect diseases such as hypertension, cancer, and diabetes, with services offered in such unlikely places as shopping centers.

Third-party insurers and governmental programs such as Medicaid and Medicare influence ambulatory care through their policies on coverage, benefits, and reimbursement levels. By increasingly paying for care provided on an ambulatory basis, they have encouraged a shift from inpatient to outpatient care for many services. Continuation of these trends is likely, with the resultant further expansion of outpatient services.

Toward an Integrated System

This chapter has discussed the current providers of ambulatory services and the characteristics that are likely to be advantageous to strengthened ambulatory care systems. The variety of services, professionals, and organizations involved in ambulatory care is immense, and no single unified structure can encompass them all. The interrelationships between providers and political realities further complicate the system. All the chapters of this book discuss issues that impinge on ambulatory care, and the relationship between ambulatory and other health services has yet to be fully elucidated. However, progress has been achieved by researchers and practitioners in developing an understanding of ambulatory care and in determining the role these services should assume in the overall health services system. The fragmented system that exists now is unlikely to continue in its present form, and many new innovations and initiatives should result in a structure that is more efficient and responsive to the needs of both consumers and providers.

REFERENCES

1. Roemer M: *Ambulatory Health Services in America*. Rockville, Md, Aspen Systems Corporation, 1981.
2. United Kingdom Ministry of Health: *Dawson Report*, interim report on the future provision of medical and allied services. London, His Majesty's Stationary Office, 1920.
3. Burton L, Smith H: *Public Health and Community Medicine*, ed 2. Baltimore, Williams and Wilkins Co, 1975.
4. Noble J (ed): *Primary Care and the Practice of Medicine*. Boston, Little, Brown, 1976.
5. Roemer M: From poor beginnings, the growth of primary care. *Hospitals* 1975; 49(5):38–43.
6. US Dept of Health, Education, and Welfare, National Center for Health Statistics: *National Ambulatory Medical Care Survey: Background and Methodology*, publication (HRA) 76-1335. Government Printing Office, 1976.
7. Lawrence L, McLemore T: 1981 summary: National ambulatory medical care survey, in *Advance Data from Vital and Health Statistics*, no 88, DHHS publication (PHS) 83-1250. Hyattsville, Md, Public Health Service, 1983.
8. Wolfe S, Badgley RF: *The Family Doctor*. New York, Milbank Memorial Fund, 1972.
9. Peterson OL, Andrews LP, Spain RS, et al: An analytical study of North Carolina general practice 1953–1954. *J Med Educ* 1956; 31(12, pt 2):1–165.
10. Petersdorf R: Internal medicine and family practice, controversies, conflict and compromise. *N Engl J Med* 1975; 293:326–332.

11. Mechanic D: *The Growth of Bureaucratic Medicine.* New York, John Wiley & Sons, Inc, 1976.

12. Becker M, Maiman L: Sociobehavioral determinants of compliance with health and medical care recommendations. *Med Care* 1975; 13:10–24.

13. Medical Group Management Association: *The Organization and Development of a Medical Group Practice.* Cambridge, Mass, Ballinger Publishing Co, 1976.

14. Rorem R: *Private Group Clinics.* Chicago, University of Chicago Press, 1931.

15. Goodman L, Bennett E, Odem R: Current status of group medical practice in the United States. *Public Health Rep* 1977; 92:430–433.

16. Freshnock L, Jensen L: The changing structure of group medical practice in the United States, 1969–1980. *JAMA* 1981; 21:2173–2176.

17. Goldfarb D (ed): *Profile of Medical Practice, 1981.* Chicago, American Medical Association, 1981.

18. Graham F: Group versus solo practice, arguments and evidence. *Inquiry* 1972; 9(2):49–60.

19. Kimball L, Lorant J: Physician productivity and returns to scale. *Health Serv Res* 1977; 12:367–379.

20. Yankauer A, Connelly J, Feldman J: Physician productivity in the delivery of ambulatory care, some findings from a survey of pediatricians. *Med Care* 1970; 8:35–46.

21. Evashwick C: The role of group practice in the distribution of physicians in nonmetropolitan areas. *Med Care* 1976; 14:808–823.

22. Egdahl R: Foundations for medical care. *N Engl J Med* 1973; 288:491–498.

23. Bauman P: The formulation and evolution of the Health Maintenance Organization policy, 1970–1973. *Social Sci Med* 1976; 10:129–142.

24. Roemer M, Shonick W: HMO performance: The recent evidence. *Milbank Mem Fund Q* 1973; 51:271–317.

25. Strumpf G, Garramone M: Why some HMOs develop slowly. *Public Health Rep* 1976; 91:496–503.

26. Meyers SM: Growth in Health Maintenance Organizations, in *Health, United States, 1981.* US Government Printing Office, 1981.

27. Luft HS: *Health Maintenance Organizations: Dimensions of Performance.* New York, John Wiley & Sons, Inc, 1981.

28. Berraducci A, Delbanco T, Rabkin M: The teaching hospital and primary care, closing down the clinic. *N Engl J Med* 1975; 292:615–620.

29. Williams S, Shortell S, Dowling W, Urban N: Hospital sponsored primary care group practice: A developing modality of care. *Health Med Care Serv Rev* 1978; 1(5/6):1–130.

30. Williams SJ: Ambulatory care: Can hospitals compete? *Hosp Health Services Admin,* in press.

31. Morehead M, Donaldson R, Seravalli M: Comparisons between OEO neighborhood health centers and other health care providers of ratings of the quality of health care. *Am J Public Health* 1971; 61:1294–1306.

32. Van Dyke F, Brown V: Organized home care: an alternative to institutions. *Inquiry* 1972; 9(2):3–16.

33. Schacter L, Elliston E: Medical care in a free community clinic. *JAMA* 1977; 237:1848–1851.

34. Anderson C, Morton R, Green L: *Community Health.* St Louis, CV Mosby Co, 1978.

35. McKinlay J, McKinlay S: The questionable contribution of medical measures to the decline of mortality in the United States in the twentieth century. *Milbank Mem Fund Q* 1977; 55:405–428.

36. Aday L, Andersen R: A framework for the study of access to medical care. *Health Serv Res* 1974; 9:208–220.
37. Starfield B, Simborg D, Horn S, et al: Continuity and coordination in primary care: Their achievement and utility. *Med Care* 1976; 14:625–632.
38. Williams S, Shortell S, LoGerfo J, et al: A causal model of health services for diabetic patients. *Med Care* 1978; 16:313–326.
39. Lebow J: Consumer assessments of the quality of medical care. *Med Care* 1974; 12:328–337.

CHAPTER 6

The Hospital

William L. Dowling

The modern hospital is the key resource and organizational hub of the American health care system, central to the delivery of patient care, to the training of health personnel, and to the conduct and dissemination of health-related research. The hospital represents the community's collective investment in health care resources, presumably available for the benefit of all, and it is often the first place people think of when they need medical care. Since the turn of the century the indispensable workshops of the physician, hospitals have become even more the economic and professional heart of medical practice as the accelerating pace of advances in medical knowledge and technology has brought medical care more and more into the institutional setting. As highly advanced, scientific institutions, hospitals manifest the complexity and detached efficiency of a clinical laboratory. As human service organizations, they are charged with the emotions of life and death and of triumphs and tragedies.

Hospitals are also big business. Collectively, they are the second or third largest industry in the United States in terms of the number of people they employ. By far the largest part of the health care system, hospitals employ about three-fourths of all health care personnel and consume more than 40% of the nation's health expenditures. About 58% of all federal expenditures for health services and about 40% of all state and local government health expenditures are for hospital care (1).

Ironically, the magnitude of the hospital sector and the central role hospitals play in the delivery of health services, both reflecting the accomplishments of hospitals in making available the benefits of medical progress, now put hospitals at the root of many of the health care system's most pressing problems—cost inflation, duplication of services, bed surpluses, overemphasis on inpatient specialized services versus ambulatory primary care services, and depersonalization of care, among others (2,3). Further, as community or quasi-public institutions heavily dependent on public dollars, hospitals are open systems, subject to influence from outside, and therefore susceptible to the efforts of community groups and external agencies to use them as instruments of social change and health system reform (4,5). Little wonder hospitals always seem to be in the middle of things.

The hospital system is a mix of public and private for-profit and not-for-profit institutions. Hospitals range from small institutions in less populated communities and isolated rural areas providing basic medical care to large regional referral centers providing a comprehensive range of sophisticated, highly specialized services. One-third belong to multiunit hospital systems. Some hospitals provide only inpatient care, whereas others have expanded their role to include ambulatory care provided through emergency rooms and outpatient clinics. A number provide home care and other outreach services as well.

The purpose of this chapter is to characterize the hospital system in the United States, emphasizing major issues and trends. Because the character of the modern hospital reflects its past, the chapter begins with a discussion of the historical development of hospitals. The second section describes the hospital system as it exists today. The third section describes the internal organization of hospitals. The last section discusses a number of major issues confronting hospitals at the present time. It should be noted that the discussion of hospitals in this chapter focuses primarily on their inpatient role. Hospitals do play, however, a substantial role in the provision of outpatient care (6,7). The number of emergency room visits and the number of outpatient referrals for diagnostic and therapeutic services in community hospitals have been increasing four times faster than the number of admissions, and the ratio of outpatient visits to inpatient admissions in community hospitals is now almost six to one. Fully 43% of the nation's community hospitals have organized outpatient departments, and 94% have emergency departments (8). Chapter 5 discusses ambulatory care in the hospital setting.

HISTORICAL DEVELOPMENT OF HOSPITALS

The history of hospitals in this country (Fig. 6-1) can be traced back to the almshouses and pesthouses that existed in some form in almost all cities of moderate size by the mid-1700s (9,10). Almshouses, also called *poorhouses* or *workhouses* were established by city governments to provide food and shelter for the homeless poor, including many aged, chronically ill, disabled, mentally ill, and orphaned people. Medical care was a secondary function of the poorhouse, but in some facilities those who became ill were isolated in infirmaries where care, such as it was before the advent of modern medicine, was provided, typically by other residents. Not until the late 1800s did the infirmaries or hospital departments of city poorhouses break away to become medical care institutions on their own—the first public hospitals.

Pesthouses were operated by local governments as isolation or quarantine stations in seaports where it was necessary to isolate people who contracted contagious diseases aboard ship. During epidemics, these institutions were used to isolate victims of cholera, smallpox, typhus, and yellow fever. Their primary purpose was to control the spread of infectious diseases by removing infected individuals from the community. As in almshouses, medical care was a secondary function—in this case, secondary to protecting the community from outbreaks of contagious diseases. Pesthouses were often established during epidemics and discontinued or closed down when the threat of disease subsided. These institutions were the predecessors of the contagious disease and tuberculosis hospitals that later emerged.

Almshouses and pesthouses were maintained for the poor and the homeless— and were avoided by everyone else. These institutions were dismal places: crowded, unsanitary, and poorly heated and ventilated. Nutrition was often inadequate, nursing care incompetent, and separation of different types of residents

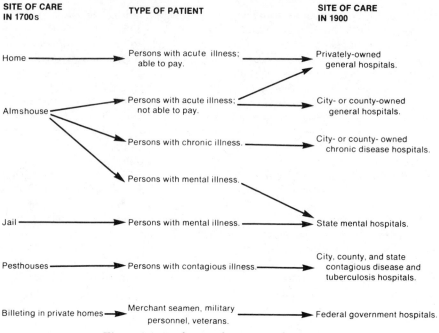

Figure 6-1. Evolution of institutional care sites.

minimal. Contagious persons, the disabled, the dying, and the insane were often crowded together. Cross-infection was rampant and mortality high. Persons who were able were cared for at home or in the homes of neighbors.

The first community-owned or voluntary hospitals in this country were established in the late 1700s and early 1800s, often at the urging of influential physicians trained in Europe who needed facilities to practice obstetrics and surgery in the manner in which they had been taught, and also to provide preceptor-type instruction for medical students. These early hospitals depended upon philanthropy, and contributions were solicited from both private citizens and the local government. Voluntary hospitals generally preceded both religious and public hospitals in the United States, representing a departure from patterns in England and Europe. Voluntary hospitals admitted both indigent and paying patients. For example, in its first year of operation (1751), the Pennsylvania Hospital admitted 24 paying patients and 40 poor patients. These hospitals were supported by community contributions and philanthropy, rather than by a church or the state. Except in the largest cities, where the concentration of poor was too great, the early voluntary hospitals cared for people in their communities who were unable to pay on a charitable basis, drawing on philanthropy and donations of time by members of the medical staff (9, 11).

The first hospitals of this type were the Pennsylvania Hospital, Philadelphia, 1751; New York Hospital, New York City, 1773; Massachusetts General Hospital, Boston, 1816; and New Haven Hospital, New Haven, Connecticut, 1826. Additional voluntary hospitals were established in Savannah, Georgia, in 1830; Lowell, Massachusetts, in 1836; and Raleigh, North Carolina, in 1839. Voluntary hospitals cared for patients with acute illnesses and injuries, but did not admit persons with contagious diseases or mental illnesses. Isolation of these unfortunates from the rest of the community was seen as a governmental responsibility. Therefore, during the same period, a number of city, county, and state mental hospitals were established. These included hospitals in Williamsburg, Virginia, 1773; Lexington, Kentucky, 1817; Columbia, South Carolina, 1829; Worcester, Massachusetts, 1832; Augusta, Maine, 1834; Brooklyn, New York, 1838; and Boston, Massachusetts, 1839.

Although voluntary hospitals provided better accommodations and care for the sick than the poorhouses that preceded them, the efficacy of care improved little, and it was not until the late 1800s that hospitals became accepted by persons of all economic strata as the best setting for the care of serious illness and injury. Before that time, most people who became ill were cared for at home. In 1873, there were only 178 hospitals with 35,604 beds in the United States. By 1909, the number of hospitals had increased to 4,359, with 421,065 beds; and by 1929, to 6,665 hospitals with 907,133 beds. This rapid growth in the number of hospitals was brought about by advances in medical science that rapidly transformed the hospital's role from a custodial institution in which to isolate and shelter the poor to a curative institution in which communities concentrated their health care resources in support of the practicing physician for the benefit of all (11,12).

Forces Affecting the Development of Hospitals

Four major developments in health care were particularly significant in transforming hospitals into the institutions of today: Advances in medical science increased the efficacy and safety of hospitals; the development of technological sophistication and specialization necessitated the institutionalization of much medical care; the development of professional nursing brought about more humane treatment of patients; and advances in medical education added teaching and research to the hospital's role (9,11,13,14).

Advances in Medical Science.   Most notable in terms of their impact on hospitals were the discovery of anesthesia and the rapid advances in surgery that followed, and the development of the germ theory of disease and the subsequent discovery of antiseptic and sterilization techniques. By the early 1800s, enough was known about anatomy and physiology so that surgeons were able to perform a variety of fairly complex surgical procedures. However, the inability to deaden pain meant that surgery had to be carried out with extreme speed. In addition, infections from surgery were common. Ether was first used as an anesthetic in surgery by Long in 1842, and then by Morton in 1846, and its use then spread rapidly. Great advances in the efficacy of surgery followed.

Before the formulation of the germ theory of disease, a few scientists, most notably Holmes in the United States and Semmelweis in Vienna, had observed and reported that fever, infection, and mortality could be reduced through cleanliness. Both concluded that childbed fever, which was the cause of high maternal mortality, was an infection transmitted by doctors, midwives, and medical students to women in labor. In 1861, Pasteur proved that bacteria were living, reproducing microorganisms that could be carried by air or on clothes and hands. It became clear that germs were the cause rather than the result of infection and could be destroyed by chemicals and heat. Lister built on Pasteur's work, and in 1867 introduced carbolic acid spray in operating rooms as an antiseptic to keep air and incisions clean. In 1886, steam sterilization was introduced, providing a means of freeing medical equipment from microorganisms. Surgical infection rates fell. Advances in surgery led to the need for skilled preoperative and postoperative care and operating room facilities, which could be provided only in hospitals. By 1900, 40% of all hospitalizations were for surgery.

Development of Specialized Technology.   By the late 1800s, medical technology began to proliferate. The first hospital laboratory opened in 1889, and x-ray films were first used for medical diagnosis in 1896. These developments greatly increased the diagnostic effectiveness of hospitals. The discovery of blood types in 1901 made blood transfusions safe; the electrocardiogram (EKG) was first used in 1903 and the electroencephalogram (EEG) in 1929. In addition to increasing the efficiency of medical care, these advances in technology affected the site and the organization of care. Since the tools of the new technology could no longer be carried around in the doctor's black bag, hospitals became the central resource where the equipment, facilities, and personnel required by modern medicine were housed. In addition, since one person could no longer be competent in all areas of medical practice, specialization began to occur within medicine, and new professional and technical occupations began to emerge. Again the hospital became a convenient place where physicians and support personnel came together to provide patient care.

Development of Professional Nursing.   Humane treatment of patients awaited the development of professional nursing. Before the late 1800s, the only humane nursing care was provided by Catholic sisters and Protestant deaconnesses, who were dedicated to caring for patients and who were fairly well trained. Some religious orders established their own hospitals, and occasionally they were called upon by city officials to provide nursing services in public institutions. Almshouses used untrained female residents to provide nursing care, and most hospitals relied on poorly paid, unskilled labor.

The transformation of nursing into a profession is credited to Florence Nightingale, who completed 4 months of nurses' training in a deaconness school in Germany. In 1854, Nightingale and 38 nurses were sent by the British government to Crimea to take charge of nursing care for wounded soldiers. The nurses found conditions deplorable and instituted cleanliness and sanitation, dietary reforms, simple but humane care, discipline, and organization. As a result, mortality dropped dramatically. Upon her return to England, Nightingale wrote of her experiences in Crimea and on the contributions of sanitation to the recovery of wounded and ill patients. In 1860, she founded the Nightingale School for Nursing in England.

In the United States, President Abraham Lincoln called upon the Catholic sisterhoods to provide nursing care for the wounded during the Civil War, but more nurses were needed. Dorothea Dix was appointed Superintendent of Nursing for the Union Army. She began a recruitment program and encouraged a 1-month hospital training program for new nurses. By the end of the war, there were 2,000 lay nurses in the country. The first permanent schools of nursing were established at Bellevue Hospital, New Haven Hospital, and Massachusetts General Hospital in 1873. Although there was some initial reluctance on the part of hospital administrators and trustees to establish nursing schools, the benefits of good nursing soon became apparent. In addition, student nurses provided better care and were less expensive than the untrained women previously employed to do this work. By 1883, there were 22 nursing schools and 600 graduates; by 1898, these totals had grown to 400 schools with 10,000 graduates.

Advances in nursing contributed to the growth of hospitals in two ways. The first was increased efficacy of treatment; cleanliness, nutritious diets, and formal treatment routines all contributed to patients' recovery. Second, considerate, skilled patient care made hospitals acceptable to all people, not just the poor. The public's fear of hospitals began to give way to an attitude of confidence and respect.

Advances in Medical Education.   Changes in medical education brought about by the Flexner Report in 1910 had a major impact on the development of hospitals. Before 1900, there was great variation in the nature and quality of medical education. There were no standards of academic training for physicians. Most medical schools were proprietary and were not connected with universities. They were dominated by influential practitioners, and most instruction was through didactic (often unscientific) lectures. Apprenticeship practices varied greatly. There was little clinical or laboratory instruction and little research.

The Flexner Report led to changes in the content and methods of instruction to emphasize the scientific basis of medicine. The standards of education established by the Flexner Report were widely accepted by both the profession and the public; as a result, schools that did not meet the standards were forced to close. State laws were established requiring graduation from a medical school accredited by the American Medical Association as the basis for a license to practice medicine. A 4-year course of study at a medical school based in a university became standard, as did clinical training in the wards of a hospital.

These changes expanded the role of the hospital to include education and research as well as patient care. The hospital's role in education became even more prominent as specialization in medicine led to a proliferation of internships and residencies in the 1920s and 1930s. The requirements of medical education necessitated the expansion of hospital facilities and services and the addition of equipment and personnel. Hospitals were called upon to assume a greater responsibility for coordinating and organizing these resources. Quality of care improved through advances in medical education, especially for patients with complex and serious illnesses. On the other hand, specialization led to a fragmentation of care among different physician specialists and ancillary personnel and a lack of interest in chronic, routine, and other "uninteresting" medical conditions.

Thus, the growth of hospitals in the United States was a direct result of advances in medical science that made hospitals effective and safe. These advances, particularly the discovery of sulfa drugs in the mid-1930s and antibiotics in the mid-1940s, changed the prevalent causes of death from acute, infectious diseases to the diseases of old age, particularly heart disease, cancer, and stroke. Hospitals have not been quick to respond to the health care problems of an aging population. Their resources continue to be concentrated on curable, short term illnesses that respond quickly to medical treatment, rather than on chronic, long term illnesses which must be managed over long periods of time. Hospitals are just now beginning to expand their role to include extended or skilled nursing care units, inpatient or outpatient rehabilitation programs, day care, home care, and other nontraditional services (15–17).

Growth of Health Insurance.   Another factor that has significantly affected the development of hospitals is the growth of health insurance. Private insurance for hospital care grew rapidly, especially between 1940 and 1960, increasing both the proportion of the population with insurance and the adequacy and scope of coverage. Today, the out-of-pocket cost of hospital care at time of use is relatively modest for most people, because most of the bill is covered by some third-party purchaser—either government or private health insurance.

A variety of factors led to the growth of hospital insurance. From the consumer's perspective, of course, a hospital stay is expensive enough to warrant the purchase of insurance protection. The hospital industry's interest in insurance began with the Depression of the 1930s, when the number of patients who could not pay their bill increased markedly and hospital use declined. The financial solvency of many hospitals was threatened, and the number of hospitals dropped from 6,852 in 1928 to 6,189 in 1937. Further, a study of nonprofit hospitals in 1935 showed that total income was 3% less than total expenses. As a result, acting through the American Hospital Association, hospitals took the initiative in actively encouraging the development of hospital insurance plans, primarily Blue Cross (13,18). These developments are discussed in detail in Chapter 11.

The growth of health insurance has had a substantial impact on hospitals. First, ensuring the financial stability of hospitals, insurance subsequently provided the flow of funds that made possible the great expansion of facilities and services and the prompt implementation of new medical technology that have characterized the hospital industry since the end of World War II. Insurance also contributed to the increased demand for health services. Since hospital services are generally better covered by insurance than services provided outside the hospital, patients are reluctant to substitute less expensive out-of-hospital services. This attitude has resulted in a bias toward hospital use versus the use of ambulatory care programs, home care programs, or nursing care facilities as sources of care and a general overuse of expensive hospital services (19,20).

Another problem in the hospital industry can be traced at least partially to cost-based reimbursement, the method of payment used by Medicare, Medicaid, and most Blue Cross plans. Cost reimbursement does not provide hospitals with an incentive to contain costs. The result has been inefficiency, duplication of services, and overbuilding (21–23). On the other hand, cost reimbursement has enabled hospitals to keep up with advances in medical technology and demands from their communities and physicians for access to a broad range of services. A key public policy issue yet unresolved is how to balance the accessibility and costliness of hospital services.

Role of Government.   Government's role in the hospital industry has changed substantially over time in both form and level. During colonial times, government involvement was mainly at the local level through ownership of almshouses and pesthouses, and grants to help construct and support voluntary hospitals. State government limited its role to running contagious disease and mental hospitals, and the federal government to running hospitals for merchant seamen, military personnel, and veterans. Gradually, the forms of involvement have multiplied and the balance has shifted to the federal level.

The initial thrust of federal involvement began in 1935, with federal categorical grants-in-aid to state and local governments to assist in the establishment of traditional public health programs: public health departments, communicable disease programs, maternal and child health programs, and public assistance for specific groups such as crippled children, the aged, blind, and disabled, and poor families with dependent children. These programs were part of the general social reform movement that came about during the Depression with the recognition that state and local government and voluntary efforts were not sufficient to meet social needs.

Direct federal involvement in the hospital industry began in 1946 with the Hill-Burton (Hospital Survey and Construction) Act. Few hospitals had been constructed during the Depression and World War II, and by the end of the war, it was generally felt that a severe shortage of hospitals existed. The Hill-Burton program was enacted to help states and communities plan for and construct hospitals and other health facilities by providing federal grants on a matching basis to supplement funds raised at the community level. The act required states to define hospital service areas, inventory existing facilities, and identify areas of greatest need. The program then provided funds for construction in priority areas. Although the initial emphasis of the program was to provide funds for the construction of new hospitals, priorities changed over time from construction to modernization and from inpatient to outpatient facilities. Funds were available through the program for the construction of nursing homes as well.

The Hill-Burton program assisted in the construction of nearly 40% of the beds in the nation's short term general hospitals and was the major single factor in the increase in the nation's bed supply from 3.5 short term beds per 1,000 population in 1946 to 4.5 beds per 1,000 today. Another positive impact of the program is that hospital facilities are more evenly distributed across rural and urban areas and high and low income states than they would have been without the program. However, the program also contributed to the overbuilding of hospitals and to the preponderance of small rural hospitals existing today.

The survey requirements in the Hill-Burton Act introduced the concepts of planning and regionalization for the first time. In 1964 the act was amended to provide federal support for the establishment and operation of comprehensive health planning agencies. In 1974, Hill-Burton was replaced by the National Health Planning and Resources Development Act, as discussed in Chapter 12. However, the idea of a functionally differentiated, integrated, regionalized hospital system first envisioned in Hill-Burton has yet to be realized; indeed, one of the lessons of Hill-Burton is that bricks and mortar alone are not enough to change the behavior of physicians and hospitals. Another provision of the Hill-Burton Act, that facilities aided by the program provide community service in the form of "a reasonable volume of care to persons unable to pay," has only recently begun to be strictly enforced amid much confusion and finger pointing (24).

From assisting with the financing of hospital construction, the federal government's involvement in the hospital industry has expanded to financing the provision of care and regulating the construction, operation, and use of hospitals. Fifty-four percent of all hospital bills are now covered by government programs, primarily Medicare and Medicaid (25), which puts the federal government in a position to exercise a great amount of control over the operation of hospitals. The regulation of hospitals is discussed later in this chapter and in Chapter 12.

CHARACTERISTICS OF THE HOSPITAL SYSTEM

The hospital industry is complex and diverse, and therefore difficult to describe simply. However, hospitals can be classified generally in one of three ways: according to length of stay, according to the predominant type of service provided, and according to ownership (26). In terms of length of stay, the most common type of hospital is the short stay or short term hospital, in which most patients suffering from acute conditions require hospital stays of less than 30 days. The average length of stay in short term hospitals is between 7 and 8 days. In long term hospitals, most of which are chronic disease, psychiatric, or tuberculosis hospitals, the average length of stay ranges from 3 to 6 months (8).

The second method of classification is by type of service. Predominant is the general hospital offering a wide range of medical, surgical, obstetric, and pediatric services. Specialty hospitals, on the other hand, provide care for a specific disease or population group. Examples of specialty hospitals are children's hospitals, maternity hospitals, chronic disease hospitals, psychiatric hospitals, and tuberculosis hospitals. During the first part of the twentieth century, the number of specialty hospitals grew substantially in areas of emerging medical specialization such as eye, ear, nose and throat diseases, obstetrics, orthopedics, and rehabilitation. These hospitals were largely the result of philanthropists responding to the initiative of prestigious physician specialists who wanted to develop their own hospitals. Due to financial difficulties and advances in medical science that make general hospitals more appropriate and efficient, specialty hospitals are less common today. Most have either closed or converted to general hospitals (9,11).

The third method of classifying hospitals is according to form of ownership: government or public ownership, private for-profit (proprietary) ownership, and private not-for-profit (religious or voluntary) ownership.

Public Hospitals

Public hospitals are owned by agencies of federal, state, or local government. Federally owned hospitals are maintained primarily for special groups of federal beneficiaries: American Indians, merchant seamen, military personnel, and veterans. State governments have generally limited themselves to the operation of mental and tuberculosis hospitals, reflecting government's early role of protecting the healthy by isolating the insane and persons with contagious diseases from the rest of society. Most local government hospitals are short term general hospitals, and these institutions comprise 31% of the nation's short term hospitals and accommodate 20% of all admissions and 26% of all outpatient visits to short term hospitals (Table 6-1). Local government hospitals can be divided into two types. The first is city, county, or hospital district institutions, mostly small or moderate in bed size, with medical staffs comprised of private physicians and serving both indigent and paying patients. These hospitals tend to be located in small cities and towns. Their costs are met primarily through third-party reimbursement, and they receive little tax support. For all practical purposes, they function the same as community-owned hospitals. The second type is large city or county hospitals in major urban areas. These hospitals serve mostly the poor, near-poor, and minorities. They are generally staffed by salaried physicians, mostly residents. Most are affiliated with medical schools. Their costs usually exceed their patient revenues, and so their deficits must be made up through tax subsidies (27).

The large urban public hospitals play an important role in the health care system. They are the place of last resort for the poor, both because they care for all patients regardless of ability to pay and because they provide services that private hospitals cannot finance or do not wish to offer: alcohol and drug abuse treatment, psychiatric services, care for persons with chronic and communicable diseases, abortion and family planning services, and so forth. They are located in areas where health resources, especially private physicians, are in short supply, and their out-

TABLE 6-1. Hospitals, Beds, Admissions, and Outpatient Visits by Ownership and Type of Service, 1981

	Hospitals		Beds		Admissions		Outpatient Visits	
	Number	Percent	Number	Percent	Number	Percent	Number	Percent
Total—all hospitals	6,933	100	1,362,000	100	39,169,000	100	265,332,000	100
Federal	348	5	116,000	8	2,032,000	5	52,555,000	18
Nonfederal								
Psychiatric	549	8	200,000	15	558,000	1	4,976,000	2
Tuberculosis	11	1	2,000	0	8,000	0	44,000	1
Long term	146	2	35,000	3	77,000	1	1,028,000	1
Short term	5,879	84	1,001,000	74	36,494,000	93	206,729,000	78
Nongovernmental								
Not-for-profit	3,356	57	706,000	70	25,955,000	71	143,953,000	70
Investor-owned for-profit	729	12	88,000	9	3,239,000	9	9,961,000	5
State and local governments	1,794	31	213,000	21	7,299,000	20	52,816,000	25

SOURCE: *Hospital Statistics*. Chicago, American Hospital Association, 1982.

patient departments are the only accessible source of ambulatory care for many inner city residents. Large urban public hospitals average 10.2 outpatient visits per inpatient admission, compared to 5.5 outpatient visits per admission in privately owned hospitals. In addition, these hospitals play a major role in medical education; 70% are affiliated with a medical school and 75% offer residency training programs (8,28). More than half of all practicing physicians received at least some of their training in public hospitals.

It was thought that enactment of the Medicare and Medicaid programs would greatly reduce the demand on public hospitals by giving the aged and the poor the means to purchase care from other sources. The expected exodus did not occur, however, probably because the gatekeepers of the community hospitals, private practitioners, are in short supply in inner city areas. In addition, some of those who are located close enough to be accessible limited the number of welfare patients they would accept. Cultural and social barriers also discouraged the poor from approaching community hospitals. As a result, inpatient and outpatient use of public hospitals dipped only slightly in 1967, the first full year of operation of both Medicare and Medicaid, and then continued a steady upward climb that continues to this day (29,30).

Despite the increasing demand that large urban public hospitals are called upon to meet, their problems are great. Characteristically, these hospitals are old and outmoded. They tend to be underequipped, underfinanced, and understaffed. They have difficulty attracting physicians and rely heavily on interns, residents, and foreign-trained physicians. Their administration is constrained by the bureaucratic red tape and rigidity of city or county government. Public hospitals have responded to these difficulties in a variety of ways. Most are affiliated with medical schools to attract faculty as supervisory physicians and to facilitate the recruitment of residents. In some areas, a special agency or commission has been created to run the public hospital in order to buffer it from government bureaucracy. In some cases, the agency is completely separate from city or county government but is empowered by enabling legislation to borrow, issue bonds, and tax, much like a school district. A number of public hospitals are attempting to improve their position by becoming the source of highly specialized tertiary services such as burn care, neonatal intensive care, or kidney dialysis for the entire community. Other aspects of this strategy include opening the medical staff to private physicians, adding amenities, and improving facilities to encourage the physicians to bring their patients to the public hospital, at least for more specialized services (31,32).

For-Profit Hospitals

For-profit, investor-owned, or proprietary hospitals are operated for the financial benefit of the individual, partnership, or corporation that owns the institution. Around the turn of the century, more than one-half of the nation's hospitals were proprietary. Most of these hospitals had been established by one or a small group of physicians who wanted a place to hospitalize their own patients, and most were quite small. Gradually, these institutions were closed or sold to community organizations. Until 1972 the number of proprietary hospitals declined steadily, although this trend was reversed around 1960 as the better-situated proprietary hospitals expanded to meet population increases and as new proprietary hospitals, typically larger than those that were closing, were built (Table 6-2). As of 1981, proprietary hospitals comprised 12% of the nation's short term hospitals, with 9% of the beds and 5% of the outpatient visits (Table 6-1) (33,34).

TABLE 6-2. Characteristics of Proprietary Short Term Hospitals, United States, Selected Years

Year	Number of Hospitals	Number of Beds	Admissions
1950	1,218	42,000	1,661,000
1960	856	37,000	1,550,000
1970	769	53,000	2,031,000
1975	775	73,000	2,646,000
1980	730	87,000	3,165,000
1981	729	88,000	3,239,000

SOURCE: *Hospital Statistics*. Chicago, American Hospital Association, 1982.

The most significant trend over the past few years has not been the number of proprietary hospitals per se but rather the building or buying up of a substantial number of hospitals by large, investor-owned corporations to form multiunit, for-profit hospital systems. At present, the five largest investor-owned corporations own or lease about 380 hospitals, totaling 60,000 beds. These corporations manage another 200 hospitals totaling 26,000 beds—most of which are nonprofit hospitals— and the growth of management contracts is now more rapid than is the number of owned hospitals. It appears that both trends will continue, at least for the foreseeable future (35).

Investor-owned hospital corporations claim that they are able to earn a profit by operating their hospitals more efficiently than nonprofit hospitals. They point to the availability of management specialists, the application of modern management techniques, cost savings in construction and maintenance, economies of scale, and group purchasing as the key factors enabling them to keep costs down enough to make a profit and pay taxes without cutting quality. For-profit hospitals have also been able to respond promptly to population shifts because of their ability to raise capital quickly (36). Critics of for-profit hospitals claim that their profits are attributable to the practice of "cream skimming": admitting only patients with less serious medical conditions and patients who are able to pay the full costs of their hospitalization. By not admitting poorly insured patients, for-profit hospitals can avoid bad debts, which may run as high as 10% of total patient charges in nonprofit and public hospitals in certain locations. By not admitting seriously ill patients, for-profit hospitals can avoid providing expensive or unprofitable services, and few offer educational programs. The quality of care in for-profit hospitals has also been criticized. The lower employee-to-bed ratio in these hospitals, for example, is pointed to as an indicator of lower quality and less sophisticated services rather than more efficient management. Another criticism is that even if for-profit hospitals are more efficient, their cost savings are not passed on to patients. Rather, it is claimed that their charges are set at the same level as other hospitals in the community, whatever their costs. Also questioned is the extent to which for-profit hospitals are willing to push the physicians on their medical staffs to be aggressive and stringent about quality and use controls when they depend on these physicians for patients. However, this argument also applies to nonprofit hospitals (37).

There is little firm evidence to support these criticisms, however, or even to accurately compare for-profit and nonprofit hospitals, although one recent study found investor-owned hospitals to be slightly more costly than nonprofit hospitals and, because of higher markups, to charge considerably more (38). What cream skimming does occur is likely to be due more to where for-profit hospitals locate (e.g., in rapidly growing suburban areas) than to the actual turning away of patients who cannot pay. The refusal to admit patients with complex conditions requiring sophisticated services and the lack of high-cost, low-use specialized services are cited by for-profit hospitals as examples of the methods they use to avoid duplication by referring outpatients requiring costly services—long a goal of those who would reform the health care system. Although the poor reputation of the small, physician-owned, proprietary hospitals of the past was often well deserved, the new investor-owned hospital corporations are most concerned about how the community views their institutions. A slightly higher proportion of for-profit hospitals are accredited by the Joint Commission on Accreditation of Hospitals than comparable-sized nonprofit hospitals. It seems appropriate to conclude that the implications of the recent growth of investor-owned hospitals are still unclear. Perhaps the greatest challenge is to determine how for-profit and nonprofit hospitals can effectively and successfully coexist in a pluralistic system (39–41). It is more likely, however, that the increasingly competitive health care environment will make the relationship between the two quite strained.

Nonprofit Hospitals

Fifty-seven percent of the nation's short term hospitals are nonprofit or voluntary institutions owned and operated by community associations or religious organizations. These hospitals accommodate more than two-thirds of all short term hospital admissions and outpatient visits (Table 6-1).

Community Hospitals

Taken together, nonfederal short term hospitals, whether for-profit, nonprofit, or public, are commonly referred to as *community* hospitals because they are typically available to the entire community and meet most of the public's need for hospital services. Community hospitals represent more than 80% of the nation's hospitals, and they provide care for more than 90% of all patients admitted to hospitals each year and accommodate 79% of all outpatient visits. In 1981 there were 5,879 community hospitals with about 1,000,000 beds (Table 6-1). The average length of stay in these hospitals is 7.6 days, down from the jump to 8.4 days that occurred in 1967 and 1968 after Medicare and Medicaid went into effect. The steady decline in length of stay since then is presumably due in part to the emphasis placed on use review in hospitals.

The major role of community hospitals is to provide short term inpatient care for patients with acute illnesses and injuries. However, their outpatient role has been growing in importance as discussed in Chapter 5. In 1981, they recorded 77,853,000 emergency room visits, and 128,876,000 clinic or outpatient department visits and ancillary service visits by patients referred to departments such as laboratory, x-ray, or physical therapy for diagnostic or therapeutic procedures. Taken together, these three types of outpatient visits totaled 206,729,000, or 5.7 outpatient visits for every inpatient admission (8).

Community hospitals are feeling pressures to expand their roles even more to become true community health centers (3,15,16). The fundamental rationale is that these hospitals represent their community's collective investment in health resources, assembled in one place and financially supported by all. Hence, access to these resources should not be limited to patients who happen to need inpatient hospitalization. Community hospitals might also play a more central and substantial role in planning and coordinating the entire range of community health services, even those services provided by other agencies and organizations (42). For a variety of reasons, including a lack of physician interest, health insurance coverage biases, poor reimbursement, the small size of the average community hospital, and resistance by nursing homes and other community health agencies to hospital encroachment, hospitals have been slow to expand their roles. However, many hospitals, especially the larger institutions, have added services in areas such as ambulatory care, long term and rehabilitation care, mental health care, and home care, which indicate a movement in the direction of a broadening role (Table 6-3). It appears that the persistent rise in the public's use of community hospitals has finally peaked, motivating many hospitals to search for new services they might offer. Perhaps this development, more than the underlying rationale, will finally give impetus to the several-decades-old concept of the hospital as a community health center (43,44).

Almost one-half of all community hospitals have fewer than 100 beds, the average size being 169 beds in 1981 (8). Small hospitals tend to care for less seriously ill patients than larger hospitals. Their average length of stay is shorter and their care less intensive and less specialized. Small hospitals cannot support as broad a range of services as larger hospitals and find it difficult to keep up with developments in medical technology. They also cannot support the range of management specialists found in larger hospitals (45). Several hundred smaller hospitals have closed since the early 1970s, and an even greater number have become part of multiunit hospital systems. In fact, the rapid growth of multihospital systems, both for-profit and nonprofit, is the most significant trend in the hospital field today.

Multihospital Systems

A total of 256 multihospital systems, defined as corporations that own, lease, or manage two or more acute care hospitals, accounted for 1,877, or 32%, of the nation's community hospitals in 1981. These 1,877 system hospitals contain 351, 408, or 36%, of the nation's community hospital beds. Of the 256 multihospital systems, 113, or 44%, are Catholic; 19, or 7%, have other religious affiliations; 93, or 36%, are secular nonprofit; and 31, or 12%, are investor owned. Although representing only 12% of the nation's multihospital systems, the investor-owned systems tend to be large, averaging 24 hospitals and 3,144 beds per system, compared to only 5 hospitals and 1,129 beds per nonprofit system. As a result, investor-owned systems contain 40% of all system hospitals, representing 28% of all system beds (35,46).

Multihospital systems are growing at a rate of about 5–7% more hospitals and 3–4% more beds each year. Growth rates of this magnitude add up quickly. It is projected that more than half of the nation's community hospitals, representing about 40% of the acute beds, will be part of multihospital systems by 1990 (46).

Two fundamental motives seem to underlie the multihospital system movement that is so dramatically changing the character of the hospital sector—organizational survival and organizational growth. Survival applies to the free-standing, single-ownership institution and explains why such a hospital decides to give up its autonomy and become part of a system. Organizational growth, on the other hand, applies to the system itself and explains why it seeks to build, buy, lease, or manage additional hospitals. For the single institution, today's increasingly complex, fast-

TABLE 6-3. Trends in Selected Hospital Facilities and Services (Community Hospitals), United States, 1960, 1981

Facility or Service	Percent of Hospitals with Facility or Providing Service		
	1960	1981	
		All hospitals	300–400-bed hospitals
Ambulatory care			
Emergency service	91	94	98
Outpatient department	54	43	66
Outpatient hemodialysis	NA[a]	13	27
Outpatient psychiatry	NA	14	32
Outpatient rehabilitation	NA	34	60
Outpatient volume	(70,700,000 visits) (1962) (2.9 visits/admission)	(206,729,000 visits) (5.7 visits/admission)	
Inpatient care			
Intensive care unit (all)	10	8	18
Neonatal care unit	NA	4	9
Pediatric care unit	NA	35	69
Cardiac care unit	NA	72	95
Mixed/other	NA	11	12
Skilled nursing care unit	NA	1	1
Self-care unit	3		
Home care program	3	11	22

186

Long term care and rehabilitation			
Physical therapy	41	88	99
Occupational therapy	9	36	73
Skilled nursing care unit	NA	11	12
Inpatient rehabilitation unit	7(1962)	5	12
Outpatient rehabilitation unit	NA	34	60
Mental health care			
Inpatient unit	11	21	47
Outpatient unit	NA	14	32
Partial hospitalization program	NA	11	21
Emergency services	NA	30	54
Foster and/or home care	NA	2	4
Consultation and education	NA	23	45
Clinical psychologist	NA	25	48
Other			
Hospice	NA	8	18
Dental	27	48	68
Social work	15	78	98
Family planning	2(1962)	9	18
Abortion service[a]	NA	29	47
Alcohol/drug dependency	NA	12	22
Speech pathology	NA	43	74

SOURCE: *Hospital Statistics*. Chicago, American Hospital Association, 1982.

[a]NA—not available, not applicable, or none.

changing, demanding, and even hostile health care environment has made survival of the fittest a stark reality. Competition, financial pressures, regulation, and other external forces so weaken or threaten many solo institutions that they turn to systems for the strength to survive, albeit under different ownership. For the established systems, acquisition of additional hospitals is a means to grow—to add new services, enter new markets, establish new referral patterns, or build more financial and political power (35, 46–48).

Patterns of Financing and Ownership

Patterns of hospital financing and ownership differ from country to country. Most countries recognize health care as an essential service in which government should have a major role. In Great Britain and many other industrialized nations, government owns and operates most of the hospitals and employs the physicians who work in them. In other countries, the government limits its role to financing care provided by private hospitals and private practitioners, but in countries such as Canada, where some form of comprehensive national health insurance is in effect, hospitals operate primarily on public funds and hence are essentially controlled by the government. In the United States, government's role has essentially been limited to financing care for needy groups such as the aged and the poor. This role has grown, however, to the point where hospitals now receive 54% of their income from government sources (primarily Medicare and Medicaid). The rest comes from private health insurance (23%), direct payments by patients (11%), and philanthropy (2%) (25). In short, the United States has a pluralistic public-private financing system with largely privately owned hospitals. However, as the portion of hospital income financed by government has increased (from about 25% in 1960 to 54% today), so has the amount of regulation, as discussed in Chapter 12.

Government's limited role in the ownership of hospitals in the United States has been shaped by four major forces. First, the government was still relatively weak in the 1800s, when the short term hospital as it exists today was evolving as a result of advances in medical science. Innovations and progress generally came from the private sector. At that time, poverty was not so severe (or was not perceived as so severe) that the needy could not be taken care of through charity and philanthropy in private hospitals. It was generally believed that the private sector could provide care for the poor as well as for those who could pay. The exception was in major cities with large concentrations of the poor. There public hospitals were established to care for the needy.

Second, government responsibility for the public's health was viewed narrowly before the Depression of the 1930s and was limited mainly to public safety (i.e., protecting healthy citizens from persons with communicable diseases and mental illnesses), to providing care for special groups such as merchant seamen, military personnel, and veterans, and to assisting the needy. State governments operated communicable disease and mental hospitals; the federal government operated hospitals for its beneficiary groups; and city and county governments in large urban areas operated hospitals for the poor.

Third, our strong tradition of reliance on the private sector means that government becomes involved only when the private sector clearly fails to provide a critical service. For example, chronic disease, mental, and tuberculosis hospital care would have been difficult to finance privately. The long stays that used to prevail would have been expensive and not readily insurable. Hospitalization generally meant loss of one's job and income, especially since the incidence of hospital-ization for these conditions was greatest among the poor. As a result, these areas of care have traditionally fallen to the public sector. The private sector proved better able to finance short term hospital care through direct payments and private health insurance, and so the government's role has been supplementary. For example, the government helped to finance the construction of hospitals through the Hill-Burton program beginning in 1946, and helped to finance care for the groups that could not afford to pay, primarily the aged and the poor.

Fourth, government involvement has been resisted by the medical profession. Physicians represent a particularly powerful group in the United States, and they have long been concerned that government involvement in the health care system would compromise their economic and professional interests.

INTERNAL ORGANIZATION OF COMMUNITY HOSPITALS

From the outside, a community hospital appears as one organization with a clear goal of providing high quality patient care to which the efforts of the professional and technical groups working there are devoted. However, from the inside, it is apparent that there are at least two different organizations with two distinct sets of goals: the administrative organization, which is responsible for the efficient man-agement and operation of the institution as a whole; and the medical staff organiza-tion, which is responsible for the patient care provided by individual physicians. Further, there are three loci of authority within a hospital—the governing board, the medical staff, and the administration—and much balancing goes on between them (49,50). Each authority group has a distinct responsibility. The board is ulti-mately responsible for everything that goes on in the hospital, both administrative and professional. It oversees the operation of the hospital and carries out its respon-sibility in three ways. First, it adopts policies and plans to guide the hospital's operation. Second, it chooses and delegates responsibility for the day-to-day man-agement of the hospital to the hospital administrator and supervises his or her performance. Third, it appoints physicians to the medical staff, approves the med-ical staff's organization for governing itself and for supervising the professional activities of its members, and delegates responsibility to the medical staff for the provision of high quality patient care (51,52).

In practice, the three areas of authority are neither so clear nor so distinct. For example, it might seem that there is a clear distinction between governance and the medical staff's responsibility for patient care. Court decisions have made it clear, however, that the hospital as an institution has a corporate responsibility or legal liability for ensuring that patients receive high quality patient care. Therefore, the governing board must make sure that only qualified physicians practice in the hospital and that quality review mechanisms are established and working (53). However, only the medical staff has the expertise to assess the qualifications and care provided by physicians. Although the medical staff is clearly subordinate to the governing board in terms of authority for the affairs of the institution, physicians are independent of strict control by the board because the board does not share their expert knowledge and special skill.

Employees of the hospital working in clinical areas often find themselves in the middle when physicians' actions conflict with hospital policy. Legally, they should follow hospital policy; however, professionally they are expected to follow the physicians' orders regarding patient care, and their day-to-day working relationships are with the medical staff (54). The independence of physicians from the hospital is emphasized because most are in private practice and not employed by the institution. On the other hand, physicians must have access to a hospital to practice modern medicine, and only the governing board has the power to grant them the privilege of practicing there. This unique relationship between physicians and hospitals is not without stresses and strains, and it makes the governance and management of hospitals a challenging responsibility (55,56).

The distinction between adopting policies to guide hospital operations and managing operations on a day-to-day basis is not always clear either. Problems arise when the governing board becomes involved in administrative matters, such as acting directly on employee grievances that come to their attention rather than referring them to the administration. On the other hand, the administration may make decisions that go beyond board policies. Thus, the community hospital is not a united front, but rather an organization with at least two separate lines of authority, administrative and medical, and with some ambiguity between what is governance and what is management. Power at the top is shared, both because the board depends on the expertise of the medical staff and because of the independent contractor status of physicians. Administrators are also becoming more and more influential because of their expertise in dealing with the increasingly complex operational and regulatory issues confronting hospitals (57). Since the internal powers do not always agree among themselves on priorities and programs, hospitals often experience internal tensions and find it difficult to respond in a systematic way to environmental conditions and changing community needs.

The Governing Board

The governing board of the community hospital has evolved in function and structure as the hospital itself has developed new roles. During the late 1800s and early 1900s, when advances in medical science were transforming hospitals from custodial institutions for the sick poor to sources of effective and safe care for the entire community, board members were mostly wealthy benefactors who had made substantial donations to establish and equip the hospital and to meet its deficits. The primary function of the board at that time was trusteeship, that is, preserving the assets they and others like them donated. The trustees' job was seen as providing the facilities and equipment and medical staff needed to care for their patients. There was little trustee involvement in medical matters. The administrator was essentially a clerk, and administrative duties were divided among the board members (9).

After World War I, the complexity and size of hospitals grew to the point where board members could no longer administer and financially support the hospital. Business managers were hired to handle administrative and financial matters; the business manager, along with the superintendent of nurses, reported to the board, and the board coordinated work between the two. As the complexity of the hospital and the competence of managers increased, the business manager gradually assumed responsibility for overseeing nursing and all other departments as well, so that only one person reported directly to the board. The manager's title became

Superintendent. The board of trustees moved into an oversight role, relinquishing day-to-day management matters to the Superintendent (58).

The governing board's role changed further as hospitals continued to grow, as management decisions took on greater complexity and significance, and as philanthropy yielded to patient revenue as the primary source of financial support. The board's role became overall policy making and planning, and board membership was used to augment and supplement the skills of the administrative staff. Boards began to be composed of fewer philanthropists and more individuals with specific management skills, such as business executives, attorneys, bankers, architects, contractors, and so forth (58,59). Even so, community hospital boards remained relatively closed to external scrutiny, with their membership essentially comprised of self-perpetuating groups of community influentials (60–62). Board decisions were mostly in the areas of finance, personnel, and physical plant, their areas of expertise, and boards typically deferred to the medical staff on medical and patient care matters, delegating fully the responsibility for the qualifications and quality of care provided by the medical staff.

During the 1960s, four major factors caused further changes in the governing board's role: 1) continuing advances in medical science, the proliferation of medical technology, and the rapid growth in the size and sophistication of hospitals gave rise to public concern about the cost of hospital care, while making the hospital even more central in the delivery of health care and valuable to the public; 2) public expectations about the hospital's responsibility to the community changed, so that hospitals began to be viewed as community resources with a definite obligation to respond to community needs; 3) regulation of hospital construction, costs, quality, and use, as well as labor relations, became more and more stringent, particularly following the establishment of Medicare and Medicaid; and 4) the Darling legal case established the concept of corporate or institutional responsibility for ensuring the quality of patient care (55,63,64).

As a result of these forces, the governing board's role broadened and became even more demanding (65,66). Boards grew active in environmental surveillance, becoming knowledgeable about community concerns and external trends and interpreting their significance for the hospital (67,68). External pressures forced hospitals to reexamine their priorities and programs, and boards found it necessary to provide clearer direction and stronger leadership in long range planning. Boards have also assumed an active role in seeing that community concerns and interests are brought into hospital decision making, and many have expanded community representation within their membership (69,70). The board has found itself in the role of balancing and mediating between the demands and pressures on the hospital from the community and external agencies, on the one hand, and from the medical staff, employees, and other internal groups, on the other (71). Finally, boards have been forced to take a more active role in quality control, rather than abdicating this responsibility to the medical staff. Although the function of quality monitoring is still delegated to the medical staff, the staff is now being held accountable for how well this function is carried out. The board is responsible for ensuring that the mechanisms for evaluating the credentials of physicians and monitoring the care they provide are established and working. Courts have held the board and the hospital responsible in malpractice cases in which reasonable precautions were not taken to ensure 1) careful selection of the medical staff; 2) establishment of high standards of care; 3) monitoring and supervision of care; and

4) enforcement of policies, rules, and regulations. In practice, board control over medical staff performance remains limited and depends more on the attitudes of the medical staff, the character of hospital-medical relations, and moral suation than on formal sanctions such as suspending or terminating a physician's privileges, an action that is very rare.

As governing boards became more actively involved in medical and patient care matters, both in determining the hospital's role and relationships with other institutions and in overseeing quality assurance mechanisms, physicians began to seek more involvement in hospital planning and policymaking. At the same time, boards felt a greater need for more direct physician participation in their deliberations (72,73). As a result, more and more boards have added physicians to their membership, although some argue against this as a conflict of interest (74). At the present time, more than half of all community hospital boards include physicians (75,76). Less frequent but emerging is the tendency of the administrator to serve on the board, generally with a change in title to President or Executive Vice President, in a corporate type of structure (68).

Today, governing boards are being challenged and scrutinized as never before. They are being called upon to demonstrate their effectiveness in ensuring that the hospitals they govern meet community needs and provide high quality care while at the same time functioning efficiently within a complex structure of guidelines and regulations, all in an environment of constant change. Not all boards are up to this task. Boards have been criticized as too inward-looking, passive, uninformed, reluctant to get involved in medical matters, and unwilling to change the status quo. It appears, however, that the pressures discussed above are causing boards to take active steps to broaden and strengthen their membership, educate themselves more fully, and streamline their structure so that they will be better equipped to provide the strong leadership that will be required in the future (77–79).

Hospital Administration

Hospital administration has grown in importance and status as hospitals have grown in size and sophistication (58,80,81). The job of implementing board policy and responsibility for the day-to-day management and supervision of the hospital is delegated by the board to the hospital administrator. The administrator has responsibility for managing the hospital's finances, acquiring and maintaining equipment and facilities, hiring and supervising hospital personnel, and coordinating hospital activities. The breadth of the administrator's responsibility is illustrated by a typical community hospital organization chart (Fig. 6-2). A key aspect of the administrator's job is to coordinate and serve as the channel of communication among the governing board, medical staff, and hospital departments. Another is planning for the future development of the hospital's services. Large hospitals have several assistant administrators who are responsible for nursing, professional services, support services, and hospital finance.

In addition to financial, personnel, and physical plant matters, administration plays an important role in patient care. For example, administration is responsible for coordinating the patient care departments with each other and with the support departments, ensuring that they are adequately equipped and staffed and technically up-to-date, and ensuring that they function smoothly. Administration must make sure that physician orders for the treatment of patients are carried out correctly and promptly by hospital personnel, but also that orders do not conflict with

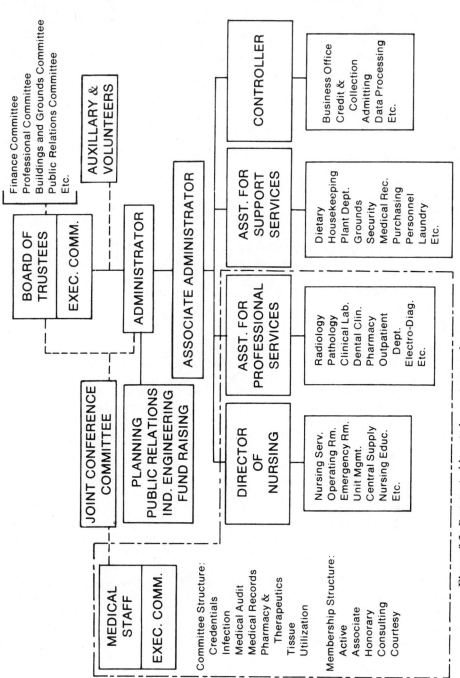

Figure 6-2. Prototypical hospital organization chart.
SOURCE: Reprinted with permission from Chamber of Commerce of the United States, *A Primer for Hospital Trustees*, Washington, DC, 1974.

governing board policies or hospital rules. The administrator is also actively involved in planning for new patient care services and in ensuring that the hospital meets accreditation, licensure, and other standards. Because the medical staff is not employed by the hospital, establishing a cooperative working relationship with its members is essential for the administrator to handle effectively the many tasks that involve both administration and medical questions. Finally, administration acts as the liaison with the community and with external agencies, both bringing information from these sources into hospital decision making and planning, and representing the hospital to these outside parties. Because of the growing impact of external and regulatory pressures on hospitals, this boundary-spanning role has become one of the most important aspects of the administrator's job. Hospital administration has advanced rapidly as a profession. Schulz and Johnson (82) describe the transition as moving from business manager (1920s–1940s), to coordinator (1950s–1960s), and now to corporate chief (with full authority for directing all aspects of the hospital's operation) and management team leader (promoting participative decision making by board, medical staff, nursing staff, and administrative representatives). Administrators are now full participants in the development of policies and plans, as well as in their implementation and in the external as well as internal affairs of the hospital (83–85).

Hospital Medical Staff

The governing board delegates responsibility for the provision of high quality patient care to the medical staff, which is formally organized to carry out this responsibility and is accountable to the board for it (86). Unlike many advanced countries, where hospital medical staffs are composed of salaried physicians, the medical staffs of community hospitals in the United States are composed mostly of private practitioners who are not employees of the hospital. The relationship between the hospital and its medical staff is a mutually dependent and sometimes stressful one. The hospital is dependent upon the medical staff to admit and care for patients and to monitor the quality of patient care. In a sense, the clients of the hospital are the physicians, since it is they who admit patients, decide how long the patients will stay, and order hospital services. On the other hand, physicians are dependent upon hospitals because to practice modern medicine they must have access to the diagnostic and therapeutic services of the hospital on behalf of their patients. This is particularly true of specialties such as obstetrics and surgery. Thus, a quid pro quo relationship exists; physicians agree to abide by hospital policies and medical staff rules and to devote time to the medical staff's quality monitoring activities (in the past, they also contributed time to care for patients who could not pay), in return for the privilege of using the community's hospital to care for their private patients (87–89).

Different categories of appointment to the medical staff carry different privileges and responsibilities (90):

Active medical staff members have full hospital privileges and provide most of the medical care in the hospital. They are responsible for the administrative activities of the organized medical staff. They can vote, hold office, and serve on committees.

Associate medical staff members consist of physicians new to the hospital. After a probationary period of 1 or 2 years, during which their work is closely watched, associate staff physicians are considered for advancement to the active medical staff. They may serve on some hospital and medical staff committees, but they cannot hold office.

Courtesy medical staff is composed of physicians who are eligible for active membership on the staff but who admit patients to the hospital only occasionally (usually because they are on the active staff of another hospital). They are not involved in any administrative functions.

Consulting medical staff are physicians who are recognized for their professional expertise and who are willing to act as consultants to the hospital's medical staff, although they practice primarily in other hospitals.

House staff are the interns and residents. They function under the supervision of attending physicians but are employees of the hospital.

In carrying out its delegated responsibility for ensuring the quality of care, the medical staff governs itself, establishes qualifications for appointment to the staff and for clinical privileges, establishes standards of care and rules and regulations to guide the provision of care, and supervises the professional performance of its members. These duties are accomplished within the medical staff bylaws, which set forth the form, functions, and responsibilities of the medical staff. The bylaws must be approved by both the medical staff and the governing board (90–92).

The administrative head of the medical staff organization is the chief of staff. The chief of staff is responsible for 1) acting as a liaison between the governing board, the administrator, and the medical staff; 2) chairing the executive committee of the medical staff and serving as an ex-officio member of all committees and usually of the governing board; 3) establishing medical staff committees and appointing their members; 4) enforcing governing board policies; 5) enforcing medical staff bylaws, rules, and regulations; 6) maintaining standards of medical care in the hospital; and 7) providing for continuing education for the medical staff (90).

Although the chief of staff is usually elected by the medical staff for a 1- or 2-year term, this position is also in a sense part of the hospital's administrative structure, directly accountable to the hospital's governing board. As such, the chief of staff is looked to by the board for advice on medical matters, as well as for assurance that the medical staff's responsibilities are being carried out. Administration of medical staff affairs can be a time-consuming job, but in most community hospitals the chief of staff fills this role in addition to pursuing a busy private medical practice. Larger hospitals often hire a full-time salaried medical director to carry out many of the administrative duties of the chief of staff; this idea is spreading although not without controversy (93–95).

Most of the organizational responsibilities of the medical staff are carried out by committees (96, 97). The *executive committee* is the key administrative and policy-making body of the medical staff. It governs the activities of the medical staff, and all other committees are advisory to it. It is composed of the chief of staff, the chiefs of the clinical departments, and members at large elected by the active medical staff. The *joint conference committee* is the formal liaison between the governing board and medical staff, and includes members from both groups plus the administrator. This committee is a forum for discussing medico-administrative matters of mutual concern. The *credentials committee* reviews the qualifications of applicants to the medical staff and makes recommendations regarding appointments, annual reappointments, and clinical privileges. Recommendations are transmitted through the executive committee of the hospital's governing board, which has final decision-making authority regarding medical staff membership and privileges.

A second type of medical staff committee advises or oversees specific functional areas or departments; examples include emergency room, nursing, pharmacy, special care, and disaster committees. A third type of committee is the evaluative or quality assurance committee responsible for monitoring the patient care provided by individual physicians. These include medical audit, use review, and tissue committees. Finally, a continuing education committee plans educational programs for the medical staff. In larger hospitals, most of these committee functions are duplicated in each clinical department.

There is a small but growing body of empirical evidence in support of the presumption that the structure of the medical staff affects quality and other aspects of hospital performance (98). Roemer and Friedman (99) studied the extent to which the degree of structure of the medical staff influences the costliness, quality, and scope of hospital services, and found that a relationship does exist. They concluded that a fairly highly structured medical staff organization functions better than a low or moderate structure. They found that effectiveness is enhanced by a core of full-time salaried physicians within the medical staff, a comprehensive department and committee structure, clearly specified policies, rules, and regulations, and thorough documentation of medical staff activities. This type of organization pattern offers the private physicians who use the hospital the benefits of full-time hospital based physicians who provide administrative support and supervision and take the leadership in developing standards of care and educational programs. An interesting finding is that a core of full-time salaried physicians tends to stimulate the other physicians to take their quality monitoring responsibilities more seriously. The mix of both salaried and private practice physicians tends to provide an environment conducive for change and improvement. It is apparent that hospitals are moving slowly, but surely, and not without conflict, toward more highly structured forms of medical staff organization that can be held more directly accountable for quality. At the same time, medical staff officers are being asked to participate more actively in governing board and management decision making. Clearly, the hospital-physician relationship of the future will be closer than in the past (100–102).

TRENDS AND ISSUES IN THE HOSPITAL INDUSTRY

The high and persistently climbing cost of hospital care is of such great concern that it is central to much public policy in the health sector. The hospital cost inflation rate since the mid-1960s has been almost three times the general economy-wide inflation rate (see Chapter 11). The key question is how to slow the trend. The special problems small and rural hospitals have in attracting resources, keeping up with advances in medicine, and maintaining their financial viability raise questions about their future role and about how they should relate to larger institutions offering the specialized services they are not able to provide. A significant trend in the hospital industry is the growth of unions, particularly professional unions, and this raises questions about the impact of collective bargaining on patient care as well as about employee-employer relations. Another trend that has had great influence on hospitals is regulation: External regulatory agencies and third-party insurers are exerting more and more control over hospitals. These trends, their impact on hospitals, and the issues they raise are discussed in this section.

Hospital Cost Inflation

The nation's health expenditures have been increasing dramatically, with hospital spending leading the way. On a per capita basis, hospital expenditures increased from $50 per person in 1960 to $500 per person in 1981. This $500 was double the per capita spending for physicians' services, more than five times what was spent for drugs or nursing home care, and more than six times what was spent for dental services. Because the cost of hospital care has been increasing so much faster than the other elements of health care, hospitals are consuming a larger and larger share of the nation's health expenditures. About 40% of our health expenditures now go for hospital care compared to about 33% in 1960 (1).

To explain the causes of the dramatic cost inflation in the hospital sector, total hospital spending can be broken down into its parts (103–105). In 1965, $9 billion was spent for care in community hospitals. By 1975, this figure had reached $39 billion, a 328% increase in 10 years. About 5% of the $30 billion increase was due to growth in the population. Another 7% was due to increases in the per capita use of hospitals: the use rate rose from 1,072 days of hospital care per 1,000 population in 1965 to 1,218 days in 1975. About 36% was due to general inflation that affected the prices of all goods and services throughout the economy. The largest component of the cost increase, however, was attributable to changes in the nature of hospital output (i.e., in the intensity, scope, sophistication, and quality of hospital care), which in turn caused hospitals to employ more and better labor inputs (accounting for 24% of the 1965–1975 expenditure increase) and more and better nonlabor inputs (accounting for the remaining 28%). In short, expenditures for hospital care have increased because more people are using hospitals more; because hospital care is more intensive and sophisticated; and because, like other businesses, hospitals must pay more for the equipment, personnel, and supplies they need (8,106). Not answered in this breakdown of the cost increase are questions about how efficiently hospitals operate and about how much of the care they provide might be provided in less expensive settings.

A wide variety of factors has caused the increase in the amount of hospital care people use (19,107). First, availability: More than 550 new community hospitals have been built since 1960, and the bed supply has increased 25% from 3.6 beds per 1,000 population in 1960 to 4.5 beds per 1,000 population today (8). Second, advances in medical science have brought new diagnostic and therapeutic services to hospitals and increased their effectiveness in dealing with injury and illness. Third, physicians are trained in sophisticated hospitals, and they learn to rely on the hospital's specialized equipment and personnel to back them up in caring for patients. Fourth, the population is aging such that the proportion of the population over age 65 increased from 9% in 1960 to almost 12% today, and the aged use about 3.5 times as much hospital care as the younger population. Another factor is urbanization: Hospitals are more accessible to people who reside in urban areas. In addition, because of the high mobility of the population, many people do not have a family physician. Instead, they turn to the hospital emergency room and the outpatient department as substitutes.

Perhaps the most important factor affecting hospital use, however, is the increase in the affluence, education, and sophistication of the population, and the resulting increase in people's ability and inclinations to seek health care. Facilitating this trend is the growth of private health insurance and the enactment of public financing programs for the aged and the poor. Insurance has removed much of the strain of paying for hospital care: Now only 10.8% of hospital bills are paid directly out of pocket by patients (1). In addition to generally increasing hospital use, insurance has biased patterns of use toward the hospital, because the costs of services tend to be covered better by insurance if the services are provided in a hospital rather than in a physician's office or nursing home (20).

Apart from the more frequent use of hospitals is the fact that the costs per inpatient day and outpatient visit have been increasing, both because of economy-wide inflation and because the care provided by hospitals is changing over time (108). Hospital services are continually increasing in intensity, scope, and sophistication as a result of advances in medical science and community and physician preferences to have available in their local hospital the widest possible range of the most up-to-date services. As a result, the cost per inpatient day increased over nine times between 1960 and 1981, from about $30 per day to $284 per day. The average hospital stay now costs more than $2,000 (8).

Regarding intensity, patients today receive more laboratory, x-ray, and other diagnostic and therapeutic services than patients who were treated for the same conditions a few years ago (19,105). Several factors have contributed to the increased intensity. Advances in medical science have made more diagnostic and therapeutic procedures available, and both patients and physicians want to take advantage of all that modern medicine has to offer. The nature of physician training in sophisticated hospitals may lead them to order more procedures. Another factor is the fear of malpractice suits, which leads to defensive medical practice: Physicians are inclined to order the extra laboratory test or x-ray procedure "just to make sure." The shortening length of stay has resulted in patients receiving more services each day than if the same services were spread over a longer period of time. Many people believe that another factor is that physicians are not directly affected financially by the costs of the services they order on behalf of their patients. A most important factor again is hospital insurance, which has led patients to want the best of care regardless of costs.

Regarding the broadening scope of services offered by community hospitals, advances in medical science have created new diagnostic and treatment technology not dreamed of a few years ago. Fetal monitoring, diagnostic radioisotope procedures, computed tomography, open heart surgery, organ transplants, microscope surgery, radiation therapy, renal dialysis, and so forth require expensive equipment, expensive facilities, and skilled personnel. Communities and physicians alike have come to expect a wide range of services to be available in their local hospitals. As a result, there has been an increase in the scope and sophistication of services being offered by even relatively small community hospitals serving limited populations (109).

The increased investment by hospitals in equipment and facilities is reflected by a substantial increase in assets per bed. In 1960, the capital investment per bed in community hospitals was about $17,000. This figure is now well over $100,000. Expenditures for equipment, facilities, and supplies have been increasing faster than expenditures for personnel. As a result, nonpayroll expenses as a portion of total expenses increased from 38% in 1960 to 43% in 1981. However, the use of personnel has increased as well, from 2.3 employees per patient in 1960 to 4.0 in 1981, an increase of more than 70%. In addition, the skill levels of hospital personnel has increased, and more hospitals are employing physicians. The average hospital salary increased 350% between 1960 and 1981, from $3,239 to $14,520 (8).

Another cost increasing factor is debt financing of capital projects. In the past, hospital construction projects were financed mostly by community fund-raising drives, philanthropy, and government programs such as Hill-Burton. As these sources of capital declined in importance, hospitals have been forced to borrow a higher proportion of the funds needed for capital projects, adding interest expense to the cost of these projects (110).

A final and increasingly significant cost-increasing factor is the administrative costs of complying with regulations. Programs now exist to regulate hospital construction, rates and reimbursement, quality and use, plant safety, and labor relations, to name a few (as discussed in Chapters 12 and 13). The array of complex and often conflicting requirements these agencies impose on hospitals contributes substantially to increased costs. The current situation is approaching the point where the solution is becoming part of the problem: Hospitals must spend money to comply with regulations, which adds to the costs that regulation was designed to control.

Shifting perspective to the prices hospitals charge private paying patients, the latter have increased even faster than costs because of the contractual adjustments hospitals are forced to grant Medicare and Medicaid as the difference between what hospitals charge to meet their full financial needs and what Medicare and Medicaid pay under current cost reimbursement regulations. These Medicare allowances, or discounts, along with the charity care and bad debts that hospitals incur but Medicare does not reimburse, are passed on to private paying patients and their insurance carriers in the form of higher prices. This cost shifting explains why hospital charges or prices have been increasing at a considerably faster rate than hospital costs in recent years.

The problem of hospital cost inflation is complex, and complex problems generally call for multifaceted solutions (21,22,108,111). It would seem that any solution must first encourage the most prudent possible hospital use consistent with good medical practice. There is growing evidence that perhaps as many as one-fourth of all patient days of care provided by hospitals are not medically necessary. This conclusion is suggested by the great variation in hospital use rates from area to area and by the substantially lower hospital use rates experienced by Health Maintenance Organizations (HMOs). Less expensive alternatives such as day surgery, ambulatory, long term, and home care can be substituted for all or some portion of the hospital stays of many patients.

The public's use of hospitals might be constrained by building higher copayment and deductible provisions into health insurance policies and limiting benefits, although the arguments against shifting more of the economic burden of health care back to the consumer are many. Other strategies include 1) attempting to counterbalance the physicians' inclination to use the hospital by changing their financial incentives and developing more HMOs; 2) attempting to strengthen external review of the appropriateness of hospital use through Professional Standards Review Organizations (PSROs); 3) encouraging the planning of more ambulatory care, day care, home care, skilled and intermediate nursing care, and other out-of-hospital care programs and improving insurance coverage for them; and 4) constraining the hospital bed supply through planning and certificate of need.

The question of how to deal with the increasing complexity and intensity of hospital care is equally difficult. It is physicians, not hospitals, who decide what diagnostic and therapeutic services to order for patients. Hence, changes in physician incentives and training must be part of the solution (112). Again, HMOs would seem to provide an appropriate set of incentives in this regard (112). Another approach would be to control malpractice insurance premiums and pressures that apparently cause physicians to practice defensive medicine. The financial incentives inherent in hospital reimbursement might be modified so as to discourage increases in the intensity of services.

Planning, and certificate of need, affiliations, mergers, and shared services among hospitals, and a movement toward regionalized hospital systems may help curtail the duplication of specialized services frequently found in multihospital communities, achieve economies of scale, and reduce the nation's bed supply (113–115). There is increasing discussion at the federal level and among third-party purchasers of offering to buy out unneeded hospitals. Finally, cost containment incentives must be brought to bear on individual institutions to encourage improvements in efficiency and productivity through modern management techniques.

A number of Blue Cross plans have experimented with incentive or prospective reimbursement schemes as an alternative to cost reimbursement in an attempt to introduce incentives to cut costs, and more than a dozen states have enacted rate regulation programs to create an environment of financial stringency that will act to slow the rate of cost increases in hospitals. Medicare waivers have been granted to a number of these states to enable Medicare reimbursement to be tailored to the state program. In addition, the Tax Equity and Fiscal Responsibility Act of 1982 established Medicare cost-per-case limits to control Medicare payments to hospitals. Evidence to date on the effectiveness of the existing incentive reimbursement and rate regulation programs is mixed, and it is unlikely that financial controls or incentives themselves are the answer to the cost inflation problem. Rather, the answer undoubtedly lies in a coordinated program of controls and incentives to contain the pace of capital investment, discourage unnecessary use, reduce existing duplication and overbedding, increase productivity, and shift some economic incentives back to consumers and physicians. The key contribution of prospective reimbursement or rate regulation may be to provide the financial environment to make these other programs work (116–119). The increasing business concern over health benefit costs, the growing price sensitivities of consumers and third-party purchasers, Medicare reimbursement reforms, and heightened competition among hospitals will impose substantially more economic discipline on hospitals in the future.

Small and Rural Hospitals

Considerable attention is being directed to the special problems of the country's many small and rural hospitals. In part because Hill-Burton priorities in the early years channeled funds to thinly populated, rural areas, the United States is a nation of many small hospitals: About one-half of all community hospitals have fewer than 100 beds. These hospitals face a number of problems that threaten their future viability. First, they are losing patients. Admissions to community hospitals with fewer than 100 beds have declined, as has their average daily census (Table 6-4). Between 1967 and 1981, the number of community hospitals with fewer than 100 beds fell from 3,442 to 2,833. Labor requirements are high in small hospitals for the services offered, and small hospitals tend to operate at less efficient levels of occupancy than larger hospitals (Table 6-5). These efficiency limitations, coupled with the limited financial means of some rural populations, have caused many small hospitals to incur substantial operating losses. Small hospitals offer a more limited range of services than larger institutions, because they have neither the patient

TABLE 6-4. Change in Average Daily Census by Hospital Size, United States, 1970–1980

	Average Daily Census		
Bed Size	1970	1980	Percent Change
6–24	3,989	2,308	−42
25–49	30,370	19,806	−35
50–99	74,093	67,630	− 8
100–199	134,117	137,774	+ 3
200–299	113,793	133,391	+17
300–399	99,404	111,144	+12
400–499	69,895	95,559	−37
500 and over	135,810	179,254	+32

SOURCE: *Hospital Statistics*. Chicago, American Hospital Association, 1982.

volume nor the physicians or specialized personnel to support much beyond the basic essential services. Small hospitals are often located in areas where they have a difficult time attracting qualified personnel. Together, all of these problems may lead to difficulty in achieving accreditation or meeting hospital certification and licensure standards.

Finally, small hospitals find it especially difficult to keep up with and respond to the increasingly complex and demanding regulatory environment without the range of management specialists common to larger institutions, and as a result, many are contracting with investor-owned corporations or larger hospitals to take over their management (40,45,120,121). It would appear that the future viability of small hospitals will depend on their adapting their mission and the services they offer to fit their resources, establishing relationships with other institutions, and seeking additional resources to support new programs to broaden their role in health care delivery in the communities they serve (122–125).

Consolidation of Community Health Resources.   Because it is especially difficult for smaller hospitals to assemble the array of equipment and personnel or to attain the patient volume needed to support a broad range of services, it is critical to consolidate around the small hospital to the greatest extent possible whatever health resources do exist in the community. Ideally, the hospital building or campus might include physicians' offices, facilities for public health nurses and health-related community organizations, a nursing home, and so forth. Consolidation would enable limited health resources to be stretched further and provide opportu-

TABLE 6-5. Selected Indicators by Hospital Size, United States, 1981

Hospital Bed Size	Full-time Equivalent Personnel per 100 Census	Percent Occupancy
6–24	377	45.4
25–49	343	52.5
50–99	308	64.5
100–199	319	71.7
200–299	334	77.8
300–399	348	79.7
400–499	365	81.7
500 and over	384	82.5

SOURCE: *Hospital Statistics*. Chicago, American Hospital Association, 1982.

nities for jointly supporting personnel such as a home care nurse, laboratory technician, or physician assistant. The hospital need not own all of these facilities; merely grouping the community's health-related activities together would be an important step. The extreme form of consolidation would be a merger of two small hospitals existing in the same or nearby communities, although there is often considerable resistance among small hospitals and their communities to a merger. A small hospital might also find the means of taking over or providing the location for an area nursing home.

Functional Differentiation.   The difficulties of providing expensive but essential services in smaller hospitals may lead to more formal functional differentiation among hospitals with regard to the levels and types of care provided. Small hospitals may drop some services and give up some types of patients they now treat, adding other services in their place. Criteria or guidelines for referrals may be developed similar to those that now exist for quality and use review. Such criteria would specify the conditions or diagnoses that would be treated in the small hospital and those that would be referred to larger hospitals. Such criteria for referral might become a formal part of accreditation and licensure standards. By limiting the types of patients they treat, small hospitals could be exempted from inapplicable equipment, facility, and personnel standards.

Functional differentiation by level of complexity or severity of illnesses would not necessarily mean reducing the role of the smaller hospital. Smaller hospitals might expand their services in the areas of ambulatory care, preventive and health maintenance services, convalescent, extended, and long term care, home care, and outreach services.

Regionalization.   The key to the future of smaller rural hospitals still seems to lie in the concept of regionalization, the much discussed but little implemented idea of formally relating small hospitals with larger urban hospitals (126,127). Regionalization begins with the concept that each level of hospital—small basic service hospitals, moderate-size community hospitals, and large regional referral centers— should provide only those services they can offer efficiently and at a high level of quality. Communities would be ensured access to a full range of services, not by each hospital attempting to provide every service, but rather by the development of closer relationships among networks of hospitals and their medical staffs to encourage the referral of patients to the institutional setting most appropriate to their needs. Such relationships could range from informal agreements to formal affiliations, jointly provided programs, or mergers of institutions into multihospital systems.

The specific objectives of regionalization include 1) a two-way flow of patients, with patients referred to larger hospitals for specialized services and returned to smaller hospitals for convalescent care, long term care, follow-up care, and home care; 2) continuing education for physicians, nurses, and other personnel from the small hospitals through participation in the educational programs of the larger hospital; 3) assistance from administrative, nursing, and professional department heads and specialists from the larger hospital representing skills not available in the small hospitals; 4) consolidation (in the larger hospital) and sharing of services the small hospitals cannot provide as efficiently or at the same level of quality as the larger hospital; 5) regularly scheduled visits by physician specialists from the larger hospitals to conduct clinics and serve as consultants in the small hospitals; 6) sharing of personnel; and 7) joint purchasing (128).

The success of regionalization depends on the support of the community, the governing board, and the medical staffs of both the small and larger hospitals (129). There are few examples of effective regional relationships. In part this situation reflects community and professional pride and a desire for independence. In part, it reflects the difficulty of working out the essential elements of regionalization: 1) the movement of referrals in both directions so that the small hospitals do not lose patients but maintain their census by providing basic, convalescent, and follow-up care; 2) granting physicians from the small hospitals privileges in the larger hospital and making them feel welcome to admit and treat their patients there when they need the specialized services of the larger hospital; and 3) broadening the role of the small hospital to include convalescent and follow-up care, long term care, home care, and so forth. In the long run, regionalization may preserve rather than threaten the independence and viability of smaller hospitals.

Unionization of Hospital Personnel

Unionization of hospital employees is growing at an increasing rate. Surveys conducted by the American Hospital Association show that in 1961, 224 hospitals, 3.2% of the nation's community hospitals, were organized and had collective bargaining agreements with one or more unions. By 1967, collective bargaining agreements existed in 555 hospitals (7.7%); by 1970, 1,046 hospitals (14.7%); by 1973, 1,197 hospitals (19.7%); and by 1976, 1,327 hospitals (23.1%) (130,131). Unionization is most common in large hospitals, particularly federal and public hospitals. California and the industrialized eastern states have the greatest number of unionized hospitals, and unionization is most common in metropolitan areas. In addition, there tend to be more unionized hospitals in states that had labor laws before 1974.

A variety of factors deterred the growth of unionization in hospitals until recently (132). Most hospitals are fairly small, and small organizations may be better able to settle employee problems informally than formally by collective bargaining. It is also more costly for unions to attempt to organize many small units rather than a few larger firms. A large number of different occupations are found in hospitals (about 125), suggesting that many unions would be necessary to represent all the interests of hospital workers. The public has tended to be less supportive of union activities in essential service organizations such as hospitals, feeling that humanitarian services should not be interrupted by strikes or work stoppages. In addition, many health professionals themselves have been ambivalent about whether unionization is consistent with their professional values. The labor force in hospitals is composed of a high proportion of women and part-time workers. High turnover rates are not unusual. Unions have been reluctant to attempt the difficult task of organizing this type of labor force. Finally, a significant barrier to unionization has been the absence of facilitating labor legislation in the hospital industry, since hospitals were exempted from the Taft-Hartley Act until 1974.

When Congress began to consider bringing hospitals under Taft-Hartley, hospitals pressed for special protection against strikes, priority for National Labor Relations Board action on disputes, and mandatory mediation requirements. Hospitals also wanted to limit the number of bargaining units, with one each for professional, technical, clinical, and maintenance and service workers (133, 134).

In 1974, hospitals became subject to Taft-Hartley, but with special provisions. A hospital or union must give 90 days' notice to the other party of a desire to change an existing contract. The Federal Mediation and Conciliation Service (FMCS) must be given 60 days' notice, and 30 days' notice if an impasse occurs in bargaining for an initial contract after the union is first recognized. A cooling-off period of at least 10 days is required before a strike can occur to enable the hospital to plan for the care of patients. The FMCS may appoint a board of inquiry to mediate among the parties if it determines that a strike would impair delivery of health care to the community. Neither the hospital nor the union are required to accept the board's recommendation, although they must provide information and witnesses called for by the board (135).

With the exemption from Taft-Hartley removed, several factors have made the hospital industry vulnerable to rapid unionization (132,136). First, many hospitals lag behind industry in personnel practices. A substantial number have no professional personnel director, and policies for resolving grievances, discipline, promotion, seniority, overtime, and night shift work are often poorly spelled out. Professional departments such as nursing often handle their own personnel matters, often ignoring the concerns of nonprofessional workers. Wages and fringe benefits in hospitals also appear to have lagged behind those of other industries.

Second, supervisory training is often insufficient. Department heads and supervisors are commonly promoted because of their professional or technical skills rather than their managerial or supervisory capabilities. In addition, supervisors and professional department heads may have divided loyalties between being part of hospital management, on the one hand, and members of professional associations that act as unions, on the other.

Third, the reluctance of professional workers to unionize has diminished. The change in attitude is attributable, in part, to the fact that their professional associations act as their unions. Professional associations are more acceptable than national trade unions might have been. In addition, the professional associations point to collective bargaining not only as a means of improving wages but also as a means of negotiating over staffing standards and work prerogatives that could affect the quality of patient care. The underlying issue of the balance between administrative and professional control over work and the work setting is especially important in professional institutions such as hospitals and adds a unique dimension to unionization in this industry. Also unique is the fear that a strike could cause harm to patients (137–140).

Regulation of Hospitals

External regulation of hospitals has grown rapidly since the mid-1960s. There are external controls over 1) institutional quality standards (licensure, certification, accreditation); 2) construction and expansion of facilities and services (Section 1122 of the 1972 Social Security Amendments, National Health Planning and Resources Development Act, state certificate of need); 3) costs or rates (Blue Cross, Medicare cost-per-case reimbursement limits, state rate regulation); and 4) use (Blue Cross, Medicare, Medicaid, PSROs). Hospital regulations come from both public agencies and private organizations. All states license hospitals, must have a certificate of need, and many have rate regulation. Many of the federal controls are tied to Medicare and Medicaid as conditions for participation or payment: certification, cost ceilings, and capital expenditure review, to name a few. The major private sector organizations that exert control over hospitals are Blue Cross plans and the Joint Commission on Accreditation of Hospitals (141,142). These and related mechanisms are discussed in Chapters 11–13; those that most directly affect hospitals are discussed below.

Controls on Quality.   The regulatory structure for controlling quality includes state licensure, federal certification, and voluntary accreditation (143–145). Licensure is a state function, generally carried out by the department of health, whereby minimum standards are established and enforced regarding the equipment, personnel, plant, and safety features an institution must have to operate. Licensing agencies are empowered to set standards, conduct inspections, issue licenses, close facilities that cannot comply with the agency's standards, and provide consultation services. In many states, however, these agencies are underfinanced and understaffed, and so standards are not enforced stringently. In addition, there is a tendency to focus on fire, safety, and physical plant standards rather than standards for medical services.

Hospitals must be certified by the designated state agency in order to participate in Medicare and Medicaid. The purpose of certification is to ensure that care for beneficiaries of these programs is purchased only from institutions that can meet acceptable minimum quality requirements. In most states, the federal Department of Health and Human Services (HHS) contracts with the health department to carry out the actual inspection process. Virtually all community hospitals are certified, so it can only be concluded that the administration of this program is not very stringent.

Accreditation is a professionally sponsored, voluntary process carried out by the Joint Commission on Accreditation of Hospitals (JCAH), a private organization formed in 1951 as a joint effort of the American College of Physicians, American College of Surgeons, American Hospital Association, and American Medical Association. The JCAH establishes quality standards and surveys hospitals that choose to seek accreditation voluntarily. Standards relate to both the structure and process aspects of quality, and considerable emphasis is given to the organization of the medical staff. About three-fourths of the nation's community hospitals, and more than 95% of those with more than 200 beds, are accredited. Accreditation is designed to encourage institutions to maintain the highest possible levels of performance rather than just minimum standards. Accredited hospitals are deemed to meet HHS's certification requirement. Although the relevance and rigor of the JCAH's standards and survey procedures are not above challenge, there is little question that from a historical perspective the JCAH has been a major force in elevating institutional standards.

Controls on Facilities and Services.   Areawide hospital planning began with Hill-Burton in 1946 (146). States were required to define hospital service areas, inventory existing facilities, and identify the areas of greatest need as determined by bed/population ratios. Hospitals not eligible for or not in need of Hill-Burton funds were not constrained by the program's plans or priorities. Voluntary areawide planning was promoted by the American Hospital Association and the U.S. Public Health Service beginning in 1959; unfortunately, it too had no clout (141). In 1965, the Regional Medical Program was established to encourage regional planning in the treatment of heart disease, cancer, and stroke. Federally sponsored health planning began in earnest in 1966 with the Comprehensive Health Planning Act. State planning agencies (314 A agencies) and areawide, private, nonprofit planning agencies (314 B agencies) were set up with federal aid to coordinate the development of health facilities and services and to discourage overbuilding and duplication. These agencies had little economic or political power, however, and no legal means of stopping capital projects, and it is generally agreed that few were effective (147).

The 1972 Social Security Amendments (Section 1122) added clout to facility and services regulation by authorizing denial of Medicare and Medicaid reimbursement for building and depreciation expenses for capital projects over $150,000 not approved by the designated state agency. Proposed projects were reviewed by area Comprehensive Health Planning (CHP) agencies, but approval powers remained with the state. There is some evidence that Section 1122 and state certificate of need programs have constrained the growth in beds, although not in equipment and other capital investments (148). These issues are discussed further in Chapter 12. The National Health Planning and Resources Development Act of 1974 established a network of state and area planning agencies. This program linked federal funding more closely with state regulation and required states to establish certificate of need programs that require prior approval by the state agency of plans to build or modernize facilities or add new services (113,114,149,150). Certificate of need thresholds were originally set at $150,000, but in 1981 they were increased to $400,000 for major medical equipment and $250,000 for new institutional services (151). The rationale was that the review process should concentrate primarily on high cost hospital capital investment. Findings of a study of certificate of need experience with computed tomography scanners suggest that these programs have not been successful in either controlling the introduction of new technology or ensuring equitable distribution of equipment among hospitals (152). Evidence that this review is costly, time-consuming, and only marginally effective in restraining hospital investments in new technologies and services has lead some health policymakers to propose that the national health planning law be repealed or substantially altered. Since current congressional sentiment appears to favor replacement of regulatory programs such as certificate of need review with a competitive market approach to cost containment, the future of national health planning is uncertain.

Cost Controls.   Programs to control hospital costs or regulate hospital rates have been introduced by federal and state agencies and by private third-party purchasers as a result of their concern over the rapid rise in their expenditures for hospital care (119,153–155). Most Blue Cross plans reimburse hospitals on the basis of costs, and so they are directly affected by cost increases, which they must pass on to subscribers in the form of premium increases. State insurance commissioners become involved because of their authority over Blue Cross premiums. Much of the pioneering work in attempting to incorporate cost containment incentives in reimbursement schemes must be credited to a number of the major Blue Cross plans. However, the impact of these incentives was limited by Blue Cross' close relationship with hospitals, its lack of mandatory sanctions, and the fact that its economic clout was limited to its share of a hospital's patients.

Public involvement in cost controls and rate regulation began in earnest after the rapid post-Medicare inflation in hospital costs in the middle to late 1960s. Medicare had adopted cost-based reimbursement and, like Blue Cross, was directly affected by cost increases. Section 223 of the 1972 Social Security Amendments authorized Medicare to set upper limits on routine inpatient service costs for reimbursement purposes, and Section 1122 limited Medicare reimbursement for capital expenditures made without approval of the designated state planning agency.

The Economic Stabilization Program (ESP), with President Richard Nixon imposed in 1971 to deal with economywide inflation, limited the amount by which hospitals could raise their rates from year to year. Hospitals were subject to ESP until 1974. It appears that this stringent program did slow rate increases and, to a lesser degree, cost increases during the 1971–1974 period, although costs soared dramatically as soon as the controls were removed. In the late 1970s, the Carter administration pushed without success for the reestablishment of federal cost and revenue controls for the hospital industry (156). In addition to federal efforts, about a dozen states concerned with controlling their Medicaid expenditures have empowered state agencies or special public utility-type commissions to regulate hospital rates. In general, these agencies approve prospectively the rates hospitals may charge for their services based on budget review or formula methods for projecting hospital costs or financial needs for the coming year. Hospitals are then reimbursed at these rates rather than on the basis of the costs they actually incur. Thus, hospitals are at risk to keep their costs below the prospectively set rates. Evidence regarding the effectiveness of state prospective rate-setting programs in containing costs is sparse but suggests that this strategy may have considerable potential. The critical question may well be whether this cost containment potential can be exploited with enough care and sensitivity so that the quality and financial viability of the hospital system are protected (116,157–159).

Recent federal cost containment efforts have been directed toward the Medicare program. Annual expenditures on Medicare increased from $3 billion in 1967 to $30.8 billion in 1980 and are projected to reach $99.1 billion by 1987 unless cost controls are added to the program (160,161). The Tax Equity and Fiscal Responsibility Act of 1982 (162) established Medicare inpatient cost-per-case reimbursement limits. These provisions extend Section 223 limits to include ancillary costs in addition to the routine costs previously covered. The legislation also establishes a growth cap on increases in Medicare costs per discharge. The cost-per-case reimbursement limits were formulated as an interim measure, to be effective until HHS designs a permanent prospective reimbursement system for Medicare that is acceptable to Congress. Indications are that HHS will model the prospective reimbursement plan for Medicare after the diagnosis-related groups (DRG) reimbursement system in New Jersey. Under this system, patients are grouped by discharge diagnosis and the hospital is paid on a per case basis, with the amount based on the diagnosis.

Control of Utilization.   The most recent form of regulation in the hospital industry is the attempt to control utilization (163–165). Medicare first required that hospitals and extended care facilities establish utilization review programs as a condition for certification as participating providers. Physician committees were to review the medical records of discharged Medicare patients to determine the necessity of the hospital care provided. This requirement was seen as a way to discourage inappropriate admissions and unnecessarily long lengths of stays, and hence as a means of keeping Medicare and Medicaid expenditures down. However, utilization review raises a number of sensitive issues, because establishing standards and monitoring physician practices with regard to hospitals may be seen as infringing on professional judgment regarding patient care.

Building on the utilization review requirements, the 1972 Social Security Amendments established Professional Standards Review Organizations (PSROs) to strengthen the appropriate monitoring process. PSROs are nonprofit associations of physicians that review the care provided Medicare and Medicaid patients in all institutions in their area under contract with HHS. PSROs establish standards of treatment against which utilization can be judged. They can delegate the actual review function to hospital medical audit and utilization review committees, but must monitor the outcome of hospital-based reviews to ensure their effectiveness.

Although the Reagan administration had originally targeted PSROs for extinction, the program was resurrected through the Tax Equity and Fiscal Responsibility Act of 1982 (166), which requires implementation of Utilization and Quality Control Peer Review Organizations (PROs). The PROs, which are scheduled to begin operation in October 1983, are closely modeled after the original PSROs in terms of staffing and operational authority. One significant difference, however, is that the new PROs will be private organizations capable of making utilization review contracts with the business community as well as Medicare and Medicaid.

The question of whether or not the hospital industry should be regulated is moot at this time because a complex regulatory environment already exists. That environment is fragmented because a great number of individual regulatory programs have evolved as specific responses to specific problems. Attempts to coordinate and rationalize the multiplicity of regulatory programs to impact on the entire delivery system in a positive manner are relatively recent (122). Regulation has become expensive for hospitals as well, calling for more careful cost-benefit analysis of regulatory requirements. The main criticisms of current external regulatory practices are 1) excessive reporting and inspection, which often takes the form of duplication and sometimes leads to conflicting requirements; 2) multiple centers of authority and accountability; 3) lack of incentives to institutions and professionals to achieve effective delivery of health care; and 4) subsidization of some groups and services by others through cost shifting (167,168). Some argue that the forces currently giving rise to a much more competitive health care environment will make extensive regulation unnecessary. These and related issues of regulation are discussed further in Chapter 12.

REFERENCES

1. Gibson RM, Waldo DR: National health expenditures, 1981. *Health Care Financing Rev* 1982; 4(1):1–36.

2. Knowles J: The hospital. *Sci Am* 1973; 229:128–137.

3. Somers AR: *Health Care in Transition: Directions for the Future.* Chicago, Hospital Research and Education Trust, 1971.

4. Schulz R, Johnson AC: *Management of Hospitals.* New York, McGraw-Hill Book Co, 1976, pp 33–36.

5. Shortell SM: Organization of hospital resources, in *Hospitals in the 1980s.* Chicago, American Hospital Association, 1977.

6. Goldsmith S: *Ambulatory Care.* Germantown, Md, Aspen Systems Corp, 1977.

7. Williams S, Shortell S, Dowling W, et al: Hospital sponsored primary care group practice: A developing modality of care. *Health Med Care Services Rev* 1978; 1(5/6):1–13).

8. *Hospital Statistics.* Chicago, American Hospital Association, 1981.

9. MacEachern MT: *Hospital Organization and Management,* ed 3. Chicago, Physicians Record Company, 1957.

10. Rosenberg S: The hospital in America: A century's perspective, in *Medicine and Society.* Philadelphia, American Philosophical Society Library, publication 4, 1971.

11. Rosen G: The hospital—historical sociology of a community institution, in Friedson E (ed): *The Hospital in Modern Society.* New York, The Free Press, 1963, pp 1–36.

12. Corwin EH: *The American Hospital*. New York, Commonwealth Fund, 1946, pp 193–213.

13. Commission on Hospital Care: Expansion of hospitals, 1840–1900, in *Hospital Care in the United States*. Cambridge, Mass, Commonwealth Fund, Harvard University Press, 1947, pp 454–526.

14. Davis K: The hospital's position in American Society, in Owen J (ed): *Modern Concepts in Hospital Administration*. Philadelphia, WB Saunders Co, 1962, pp 6–16.

15. Brown RE: The general hospital has a general responsibility. *Hospitals* 1965; 39(12):47–54.

16. McKeown T: Medical education and medical care: An examination of traditional concepts and suggestions for change, in Knowles J (ed): *Doctors, Hospitals, and the Public Interest*. Cambridge, Mass, Harvard University Press, 1965, pp 254–270.

17. Somers AR: *Health Care in Transition: Directions for the Future*. Chicago, Hospital Research and Education Trust, 1971, pp 27–38.

18. Somers AR: *Health Care in Transition: Directions for the Future*. Chicago, Hospital Research and Education Trust, 1971, pp 39–72.

19. Feldstein M: *The Rising Cost of Hospital Care*. Washington, DC, Information Resources Press, 1971.

20. *Trends Affecting the U.S. Health Care System*, DHEW publication (HRA) 76-14503. Bureau of Health Planning and Resource Development, Health Planning Information Service, 1976, pp 195–199.

21. Davis K: Rising hospital costs: Possible causes and cures. *Bull NY Acad Med* 1972; 48:1354–1371.

22. McCarthy CM: Supply and demand and hospital cost inflation. *Med Care Rev* 1976; 33:923–948.

23. *Trends Affecting the U.S. Health Care System*, DHEW publication (HRA) 76-14503. Bureau of Health Planning and Resource Development, Health Planning Information Service, 1976, pp 124, 173–175.

24. *Trends Affecting the U.S. Health Care System*, DHEW publication (HRA) 76-14503. Bureau of Health Planning and Resource Development, Health Planning Information Service, 1976, pp 91–95.

25. Gibson RM, Waldo DR: National health expenditures, 1981. *Health Care Financing Rev* 1982; 4(1):24.

26. Schulz R, Johnson AC: *Management of Hospitals*. New York, McGraw-Hill Book Co, 1976, pp 30–43.

27. Cooney J: Public hospitals: We must love them or leave them, study says. *Mod Hosp* 1972; 118(5):87–92.

28. Dumbaugh K, Bentkover J, Neuhauser D: Public hospitals: An evolution, in Levin A (ed): *Health Services: The Local Perspective, Proceedings of the Academy of Political Science* 32(3):148–158. New York, The Academy, 1977.

29. Conference Report: Impact of government programs on public hospitals—directions for the future. *Public Health Rep* 1968; 83:53–60.

30. Tetelman A: Public hospitals—critical or recovering? *Health Serv Rep* 1973; 88:295–304.

31. Levin PJ: Public hospitals must adapt to changes in the delivery system. *Hospitals* 1977; 51(8):81–88.

32. *The Future of the Public General Hospital—An Agenda for Transition*. Report of the Commission on Public General Hospitals (R. Nelson, chairman). Chicago, Hospital Education and Research Trust, 1978.

33. Steinwald B, Neuhauser D: The role of the proprietary hospital. *Law Contemp Probl* 1970; 35:817–838.

34. Stewart DA: The history and status of proprietary hospitals. *Blue Cross Reports*, research series 9, Chicago, Blue Cross Association, 1973.

35. Annual survey of multihospital systems. *Mod Health Care* 1982; 12(5):67–130.

36. Kushman JE, Nuckton CF: Further evidence on the relative performance of proprietary and nonprofit hospitals. *Med Care* 1977; 15:189–204.

37. *Trends Affecting the U.S. Health Care System*, DHEW publication (HRA) 76-14503. Bureau of Health Planning and Resource Development, Health Planning Information Service, 1976, pp 299–305.

38. Lewin LS, Dermon RA, Maugulies R: Investor-owneds and non-profits differ in economic performance. *Hospitals* 1981; 55(13):52–58.

39. Hill DB, Stewart DA: Proprietary hospitals versus non-profit hospitals: A matched sample analysis in California. *Blue Cross Reports*, research series 9. Chicago, Blue Cross Association, 1973.

40. Ruchlin H, Pointer D, Cannedy L: A comparison of for-profit investor-owned chain and nonprofit hospitals. *Inquiry* 1973; 10(4):13–23.

41. Schweitzer SO, Rafferty J: Variations in hospital product: A comparative analysis of proprietary and voluntary hospitals. *Inquiry* 1976; 13:158–166.

42. Terris M: The comprehensive health center. *Public Health Rep* 1963; 78:861:866.

43. Somers AR: *Health Care in Transition: Directions for the Future*. Chicago, Hospital and Research and Education Trust, 1971, pp 99–126.

44. Somers AR: Towards a rationale community health care system: The Hunterdon model. *Hosp Progr* 1973; 54(4):46–54.

45. Spitzer WD: The small general hospital: Problems and solutions. *Milbank Mem Fund Q* 1970; 48:413–477.

46. Dowling WL: Multihospital systems—present status and future prospects. *Hosp Progr* 1983; 64(4).

47. Zuckerman HS: Multi-institutional systems: Promise and performances. *Inquiry* 1979; 16(4):291–314.

48. Brown M, McCool B (eds): *Multihospital Systems*. Germantown, Md, Aspen Systems Corp, 1981.

49. Coe R: *Sociology and Medicine*. New York, McGraw-Hill Book Co, 1970, pp 264–288.

50. Georgopoulos BA (ed.) *Organizational Research in Hospitals*. Ann Arbor, University of Michigan Press, 1973.

51. Broehl WD: Policy formulation and implementation: The governing board, in Moss AB, Broehl WG, Guest RH (eds): *Hospital Policy Decisions: Process and Action*. New York, GP Putnam's Sons, 1966, pp 23–79.

52. Melkonian D, Raichel T: Organization of a hospital. *Provider Rev Manual*. Chicago, Blue Cross Association, 1974, pp 18–50.

53. Southwick A: The hospital as an institution—expanding responsibilities change its relationship with the staff physician. *California West Law Rev* 1973; 9:429–467.

54. Smith HL: Two lines of authority are one too many: The hospital dilemma. *Mod Hosp* 1955; 84:59–64.

55. Perkins R: The physician's view of the hospital: A love-hate relationship. Parts 1 and 2. *Hosp Med Staff* 1975; 4(4):1–7; 1975; 4(5):10–14.

56. Scott WR: The medical staff and the hospital: An organizational perspective. *Hosp Med Staff* 1973; 1:33–38.

57. Perrow C: Goals and power structure: A historical care study, in Friedson E (ed): *The Hospital in Modern Society*. New York, Free Press, 1963.

58. Johnson EL: Changing role of the hospital's chief executive officer. *Hosp Adm* 1970; 15:21–34.

59. Gilmore K, Wheeler J: A national profile of governing boards. *Hospitals* 1972; 46:105–108.

60. Blankenship LV, Elling RH: Organizational support and community power structure: The hospital. *J Health Hum Behav* 1962; 3:257–369.

61. Burling T, Lentz EM, Wilson RN: The board of trustees, in *The Give and Take in Hospitals*. New York, GP Putnam's Sons, 1956, pp 39–50.

62. *Trends Affecting the U.S. Health Care System*, DHEW publication (HRA) 76-14503. Bureau of Health Planning and Resource Development, Health Planning Information Service, 1976, pp 339–341.

63. Perloff E: Health care issues for the 70s: For the trustee, deepening responsibilities. *Hospitals* 1970; 44(1):84–89.

64. Springer E: The Darling case: Ten years later. *Hosp Med Staff* 1975; 4(6):1–7.

65. Schulz R, Johnson AC: *Management of Hospitals*. New York, McGraw-Hill Book Co, 1976, pp. 47–67.

66. Willits RD: What boards of trustees do. *Trustee* 1974; 27(5):1–8.

67. Marmor T: Public accountability and consumerism, in *Hospitals in the 1980s*. Chicago, American Hospital Association, pp 189–202.

68. Pfeffer J: Size, composition and function of hospital boards of directors: A study of organization-environment linkage. *Adm Sci Q* 1973; 18:349–364.

69. Bellin L: Changing composition of voluntary hospital boards—an inevitable prospect for the 1970s. *HSMHA Health Rep* 1971; 86:674–681.

70. Cathcart HR: Including the community in hospital governance. *Hosp Progr* 1970; 51(10):72–76.

71. Kovner A: Hospital board members as policy-makers. *Med Care* 1974; 12:971–982.

72. Jorgenson CJ: Should doctors be on your board? *Hosp Adm* 1970; 15(4):6–13.

73. Guest R: The role of the doctor in institutional management, in Georgopoulos B (ed): *Organizational Research in Health Institutions*. Ann Arbor, University of Michigan Press, 1972.

74. Hahn JA, Bornemeier W: AHA, AMA leaders present views on physician board membership. *Hosp Topics* 1970; 48(7):24–25.

75. Schulz R: Does staff representation equal active participation? *Hospitals* 1972; 46(24):31–35.

76. A profile of the hospital trustee. *Trustee* 1975; 28(1):21–23, 26.

77. Kovner A: Improving community hospital board performance. *Med Care* 1978; 16:79–89.

78. Prybil LD, Starkweather DB: Current perspectives on hospital governance. *Hosp Health Serv Adm* 21:67–75, 1976; 21:67–75.

79. Study points way to better governance. *Hospitals* 1974; 48(19):35–38.

80. Schulz R, Johnson AC: *Management of Hospitals*. New York, McGraw-Hill Book Co, 1976, pp. 129–164.

81. Thompson J, Filerman G: Trends and developments in education for hospital administration. *Hosp Adm* 1967; 12:13–32.

82. Schulz R, Johnson AC: *Management of Hospitals*. New York, McGraw-Hill Book Co, 1976, pp 147–164.

83. Kovner A: The hospital administrator and organizational effectiveness, in Georgopoulos B (ed): *Organization Research in Health Institutions*. Ann Arbor, University of Michigan Press, 1972, pp 355–376.

84. Kuhl IK: *The Executive Role in Health Services Delivery Organization*. Washington, DC, Association of University Program in Health Administration, 1977.

85. White R: The hospital administrator's emerging professional role, in Arnold MF, Blank-

enship LV, Hess JM (eds): *Administering Health Systems*. Chicago, Aldine-Atherton, 1971.

86. Williams KJ: Basic principles of medical staff organization. *Hosp Progr* 1970; 51(3):50–55.

87. Perkins R: The physician's view of the hospital: A love-hate relationship. Part 2. *Hosp Med Staff* 1975; 4(5):12.

88. Schulz R, Johnson AC: *Management of Hospitals*. New York, McGraw-Hill Book Co, 1976, pp 68–69.

89. Williams KJ: Medical staff issues—past and present. *Hosp Med Staff* 1972; 1(1):2–13.

90. *Accreditation Manual for Hospitals*. Chicago, Joint Commission on Accreditation of Hospitals, 1978, pp 78–89.

91. Blaes SM: Why and how should medical staff laws be revised? *Hospitals* 1973; 47(23):100–106.

92. Mills DH: Staff bylaws: An internal code of conduct. *Hosp Med Staff* 1976; 5(8):7–9.

93. Fischer DC: Catholic Hospital Guidelines—Physician-directors: Logical next step. *Hosp Progr* 1975; 56(3):28–33.

94. Harvey JD: The hospital medical director: An administrator's view. *Hosp Progr* 1970; 51(11):80–84.

95. Williams KJ: Does your hospital need a medical director? *Med Economics* 1973; 15(22):228–236.

96. Jack WW: Medical staff functions and leadership. *Hosp Progr* 1970; 51(11):76–79.

97. Roemer M, Friedman E: *Doctors in Hospitals*. Baltimore, Johns Hopkins University Press, 1971, pp 29–48.

98. Shortell SM: Hospital medical staff organization: Structure, process, and outcome. *Hosp Adm* 1974; 19:96–107.

99. Roemer M, Friedman E: *Doctors in Hospitals*. Baltimore, Johns Hopkins University Press, 1971.

100. Johnson EA: An emerging medical staff organization. *Hosp Adm* 1972; 17:26–38.

101. Paxton HT: No more autonomy for hospital medical staffs. *Med Economics* 1971; 48(Nov 22):35–44.

102. *Trends Affecting the U.S. Health Care System*. DHEW publication (HRA) 76-14503. Bureau of Health Planning and Resource Development, Health Planning Information Service, 1976, pp 333–338.

103. Altman SH, Eichenholz J: Inflation in the health industry: Causes and cures, in Zubkoff M (ed): *Health: A Victim or Cause of Inflation?* New York, Milbank Memorial Fund, 1976, pp 7–30.

104. McMahon JA, Drake DF: Inflation and the hospital, in Zubkoff M (ed): *Health: A Victim or Cause of Inflation?* New York, Milbank Memorial Fund, 1976, pp 130–148.

105. Raske K: Components of inflation: An analysis of the causes of increases in hospital cost. *Hospitals* 1974; 48(13):67–70.

106. Drake DF, Raske KE: The changing hospital economy. *Hospitals*. 1974; 48(22):34–40.

107. *Trends Affecting the U.S. Health Care System*. DHEW publication (HRA) 76-14503. Bureau of Health Planning and Resource Development, Health Planning Information Service, 1976, pp 162–176.

108. Schulz R, Johnson AC: *Management of Hospitals*. New York, McGraw-Hill Book Co, 1976, pp 202–222.

109. *Trends Affecting the U.S. Health Care System*. DHEW publication (HRA) 76-14503. Bureau of Health Planning and Resource Development, Health Planning Information Service, 1976, pp 321–328.

110. *Trends Affecting the U.S. Health Care System.* DHEW publication (HRA) 76-14503. Bureau of Health Planning and Resource Development, Health Planning Information Service, 1976, pp 179–181.

111. McMahon JA, Drake DF: Inflation and the hospital, in Zubkoff M (ed): *Health: A Victim or Cause of Inflation?* New York, Milbank Memorial Fund, 1976, pp 130–148.

112. Redisch MA: Physician involvement in hospital decision making, in Zubkoff M, Raskin E, Hauft RS (eds): *Hospital Cost Containment—Selected Notes for Future Policy.* New York, Milbank Memorial Fund, 1978, pp 217–243.

113. Institute of Medicine: *A Policy Statement—Controlling the Supply of Hospital Beds.* Washington, DC, National Academy of Sciences, 1976.

114. McClure W: *Reducing Excess Hospital Capacity.* Minneapolis, Interstudy, 1976.

115. *Trends Affecting the U.S. Health Care System.* DHEW publication (HRA) 76-14503. Bureau of Health Planning and Resource Development, Health Planning Information Service, 1976, pp 99–108.

116. Dowling WL: Prospective rate setting—concept and practice. *Top Health Care Financing* 1976; 2:1–37.

117. Griffith JR, Hancock W, Munson FC: Practical ways to contain hospital costs. *Harvard Business Rev* 1973; 51(6):131–139.

118. Thueson J: Hospitals' programs and progress in cost containment reported. *Hospitals* 1977; 51(18):131–138.

119. *Trends Affecting the U.S. Health Care System.* DHEW publication (HRA) 76-14503. Bureau of Health Planning and Resource Development, Health Planning Information Service, 1976, pp 137–140, 200–210.

120. Kernaghan SG: Legislation: the painful shot in the arm. *Hospitals* 1974; 48:65–75.

121. Cooper JK, Heald K, Samuel SM, et al: Rural or urban practice: Factors influencing the location decision of primary care physicians. *Inquiry* 1975; 12:18–25.

122. *Delivery of Health Care in Rural America.* Chicago, American Hospital Association, 1977, pp 38–61.

123. *Health Care Delivery in Rural Areas.* Chicago, American Medical Association, 1976.

124. Madison DL: Recruiting physicians for rural practice. *Health Serv Rep* 1973; 88:758–762.

125. US Public Health Service: *Building a Rural Health System,* DHEW publication No. (HSA) 76-15028. Rockville, MD, Bureau of Community Health Services, 1976.

126. Phillips D: Reaching out to rural communities: Hospital's expanding role as a social agency, parts 1 and 2. *Hospitals* 1972; 46(11):33–38; 1972; 46(12):53–57.

127. Rannels HW, Ross DE, Waxman CR: The community hospital and regional health care responsibilities—how to do it! *Med Care* 1975; 13:885–896.

128. McNerney WJ, Riedel D: *Regionalization and Rural Health Care,* research series 2. Ann Arbor, Bureau of Hospital Administration, University of Michigan, 1962.

129. Strowbridge RH: How to cope with the big problems of a small or rural hospital. *Trustee* 1973; 26(8):3–7.

130. Frenzen PD: Survey updates unionization activities. *Hospitals* 1978; 52(15):93–98.

131. Juris, H Rosmann, Maxey C, et al: Nationwide survey shows growth in union contracts. *Hospitals* 1977; 51(6):122–130.

132. Schulz R, Johnson AC: *Management of Hospitals.* New York, McGraw-Hill Book Co, 1976, pp 237–255.

133. *Taft Hartley Amendments: Implications for the Health Care Field, Report of a Symposium.* Chicago, American Hospital Association, 1976.

134. Rosmann J: One year under Taft-Hartley. *Hospitals* 1975; 49(24):64–68.

135. Pointer D, Metzger N: *The National Labor Relations Act: A Guidebook for Health Care Facility Administrators.* New York, Spectrum Publications, 1975, pp 41–60.

136. Rakich, JS: Hospital unionization: Causes and effects. *Hosp Adm* 1973; 18(1):7–18.

137. Davis LJ, Foner M: Organization and unionization of health workers in the United States—the trade union perspective. *Int J Health Serv* 1975; 5:19–36.

138. Phillips DF: New demands of nurses: San Francisco area nurses' strike, parts 1 and 2. *Hospitals* 1974; 48(16):33–38; 1974; 48(18):41–44.

139. Bloom BS: Collective action by professionals poses problems for administrators. *Hospitals* 1977; 51(6):167–174.

140. Wilmot IG: Management's viewpoint, in *Taft-Hartley Amendments: Implications for the Health Care Field.* Chicago, American Medical Association, 1976, pp 78–94.

141. Somers AR: *Hospital Regulation: The Dilemma of Public Policy.* Princeton, NJ, Princeton University, Industrial Relations Section, 1969.

142. Schulz R, Johnson AC: *Management of Hospitals.* New York, McGraw-Hill, 1976, pp 256–271.

143. Somers AR: *Health Care in Transition: Directions for the Future.* Chicago, Hospital Research and Education Trust, 1971, pp 101–131.

144. Schulz R, Johnson AC: *Management of Hospitals.* New York, McGraw-Hill, 1976, pp 185–201.

145. Schlicke CP: American surgery's noblest experiment: The story of hospital accreditation. *Arch Surg* 1973; 106:379–385.

146. Somers, AR: *Health Care in Transition: Directions for the Future.* Chicago, Hospital Research and Education Trust, 1971, pp 132–161.

147. *Trends Affecting the U.S. Health Care System.* DHEW publication (HRA) 76-14503. Bureau of Health Planning and Resource Development, Health Planning Information Service, 1976, pp 91–109.

148. Salkever DS, Bice TW: Certificate-of-need legislation and hospital costs, in Zubkoff M, Raskin E, Hanft RS (eds): *Hospital Cost Containment: Selected Notes for Future Policy.* New York, Milbank Memorial Fund, 1978, pp 429–460.

149. Chassin MR: The containment of hospital costs: a strategic assessment. *Med Care* 1978; 16(suppl):21–26.

150. *Trends Affecting the U.S. Health Care System.* DHEW publication (HRA) 76-14503. Bureau of Health Planning and Resource Development, Health Planning Information Service, 1976, pp 91–109.

151. Public Law 97-35. The Omnibus Budget Reconciliation Act of 1981. US Government Printing Office, 1981.

152. Pardini AP, Cohodes DR, Cohen AB: Certificate of need and high capital cost technology: The case of computerized axial tomographic scanners. Report to the Bureau of Health Planning, HRA, DHHS. HRA Contract 231-77-1004. Cambridge, Mass: Urban Systems Research and Engineering, 1980.

153. *Controlling the Cost of Health Care.* DHEW publication (HRA) 77-3182. NCHSR Policy Research Services, 1977.

154. Zubkoff M, Rankin IE, Hanft RS (eds): *Hospital Cost Containment: Selected Notes for Future Policy.* New York, Milbank Memorial Fund, 1978.

155. Somers AR: *Hospital Regulation: The Dilemma of Public Policy.* Princeton, NJ, Princeton University, Industrial Relations Section, 1969, pp 162–191.

156. Dunn W, Lefkowitz B: The hospital cost containment act of 1977: An analysis of the administration's proposal, in Zubkoff M, Raskin E, Hanft RS (eds): *Hospital Cost Con-*

tainment: Selected Notes for Future Policy. New York, Milbank Memorial Fund, 1978, pp 166–214.

157. Bauer K: Hospital rate setting—this way to salvation? in Zubkoff M, Raskin E, Hanft RS (eds): *Hospital Cost Containment: Selected Notes for Future Policy*. New York, Milbank Memorial Fund, 1978, pp 324–369.

158. Chassin MR: The containment of hospital costs: A strategic assessment. *Med Care* 1978; 16(suppl):36–45.

159. Hellinger FJ: An empirical analysis of several prospective reimbursement systems, in Zubkoff M, Raskin E, Hauft RS (eds): *Hospital Cost Containment: Selected Notes for Future Policy*. New York, Milbank Memorial Fund, 1978, pp 370–400.

160. Iglehardt JK: Will Medicare's successes spoil its chance to survive spending cuts? *Natl J:* 1982; 14(18):772–775.

161. US Senate, Special Committee on Aging, Health Care Expenditures for the Elderly: How much protection does Medicare provide? 97th Congress, Second Session. US Government Printing Office, April 1982.

162. Public Law 97-248. The Tax Equity and Fiscal Responsibility Act of 1982. US Government Printing Office, 1982.

163. Chassin MR: The containment of hospital costs: a strategic assessment. *Med Care* 1978; 16(suppl):27–35.

164. Goran MJ, Roberts JS, Kellogg M, et al: The PSRO hospital review system. *Med Care* 1975;13(suppl):1–33.

165. *Trends Affecting the U.S. Health Care System*. DHEW publication (HRA) 76-14503. Bureau of Health Planning and Resource Development, Health Planning Information Service, 1976, pp 131–136.

166. Public Law 97-248. The Tax Equity and Fiscal Responsibility Act of 1982. US Government Printing Office, 1982.

167. *Hospital Regulation*. Report of the Special Committee on the Regulatory Process. Chicago, American Hospital Association, 1977, pp 17–26.

168. O'Donoghue P: *Evidence about the Effects of Health Care Regulation: An Evaluation and Synthesis of Policy Relevant Research*. Denver, Spectrum Research, Inc, 1974.

CHAPTER 7

Long Term Care Versus Tender Loving Care

Robert L. Kane

Rosalie A. Kane

This chapter provides an overview of that amorphous field referred to as *long term care (LTC)*. The term confuses as much as it clarifies. Like many labels, it is defined by exclusion, in this case implying a distinction from the acute services available in the hospital and physicians' offices. But the division is not clear. For instance, when a patient receiving LTC, perhaps in a nursing home, has an acute illness, is the care acute or long term? Such questions become relevant only when they affect the care available or the resources to pay for it. As will be seen, these are both major issues for LTC.

As might be expected, there is no uniform definition for LTC. The following description is perhaps preferable to most because it highlights important aspects of the problem:

> Long term care: A range of services that addresses the health, personal care, and social needs of individuals who lack some capacity for self-care. Services may be continuous or intermittent, but are delivered over sustained periods to individuals who have a demonstrated need, usually measured by some index of functional incapacity.

This statement emphasizes the common theme of most discussions of LTC: the dependence of an individual on the services of another for a substantial period. The definition is carefully unspecific about who provides these services or what they are. LTC is certainly not the exclusive purview of the medical professions. Indeed, most of the long term care in this country is provided not by paid personnel but by a host of individuals loosely referred to as *informal support*. These persons may be family, friends, or neighbors. The services include whatever pragmatic blend is needed to maximize functioning. Although the nursing home is the major recipient of public dollars for LTC, this care can also be delivered through home health or homemaking agencies, day centers, and a variety of socially oriented programs (e.g., friendly visiting, respite services for family caregivers, telephone reassurance, and service centers in senior housing units). Addressing functional dependency as it does, LTC requires substantial labor, both paid and volunteer. Some authorities, however, suggest that the functional dependency triggering LTC could be ameliorated through structural changes in environmental arrangements ranging from specific home improvements to compensate for disability to provision of appropriate, affordable housing built specifically for the frail and elderly.

LTC lies in an indefinite no-man's-land between professional and nonprofessional support. For many years, it was undisputed territory, more noted for avoidance than for competition to enter it. But recently, interest in the plight of the aged has grown. There have been signs of recognition that the dependent elderly represent both a need and a market for a variety of services.

To illuminate the current state of LTC, five major questions are addressed in this chapter: 1) Why is LTC such an issue? 2) Who is at risk? 3) What is the role of the nursing home? 4) How did we get where we are? 5) What can be done about it?

WHY IS LTC SUCH AN ISSUE?

The growing concern about LTC can be traced to the confluence of two forces: the growth of both the elderly population and the cost of care, particularly the public cost of care. Both are the source and the product of social policies. Although the demographic trends have been known for years, they are suddenly a cause for alarm. The sense of crisis can be attributed to a perception that the growth in the population over age 65 is occurring in that segment that disproportionately consumes health services. The greatest concern focuses on the post-World War II baby boom cohort moving through time; the disruption of social institutions that cohort creates will be magnified when it becomes elderly after the turn of the century.

Even at present, with only about 11% of the population over age 65, financial problems are evident. Figure 7-1 shows where medical care funds for the elderly come from and where they go. The elderly consume a disproportionate share of the health care dollar, especially the public part of that dollar. In 1978, the elderly accounted for just over $2,000 per capita for health care expenditures (compared with $765 for younger adults and $285 for youths); moreover, 65% of the health care dollar for the elderly came from public funds.

For LTC expenditures, the picture is less clear because so many sources are involved. In the major locus of expenditure, the nursing home, several contrasts with overall health care expenditures exist. As seen in Figure 7-2, the largest source of LTC funding comes from Medicaid, a welfare program. Medicare contributes surprisingly little, and the role of private sources is larger. Since Medicare and Medicaid are open-ended funding sources (i.e., their budgets are essentially determined by the demands placed on them, with no fixed ceilings), they are prime targets for growing expenditures. Despite the complaints of providers about the parsimony of federal and state programs, since 1965 (when Medicare and Medicaid were introduced) the per capita expenditure for both hospitals and physicians (after adjusting for inflation and population growth) has increased more for the elderly than for those under age 65.

LTC thus represents a growing expense from both private and public sources.

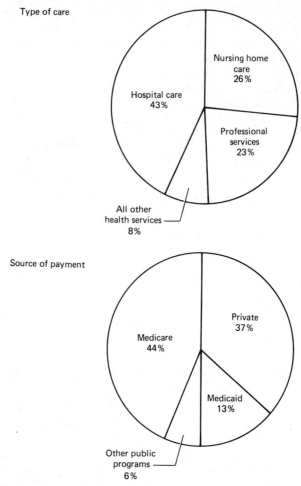

Type of care

Source of payment

Figure 7-1. Per capita health care expenditures for the elderly by type of care and source of payment: United States, 1978. Note: Other health services include drugs and drug sundries, eyeglasses and appliances, and other health services.

SOURCE: Federal Council on Aging: *The Need for Long-Term Care: A Chartbook of the Federal Council on the Aging,* publication (OHDS) 81-20704. US Government Printing Office, 1981.

The demographic forecasts suggest that, as the baby boom cohort ages by the early part of the next century, there will be more dependent old people and fewer young working people for them to depend on. When changes in social mores are added to this picture—less stable marriages, more working women, decreased birth rate—this dependency forecast becomes even grimmer. Finally, it must be acknowledged that few are pleased with what is currently purchased with LTC dollars. The nursing home is shunned by professionals, patients, and families. There is no reason to expect improvements unless there are some very serious commitments toward new national goals. It is thus scarcely surprising that so many people are actively pursuing alternative forms of LTC.

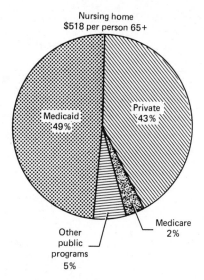

Figure 7-2. Sources of nursing home expenditures.
SOURCE: Adapted from *Long Term Care: Background and Future Directions*, publication 81-20047. US Government Printing Office, 1981.

WHO IS AT RISK?

Before nursing homes can be avoided or used more appropriately, it must be understood who is at risk for nursing home care. The answer depends on how the question is asked. At the simplest level, it can be reported that, at any given point in time, one person out of 20 aged 65 years or older is a resident in a nursing home. But this 5% figure is misleading on several counts. The use of age 65 to signal the onset of old age is arbitrary and capricious. As one social program begat the next, this definition was handed down from the time of Bismarck's social insurance scheme in the nineteenth century. Unfortunately, the phrase "65 and older" hides important differences.

Consider, for example, the rate of nursing home use, which is 5% of the population aged 65 and over; this figure must be disaggregated to be understood. Of those aged 65 to 69, only about 1% are in nursing homes; of those aged 75 to 79, only about 6%; but of those aged 85 and over, more than 20% are in nursing homes. In fact, the average age of nursing home residents is over 80.

The 5% figure is misleading in another sense as well. It is static; it counts people at only one point in time. When more dynamic data are examined to estimate the total risk of nursing home placement over a lifetime, the figure rises considerably. Simply using the proportion of deaths among those over age 65 that occur in nursing homes, estimates of about 25% result (1,2). The studies that have followed an aged cohort over time report that 25% to 40% of 65-year-olds will spend some time in a nursing home before their death (3,4).

Another simple approach to identifying the risk factors is simply to compare the persons in nursing homes with those in the community (Table 7-1). Persons in nursing homes are older, less likely to be married, and more likely to be female and white.

TABLE 7-1. Number of Nursing Home Residents and the Noninstitutionalized Population Aged 65 Years and Over and Percent Distribution, by Age, Sex, Race, and Marital Status: United States, 1977

Age, Sex, Race, and Marital Status	Nursing Home Residents	Noninstitutionalized Population
	Number	
All residents	1,126,000	22,100,000
	Percent distribution	
Total	100.0	100.0
Age		
65–74 years	18.8	64.0
75 years and over	81.2	36.0
Sex		
Male	26.1	41.3
Female	73.9	58.7
Race		
White and Hispanic	93.3	90.6
Black and other	6.7	9.4
Marital status		
Married	12.1	53.2
Widowed	69.3	36.4
Divorced or separated	4.5	4.2
Never married	14.2	6.2

SOURCE: *Characteristics of Nursing Home Residents, Health Status and Care Received: National Nursing Home Survey, United States, May–December 1977*, publication (PHS) 81-1712 (*Vital and Health Statistics*, series 13, no 51, Table D). Hyattsville, Md, National Center for Health Statistics, 1981.

Note: Figures may not add to totals due to rounding.

How important is physical health? Butler and Newacheck (5) argue that social support is more critical than disability in determining the likelihood of nursing home admission. Using cross-sectional data, they have shown that persons who are unmarried and living alone or with relatives are at greatest risk. This does not mean, as some have suggested, that this is an era in which children abandon their parents. Brody (6) and Shanas (7) have shown that children continue to provide strong support for older persons, but there is some reason to suspect that fatigue sets in. Eggert and his colleagues (8) describe the archetypal situation wherein the family that can no longer cope with repeated illness and disruption turns to the nursing home as a last resort. Callahan and his colleagues (9) suggest that families might be encouraged to do more. They urge stronger incentives to support families in providing more care for dependent elderly relatives.

The use of nursing homes should not be interpreted as a lack of informal social support. Studies like those by the Government Accounting Office (10,11) suggest that family and friends provide the bulk of nonmedical services to dependent older persons living in the community. Looked at another way, 9 out of 10 such individuals have someone to rely on for such help. This help may be the critical factor in avoiding or delaying nursing home placement. Using a multidimensional rating scale, which sums disabilities along five dimensions (physical, mental, social, economic, and activities of daily living), researchers found 87% of a nursing home sample to be at least mildly or moderately impaired in all five areas; 14% of a community sample of elderly were equally impaired (12).

Using a rough 5% estimate of nursing home prevalence, a crude estimate of the ratio of the total number of impaired elderly in the community compared to the number in nursing homes is: $[(0.14) \times (0.95)]/[(0.87) \times (0.05)] = .13/.04 = 3.25$. Thus, by this estimate, there are about three equally disabled elderly persons in the community for every one in a nursing home. (One may still argue that those in the nursing home are *more* disabled because the measure is not sensitive enough to distinguish that end of the spectrum, but at least, up to a dramatic threshold, the ratio holds.)

Another calculation confirms the excess of community-dwelling disabled but suggests that it may be more modest. A 1977 national survey identified almost 1.6 million individuals living in the community who required assistance with at least one out of four activities of daily living (ADL): bathing, dressing, eating, or toileting. This number exceeded the number in nursing homes during the same year with comparable limitation of function (1.2 million) (13). That ratio suggests four disabled persons in the community for every three persons in a nursing home.

What, then, are the factors that allow these disabled people to remain in the community, and how malleable are they? The critical role of social support, especially family and friends, has already been acknowledged. To plan rationally for an LTC program, better data are needed to identify those at highest risk of institutionalization. Table 7-2 summarizes some of the reports of various investigators who have looked at this question.

Vicente and her colleagues (3) used data from the Human Population Laboratory Longitudinal Study to follow those aged 55 and over for 9 years in order to assess their rate of nursing home use. Common factors in those with at least one admission were advanced age, low income, female gender, white race, and lack of social supports. Health status, measured as chronic limitation of activity, did not differentiate users from nonusers.

Palmore (4) followed a group of 207 elderly persons in the Durham area for 20 years. He found that the probability of spending some time in a nursing home was greater for women, whites, those never married, those without living children, and those with 6 or fewer years of schooling.

Weissert et al.'s (14) analysis of the day care experiment over the study year suggested that the patient characteristics significantly associated with entering institutions were being white, having fewer social activities and more bed disability days, and having a diagnosis of a circulatory disorder or an injury, having functional limitations as measured by the Katz ADL scale (a six-item measure of independence in feeding, bathing, dressing, toileting, transferring, and a measure of continence). A similar analysis of persons from the homemaker portion of the experiment showed no significant associations, but this lack may be explained by the fact that all participants had to have been hospitalized for at least 3 days during the 2 weeks immediately before entering the study.

McCoy and Edwards (15) used data from the 1973 Survey of Low-Income Aged and Disabled to predict 1974 institutionalization rates among welfare recipients aged 65 and over. They found the probability of institutionalization to be increased with functional impairment (measured by a modified Katz ADL scale), advanced age, household isolation, presence in the household of nonrelatives, and white race. Institutionalization was decreased in association with measurable social support, including frequent contact with friends and relatives and the propinquity of children.

TABLE 7-2. Risk Factors for Nursing Home Admission

Source	Sample	Risk Factors
National Center for Health Statistics (81)	Survey of nursing home residents in 1977 (compared to those aged 65+ living in the community)	Age, female, white, unmarried
Vicente et al. (3)	Nine-year follow-up of residents aged 55+ in Alameda County, Calif.	Age, poverty, white, lack of social supports
Palmore (4)	Twenty-year follow-up of residents aged 60+ in the Piedmont, N.C., area	Unmarried, white
Weissert et al. (82)	One-year study of day care recipients and controls in six sites	Primary diagnostic conditions, impairment prognosis, hospital outpatient or other use of ambulatory care
Weissert et al. (14)	One-year study of homemaker recipients and controls in four sites; patients were hospitalized for at least 3 days during the 2 weeks before the study	Primary diagnostic conditions, ADL prognosis, bed disability prognosis, hospital outpatient or other use of ambulatory care
McCoy and Edwards (15)	National sample of welfare recipients aged 65+	Age, functional impairment, white, living alone or with nonrelatives, lack of social supports

Risk factors are intimately associated with social support and social resources. A problem in targeting services on that basis, however, is that social support levels are unpredictable and subject to change. Little work has been done to assist us in targeting those individuals with fragile social support systems. Kulys and Tobin (16) studied a population of community-based elderly and pointed to a group whose support system was "one deep," meaning that if the current assistant were not available, no obvious backup could be identified.

Katz and Papsidero (17) have proposed a Social Functioning Index (SFI) composed of varying combinations of items covering five principal categories: social living environment (living alone or with others); ADL; diagnosis (life-threatening or not); mental status; and age. These factors have been used to predict 1-year survival.

WHAT IS THE ROLE OF THE NURSING HOME?

The Homes and the Patients

The nursing home is indeed the touchstone of LTC; all other modalities seem to be compared to it. Table 7-3 presents data on nursing homes in terms of the number of

TABLE 7-3. Characteristics of Nursing Homes

| | Percent of: | |
Characteristic	Homes	Beds
Ownership		
Proprietary	76.8	69.3
Voluntary nonprofit	17.7	21.1
Government	5.5	9.7
Level of care		
Skilled	19.2	21.0
Skilled and intermediate	24.2	39.2
Intermediate	31.6	27.9
Other (not certified)	25.0	11.9
Bed size		
Fewer than 50	42.3	13.0
50–99	30.8	29.8
100–199	22.3	39.0
200+	4.6	18.2

SOURCE: *The National Nursing Home Residents, Health Status and Care Received: National Nursing Home Survey, United States, May–December 1977*, publication (PHS) 81-1712 (*Vital and Health Statistics*, series 13, no 51, Table 43). Hyattsville, Md, National Center for Health Statistics, 1979.

homes and of beds; because larger homes are different from smaller ones, this distinction is useful. As seen in the table, more than three-fourths of nursing homes are run for profit; nonprofit homes tend to be larger than for-profit ones. Level of care is traditionally divided into skilled and intermediate, reflecting the amount of professional nursing care provided. However, only those patients covered by public funds need be classified in this way. Therefore, those homes that choose not to become certified to accept public patients need not be rated. More than two-thirds of nursing homes have fewer than 100 beds, although the trend is toward larger homes.

As shown in Table 7-4, three-fourths of the homes are more than 10 years old; almost 40% are more than 20 years old. More than 60% were purposely built; converted hospitals are rare. Most homes contain a mixture of private and semiprivate rooms. Fewer than one-third of the homes reporting in the 1977 survey identified themselves as part of a chain. Another 13% were tied to a health care or retirement facility. Interestingly, a substantial number of homes offer services to nonresidents, suggesting a possible role for nursing homes as a locus of varied modalities of LTC in a community.

Nursing homes are not staffed like hospitals. Whereas a community hospital maintains a staff of almost 300 full-time equivalents (FTEs) per 100 beds, the nursing home has less than one-sixth of that ratio. Table 7-5 demonstrates that staff in general, and especially skilled nursing staff, drops with lower levels of care.

The nursing home remains a relatively inexpensive form of care. In 1976, the average cost per patient day was almost $24. Proprietary homes cost somewhat less than nonprofit or government homes. Skilled facilities cost substantially more than intermediate care ($30 vs. $18.50) (18, Table 15). (In 1981, daily rates for skilled care in California ranged from $35 to $38; in other states, rates are substantially higher.)

TABLE 7-4. Facility and Operating Characteristics of Nursing Homes

Characteristic	Percent of Homes
Age of building	
less than 5 years	7
5–10 years	19
10–20 years	36
21+ years	38
Original purpose	
Nursing home	62
Hospital or health-related facility	6
Private home, apartment, or hotel	25
Average number of beds per room	
Fewer than 2	49
2 to fewer than 3	47
3 to fewer than 4	4
Type of operation	
Member of group or chain	28
Distinct unit of hospital, other health care facility, or retirement center	13
Services provided to nonresidents	
Home health care	13
Adult day care	24
Physical therapy	31
Occupational/recreational therapy	23
Meal delivery	54
Homemaking/chore service	2

SOURCE: *The National Nursing Home Residents, Health Status and Care Received: National Nursing Home Survey, United States, May–December 1977*, publication (PHS) 81-1712 (*Vital and Health Statistics*, series 13, no 51, Tables 5, 6, and 7). Hyattsville, Md, National Center for Health Statistics, 1979.

TABLE 7-5. Staffing Characteristics of Nursing Homes[a]

	Level of Care			
Employees	Skilled	Skilled and Intermediate	Intermediate	Not Certified
Total	52.7	51.8	40.7	29.2
Administrative, therapeutic, and medical	5.9	4.9	4.7	29.2
Nursing	46.8	46.9	36.0	24.1
Registered nurse	(7.1)	(5.9)	(2.4)	(2.8)
Licensed practical nurse	(6.6)	(6.5)	(6.3)	(3.0)
Aide	(33.1)	(34.6)	(27.3)	(18.4)

SOURCE: *The National Nursing Home Residents, Health Status and Care Received: National Nursing Home Survey, United States, May–December 1977*, publication (PSH) 81-1712 (*Vital and Health Statistics*, series 13, no 51, Table 8). Hyattsville, Md, National Center for Health Statistics, 1979.

[a]Full-time equivalents per 100 beds.

Admission Statistics Versus Resident Statistics

When talking about nursing home patients, data based on a study of those residing in a facility at a given time must be distinguished from data for those entering or leaving the facility. The former are equivalent to a point prevalence measure; the latter represent a type of incidence data. The conclusions reached about nursing home patients may be quite different, depending on this distinction. Keeler and his colleagues (19) have identified two streams of patients entering the nursing home. One group will leave fairly quickly (within 3 to 6 months); the other will stay for several years. The short stayers tend to be younger, have more physical problems, and enter from the hospital. The long stayers are more likely to be older, confused, and incontinent. At admission, the patients are about equally distributed between short stayers and long stayers, but a study of residents will find about nine times as many long stayers.

Table 7-6 compares selected characteristics of patients discharged from nursing homes to those of residents. As expected, residents are more likely to be female, older, and unmarried. Discharged patients had higher rates of impaired mobility and incontinence. Residents evidence more dementia and less somatic illness.

As seen in Table 7-7, nursing homes experience higher rates of patient turnover than might be expected. More than one-half of the discharges occur within 3 months of admission. Median length of stay is 60 days for live discharges and 130 days for the dead. One-quarter of those discharged are dead, and at least another 8% are known to die in the hospital. However, more than 25% of discharged nursing

TABLE 7-6. Comparison of Selected Characteristics of Nursing Home Discharges and Residents

Characteristic	Percent of 1976 Discharges	Percent of 1977 Residents
Female	63.5	71.2
Age 85+	29.7	34.5
Married	23.5	11.9
Bedfast/chair fast	50.0	37.3
Incontinent of bladder or bowel	48.9	45.3
Chronic brain syndrome/ senility[a]	38.7	56.9
Congestive heart failure[b]	5.0	4.0
Stroke[b]	12.5	7.9
Cancer[b]	8.2	2.2
Arteriosclerosis[b]	17.6	20.3

SOURCES: *Characteristics of Nursing Home Residents, Health Status and Care Received: National Nursing Home Survey, United States, May–December 1977,* publication (PHS) 81-1712 (*Vital and Health Statistics,* series 13, no 51, Tables 5, 8, and 10). Hyattsville, Md, National Center for Health Statistics, 1979. *Discharges from Nursing Homes: 1977 National Nursing Home Survey,* publication (PHS) 81-1715 (*Vital and Health Statistics,* series 13, no 54, Tables 3–5). Hyattsville, Md, National Center for Health Statistics, 1981.

[a]Listed as a chronic condition or impairment.

[b]Listed as a primary diagnosis.

TABLE 7-7. Discharges from Nursing Homes

Characteristic	Percent
Length of stay	
less than 1 month	33.6
1–3 months	20.1
3–6 months	12.1
6–12 months	10.0
1–3 years	14.0
3–5 years	6.1
5+ years	4.1
Discharged to:	
Dead	25.9
Community	27.4
Acute hospital	30.4[a]
Another nursing home	9.7
Other/unknown	6.6

SOURCE: *Discharges from Nursing Homes: 1977 National Nursing Home Survey*, publication (PHS) 81-1715 (*Vital and Health Statistics*, series 13, no 54, Table 3). Hyattsville, Md, National Center for Health Statistics, 1981.

[a]8.1% known to have died in the hospital.

home patients return to the community; the shorter the length of stay, the better the chance of returning to the community.

Nursing homes present yet another paradox and dilemma. Although physicians are reluctant to enter patients, the physician's signature is required for payment under Medicaid and Medicare. One might readily predict a pattern of perfunctory physician visits that comply with regulations but do not necessarily lead to careful patient assessment (20–23).

The nursing home itself can be a depressing environment, imposing the worst features of institutional care on those least able to resist. A series of fictionalized autobiographic works and participant observer studies provides some insight into what living in a nursing home means to an individual (24–28).

HOW DID WE GET WHERE WE ARE?

The United States now has enormous investments in institutional LTC. Not only are buildings in place, but programs and policies have been developed with the nursing home in mind. New proposals are offered in terms of how they will affect the demand for nursing home care. Many of the payment schemes and eligibility criteria encourage nursing home usage over other forms of LTC.

Some of the highlights of LTC have already been discussed. Its major public funding comes from a welfare program to support medical care for the needy and indigent. One obvious incentive is thus to create need and indigency. This spend-down necessity leaves the client without resources and thus threatens his or her chances of returning to the community once institutionalized. The question of need becomes one of defining eligibility in sufficiently medical terms, even though much of the basis for the need is social.

The medical basis for the LTC program puts the physician in an awkward position. As society's gatekeeper, the physician must certify the patient's need for services. As the patient's advocate, the physician must seek ways to ensure that the client obtains needed services. To the extent that the critical difference in need for LTC is determined by social rather than medical factors, the concerned physician may well lack the requisite skills and knowledge to make an informed judgment about the most appropriate resources for care. If physicians are less interested in the dependent elderly patient, they are still less likely to make good decisions, hence the frequently heard criticism that our society has medicalized a social phenomenon. Physicians may react with discomfort at the need to identify physical limitations to legitimate the need for social care.

Funding for LTC

The current resources for LTC are in large measure the result of public programs. Dunlop (29) traces the growth of the nursing home industry to the initiation of vendor payments, which antedate Medicaid. The fiscal payment (per diem) system tied to level of care (LOC) creates incentives to skim the patient pool—to admit those just over the threshold of eligibility in a care level and to reject the heavy-care patient who costs more but is reimbursed at the same skilled rate. (Unfortunately, the science of assigning patients to an LOC is imprecise [30], but only those decisions adverse to the nursing home are likely to be challenged.)

Fearing the further evolution of Medicaid mills, Congress has been unwilling to authorize reimbursement under Medicare Part B for nonphysician providers (physician assistants and geriatric nurse practitioners) without onsite supervision, thus eliminating a potentially effective and efficient source of primary care for institutionalized and homebound elderly. Although mandated to ensure the quality of care under federal programs, government officials and their designees have had difficulty finding an appropriate technology with which to assess quality (31). The regulatory approach has not worked well (32).

LTC is primarily supported under four public programs: Titles XVIII, XIX, and XX of the Social Security Act and Title III of the Older Americans Act. The first two can be thought of as medical programs and the last two as social programs, although this distinction is often imprecise. The benefits under these programs are summarized in Table 7-8.

Title XVIII (Medicare) is essentially a medical program that places major emphasis on hospital care. Its coverage of LTC was intended to encourage use of less expensive nonhospital care for patients who were still convalescing. Recent shifts indicate a move to allow use of benefits without prior hospitalization. Part B of Medicare funds medical care, including some ancillary services. Specifically excluded are preventive services, drugs, eyeglasses, and hearing aids (items that may be critical to effective functioning in an elderly patient). Both parts of Medicare use a "reasonable cost" reimbursement. For physician fees, this becomes "usual, customary and reasonable," a norming approach based on a percentage of the average fee for a physician class in a given area. Although Medicare home care benefits have been liberalized over time, they are still too tied to requirements of homeboundedness, need for skilled service, and intermittency to form consistent bases for a home health benefit.

TABLE 7-8. Summary of Major Federal Programs for the Elderly[a]

Program	Eligible Population	Services Covered	Deductibles and Copayments
Medicare (Title XVIII of the Social Security Act)			
Part A: hospital insurance	All persons eligible for Social Security and others with chronic disabilities, such as end-stage renal disease, plus voluntary enrollees 65+.	Per benefit period, "reasonable cost" for 90 days of hospital care plus 60 lifetime reserve days; 100 days of skilled nursing facility (SNF); home health visits (see text).	$260 deductible and copayments of $65/day for hospital days 61–90; $130/day for lifetime reserve days; $32.50 for SNF days 21–100.
Part B: supplemental medical insurance	All those covered under Part A who elect coverage. Participants pay a monthly premium of about $12.	80% of "reasonable cost" for physician services; supplies and services related to physician services; outpatient, physical, and speech therapy; diagnostic tests and x-ray films; surgical dressings; prostheses; ambulance; home health visits.	
Medicaid (Title XIX of the Social Security Act)	Persons receiving Supplemental Security Income (SSI) (such as welfare) or receiving SSI and a state supplement, or who meet lower eligibility standards used for medical assistance criteria in 1972, or who were eligible for	Mandatory services for the categorically needy: inpatient hospital services; outpatient services; SNF; limited home health care; laboratory tests and x-ray films; family planning; early and periodic	None, once patient spends down to eligibility level.

	Eligibility	Services	Fees
	SSI or were in institutions and eligible for Medicaid in 1973. Medically needy persons who do not qualify for SSI but have high medical expenses are eligible for Medicaid in some states; eligibility criteria vary from state to state.	screening, diagnosis, and treatment for children through age 20. Optional services vary from state to state: dental care; therapies; drugs; intermediate care facilities; extended home health care; private duty nurse; eyeglasses; prostheses; personal care services; medical transportation and home health care services. (States can limit the amount and duration of services.)	Fees are charged to those with incomes of more than 80% of the state's median income.
Title XX of the Social Security Act	All recipients of Aid to Families with Dependent Children (AFDC) and SSI. Optionally, those earning up to 115% of state median income and residents of specific geographic areas.	Day care; substitute care; protective services; family counseling; home-based services; employment, education, and training; health-related services; information and referral; transportation; day services; family planning; legal services; home-delivered and congregate meals.	
Title III of the Older Americans Act	All persons 60 years and older. Low income minority and isolated older persons are special targets.	Homemaker; home-delivered meals; home health aides; transportation; legal services; counseling; information and referral plus 19 others. (Fifty percent of funds must go to those services listed.)	Some payment may be requested.

[a]Information applies as of July 1982. Medicare deductibles are subject to change.

Medicaid, a welfare program authorized under Title XIX of the Social Security Act, is operated jointly by federal and state governments. The federal government provides between 50% and 78% of the state's costs of underwriting health services to the poor. Federal guidelines set minimum standards; the state has the option to go beyond this threshold by increasing benefits or broadening eligibility. The principal targets of the program are those persons covered under categorical welfare programs (such as families with dependent children, the aged, blind, permanently disabled, and medically needy). The categorically needy components of the aged, blind, and disabled were combined under a federally sponsored program, Supplemental Security Income (SSI), in 1974. The elderly are thus identified as being either SSI recipients or medically needy. Because Medicaid is a program designed to serve people with inadequate financial resources, there are no deductibles or copayments. However, many critics of the program have pointed out that it imposes a burden of poverty as a condition of eligibility. Persons are required to divest themselves of their own resources (the so-called spend-down requirement) before becoming eligible for Medicaid assistance. The program consists of two groups of services: mandatory services and a larger set of optional services provided at the discretion of the state, which can set limits on the amount and duration of such care. Even the mandatory services can be expanded or contracted at the option of a state government. The states also have the ability to set payment levels, which cannot exceed what is paid for private care. At present, approximately 40% of the Medicaid budget goes to nursing homes. An all too frequent pattern begins with an individual entering a nursing home under Medicare coverage. After the coverage lapses or the patient no longer meets the more stringent Medicare requirements, he or she exhausts private funds until eligible for Medicaid coverage. Medicaid can cover a wide array of home health services, but only a few states (most notably New York) have chosen to invest substantial Medicaid dollars in home care.

In contrast to the two programs just described, the two additional programs are primarily for social services with some medical components. Under *Title XX of the Social Security Act* (known as the *Social Service Amendments*), federal funds are paid to state government agencies as block grants based on state populations. The states are paid 75% of social service program costs up to their respective Title XX ceilings (90% for family planning costs). The eligible population includes persons covered under categorical welfare programs and, at the state's option, other groups identified on the basis of income or special needs. A wide variety of services is available under the program. General mandates of the program can be summarized under five broad goals: 1) to help people become or remain economically self-supporting; 2) to help people become or remain self-sufficient; 3) to protect children and adults who cannot protect themselves from abuse, neglect, and exploitation and to help families stay together; 4) to prevent and reduce inappropriate institutional care as much as possible by making home and community services available; and 5) to arrange for appropriate placement and services in an institution when this is in a person's best interest.

Title III of the Older Americans Act mandates a series of services targeted at older people (here defined as those who are 60 years or older). This program is supported by federal grants to state and then to local agencies to plan and coordinate services to older persons comprehensively. There are no income criteria, although some payment can be requested for those with income exceeding a threshold set by the local agency.

Under recent legislation, states can apply for federal waivers to allow more

TABLE 7-9. Resources for Home Care in Four Federal Programs

Program	Expenditures for Home Care (millions of dollars)	Percent of Total Program Budget	Time Period
Title XVIII (Medicare)	600	2.1	CY 1979
Title XIX (Medicaid)	211	1.2	FY 1978
Title XX	530	16	FY 1980
Title III (Older Americans Act)	43	15	FY 1980

SOURCE: *Medicare Home Health Services: A Difficult Program to Control*, publication (HRE) 81-155. General Accounting Office, 1981.

discretion in the use of Medicaid funds for LTC. Such waivers require a statewide plan that includes case management to assess the needs of clients and to match them with appropriate sources.

Unquestionably, the pattern of LTC in the United States has evolved around the institution, primarily the nursing home. More than 90% of expenditures for LTC go to nursing homes. As shown in Table 7-9, Medicare and Medicaid, the two largest federal LTC programs, spent only 2% and 1% of their respective budgets for home care. Much discussion has focused on the need to redress the balance. Unfortunately, the unplanned evolution of home care coverage has created a number of inconsistencies across programs. Table 7-10 portrays the variation in services and eligibility for the four major federal programs that support home care. Even a well-motivated broker of services would have difficulty assembling a package of services in the face of such a diverse collection of rules.

Each new service introduced creates its own set of incentives for misuse. The home health care benefit under Medicare was liberalized in 1981; the 100-visit

TABLE 7-10. In-home Services Provided Under Four Federal Programs

Items	Social Security Act			Older Americans Act, Title III
	(Medicare) Title VIII	(Medicaid) Title XIX	Title XX	
Services authorized				
Nursing	X	X		X
Therapy	X	X		X
Home health aide	X	X	X	X
Homemaker			X	X
Chore			X	X
Medical supplies and appliances	X	X		
Eligibility requirements				
Age	X			X
Income		X	X	
Need for skilled nursing	X			
Homebound	X			
Physician authorization	X	X		

SOURCE: *Medicare Home Health Services: A Difficult Program to Control*, publication (HRE) 81-155, Appendix I. General Accounting Office, 1981.

limitation, the required prior hospitalization, and the deductible were eliminated. Fears that this broadened benefit might prompt misuse led to a mandated Government Accounting Office (GAO) study (33). The report indicated that more than one-fourth of the claims reviewed showed evidence of misuse. Clients were not clearly homebound; need for services was not clearly indicated. Moreover, the GAO found evidence of displacement; home health aides were performing chores previously done by family members. This study should not be interpreted as exposing fraud. Rather, it indicates how market forces can motivate providers to use the program coverage to the fullest extent possible.

WHAT CAN BE DONE ABOUT IT?

The cry has been heard, but what action should we take? Reformers in LTC are quick to make claims and recommendations but short of data demonstrating the efficacy of alternative approaches. A problem in assessing the cost/benefit ratio of any intervention in LTC is the possibility that the experimental treatment may reduce the mortality of recipients. Even in a truly randomized design, differential attrition from mortality may leave different experimental and control groups. The group with the lower mortality is likely to have a commensurately higher morbidity. Nor is our attitude toward the mortality of LTC recipients clear. There is evidence of willingness to allow some patients to die without dramatic interventions (34). Mortality may not always be the worst program outcome.

The instinctive response against nursing home care is to move the services into the community—the home or the ambulatory center. The arguments in favor of such a move are several: people prefer to live in their own home; people do better in their own home; and care is less expensive at home. Weissert et al.'s (35) analysis of the homemaker and day care experiments calls into question the last two contentions. As noted in a previous section, persons assigned to day care showed less deterioration in function, but their use of services was no less than that of the controls; those receiving homemaker services demonstrated neither a functional nor a fiscal benefit. Weissert (36) attributes part of this lack of impact on costs to the low rate of nursing home use by controls.

The question of how to intervene depends on what is to be accomplished. There are many points along the spectrum of LTC toward which interventions can be targeted. Figure 7-3 portrays this spectrum from community to grave and indicates where these various types of interventions might occur. The farther to the left, the more highly functional community-dwelling persons are dealt with. A strategy designed to provide this group with better services could be considered a form of prevention, based on the idea that better service now will protect the individual against the need for institutionalization some time in the future. The probability of such a modus operandi depends greatly on the extent to which those at future risk can be identified and on the ability to intervene effectively. As noted earlier, the overall probability of entering a nursing home is about one in four. Thus, any intervention must be able to lower the rate of institutionalization below this 25% level. Looked at another way, three out of four persons would not enter a nursing home anyway.

The farther to the right in Figure 7-3, the greater is the risk of nursing home admission. Several points of intervention are easily identifiable. Consider patients

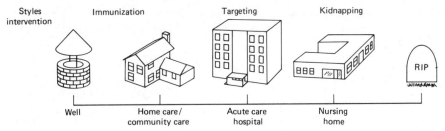

Figure 7-3. The spectrum of long term care.

discharged from an acute care hospital. Some diversionary activity can be inter-
posed at the point just before the patient's actual admission to a nursing home. In
the nursing home, individuals more appropriately cared for in the community can
be identified. Each of these strategies has in fact been tried (37). Table 7-11 summarizes some of the programs testing different approaches to using community
alternatives.

Case Management

Common to many of these programs is the need to assess potential clients to determine their need for care (i.e., types and frequency of care needed), to design an
appropriate package of services, and to ensure that such services are actually provided. This assessment and brokerage function is referred to as *case management.*
Case management comes in various forms; in its most complete state, the case
manager controls the resources available to the client, purchasing services on the
client's behalf or authorizing any such expenditures. Certainly, the effective case
manager must have resources to manage and sufficient influence over how those
resources are used.

   Despite the enthusiasm for case management, its role is not yet established.
Some observers of available data argue that the case for such services is established
(37). Others are less convinced. A large-scale national effort has been mounted to
test the cost effectiveness of case management. The National Channeling Demonstration project will test two models in several states. One model essentially coordi-
nates existing resources. The other can draw upon new funds to purchase needed
services without the restrictions usually imposed by program regulations.

Geriatric Assessment Units

Somewhere between hospital discharge planning and case management is the
geriatric evaluation unit (GEU). Such units are usually based in a hospital, but can
be either inpatient or outpatient operations. They differ from case management in
the thoroughness of their evaluation. Rather than gathering information to determine simply the needed mix of services, they are intended to provide a thorough
evaluation of the patient's problems with the goal of identifying remediable conditions, simplifying treatment regimens, assessing function in homelike surroundings, and developing a treatment program to maximize function. The primary
targets of GEUs are patients discharged from the acute care hospital and destined
for nursing homes, but such programs can also serve community dwellers considered to be at high risk. Although no carefully controlled studies have established

TABLE 7-11. Examples of Alternative LTC Programs

Project	Description	Results
Case management		
Triage (83)	Quasi-experimental design • 307 clients from community • 195 controls from another community Services authorized by triage under Medicare waivers	Use of services and costs higher for triage Mental status outcome better for triage Physical and social outcomes no different
Access (84)	Descriptive report with comparisons to other counties in New York Preadmission screening of patients referred for institutional care Implemented and monitored service under Medicaid waiver; now Medicare, too	1979: of patients from hospital, 57% of Medicaid and 20% of paying patients went home; of patients from community, 96% and 89%, respectively, stayed home Costs less than equivalent institutional care, but no real control group
Wisconsin Community Care Organization (85)	Experimental design attempted; 71 of 283 experimentals excluded Medicaid waivers used to serve clients from hospital and community	Experimentals cost less Rate of admission to hospital and nursing home no different, but total number of days less
Georgia Alternative Health Services Project (86)	Experimental design • 572 experimentals • 172 controls • 1-year follow-up Services included alternative living arrangements, day care, and home care	Experimentals had lower mortality and higher costs, but fewer nursing home days
Multipurpose Senior Services Project	Eight sites in California Clients from community, hospital, and nursing home Medicaid waivers used to purchase needed services after extensive assessment Comparison group identified separately	None available yet
Long-Term Care Channeling Demonstration	Sites in 10 states Two levels of program: case management only, and with additional funds and authorization control Random allocation possible in most places	None available yet

TABLE 7-11. (Continued)

Project	Description	Results
Geriatric evaluation units Evaluation units (38)	Units usually in hospital Most inpatient, but can be ambulatory Usually take patients discharged from acute service facility, but may come from community	No clear demonstration of efficacy, but reports are very positive Less use of nursing home New problems uncovered Regimens simplified
Housing Community Housing for the Elderly (42)	Experimental design Clients aged 62+, not functionally impaired 24 clients offered and accepted purposely built community housing Of 63 controls, 22 moved on their own 3-year follow-up	Mortality lower and satisfac- tion higher among experimen- tals Movers did better than non- movers among controls
Highland Heights (41)	228 elderly, physically impaired experimentals admitted to special housing unit Matched to 228 controls 5-year follow-up	Experimentals had lower mor- tality and lower rate of nursing home entry Generally fewer hospital and nursing home days 51 clients admitted from nurs- ing home (i.e., deinstitution- alized)
Support services Lifeline (45)	Emergency alarm sys- tem linked to emergency response station Matched pairs of experi- mentals and controls drawn from public hous- ing • 35 severely func- tionally impaired and socially isolated (I) • 46 severely func- tionally impaired and not socially isolated (II) • 58 socially isolated and moderately func- tionally impaired or medically vulnerable (III)	30% refused the service Fewer experimentals entered a hospital or nursing home Costs of formal and informal community services less for controls Benefit/cost ratio highest for group II

TABLE 7-11. (Continued)

Project	Description	Results
Capitation Social HMO	Four demonstration projects just getting under way Single rate covers case management, physician care, home care, hospital, and limited nursing home care, plus social services Method of calculating capitation rates not yet fixed Marketing not established	Not yet available

the cost effectiveness of these programs, the reports from early GEUs are positive (38).

Capitation

The logical extension of the case management concept is a fully capitated (i.e., prepaid) system that will operate from a fixed budget. Some experiments along these lines have already been tried; more are under way. Among the several issues to be determined is how broad the coverage can (or should) be. Medicare already provides for purchase of Health Maintenance Organization (HMO) services for elderly clients at a rate higher than that for younger persons enrolled in the HMO. But this type of coverage is restricted to little more than the narrow medical (especially acute medical) package of services under Medicare. Enthusiasts for capitation agree that its real potential will not be tapped until it combines social and medical services, presumably using savings from expensive medical care to finance effective social interventions (39). A Social HMO (SHMO) model is now in the early development stage in several areas (40); it is certainly too early to draw conclusions about feasibility, to say nothing of effectiveness. Still unsettled are basic questions such as the following: How should rates be set (by risk level)? Who will be interested in enrolling? How can risks be shared among providers of service, the SHMO, and the consumer?

Where does LTC end? Entertaining the idea of including all LTC under a single capitation rate requires serious thought about what should be included. This is no easy task. Arguments can be advanced for including various forms of housing (retirement homes, sheltered housing with general supervision), perhaps even housing subsidies. Several studies have suggested that housing improvement is associated with decreased mortality in the elderly (41–44). Close cooperation with housing authorities is needed in any LTC planning.

The elderly person may well turn out to be much more responsive to a variety of interventions than has been suspected. Each new report of a success suggests another candidate for inclusion under LTC. For example, an experiment with an in-home emergency call system seems to have had dramatic results in relieving anxiety and reducing use of health care services in some older persons (45).

LTC lacks a clear method for linking what is hoped to be achieved to what society is willing to pay. Capitation offers one response to that dilemma; it avoids the common pitfall of the perverse incentives of fee-for-service reimbursement (wherein the worse a patient gets, the more the provider is paid) and offers a flexible means for using available resources. However, critics of capitation argue that providers may selectively market their services to those least in need, and may take shortcuts and eliminate or delay important services in order to save money. The elderly, especially the dependent elderly, may be the consumers least able to vote with their feet.

Our societal goals have not been articulated clearly. If the ends society seeks to achieve can be better defined, appropriate incentive systems to achieve them can be developed. Techniques for outcome-based reimbursement in LTC are not difficult to envision (46); more perplexing is the task of elucidating societal value preferences for what is truly sought from LTC (47). Perhaps the way we approach LTC tells us more about ourselves than we want to know.

THE MEDICAL COMPONENT OF LTC AND QUALITY OF CARE

Nursing homes are not the favorite haunts of physicians. In one study, only 14% of the active physicians in a metropolitan area participated in nursing home care (48). Closer scrutiny of the care that is provided offers little solace (20). A review of the medical records of nursing home patients in a metropolitan area revealed a substantial number of charts with no evidence of a new observation or physical examination for 6 months or more (21).

Several studies have documented the inadequacy of geriatric care and the need for more and better medical care for the elderly (49,50). The equation is one of strategy. Does society train existing doctors better, develop a new cadre of geriatric specialists, or use other types of caregivers?

Other disciplines may be appropriate primary caregivers for LTC. The growth of the nurse practitioner movement offers an attractive alternative to sole reliance on physicians. The philosophy of nursing places emphasis on care rather than on curing, and its traditions encourage nurses to work more comfortably with nursing home staffs to upgrade their skills. Geriatric nurse practitioners would thus appear to be an ideal solution to the problem of how to improve the care provided to LTC patients (51). One demonstration project using a team of geriatric nurse practitioners and social workers provides cause for enthusiasm. The care rendered by the team, supported by physician and clinical pharmacist consultants, was not only better than the alternatives but was also cost effective. The savings in other care costs were greater than the entire cost of fielding the team (52). This experience has been replicated (53); the need to modify Medicare regulations to permit wider use of nonphysician providers is clear. The reluctance to do so can be traced to a fear of exploitation. It is not yet known how to ensure quality and prevent fraud in medical care. The elderly are an especially vulnerable group.

Quality of Care

There is a disappointing dearth of useful data on the quality of nursing home care. What little light is shed tends to be diffuse; a number of problems remain unresolved. Despite a plethora of instruments to measure various aspects of patient functioning, few are well standardized with known measures of validity and reliability (54). Few instruments have been applied across large cross sections of nursing homes. There is little agreement about what constitutes good care. Advocates of the medical and social models continually debate the respective merits of these approaches. Without a consensus about goals, evaluation is impossible. Not surprisingly, those studies of quality that are available are not always consistent in their findings, especially when different measures are used. Related issues concerning the quality of medical care are presented in Chapter 13.

One can discern a certain hierarchy in these studies. Several reports deal with the question of whether nursing home patients really need the level of care they are receiving. This question is generally couched in terms of those needing less, or at least less expensive, care, but occasionally patients are found to need more care. The judgment about need is most often implicit, based on clinical expertise, but there have also been attempts to develop explicit criteria (31).

More researchers have addressed the assessment of quality by examining the structure of care provided by nursing homes. Using essentially unvalidated measures based on assumptions of what constitutes good care, these investigators have ranked nursing homes based on such factors as amount of care or nurse/patient ratios, types and variety of programs, and impressions about the physical facilities.

Mandated programs to assess the need for care and appropriate length of stay of Medicaid and Medicare patients have been conducted by state agencies. The model for such assessments is the hospital use review (UR) procedure, which may not be directly transferable to the nursing home. These reviews correspond to process measures in the more common parlance of quality of care assessment as presented in Chapter 13. Several investigators have attempted to take advantage of this set of data to describe nursing home care (31).

In only rare instances have researchers examined changes in patients over time to observe the outcomes of nursing home care (55). Outcome assessments are critical in an area such as nursing home care, where the relationship between what is done and what happens to patients is so poorly delineated. The continued trend toward increasingly rigorous regulations with no demonstrated efficacy is likely to increase tension and costs but may not necessarily lead to improved care. The posture of the regulators comes increasingly to resemble that of the edentulous lion who roars for attention but soon frightens only the uninitiated. The frustration over the inability to regulate nursing homes effectively and the growing cost of regulation have led the federal government to propose a relaxation of rules at a time when *better*, not *fewer*, rules are needed. Haunting our concerns about quality is the ever-present question of how to ensure quality in even more decentralized programs such as home care.

Quality of care is directly linked to questions of costs and payment. A few innovative reimbursement proposals have been suggested to create climates conducive to better nursing care. One proposal is for a prospective incentive reimbursement scheme in which facilities would be grouped into homogeneous peer categories and paid a mean per diem rate based on four factors: dollar ceiling for the peer group, occupancy rate, health status of patients, and facility evaluation (56). Reimbursement above a fixed range of the group mean would require documentation that these additional funds contribute to quality-related services. Operating surpluses for fully compliant homes would be partially distributed to the owners and employees and partially used to purchase capital expansion rights.

Another proposal for achieving quality care at the appropriate level is to hold nursing homes responsible for the provision of minimum custodial care only, and to permit residents to purchase all other services on the open market (57). Such a system would, according to its advocates, end placement at an inappropriate level and have the added psychologic benefit of permitting the resident to control his or her medical care and make personal decisions. The nursing home would become a more homelike environment under these conditions. This model is attractive theoretically but there are many potential problems that would need to be addressed in the pilot tests of the plan. How is custodial care to be defined? If it includes necessary bedside nursing, would a level-of-care system again become necessary, or would the patient also purchase intensive nursing services on the open market? Would the services be available on the open market? And, perhaps most crucial, what safeguards would be developed to protect those residents who do not have the capacity to exercise their purchasing power and who do not have family members as guardians? A rather complex administrative system with guardianship mechanisms would surely be necessary.

Kane (46) has proposed a model whereby nursing homes would be paid in proportion to the degree that their patients achieved good outcomes. Each patient's outcome would be compared with an individualized prognosis generated from data collected by independent reviewers. Payment would be based on average costs for that class of patient multiplied by a prognostic adjustment factor (PAF). Where a patient did better than expected, the PAF would be greater than 1; where the outcome was worse than expected, the PAF would be less than 1. Such a system is compatible with both prospective and retrospective reimbursement procedures. Its major virtue is the focus on the results of care, thereby minimizing the need for rules and regulations.

QUALITY OF LIFE

In an ideal situation, quality of care and quality of life should be highly overlapping concepts. The facility achieving a high level of quality of care should, by definition, ensure residents a good quality of life. As noted above and in Chapter 13, quality of care is difficult to achieve and to measure. But quality of life is an even more elusive concept, dependent on individual preferences and limited by individual health, regardless of residence in a nursing home. To the extent that particular nursing home settings have been related to the quality of life of the residents, positive ratings of quality may also be independent of highly competent technical care. In some ways, medical technology may produce a well-ordered, hospital-style environment that is most unattractive for a long term resident.

A fairly safe generalization is that few persons perceive nursing home admission as a positive event. Dread and despair are the reactions most frequently associated with nursing homes among the prospective client population. It is difficult to assess the facility's role in providing a high quality of life for residents in the face of all the negative connotations that the home carries in the minds of its clientele.

More is known about what is wrong with life in a nursing home than how a program may go about remedying the situation. The books by nursing home residents or by participant observers in long term care institutions mentioned above cite the loss of personal freedom inherent in the role and the extreme difficulty residents may encounter in completing simple actions, such as making a telephone call. The former identity of the nursing home residents tends to become subsumed under the classification "patient." In a demonstration project that attempted to meet the social needs of the patients, Jorgensen and Kane (58) noted that the interests and skills of the residents (such as piano playing) were unknown to nursing home staff before the beginning of the project.

Brody cataloged what she called the "iatrogenic diseases of institutional life" as follows (59):

> dependency; depersonalization; low self-esteem; lack of occupation or fruitful use of time; geographic and social distance from family and friends and cultural milieu; inflexibility of routines and menus; loneliness; lack of privacy, identity, own clothing, possessions, and furniture; lack of freedom; desexualization and infantilization; crowded conditions; and negative, disrespectful, or belittling staff attitudes.

It is with such criteria that quality of life can be measured. Some of the items, such as inflexibility of routines and menus, lack of privacy, and negative staff attitudes, may be directly attributable to institutional life, whereas others, such as loneliness and geographic distance from family and friends, may also characterize the lives of many elderly persons outside the nursing home. Nor are there before/after studies to show how the quality of particular patients' lives deteriorate upon admission to a nursing home.

The nursing home has sometimes been called a decision-free environment for its residents. This quality has taken on an extremely ominous note because of our current understanding of the phenomenon called *learned helplessness* (60). According to this theory, when a person perceives that his or her actions no longer elicit responses, a syndrome develops characterized by depression, cessation of efforts to influence events, and inability to determine when one's actions have actually elicited a response. Learned helplessness has been documented in nursing home residents, and a number of field studies have demonstrated that startling changes may occur in both effective state and level of activity when small changes are made that increase actual or perceived control among nursing home residents. In one of these studies, regular visits from volunteers, coupled with the residents' power to decide the timing of the visits, produced beneficial effects (61). Two other studies demonstrated that the ability to make small decisions, such as the timing of visits or the selection of and care for a plant, led to lessened depression and an improved level of activity compared to a control group that received similar attention, but in a paternalistic way that offered no decision-making opportunities (62,63).

Ferrari studied the effect of perceived control among those on a waiting list for admission to a nursing home (64). After controlling for level of health, she found that those patients who perceived that they themselves had decided to enter the facility before admission were significantly more likely to survive after admission than those who perceived that they had no choice. This study suggests, first, that the repercussions of perceived helplessness are actually life-threatening and, second, that quality of life in a nursing home may be partially related to procedures of selection, referral, and decision making before admission.

Because individual control is an important dimension affecting the quality of a nursing home resident's life, information is necessary about the preferences of particular groups of elderly persons and about which patients fare best under what kinds of conditions. Few data of this nature are available, in part because controlled clinical trials of nursing home conditions raise ethical questions and in part because, in many areas, beds are limited and few choices of placement are possible. Unlike free market industries, it is impossible to study nursing home preferences by observing the movement of patients from facilities with which they are dissatisfied to other facilities. There is some evidence to suggest, however, that the widely known negative effects of relocation of nursing home patients do not occur when the patient requests the transfer and is prepared for the move (65).

Fragmentary findings exist to suggest conditions that may be desirable in nursing homes from a quality of life standpoint. Jorgensen and Kane found that patients were mostly willing to accept nursing home placement if some continuation of their previous life style was possible (58). In another study, a change to heterosexual living spaces improved adjustment to the nursing home and social behavior in male residents (66). The factors most clearly associated with negative adjustment to nursing homes in a group of 20 women were lack of privacy, lack of independence, and distance from family and friends (67). A comparison of institutionalized and noninstitutionalized elderly found an association between future commitments (measured by number of planned appointments in the week ahead) and successful aging; those in nursing homes tended to have fewer future commitments (68). Jones hypothesized that crowded conditions caused interpersonal conflict and that friendships tended to be formed not with people in the same room but with people several doors away (69). Some of these finding are consistent with the impressions from a study of nursing homes abroad that homogeneous populations, based on ethnicity and culture, single rooms, separation of the mentally alert from the disorganized, and opportunity to pursue former interests are associated with a higher quality nursing home environment (70). Studies such as those cited above, however, are not useful for forming guidelines to assess quality of life because they are isolated pieces of work that have not generally been repeated and do not form a coherent knowledge base.

MEDICAL VERSUS SOCIAL MODELS

How, then, can measures of quality of care and quality of life be combined? Inevitably, one is led back to the distinction between the social and medical models for LTC.

If the nursing home is not the natural heir to social responsibility for the elderly, it has at least become the de facto answer to fill a void formerly filled by family members in a less complex and less mobile era, a void partially filled by government social services and personal health services in European countries. Like many products of mixed marriages, the nursing home faces a severe identity crisis. It is far from clear whether its dominant lineage is medical or social. Although most of the regulations for nursing homes seem to cast the facilities as miniature hospitals, most of the problems are more social than medical.

The question of eminent domain has not been resolved. The issue of predominance between the medical and social models for LTC is not merely a battle for bureaucratic supremacy between two factions of government. It is a fundamental clash of beliefs regarding the style of life to be pursued and the appropriate manner of its pursuit. This conflict of credos involves questions of both ends and means— the goals and expectations generated by different perspectives and the paths deemed most approachable to reach them. Under the growing pressure of enforced fiscal austerity, a choice is increasingly necessary. No longer can providers and consumers tolerate the ambiguity resulting from assigning equal weight to both approaches.

The social model is attractive because it emphasizes that health care, albeit crucial, is just one of many services needed to raise the quality of life of the aged. Especially with an elderly population, the often dwindling benefits of heroic medical measures must be balanced against the heavy social and psychologic costs. Morbidity and disability are conditions of life for the majority of aged people. A medical model allows the conditions to define a range of life circumstances. The permanence and intractability of these problems argue for societal provisions to protect the elderly from a permanent patient role for decades before their death.

Meeting Health Care Needs

Although long term institutional care should be perceived and organized as a social program, medical nihilism cannot be advocated. Clearly, medical services are needed for nursing home patients, and perceptive, responsive, skilled practitioners are needed to fill those roles. But first, physician uninterest in elderly patients in general and nursing home patients in particular must be overcome. There are two quite distinct approaches to redressing this situation: 1) to elevate medical practice with the elderly through education, credentialing, and research money into a prestigious specialty; and 2) to train and use nonphysician primary care personnel to serve the institutionalized aged. The effectiveness of the nurse practitioner as a deliverer of care in nursing homes was described above. These approaches are two extremes on a continuum; a midpoint approach would be sensitization of family practitioners and internists to the particular needs of the elderly. Another solution would be a simultaneous emphasis on the development of geriatric medical specialists for differential diagnosis while other personnel are used for ongoing care. This approach has been used in a number of European countries, particularly Great Britain (70).

What are the advantages and disadvantages of various models for medical care in nursing homes? The geriatrician emphasis carries with it the likelihood of increasingly sophisticated differential diagnosis but has the pitfalls of accentuating the hospital mode of nursing home life (71). On the other hand, it is important that nursing personnel who work on a daily basis with residents and physicians in nursing homes be alert to physical problems and be able to differentiate the disorientation accompanying an acute illness from the disorientation of old age. Whether a cadre of geriatricians is needed to spearhead training and research for such awareness is not yet certain.

One can assert more safely that a team approach is required for providing health services to the elderly. Many of the interventions that are most effective in terms of increasing comfort and reducing functional disability are provided by physical therapists, dentists, optometrists, podiatrists, and hearing aid specialists. A pharmacist, too, is invaluable for monitoring the drug use of patients. Although there is often overdependence on the magic of teamwork, health care to long term institutional residents has the ingredients necessary to justify a team approach. There are clearly differentiated functional tasks for the different team members and, because the mobility of the patient group is limited, the importance of assembling a comprehensive service in a convenient manner is increased. Indeed, in most instances, many health care personnel are not available to residents of nursing homes, nor is there any mechanism for reimbursing many needed services. Data from the National Center for Health Statistics 1973–1974 Nursing Home Survey indicates that only 9.9% of nursing home patients receive physical therapy, 15.2% recreational therapy, 5.7% occupational therapy, 0.5% speech therapy, and only 8% any form of professional counseling (72).

If, in the face of finite resources, a choice is required between geriatric specialists or geriatric nurse practitioners mobilizing a team of providers as needed, the latter would seem to offer the greater possible benefit. Perhaps if the nursing home is really a "home," as the designation implies, it would not be too far fetched to consider that home health services should be developed to serve nursing home residents as well as those in their own dwelling.

Regardless of the medical resources adopted, there is great value in maintaining some balance of forces separate from the nursing home itself. The providers of medical services should have an entity distinct from the nursing home if they are to offer a set of standards independent of the institution's. The resultant dynamic tension is not intended to be a source of conflict, but to provide an outside influence that will promote improved quality. This approach represents a segment of the hospital model worthy of adoption.

Meeting Social Needs

Gottesman and Brody have suggested three general approaches to improving the quality of life in a nursing home through psychosocial interventions (73). The first is the use of a variety of therapeutic approaches with explicit goals to change or improve the patient. The second requires structural changes in organization, staffing patterns, and relationships in the nursing home community; these changes would be designed to facilitate individualized care while developing a sense of community. The third refers to changes in the relationship between the nursing home and the community designed to break down communication barriers, increase the visibility of nursing homes, and develop more flexible programs to serve the community.

The first approach, the therapeutic one, has been a partial response to the lack of mental health services for the elderly, particularly those in institutions. Reactive depressions are endemic among elderly nursing home residents, and paranoid responses are also prevalent. Sometimes these psychiatric disturbances have been lumped together into the catchall concept of *senility*. Senile disorientation is itself often considered hopeless, and frequently no treatment is offered. Among the more popular treatments are various talking therapies ranging from reminiscence groups to current events clubs, more traditional drug and convulsive therapy for depression, and reality orientation therapy to combat and stem disorientation. The last of these treatments consists of short daily group sessions directed to reinforcing awareness of time, place, and names, with reinforcement from staff on a 24-hour basis. Controlled studies of these various and sometimes conflicting (compare reality orientation to reminiscing) interventions are rare, and it is difficult to separate the Hawthorne effect (changes in behavior due to the experiment) for a population that has notoriously been neglected. Another therapeutic approach is general behavior modification, sometimes complete with token economies to reinforce desired behaviors.

The shortcoming of all the therapeutic approaches is that they do not compensate for a deficient environment. What good is reality orientation if reality itself is bleak? What use is reminiscing if the elderly perceive it as an exercise in humoring them rather than a genuine interest in and social use for their experiences? What use is counseling to alleviate depression if, as noted earlier, depression is a by-product of the helplessness and perceived lack of control inculcated by the nursing home itself? Austin and Kosberg interviewed the administrators and head nurses of 27 Florida nursing homes and found that the opportunities for patient autonomy and decision making were minimal (74). For example, in one-half of the homes, patients were not allowed to visit patients of the opposite sex with their doors closed; in one-third of the homes, bedtimes could not be determined by the patients; in no instance could patients determine waking hours; and there was almost never a choice of roommate. Contrast this to the assertion that the most desirable environment for LTC is a naturalistic environment designed by the clientele (75).

The second general approach involves the creation of a sense of community through various adjustments of resident/staff mix and development of community councils for decision making, creation of an active recreational program, and elevation of staff competency by training as well as by adding professionals. There are certainly some nursing homes in the country that are especially attractive environments, and this fact can readily be perceived by visitors. Former U.S. Senator Frank Moss, previously chairperson of a Senate Long-Term Care Subcommittee, documented some of the ingredients of a good nursing home based on staffing, facilities, and programs, and encouraged family members to approach nursing home selection with a checklist of requirements (76).

The third approach, bridging the gap between nursing home and community, is quite promising. In this general category are included a variety of emphases: encouraging volunteers from the community to enter the nursing home; encouraging volunteer nursing home residents to offer service in the community; integrating day centers with nursing homes; encouraging brief admissions to relieve families; and combining programs for children with those of LTC facilities. Innovations that increase the visibility of the nursing home in the community not only create opportunities for residents to fulfill community roles but also reduce potential abuses through the protection of public scrutiny.

Although there is much evidence that the aged are not readily abandoned by family members (77,78), but rather are placed in nursing homes when the family has exhausted its own resources (79), there is nevertheless a withdrawal of many family members after admission to a home. As Gottesman indicates, the relative of the patient will not hold the nursing home accountable if most contact ceases after the initial referral, especially if "the implicit contract between the nursing home and relatives is one of noninterference by the other from whom the home takes over a difficult burden" (80). Additionally, of course, those who have no remaining families are overrepresented among nursing home residents. Therefore, the public attention to nursing homes created by a variety of community-based strategies may be essential to create a public that holds the nursing home responsible.

REFERENCES

1. Kastenbaum R, Candy SE: The 4% fallacy: A methodological and empirical critique of extended care facility population statistics. *Aging Hum Dev* 1973; 4:15–21.

2. Kane RL, Kane RA: Care of the aged: Old problems in need of new solutions. *Science* 1978; 200:913–919.

3. Vicente L, Wiley JA, Carrington RA: The risk of institutionalization before death. *The Gerontologist* 1979; 19:361–366.

4. Palmore E: Total chance of institutionalization among the aged. *Gerontologist* 1976; 16:504–507.

5. Butler LH, Newacheck PW: Health and social factors relevant to long-term care policy, in Meltzer J, Farrow F, Richman H (eds). *Policy Options in Long-Term Care.* Chicago, University of Chicago Press, 1981.

6. Brody EM: Aging of the family. *Ann Am Acad Political Social Sci* 1978; 438:13–27.

7. Shanas E: The family as a social support system in old age. *Gerontologist* 1979; 19:169–174.

8. Eggert GM, Granger CV, Morris R, et al: Caring for the patient with long-term disability. *Geriatrics* 1977; 32:102–113.

9. Callahan JJ, Diamond LD, Giele JZ, et al: Responsibility of families for their severely disabled elders. *Health Care Financing Rev* Winter 1980; 29–73.

10. US Comptroller General: *The Well-Being of Older People in Cleveland, Ohio,* publication (HRD) 77-70. US Government Accounting Office, 1977.

11. US Comptroller General: *Conditions of Older People: National Information System Needed,* publication (HRD) 79-95. US Government Accounting Office, 1979.

12. US Comptroller General: *Report to Congress on Home Health—The Need for a National Policy to Better Provide for the Elderly,* publication (HRD) 78-19. US Government Accounting Office, 1977.

13. Willging PR, Neuschler E: Debate continues on future of federal financing of long-term care. *Hospitals,* July 1982, pp 61–66.

14. Weissert WG, Wan TTH, Livieratos BB, et al: Cost-effectiveness of homemaker services for the chronically ill. *Inquiry* 1980; 17:230–243.

15. McCoy JL, Edwards BE: Contextual and socio-demographic antecedents of institutionalization among aged welfare recipients. *Med Care* 1981; 19:907–921.

16. Kulys R, Tobin SS: Older people and their "responsible others." *Soci Work* 1980; 25:138–145.

17. Katz S, Papsidero J: *A Data Archive for Use in Long-Term Care Policy Analysis: Final Report.* East Lansing, Mich, Michigan State University, 1981.

18. *The National Nursing Home Residents, Health Status and Care Received: National Nursing Home Survey, United States, May–December 1977,* publication (PHS) 81-1712 (*Vital and Health Statistics,* Series 13, no 51). Hyattsville, Md, National Center for Health Statistics.

19. Keeler EB, Kane RL, Solomon DH: Short- and long-term residents of nursing homes. *Med Care* 1981; 19:363–369.

20. US Congress, Senate Subcommittee on Long-Term Care of the Special Committee on Aging: *Doctors in Nursing Homes: The Shunned Responsibility* (supporting paper no 3 in *Nursing Home Care in the United States: Failure in Public Policy*). US Government Printing Office, 1975.

21. Kane RL, Hammer D, Byrnes N: Getting care to nursing home patients: A problem and a proposal. *Med Care* 1977; 15:174–180.

22. Keeler EB, Solomon DH, Beck JC, et al: Effect of patient age on duration of medical encounters with physicians. *Med Care* (in press).

23. Willemain T, Mark RB: The distribution of intervals between visits as a basis for assessing and regulating physician services in nursing homes. *Med Care* 1980; 18:427–441.

24. Tulloch J: *A Home Is Not a Home.* New York, Seabury Press, 1975.

25. Laird C: *Limbo*. Novato, Calif, Chandler and Sharp Publishers, Inc, 1979.

26. Gubrium JF: *Living and Dying at Murray Manor*. New York, St. Martin's Press, 1975.

27. Bennett C: *Nursing Home Life: What It Is and What It Could Be*. New York, Tiresias Press, Inc, 1980.

28. Newton E: *This Bed My Centre*. Melbourne, Australia, McPhee Gribble Publishers, 1979.

29. Dunlop BD: *The Growth of Nursing Home Care*. Lexington, Mass, Lexington Books, 1979.

30. Foley WE, Schneider DP: A comparison of the level of care predictions of six long-term care patient assessment systems. *Am J Public Health* 1980; 70:1152–1161.

31. Kane RA, Kane RL, Kleffel D, et al: *The PSRO and the Nursing Home, vol 1: An Assessment of PSRO Long-Term Care Review* (R-2459/1-HCFA). Santa Monica, Calif, Rand Corporation, 1979.

32. Vladek BG: *Unloving Care: The Nursing Home Tragedy*. New York, Basic Books, 1980.

33. *Medicare Home Health Services: A Difficult Program to Control*, publication (HRD) 81-155. US General Accounting Office, 1981.

34. Brown NK, Thompson DJ: Nontreatment of fever in extended-care facilities. *N Engl J Med* 1979; 300:1246–1250.

35. Weissert WG, Wan TH, Livieratos BB: *Effects and Costs of Day Care and Homemaker Services for the Chronically Ill: A Randomized Experiment*, publication no (PHS) 79-3258. Hyattsville, Md, US Dept of Health, Education and Welfare, 1980.

36. Weissert WG: Toward a continuum of care for the elderly: A note of caution. *Public Policy* 1981; 29:331–340.

37. US Comptroller General: *Entering a Nursing Home—Costly Implications for Medicaid and the Elderly*, publication (PAD) 80-12. US Government Accounting Office, 1979.

38. Rubenstein LZ, Rhee L, Kane RL: The role of geriatric assessment units in caring for the elderly: An analytic review. *J Gerontol* (in press).

39. Ruchlin HS, Morris JN, Eggert GM: Management and financing of long-term care services: A new approach to a chronic problem. *N Engl J Med* 1982; 306:101–106.

40. Diamond L, Berman D: The social/health maintenance organization: A single entry, prepaid long-term delivery system, in Callahan JJ Jr, Wallek S (eds): *Reforming the Long-Term Care System: Financial and Organizational Options*, Lexington, Mass, Lexington Press, 1980.

41. Sherwood S, Greer DS, Morris JN, et al: *An Alternative to Institutionalization: The Highland Heights Experiment*. Cambridge, Mass, Ballinger Publishing Co, 1981.

42. Brody EM: Community housing for the elderly: The program, the people, the decision-making process and the research. *Gerontologist* 1978; 18:121–129.

43. Carp FM: Impact of improved living environment on health and life expectancy. *Gerontologist* 1977; 17:242–249.

44. Lawton MP: *Social and Medical Services in Housing for the Aged*, publication no (ADM) 80-861. US Government Printing Office, 1980.

45. Ruchlin HS, Morris JN: Cost-benefit analysis of an emergency alarm and response system: A case study of a long-term care program. *Health Serv Res* 1981; 16:65–80.

46. Kane RL: Paying nursing homes for better care. *J Community Health* 1976; 2:1–4.

47. Kane RL, Kane RA: *Value Preferences and Long-Term Care*. Lexington, Mass, DC Heath, 1982.

48. Solon JA, Greenawalt LF: Physicians' participation in nursing homes. *Med Care* 1974; 12:486–495.

49. Institute of Medicine: *Aging and Medical Education*. Washington, DC, National Academy of Sciences, 1978.

50. Kane RL, Solomon DH, Beck JC, et al: *Geriatrics in the United States: Manpower Projects and Training Considerations.* Lexington, Mass, DC Heath, 1981.

51. Pepper GA, Kane RL, Teteberg B: Geriatric nurse practitioner in nursing homes. *Am J Nurs* 1976; 76:62–64.

52. Kane RL, Jorgensen L, Teteberg B, et al: Is good nursing-home care feasible? *JAMA* 1976; 235:516–519.

53. Master RJ, Feltin M, Jainchill J, et al: A continuum of care for the inner city: Assessment of its benefits for Boston's elderly and high-risk populations. *N Engl J Med* 1980; 302:1434–1440.

54. Kane RA, Kane RL: *Assessing the Elderly: A Practical Guide to Measurement.* Lexington, Mass, DC Heath, 1981.

55. Kane RL, Riegler S, Bell R, et al: *Predicting the Course of Nursing Home Patients: A Progress Report* (N-1786-NCHSR). Santa Monica, Calif, Rand Corp, 1982.

56. Ruchlin HS, Levey S, Muller C: The long-term care marketplace: An analysis of deficiencies and potential reform by means of incentive reimbursement. *Med Care* 1975; 13:979–991.

57. Ruchlin HS, Levey S: An economic perspective of long-term care, in Sherwood S (ed): *Long-Term Care: A Handbook for Researchers, Planners, and Providers.* New York, Spectrum Publications, Inc, 1975.

58. Jorgensen LA, Kane RL: Social work in the nursing home: A need and an opportunity. *Soc Work Health Care* 1976; 1:471–482.

59. Brody E: A million procrustean beds. Gerontologist 1973; 13:430–435.

60. Seligman M: *Helplessness: On Depression, Development and Death.* San Francisco, WH Freeman & Co, 1975.

61. Schulz R: Effects of control and predictability on the physical and psychological well-being of the institutionalized aged. *J Pers Soc Psychol* 1976; 33:563–573.

62. Langer E, Rodin J: Effects of choice and enhanced personal responsibility for the aged: A field experiment in an institutional setting. *J Pers Soc Psychol* 1976; 34:191–198.

63. Mercer S, Kane RA: Helplessness and hopelessness in the institutionalized elderly. *Health Soc Work* 1979; 4:90–116.

64. Ferrari N: *Institutionalization and Attitude Change in an Aged Population: A Field Study in Dissonance Theory,* dissertation. Western Reserve University, Cleveland, 1962 (mimeo).

65. Ogren E, Linn M: Male nursing home patients: Relocation and mortality. *J Am Geriatr Soc* 1971; 19:229–239.

66. Silverstone B, Wynter L: The effects of introducing a heterosexual living space. Gerontologist 1975; 15:83–87.

67. Abdo E, Dills J, Schectman H, et al: Elderly women in institutions vs. those in public housing: Comparison of personal and social adjustments. *J Am Geriatr Soc* 1973; 21:81–87.

68. Schonfield D, Hooper A: Future commitments and successful aging: I. Random sample, II. Special groups. *J Gerontol* 1973; 28:189–196, 197–201.

69. Jones DC: Spatial proximity, interpersonal conflict and friendship formation in the intermediate care facility. Gerontologist 1975; 15:150–154.

70. Kane RL, Kane RA: *Long-Term Care in Six Countries: Implications for the United States.* US Government Printing Office, 1976.

71. Anderson N, Hopkins RH, Schneider R, et al: *Policy Issues Regarding Nursing Homes: Findings from a Minnesota Survey.* Minneapolis, Institute for Interdisciplinary Studies, 1969.

72. Knee R: The long-term care facility, in Dobroff R (ed): *Social Work Consultation in Long-Term Care Facilities*. US Government Printing Office, 1978.

73. Gottesman L, Brody E: Psycho-social intervention programs within the institutional setting, in Sherwood S (ed): *Long-Term Care: A Handbook for Researchers, Planners and Providers*. New York, Spectrum Publications, Inc, 1975.

74. Austin M, Kosberg J: Nursing home decisionmakers and the social service needs of residents. *Soc Work Health Care* 1976; 1:447–456.

75. Gottesman L, Quarterman C, Cohn G: Psycho-social treatment of the aged, in Eisdorfer C (ed): *The Psychology of Adult Development and Aging*. Washington, DC, American Psychological Association, 1973.

76. Moss FE, Halamandaris VJ: *Too Old, Too Sick, Too Bad*, Germantown, Aspen Systems Corp, 1977.

77. Shanas E: Family responsibility and the health of older people. *J Gerontol* 1960; 15:408–411.

78. Brody E: *A Social Work Guide for Long-Term Care Facilities*. US Government Printing Office, 1974.

79. Eggert G, Granger CV, Morris R, et al: *Community-Based Maintenance Care for the Long-Term Patient*. Waltham, Mass, Levinson Policy Institute, Brandeis University, 1975.

80. Gottesman L: Organizing rehabilitation services for the elderly. *Gerontologist* 1970; 10:287–293.

81. *Characteristics of Nursing Home Residents, Health Status and Care Received: National Nursing Home Survey, United States, May–December 1977*, publication (PHS) 81-1712 (*Vital and Health Statistics*, series 13, no 51). Hyattsville, Md, National Center for Health Statistics, 1981.

82. Weissert W, Wan TH, Livieratos B, et al: Effects and costs of day care services for the chronically ill: A randomized experiment. *Med Care* 1980; 18:567–583.

83. Hicks B, Raisz H, Segal J, et al: The triage experiment in coordinated care for the elderly. *Am J Public Health* 1981; 71:991–1003.

84. Eggert GM, Bowlyow JE, Nichols CW: Gaining control of the long-term care systems: First returns from the access experiment. *Gerontologist* 1980; 20:356–363.

85. Applebaum R, Seidl FW, Austin CD: The Wisconsin community care organization: Preliminary findings from the Milwaukee Experiment. *Gerontologist* 1980; 20:350–355.

86. Skellie FA, Mobley GM, Coan RE: Cost-effectiveness of community-based long-term care: Current findings of Georgia's alternative health services project. *Am J Public Health* 1982; 72:353–358.

CHAPTER 8

Mental Health Services: Growth and Development of a System

Mary Richardson

Mental health services have experienced considerable growth and change over the last several decades. Who is treated, and the problems they are treated for, have altered with changing definitions of mental illness, changing viewpoints about the appropriate response to mental health problems, and increasing social recognition and acceptance of mental health services as a treatment rather than a custodial function. This chapter describes the development of mental health services in this country, the users and reasons for use, the organization and financing of services, recent trends, and the problems of providing care.

HISTORICAL PERSPECTIVES ON DEFINITIONS OF MENTAL ILLNESS

Societies have always defined and classified human behavior in ways that differentiated what was acceptable and what was not. Describing the more subtle maladaptations of human beings to society involves social and cultural values; as value systems change, so do conceptions of deviant behavior. Societal tolerance of deviant behavior partially determines what constitutes mental illness. In more recent times, psychiatric or emotional disability has been defined within biologic, sociologic, and cultural frameworks. However, scientific definitions have their philosophic roots in a history that predates much current scientific thought.

During the Middle Ages, aberrant behavior was attributed to demonic influences, evil spirits, and the like. In an agrarian feudal society, deviance had to do with the ability to work and sustain oneself. People thought of as mad were allowed to wander about if they were not too troublesome (1). Communities were able to offer them some basic support; if they became troublesome, they were driven away.

With the rise of a mercantile society in Europe and a breakdown of feudal estates, major social and political upheavals occurred. Many people were left homeless, with no means of support. Groups of unemployed people and disbanded soldiers drifted around the countryside. Persons who had previously been defined as mad or insane were classified with those who were poor and homeless. They were grouped together in a much larger category of people considered to be socially destitute. Small communities quickly lost the ability to offer even minimal support to these people.

In England, the Elizabethan Poor Laws of 1601 heralded a recognition of the responsibility of government, and society as a whole, in addressing the problems of the destitute and the ill. In each community parish, overseers were assigned to provide care for these sick and disaffected members of society. Later, lunatic hospitals were opened throughout England. These hospitals existed more to protect the citizenry by isolating social misfits than to provide even a minimum of care. Conditions in these institutions were generally abominable. Inmates were often chained and provided only the barest essentials of survival.

In 1656, the French Parliament authorized the construction of the Hôpital Generale. The poor, the sick, and the insane were confined in circumstances much like those of the English lunatic hospitals. However, with the eighteenth century came the Age of Enlightenment and a revolution in scientific thought. In France, Philippe Pinel introduced the idea of mental illness within a medical framework (2). Pinel was initially the physician of the Infirmaries at the Hospice de Bicêtre in Paris. Although he was historically given credit for unchaining the inmates and introducing humanistic treatment, writings discovered more recently reveal that it was actually Jean-Baptiste Pussin, the governor of mental patients, who had actually begun this more humane treatment (2). The ideas of both Pinel and Pussin, who had once been a patient at Bicêtre, spread throughout Europe and later to the United States.

In the late 1800s, Kraepelin, a German physician, outlined a concise system of classification establishing mental illness as a separate and distinct disease entity subject to the rules that applied to physical or somatic diseases. His work legitimized psychiatry as a branch of medicine. Kraepelin described in detail the symptoms, course of the disease, and prognosis of dementia praecox and manic-depressive psychoses. Sigmund Freud, the father of psychoanalysis, described neuroses in a deterministic fashion by proposing that all events could be traced to a specific origin. He described mental illness as related to disturbances and distortions from unconscious developmental difficulties in psychic growth and maturation, and traumatic experiences and conflicts over sexual and self-destructive instincts. Although psychotherapy came to be regarded as a medical and psychiatric specialty, Freud established the psychologic viewpoint.

Continuing biomedical research in the twentieth century produced evidence that supported the concept of organic causations for mental illness. The discovery of the spirochete that causes syphilis and general paresis, and discoveries of chromosomal aberrations in mental retardation, were cited as such evidence. Studies of schizophrenia, defined as a diagnosis by Bleuler in the early 1900s (replacing dementia praecox), and manic-depressive syndromes have suggested possible familial tendencies. For example, 10% of siblings and children of schizophrenic patients are also diagnosed as schizophrenic, possibly indicating a biologic basis for this illness. Transcultural studies of mental illness have demonstrated remarkably uniform prevalence rates for schizophrenia in different countries and cultures.

However, modern techniques for the study of chromosomal aberrations do not isolate genetic differences, and even with clinical evidence suggesting a biologic component, critics would argue that a diagnosis of schizophrenia is highly subjective, and that the perception of behavior as being schizophrenic is relative to the environmental context. Studies of other illnesses such as the neurotic or drug abuse syndromes have so far been unable to identify biogenetic factors.

Social Psychiatric and Behavioral Definitions

During the twentieth century there has been increasing acceptance of pluralistic determinants of mental illness, including biologic, sociologic, and social factors. Harry Sullivan was the first American psychiatrist to develop a theory stressing the importance of interpersonal relations in disease etiology. Concurrent with the development of social psychiatric definitions were new psychologic and behavioral concepts of mental illness. Carl Jung broke away from the Freudian approach and formed the field of analytic psychology. Erich Fromm, a psychoanalyst never trained in medicine, and others applied anthropologic and sociologic concepts to Freud's theories. Later, John B. Watson discarded Freudian theory and developed behaviorism, which recognized only observable behavior as critical to the diagnosis of mental illness. He believed that all behavior was predictable based on environmental stimuli. Psychologists introduced classic conditioning and learning theory to psychiatrists and other psychopathologists.

Social psychiatric and behavioral definitions of mental health reduced reliance on the disease concept of mental illness as internally manifested by the client; rather, social and cultural relativity and personality development were emphasized as significant factors in mental health. The development of humanistic psychology also had origins in the behavioral movements. The Freudian approach was considered too pessimistic and the behavioral approaches too mechanistic. Carl Rogers developed the technique of client-centered therapy, which recognized the client's role in affecting his or her own rehabilitation. Using this approach, client behavior is compared to expected behavior for the culture or environment of the patient. Differences between adaptive and maladaptive functioning vary from culture to culture and are more or less acceptable according to one's economic or social status. The validity of these broader environmentally based approaches are supported by transcultural psychiatric research that documents mental illness in all cultures and suggests that outward manifestations of these illnesses are shaped by the childrearing practices, indoctrinations, sanctions, encouragements and discouragements of each culture.

Definitions of mental illness may also be predicated on the social and cultural values of the care provider and may be in conflict with the accepted norms of the recipient. This problem can be difficult if care providers are representative of the majority group within a population and the potential recipient is a member of a minority group. Behavior that is tolerated, accepted, or even encouraged within the minority group may be seen as deviant or sick behavior by the majority group. For example, an epidemiologic study of psychiatric disorders in a Pacific Northwest coastal Indian village found differing symptom patterns in men and women (3). Women, suffering more from psychoneuroses, were viewed as ill within this society, whereas men, generally suffering from alcoholism, not only did not seek treatment but were not even considered ill by their community. Hence, treatment for women was accepted and even encouraged, whereas treatment for men was not.

Finally, defining the overlap between social problems and mental illness is difficult. Are deviations such as delinquency or criminal behavior a mental health problem? What about poverty, discrimination, and unemployment? Mental health professionals must determine the extent of their roles as caregivers and as agents of social change.

EXTENT OF MENTAL DISORDERS

The American Psychiatric Association classifies mental illness within three general categories: impairment of brain tissue, mental deficiency, and disorders without a clearly defined clinical cause. Most disorders treated by mental health professionals fall in the third category, but diagnosis of these problems is subjective in actual clinical practice. The *Diagnostic and Statistical Manual (DSM)* (4), published by the American Psychiatric Association, contains this classification system, which is used extensively in diagnosing mental illness. These classifications are generally used in measuring incidence and prevalence of mental illness, as well as the use of services.

Incidence and Prevalence of Mental Illness

Schizophrenia continues to be a major mental health problem in this country. The affective disorders, which include psychotic depression, mania, and manic depression, are another primary component of mental illness in our society. Drug abuse and alcohol-related problems form a third major category. Many people suffer from anxiety, moderate depression, and other emotional disorders. There is some evidence that only about one-fourth of those suffering from a clinically significant disorder have been in treatment (5). Table 8-1 presents the estimated distribution of people with mental disorders by treatment facility. Note that 54.1% of those seeking treatment do so in a primary care medical setting. Figure 8-1 shows the distribution

TABLE 8-1. Estimated Percent Distribution of Persons with Mental Disorders, by Treatment Setting, United States, 1975

Treatment Setting	Percent of People
Primary care/outpatient medical sector	54.1
Not in treatment/other human services sector[a]	21.5
Specialty mental health sector	15.0
Both specialty mental health sector and primary care/outpatient medical sector (overlap)	6.0
General hospital inpatient/nursing home sector[a]	3.4

SOURCE: President's Commission on Mental Health: *Final Report*, vol II, *Task Panel Reports*. US Government Printing Office, 1978.

[a]Excludes overlap of an unknown percentage of persons also seen in other sectors.

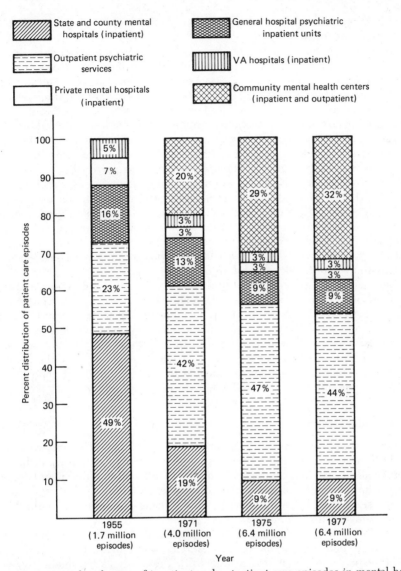

Figure 8-1. Percent distribution of inpatient and outpatient care episodes in mental health facilities by type of facility: United States, 1955, 1971, 1975, 1977.
SOURCE: Mental Health Statistical Note No. 154. Trends in patient care episodes in mental health facilities. US Department of Health and Human Services, Alcohol, Drug Abuse and Mental Health Administration, September, 1980.

of people seeking care by mental health settings; the majority of contacts now occur in outpatient facilities.

There have been a number of attempts to measure the prevalence of mental illness in American society. An estimated 10 million Americans experience one or more episodes of serious mental illness before reaching old age. The President's Commission on Mental Health also estimated that 20–32 million Americans are in need of mental health services (5). The President's Commission on Mental Health, on the basis of an analysis of available epidemiologic studies, reported the following prevalence rates for functional psychiatric disorders as a percentage of the total U.S. population: schizophrenia, 0.5–3.0; manic-depressive psychosis, 0.3; neurosis (including other depressive disorders), 8.0–13.0; and personality disorders, 7.0. Most reporting of mental illness is done by public agencies as a requirement of funding, and little information is available from private practitioners and nonpublic facilities. As a result, even the most valiant attempts to estimate the incidence and prevalence of mental illness are at best approximations. Many studies use such vague terms as *psychiatric impairment* rather than a more definitive diagnosis. Even diagnoses recorded on insurance claims forms are subject to considerable bias since reimbursement is dependent on diagnosis.

The Center for Epidemiologic Studies of the Division of Biometry and Epidemiology, National Institute of Mental Health, has sponsored an Epidemiologic Catchment Area (ECA) program (6). A Diagnostic Interview Schedule has been developed, which focuses on specific disorders using psychiatric diagnostic categories, and is being administered in defined catchment areas throughout the country. Because multiple sites and a common survey instrument are used, the results are comparable. The ECA program is expected to make a significant contribution to psychiatric epidemiologic knowledge.

Use of Mental Health Services

Data concerning the use of mental health services also tend to be somewhat unreliable. Definitive diagnoses are often not reported. Most data are from the public sector. In addition, since studies are not often based on enrolled populations, the denominator for determining use rates is elusive. However, federal reporting does provide information on admissions by disorder, as presented in Table 8-2, and patient characteristics (Table 8-3).

From the available evidence, women are slightly higher users of mental health services than men; adolescent boys use services more often than adolescent girls (7). The response to symptoms and the willingness to seek treatment vary within the population and affect use of services. For instance, adolescent boys may act out in a more visible manner than adolescent girls and therefore be referred more often for care. Attitudes of society toward men or women seeking services may create a more comfortable climate for women to do so.

Psychologically oriented illness accounts for a significant proportion of ambulatory medical services and prescribed drugs. An estimated 54% of people suffering from mental disorders are seen by primary care physicians in an outpatient setting (Table 8-1). People with mental or emotional distress often seek care from their family physician, a hospital outpatient clinic, or an emergency room. Various studies of the prevalence of psychosomatic illnesses of patients with physical symptoms and no apparent organic explanation in primary care medical practices suggest that from 15% to 50% of visits are for such illnesses.

Substantial differences exist in use among racial and ethnic groups. The effect

TABLE 8-2. Number and Percent Distribution of Admissions to Selected Mental Health Facilities, by Mental Disorder, United States, 1975

Diagnosis	State and County Mental Hospital	Private Mental Hospital	General Hospital Psychiatric Inpatient Unit	Outpatient Psychiatric Services	Community Mental Health Centers	Total: All Facilities
Total	385,237	128,832	515,537	1,406,065	919,037	3,355,708
Alcohol disorders	106,615	10,827	35,932	53,125	89,338	295,837
Drug disorders	14,435	3,077	17,849	22,094	28,638	86,093
Organic brain syndromes	20,372	5,195	18,981	30,821	22,443	97,812
Depressive disorders	44,965	55,068	194,399	180,735	122,948	598,115
Schizophrenia	129,425	28,315	124,458	148,303	91,914	522,415
Childhood disorders	5,987	1,564	4,625	143,462	120,642	276,280
Social maladjustments	1,139	164	1,818	143,278	66,395	212,794
All other diagnoses	57,163	24,783	114,622	526,926	242,155	965,649
No mental disorder	5,136	839	2,853	157,321	134,564	300,713
Percent distribution by diagnosis						
Total	100.0	100.0	100.0	100.0	100.0	100.0
Alcohol disorders	27.0	8.3	7.0	3.8	9.7	8.8
Drug disorders	3.7	2.4	3.5	1.6	3.1	2.6
Organic brain syndromes	5.3	4.0	3.7	2.2	2.4	2.9
Depressive disorders	11.7	42.5	37.7	12.9	13.4	17.8
Schizophrenia	33.6	21.8	24.1	10.5	10.0	15.6
Childhood disorders	1.6	1.2	0.9	10.2	13.1	8.2
Social maladjustments	0.3	0.1	0.4	10.2	7.2	6.3
All other diagnoses	14.8	19.1	22.1	37.4	26.6	28.8
No mental disorder	1.3	0.6	0.6	11.2	14.6	9.0

SOURCE: President's Commission on Mental Health: *Final Report*, vol II, *Task Panel Reports*. US Government Printing Office, 1978, p 102.

TABLE 8-3. Age-Adjusted Admission Rates By Race, Sex and Type of Facility, Selected Mental Health Facilities, United States, 1975[a]

Race and Sex	State and County Mental Hospitals	Private Mental Hospitals	Inpatient Psychiatric Services			Federally Funded CMHCs	Outpatient Psychiatric Services
			Non-federal General Hospitals				
			Total	Public	Nonpublic		
Total—all races	182	61	244	66	178	435	665
Male	245	55	209	70	139	427	611
Female	124	67	276	62	214	441	709
White	160	65	243	61	182	415	639
Male	213	57	206	64	142	404	588
Female	110	71	278	58	220	425	683
All other races	340	39	238	98	140	571	834
Male	477	40	219	108	111	593	747
Female	226	39	253	89	165	550	890

SOURCE: President's Commission on Mental Health: *Final Report*, vol II, *Task Panel Reports*. US Government Printing Office, 1978, p 103.

[a]Denominator is estimated 1975 United States population.

of client and organizational variables, such as patient socioeconomic status, the racial and cultural background of the therapist, and the organizational setting in which services are provided, on use of services has yet to be determined. Mexican-Americans have been shown to use mental health services when they are available in a community setting (8). Studies of the use of services in a community mental health center indicate that members of minorities are hospitalized more often than whites (9). Differences in the volume of services received by blacks, Chicanos, and other minority groups as compared to whites have also been reported. For example, in a study of patients admitted to Los Angeles County General Hospital for psychiatric treatment, 11% of whites as compared to 3% of blacks had more than 10 visits per illness episode (10). White clients also received more psychotherapy services; minority clients, unlike white clients, sometimes received medication but no therapy.

Rates of institutionalization, when correctional institutions are included, differ for whites and nonwhites. In 1960, although mental hospitalization rates were only 20% higher for nonwhites than for whites, nonwhites were institutionalized primarily in correctional institutions and whites in medical care facilities. By 1970, the rate of institutionalization in correctional facilities was even greater for nonwhites (11). The social nature of many mental illnesses raises questions as to whether these patterns reflect biases in society.

The use of private versus public facilities varies by income. Higher income people use private practitioners predominantly, whereas lower income people rely more heavily on public sources of care. Race is also a factor, perhaps interacting with income, related to the location in which services are received. Approximately 36% of whites and 11% of nonwhites in a recent national survey of the use of mental health facilities received services in a private inpatient setting. This difference was moderated for outpatient services; 32% of whites and 26% of nonwhites were treated in private facilities (11).

Minorities are more likely to be from lower economic groups, to have less education, and perhaps also to have a language barrier. Studies of blacks using mental health services refer to "black English" and report miscommunications between white therapists and black patients. Also, blacks are less likely to receive individual psychotherapy, which is often biased toward educated, verbal clients from a culture similar to that of the therapists. Mexican-Americans and native Americans encounter language, education, and economic stumbling blocks as well. Command of English and understanding how to access the formal mental health services system affect the type of treatment obtained. In response to these barriers and for traditional reasons, some people also rely on alternative sources of care within their own culture. For example, the Mexican-American may seek help from the Curandero and the native American from the medicine man. The formal mental health system is slowly learning to view these alternative systems with respect and to seek their advice in the treatment of people from different cultural backgrounds.

DEVELOPMENT OF THE MENTAL HEALTH SERVICES SYSTEM IN THE UNITED STATES

Early Mental Health System

The development of American psychiatry in the nineteenth century was strongly influenced by Dr. Benjamin Rush, long considered the father of American psychiatry, who was also a pioneer in hospital reform. Before the nineteenth century, formal treatment centers were nonexistent. Private physician services were available to those with money. The rest faced imprisonment or hospitalization, one being not much different from the other. The hospital reform spearheaded by Pinel in the late 1700s in France was paralleled in this country by Rush's activities. The American Psychiatric Association was started through the efforts of affiliated hospital superintendents who, like Rush, were concerned with hospital conditions. Even into the early twentieth century, treatment of mental illness based on medical-clinical approaches occurred in state-supported hospitals, which were often located in remote areas and functioned as large human warehouses.

The disease concept of mental illness implies that the patient can become "well" and generally assumes that the therapist, historically a psychiatrist, will diagnose the illness and define subsequent treatment. The Freudian model has led to long term and intensive psychotherapy, and to therapeutic and personnel requirements that are beyond the resources available to the state hospitals. Mental illness was also highly stigmatized and subject to funding limitations by state legislatures, the primary purpose being to provide public protection from "crazy people" rather than to provide a public good for people with psychiatric problems.

The National Mental Health Act of 1946 (PL 79-487) signified an increased federal interest in the plight of the mentally ill. The law created the National Institute of Mental Health and increased appropriations for therapy and research. In addition, recognition of the psychologic problems of soldiers during World War II motivated Veterans Administration hospitals to provide expanded mental health services.

Development of Outpatient Services

The development of psychopharmacology in the 1950s had a profound impact on the field of mental health. Psychotropic drugs led to dramatic breakthroughs in the treatment of mental illness and enabled thousands of patients previously considered incurable to be effectively treated on an outpatient basis. The use of these drugs also created a climate that encouraged the development of various innovative therapeutic approaches.

Before World War II, few outpatient mental health facilities existed. With growing federal interest, the number of outpatient facilities increased. At the same time, the prognosis for the thousands of patients in mental hospitals, many of whom suffered from schizophrenia, depression, and mania, remained dismal. However, the use of antipsychotic medications for schizophrenia, antidepressants for depression, and, more recently, lithium in the treatment of mania rapidly improved the prognosis for these patients. With the development of psychotropic medications, medical-clinical models of treatment continued to be the major influence on hospital treatment of mental illness. Psychotropic drugs also led to a radical decline in hospital length of stays for patients with psychiatric diagnoses. Patients now could control their behavior through the use of these drugs and, it was hoped, could function in the community. Thus, a mental health system previously based primarily on inpatient facilities had to develop new approaches to serving patients who no longer needed to be hospitalized.

Although mental health professionals continued to expand their understanding of mental and emotional disorders, the general public was still distrustful of and misinformed about the nature of mental illness, and there was little advocacy for improvement except from the mental health community. Nevertheless, there was a dramatic increase in outpatient clinics from 400 before World War II to 1,234 by 1954 (12). Finally, in 1955 the National Mental Health Study Act (PL84-182) was passed, which authorized $750,000 for a 3-year study of the entire mental health system. The result was the *Action for Mental Health Report*, published in 1961. Although this report covered many issues in the provision of mental health services, the primary emphasis of the legislation that followed, during the Kennedy administration, was on outpatient services. Concern was increasingly focused on providing comprehensive mental health services to people not requiring hospitalization as well as to those not previously having access to mental health services. The Mental Retardation Facilities and Community Mental Health Centers Construction Act of 1964 (PL 88-164) provided construction monies for community mental health centers that were to serve designated catchment areas of 75,000 to 200,000 people. The five basic services that the centers were required to provide included inpatient, outpatient, emergency, day treatment, and consultation and education services. Significantly, the legislation mandated that services be provided regardless of the patient's ability to pay.

Many centers were built with the newly available funding for construction, but money for staffing and operations continued to be scarce. Finally, in 1967, an amendment to the legislation provided the necessary operations money on a matching basis, with funding for each center declining over an 8-year period. This was the "seed money" concept, and it was hoped that the construction and development of a community mental health center would encourage the community gradually to assume financial responsibility for services. Since catchment areas varied in their ability to provide matching funds, the subsidy for services in different areas also varied considerably. And although there was an allowance for the poorer communities, the capability readily to obtain local matching funds was a distinct advantage for some centers. In retrospect, the whole notion of matching local funds ignored the inability of some communities to assume the associated financial burden, especially in areas of greatest need. Since many centers faced closure or significant reduction in services, additional legislation (PL 94-63) was passed in 1975. This law included provision for a 1-year distress grant at the end of the 8 years of operational support if alternate funding was not obtained. This legislation was designed to overhaul the Community Mental Health Center network and also to increase the original five required services to 12, including care for drug abuse problems, children, and the aged, as well as screening, follow-up, and community living services. In addition, the National Center for Prevention and Control of Rape was created. Planning and evaluation of local community mental health services was mandated; 2% of each center's budget was to be used for these purposes.

Community Mental Health Centers are also required to operate under the authority of a board of directors that represents the local community. These boards, however, are often composed of well-educated, upper middle income people who are frequently health care providers despite the location of many mental health centers in lower income communities.

Although Community Mental Health Services have notably expanded the outpatient mental health services system in the United States, they have fallen short of many of the original goals. As a result, alternative sources of care have developed in many communities. These sources are often grass roots movements, funded on shoestring budgets, and organized by people who perceive unmet mental health needs. Examples include more than 2,000 hot lines, 200 houses for runaways, and 400 free clinics that operate throughout the nation (5).

Concern for the inadequacies of the current mental health system led President

Jimmy Carter to establish the President's Commission on Mental Health in 1977. The president's wife, Rosalynn, served as honorary chairperson, indicating her active interest in mental health services in Georgia during Carter's tenure as governor. The report produced by the commission went on to influence policy formation and in many ways became the heart of the Carter administration's Mental Health Systems Act, passed by Congress in 1980 (PL 96-398) (1). Although the Systems Act authorized continuation of provisions to establish additional Community Mental Health Centers and authorized spending for many new initiatives, it was never implemented. With the coming of a new, conservative administration under President Ronald Reagan, monies authorized were never appropriated.

MENTAL HEALTH PERSONNEL

Psychiatrists

Psychiatry is the medical specialty dealing with mental disorders. Traditional psychiatry offers medical-clinical definitions of mental illness. Social psychiatry, in contrast, is concerned with the environmental and societal phenomena involved in mental and emotional disorders and the use of social forces in the treatment of such disorders. Much of the scientific work of social psychiatry has been in the area of epidemiology, particularly estimation of the incidence and prevalence of mental illness in community and hospital settings. Growing concern for the environment in large mental hospitals during and after World War II also added impetus to the social psychiatric movement, and as early as 1946, the American Psychiatric Association adopted a strict set of standards for mental hospitals and appointed a Central Inspection Board for enforcement of these standards. Social psychiatry, in an effort to transform these large institutions from custodial care to treatment centers, developed the concept of the therapeutic community, the fundamental tenet of which is that patients can assist in their own rehabilitation as well as in the rehabilitation of other patients. Social psychiatry also includes transcultural and community psychiatry. Transcultural psychiatry studies the incidence and prevalence of mental disease across societies and delineates the social forces that affect the manifestations of these illnesses. Community psychiatry has been described as "social psychiatry in action" (13) and is involved in the development, planning, and organization of community mental health programs and consultation to local agencies.

The number of psychiatrists in the United States has increased from approximately 7,000 in 1950 to more than 27,000 today, including those working primarily in administration (5). Psychiatrists are distributed approximately equally between private practice and public service in state mental hospitals and community facilities. Some psychiatrists work in both public and private settings.

Psychologists

Psychiatrists have traditionally assumed clinical leadership roles. Psychologists, psychiatric nurses, and social workers are, however, seeking more equal status with physicians. Psychology, which struggled to create its own professional identity in the early years of this century, has emphasized scientific research in academic settings. Beginning as a philosophy, psychology has become firmly established as a social science, and psychologists have promoted and conducted research on the functioning of the human mind, especially through development of scientific testing instruments. Beginning in the early twentieth century, psychologic testing began to be used in conjunction with psychiatric treatment. Research by psychologists in classic conditioning and behavior theory also aided psychiatrists, who still provided most therapeutic care.

During World War II, psychologists began to seek an increased role in clinical practice. With the expansion of mental health services in Veterans Administration hospitals, the training of clinical psychologists began in earnest. In 1946, the Veterans Administration, in conjunction with the American Psychological Association, began the Veterans Administration Psychology Training Program which is still a major source of training for clinical and counseling psychologists. The professional application of psychology received further endorsement in the American Psychological Association Vail Conference of 1973, which emphasized the continued training of clinicians and scientists in psychology.

Psychologists are licensed or certified in all states and the District of Columbia. In almost all states, the training required for licensure is a doctoral degree, although a few states allow limited licensure for graduates of master's degree programs; however, independent private practice is prohibited. Licensure is not required for practice in some settings, however, and unlicensed psychologists most often practice in school or community mental health facilities. In early 1977, the American Psychological Association reported a membership of 47,000 (14), although there may be as many as 70,000 master's and doctoral level psychologists (5).

Social Workers

The history of social work dates back to the late nineteenth century and the volunteer mothers who provided disadvantaged persons with charitable aid through the Charity Organization Societies. Social work began to develop as a profession during the early twentieth century. Reform-minded women, struggling for equality, became social workers and began working in medical and psychiatric settings, schools, and correctional institutions. The development of social psychiatry also prompted the formation of a professional identity for social workers. Adopting the Freudian psychoanalytic model of many psychiatrists, social workers struggled for increasing responsibility in the treatment of mental and emotional disorders. The practice of psychotherapy expanded the social worker's domain from providing charitable assistance to the poor to providing a therapy that was viewed as legitimate by middle and upper class people. Since psychoanalysis and psychotherapy remained medical specialties, social workers were not too successful in developing a separate professional identity, and their practice continued in the shadow of psychiatry.

Social work continues to struggle for an independent identity and a more equal role in the delivery of mental health services. Training includes 2-year associate degree programs graduating human services workers, baccalaureate programs in social work, currently recognized as the beginning professional level, master's level degrees in social work, and doctoral programs. In addition to the basic training of the discipline, social work education offers specialized training in mental health and in human services administration. The National Association of Social Workers lists about 70,000 members, but there may be as many as 300,000 social service workers (5). Social workers are licensed in 23 states, and efforts toward social work licensure are under way in many other states.

Psychiatric Nurses

The professional training of nurses in this country began in the 1860s and consisted primarily of apprenticeships. The first training program that prepared nurses to care for the mentally ill was started in 1882 at McLean Hospital, a private psychiatric facility in Waverly, Massachusetts. Although there was a growing appreciation of nurses who received this type of training, poorly funded psychiatric hospitals continued to employ lesser-trained aides at very low pay. Whatever nursing care did exist in these hospitals consisted mainly of custodial care focusing on the physical needs of the patient, and the nurse continued to practice in a dependent relationship with a physician.

The development in the 1930s of somatic treatments for mental illness, such as insulin shock therapy, psychosurgery, and electroshock therapy, required the services of highly skilled nurses and established a more significant role for nurses in psychiatric treatment. The advent of the therapeutic community in psychiatric hospitals broadened the role of the nurse even further. As the 24-hour care necessary for developing and maintaining the therapeutic milieu was recognized, the nurse became a valuable member of the therapeutic team. The involvement of nurses in group psychotherapy after World War II resulted in federal appropriations for training nurses. However, despite the recognition of psychiatric nursing as a legitimate nursing role, the exact function of the nurse in mental health care remained only vaguely delineated.

Nursing education has become much more academically based over the past 20 years as the need for college level training programs and nursing research was recognized. Graduates of nursing schools obtained an increasingly strong professional and academic education, often training side by side with psychiatrists, psychologists, and social workers. Nurses who earned advanced degrees were often recruited for teaching, however, and the 2-year associate degree and diploma nurses were more prevalent in clinical practice. As nurses began to move into the role of psychotherapists, partially in response to the shortage of psychiatrists in most hospitals, interprofessional conflicts developed. But the exploding demand for psychotherapists further legitimized the nurse's role in therapy and, by the late 1960s, the clinical specialty of psychiatric nursing was firmly established. The first organization to certify clinical specialists in psychiatric nursing, in 1972, was the New Jersey State Nurses Association.

Nursing education includes training in psychiatric nursing at all academic levels. The associate degree nurse with 2 years of training in an academic program and the diploma nurse trained in a hospital program most often provide clinical services. The baccalaureate and master's level nurses often work in supervisory positions or in teaching, and doctorate level nurses usually teach rather than provide clinical services. The majority of clinically active psychiatric nurses work in hospital settings.

Clinical psychiatric nurses have not been received with overwhelming enthusiasm by other mental health professionals, partially as a result of controversies over professional status and duties within the nursing profession itself. Nursing has yet to define clearly the appropriate roles of nurses and their relation to other mental health professionals. In addition, paraprofessionals such as mental health workers and psychiatric aides want nurses to perform supervision and management roles so as to leave a wider territory for their own struggle for psychotherapeutic practice rights. In community settings, social workers want to perform psychotherapy and have psychiatric nurses perform more in the tradition of the public health nurse. Currently, many psychiatric nurses in mental health settings do not have the specialized graduate level training that the title implies. There are approximately 1 million nurses in the United States (5); of the 177,000 nurses in the American Nurses Association, 29,000 are categorized as psychiatric nurses.

Other Mental Health Personnel Concerns

The roles of the various mental health service providers vary with the setting in which they practice. Inpatient psychiatric services are oriented toward the more traditional medical-clinical model, with the psychiatrist assuming the primary role and nurses, psychologists, and social workers offering support services. The growth of community services provided some impetus for change toward a more egalitarian role for all mental health professionals, particularly in the Community Mental Health Centers, which were intended to operate within the social and behavioral models of treatment. However, the more traditional therapies persist even in these centers, and all professionals practice similarly. Differences in professional training are reflected more in incomes than in professional activity, and most mental health professionals jockey for the same narrow therapeutic territory. Psychiatrists many times also assume consulting and supervisory roles in addition to providing care and supervising medications.

Administration in mental health has been largely performed by psychiatrists in mental hospitals. Community Mental Health Centers, although originally envisioned to have psychiatrists as directors, tend to use primarily psychologists and social workers as administrators. Since clinical skills alone are inadequate for administration, educational programs have been developed to offer some training in administration and management for mental health professionals, especially in social work and community psychiatry. In addition, there is a growing trend toward professionally trained mental health administrators without a clinical background.

Tables 8-4 and 8-5 present the supply and distribution of personnel among mental health facilities. The growth in personnel since 1950 reflects the increase in

TABLE 8-4. Estimated Number of Professional Mental Health Personnel, by Discipline, United States, Selected Years

Year	Psychiatrists	Psychologists	Social Workers	Registered Nurses
1950	7,100	7,300	NA[a]	NA
1955	10,600	13,500	20,000	NA
1960	14,100	18,200	26,200	504,000
1965	18,500	23,600	41,600	600,000
1970	23,200	30,800	49,600	722,000
1975	25,700	39,400	64,500	906,000
1976	26,500	42,000	69,600	961,000

SOURCE: President's Commission on Mental Health: *Final Report*, vol II, *Task Panel Reports*. US Government Printing Office, 1978, p 488.

[a]NA—not available.

TABLE 8-5. Full-Time Equivalent Positions, by Discipline, All Mental Health Facilities, United States, Selected Years[a]

Discipline	Year			
	1968	1972	1974	1976
Psychiatrists	9,891	12,938	14,947	15,339
Other physicians	2,736	3,991	3,548	3,356
Psychologists	5,212	9,443	12,597	15,251
Social workers	9,755	17,687	22,147	25,887
Registered nurses	24,256	31,110	34,089	39,392
Other mental health professionals	12,136	17,514	29,325	34,249
Physical health	NA[b]	8,203	10,507	9,631
Total professional patient care staff	63,986	100,886	127,160	143,105
Licensed practical nurses	NA	19,616	17,193	15,337
Mental health workers	NA	120,753	128,529	130,021
Total patient care staff	NA	241,255	272,882	288,463
Administrative, clerical, maintenance	NA	134,719	130,142	134,795
Total	NA	375,974	403,024	423,258

SOURCE: President's Commission on Mental Health: *Final Report*, vol II, *Task Panel Reports*. US Government Printing Office, 1978, p 484.

[a]Excludes private practice.

[b]NA—not available.

mental health concerns and increased appropriations for training. Equally important to note is the increase in personnel with baccalaureate degree or lower levels of education. The mental health system experienced an explosion in the demand for practitioners as increased federal funding was authorized by the Congress. In addition to increased demand for psychiatrists, psychologists, social workers, and psychiatric nurses, a number of allied mental health fields developed; these fields represent 12% of all mental health personnel (5).

Schools of education are training counseling and guidance personnel as well as special education teachers who work in schools and other settings. The special needs of people recovering from mental and emotional disabilities have been recognized by such professional groups as occupational and recreational therapists and vocational counselors. Practitioners in marriage counseling, art, music, dance therapy, and religion provide counseling and therapy in many mental health settings. Training for these allied professionals varies tremendously. These personnel serve as mental health workers, alcohol and drug abuse counselors, day care workers, board and home care providers, foster parents, patient advocates, and hospital psychiatric aides. In some mental health centers, half of the positions are filled by these individuals.

Indigenous healers are rarely recognized by traditional mental health service providers but have an important role in caring for physical and emotional disturbances in many minority cultures. Community volunteers are also an important component of the mental health work force. Thousands of people offer their time and services, performing tasks ranging from assisting with clerical needs to working directly with patients.

Issues of access to care raise concerns over the racial and economic mix of mental health professionals and the predominance of male practitioners. Speculation about the capability of many providers to respond to different cultural groups, and especially the poor, fosters much of this concern, particularly since the poor and minorities often have lower use rates for mental health services. Psychiatry, in particular, includes few minority practitioners, and foreign medical graduates often staff state and county hospitals. Foreign graduates may have difficulty adapting to the culture and language of their American clientele. Psychology also has few minority practitioners, but graduate programs are now increasing the number of minority and women students. About 10% of graduate students currently are minorities, and 33% of psychology doctorates in 1976 were awarded to women (5). Social work has long recognized the importance of training in different social and cultural systems, has many minority practitioners, and, indeed, has traditionally been considered a woman's field. Men have now been increasingly entering social work and nursing.

THE ORGANIZATION OF SERVICES

Financing Care

Many mental health services are provided in the public sector, funded by public money, and as a result are subject to the whims of legislatures and special interest groups. Unfortunately, advocacy for mental health has been weak and state legislatures generally have not placed high priority on these services. Public funding in mental health has been likened to a "floating crap game." The money moves from one priority to another depending upon popular therapies and modalities and the source of funds; provider agencies must try to stay ahead of the game. In addition to federal programs, state support has gradually increased but has remained inadequate. Local governments, through various taxing mechanisms, also provide some support. Reimbursement from private health insurance has provided only a small percentage of the total revenue for public agencies but most of the revenue for private care. Philanthropy remains a negligible funding source.

Community Mental Health Centers face a variety of cost problems. Some of the local money for services was to have come from resources no longer needed because of the deinstitutionalization of hospital patients. As patients moved from hospital to community care, it seemed that money no longer needed for their hospital care could be transferred to support community care. However, most state hospitals did not close, as originally hoped, with the introduction of psychotropic medications. More and more, it is becoming evident that there is a group of people who simply cannot be supported by community resources and must remain in institutions. In addition, the dollars have not always followed the patient, and those that have seem not to go as far. The centers are required to provide a wide range of services and do not qualify for reimbursement for all of them. Multiple funding sources also require multiple reporting and extra administrative effort. Demand for services has increased from both hospitalized patients and an increased number of people seeking care, not all of whom have the financial resources to do so. Centers are mandated to provide services to everyone, including the poor and working poor, regardless of ability to pay. As federal dollars become more scarce and states fail to replace federal funding completely, fewer resources must be spread more thinly.

Financing of services provided by private practitioners and private facilities is provided largely from third-party insurance or from out-of-pocket payments by patients. Most third-party payers reimburse only psychiatrists, although, in limited instances, some will reimburse psychologists and social workers.

Insurance Coverage for Mental Health Services

As discussed in Chapter 11, voluntary insurance coverage developed initially for acute care hospital services, and primarily for surgical care. Gradually, ancillary and outpatient services were added, although not to the extent that inpatient care was covered. Throughout this process, mental health services were simply not considered. Before World War II, treatment for mental illness consisted primarily of removing afflicted persons from society and placing them in state mental hospitals. With the exception of limited private psychiatric services, state hospitals were the only source of care available and were not included in insurance plans.

Few incentives existed for insurers to add mental health benefits, especially since they were poorly defined, had few precise diagnoses, used controversial and changing therapies, and could not be demonstrated to have efficacious treatments. Demand was not predictable, and the users of services were unable to provide strong advocacy. Mental health benefits are often considered a low priority by people who do not believe that they are at potential risk. Mental illness has a stigma and is something that happens to someone else.

Eventually, some mental health benefits began to be included in insurance contracts. Short term inpatient mental health services were covered initially, although not as extensively as inpatient medical and surgical services, and often had a high coinsurance provision (such as 50%) and a low total dollar benefit limitation. Outpatient benefits for mental health services are less comprehensive than for other types of ambulatory care and sometimes are nonexistent. The Federal Employees Health Insurance Plan was the first to experiment with comprehensive mental health benefits, and reported high costs, lengthy treatment times, and questionable outcomes for psychoanalysis, the most commonly sought treatment. The United Auto Workers was the next major group to provide comprehensive coverage, and experienced reasonable costs.

As Medicare and Medicaid were developed, they included limitations for mental health services despite the verbal support from federal officials for more comprehensive coverage. Medicare has dollar restrictions and coinsurance requirements. Medicaid, although originally intending to prohibit discrimination on the basis of diagnosis, required the states to specify mental health clinics as providers if mental health services were to be a covered benefit. Many states did not specify mental health clinics in their legislation and consequently do not provide benefits under Medicaid for mental health care.

Federally funded Health Maintenance Organizations, originally mandated to include mental health benefits, are no longer required to do so. The emphasis in this setting is on short term psychiatric intervention designed to stabilize and return the patient to work or other prior activity. Other prepaid group practice plans generally do not cover chronic mental illness or organic psychiatric problems. Often, the terms of coverage specify that the mental illness must be amenable to short term treatment, with the likelihood of significant improvement in the patient's condition. A study of the use of mental health services in one large prepaid group practice plan indicated that the mental health visits for two-thirds of the patients were also the first exposure to any type of formal counseling for them. Diagnoses consisted primarily of acute crisis situations, marital maladjustment, or situational adjustment reactions, and the enrolled population consisted primarily of stable middle class employees and their families (15). The average annual number of services per patient was 3.6, reflecting an orientation toward crisis intervention and short term counseling.

Services in the Private Sector

Services in the private sector include those provided by private psychiatric hospitals, psychiatric units in private acute care hospitals, private clinics offering outpatient services, and a proliferation of private practitioners operating in solo and group practice settings. Only very limited data are available on the providers and patients in private settings. Perhaps 10,000 psychiatrists were in private practice by the early 1980s. In one survey, nearly one-third of the psychiatrists who responded indicated that their subspecialty was psychoanalysis, 10% child psychiatry, and 6% other subspecialties; the remaining 51% indicated no psychiatric subspecialty (16). The responding psychiatrists reported that 5% of patients were very mildly impaired, 18% mildly impaired, 50% moderately impaired, and 27% were considered severely impaired. Fifty percent of the patients of these private psychiatrists had at least some insurance coverage, and most patients were from families with incomes in the $10,000–$30,000 range. In contrast, a study of patients seeking services in the public sector indicated that nearly all had incomes under $15,000.

Approximately 40% of patients seeking mental health services use the private sector, but their use represents only 15% of the total mental health visits in the country. This is explainable since 44% of those seeking services in the private sector are diagnosed and then referred for treatment elsewhere. In addition, private psychiatrists treat a much less diverse population than do community clinics and have little contact with alcoholic or drug abuse patients, or with children and the aged.

A recent trend in the private sector is an increase in the number of private psychiatric hospitals owned and operated by hospital corporations. Additionally, many acute care hospitals, both private and public, are adding or expanding psychiatric services as part of their overall operation. Management services for these psychiatric inpatient units in general hospitals are often contracted from private psychiatric hospital corporations.

Services in the Public Sector

A wide range of ambulatory public services are provided in outpatient psychiatric clinics, community mental health centers, halfway houses, transitional care facilities, and alternative care sources. Inpatient services include both state and county psychiatric hospitals, psychiatric units in public hospitals, and residential treatment centers for both children and adults. Other services are sought outside the mental health system. Psychologic and emotional problems account for many visits to general medical facilities. Family service agencies provide mental health services as well as other social services. Limited mental health services can be obtained in school systems, colleges, and universities.

Alternative services that have developed within the last 10 years address mental health, economic, environmental, and social issues. Hot lines, developed to handle crisis situations, offer anonymous and instant accessibility, and their personnel have up-to-date knowledge of the needs and problems of the communities they serve. Services for runaway young people started with little financial support beyond community philanthropy. Federal and state funding was later accepted by some but rejected by others due to confining mandated service requirements imposed by these sources. Other programs include long term residential programs, pioneering programs offering women's mental health services, rape crisis centers, shelters for battered women, and service programs for older people. Many of the free clinics offering primary medical care also include social and psychologic services. The holistic health clinics emphasize physical and mental illness, in addition to "wellness" in a broader context than traditional medical and mental health services. Many of these alternative services use mental health providers and techniques, but often depend on paraprofessionals and less well trained persons to provide care. These alternative services may appear and disappear overnight. They tend to be very responsive to immediate needs and often pave the way for innovation and change by more traditional providers. This care is considered by many to be equal, if not superior, to that offered by the more traditional mental health centers and is often much less expensive to provide (5).

ISSUES AND TRENDS IN MENTAL HEALTH

The struggle to understand complex human processes more fully has resulted in differentiation and specialization in addressing problems in physical and mental functioning. Mental health services, although part of the larger health care system, remain different in many ways. There is still a tendency to view the problems of mind and body as distinctly separate. Yet the problems of those who seek services within the mental health system often require a blend of medical, psychiatric, psychologic, and social services. Increasingly, medical, social, and behavioral experts are coming together to seek solutions to complex human problems. An excellent example is recent research into the relationship between stress and heart disease. Health promotion efforts and the treatment of heart disease are beginning to incorporate the ideas not only of medical science but of behaviorism and sociology as well. Another example is loss of functioning in the elderly, which has long been labeled senility and often ignored. Now the variety of physical, psychologic, and social problems that affect people during the aging process are being recognized. Mental health service providers, working in concert with medical care specialists and other human service providers, are better able to address the needs of this population. The relationships in mind-body interaction will require greater integration of medical, mental health, and other human service providers. Hence, there will be a continuing emphasis on interdisciplinary training and service provision for those professionals entering the mental health system. Interdisciplinary service teams are growing in number. Community Mental Health Centers have, in the past, been more likely to function as interdisciplinary teams. Now this model is spreading to other settings as well.

Coordinating Services

Numerous variables affect the use of mental health services. The recognition of psychologic or emotional distress as a problem is necessary if people are to seek services voluntarily. What may be viewed as mental illness by professionals or family may not be viewed as such by the patient. Since mental illness is still stigmatized, patients may not acknowledge their problems to the extent of seeking services, or are deterred from doing so by family or friends concerned with the reaction of others. And as discussed above, what is illness to society or professionals may be acceptable behavior to the mentally ill person's social group. The lack of accessible sources of care may preclude seeking services from the formal mental health system.

Knowing where to seek care is essential. A study in Australia that compared a middle class and a working class neighborhood indicated that people from the higher socioeconomic group were more likely to know where to find help in times of stress (17). Often, professionals themselves do not know all of the available resources. School and social welfare agency personnel and mental health and other health care professionals may not know of each other's services or have any formal communication channels through which to share information about resources. One report noted that 60% of the people who seek social services are turned away from agencies; only 17% of the remaining 40% are actually served, and only one out of five persons referred from one service to another even reach the agency to whom they are referred (18).

Barriers to Service

Concern about financial barriers in Community Mental Health Centers has focused on federally mandated services that were to be provided regardless of the patient's ability to pay. Access to and availability of care have encouraged the development of networks of outpatient facilities. The social status and racial or ethnic background of therapists as compared to patients, as noted previously, is an issue that continues to be addressed by training professionals from diverse economic, racial, and cultural backgrounds. Education of the public about mental illness and sources of care helps to remove attitude and knowledge barriers. Research continues into the causes, treatments, and possible remedies for psychiatric and emotional problems. Yet many people still do not receive needed care.

Inpatient and outpatient mental health services are still more available in urban than in rural areas. Funding for mental health is increasingly inadequate to meet the need for care. Although public services are available to moderate and low income people, they are not adequate to meet their needs. The concept of providing services to all people regardless of their ability to pay is rendered less than effective by long waiting lists in many centers. If you can pay, you can buy services. If you can't, you may end up on a waiting list.

Outpatient services continue to be more heavily used by whites than by blacks and other minorities, whereas hospitalization rates for nonwhites are higher. For example, in one study blacks were perceived as having more symptoms and complaints of persecution, suspiciousness, drug and alcohol abuse, and seizures than nonblack patients; yet in this study, median length of stay was 16 days for blacks and 26 days for nonblacks (9). Only 25% of black patients received individual psychotherapy compared with 80% of nonblack patients. Care may indeed differ, psychosocial variables modify how symptoms are perceived and recorded, and treatment may be influenced by provider attitudes, values, and administrative policy. Blacks use Community Mental Health Center services much the same as people of lower socioeconomic status use emergency rooms in general hospitals. They visit a community clinic in an emergency but do not continue ongoing treatment once they are stabilized.

Services for the aged and children remain dismally lacking. Although many people below age 15 and over age 65 suffer from psychiatric and emotional disorders, most services are oriented toward young and middle-aged adults.

Deinstitutionalization has been an aim of federal legislation and of legal cases relating to a person's right to be treated in the least restrictive environment. In reality, few state hospitals have closed. New admissions to psychiatric hospitals have increased approximately 90% since 1950, and readmission rates have increased almost 600%. Average length of stay has declined from 20 years for psychoses and 9 years for neuroses to an average overall length of stay of 5 months (19). Censuses are lower, but people are returning for readmission after they are discharged. The chronically mentally ill patient is still caught in a revolving door, wandering in and out of the mental health system.

Despite efforts toward better case management for patients leaving the hospital and needing outpatient services, previously hospitalized people often "fall through the cracks" and do not seek services again until a crisis occurs. When this happens, they will often visit an emergency room at a general hospital. This practice has partially resulted in a significant increase in the availability of psychiatric services in acute care settings. Nursing homes also receive many previously hospitalized psychiatric patients. Discharges of state hospital patients to nursing homes increased from 196 per 100,000 in 1950 to 456 per 100,000 in 1970 (19). Many patients leave the hospital, receive only occasional and fragmented services, and end up in communities of ex-hospital patients who are dependent upon other parts of the social welfare system for survival. Those patients who find their way into transitional care may end up in boarding house situations where few services are offered and continued dependence is fostered instead of integration into the community. Families may be ill equipped to deal with relatives returning from the hospital and may provide little or no support, either emotional or financial, in helping the ex-patient find a job, other housing, ongoing mental health care, or other necessary services.

Mental Health Law

Over the years, the focus on laws relating to mental health has shifted along with changing attitudes, treatments, and services. In the past, public safety issues rather than patient rights were reflected in laws and legal decisions about mental health issues. As the dysfunctional effects of long term institutionalization became more evident and a greater concern for individual rights was expressed, legislation began to recognize minimum criteria for treatment, alternatives to institutionalization, and a greater acknowledgment of patient rights. It is interesting to note that lawyers rather than mental health professionals led the way in the struggle for patients' rights in the mental health field. The right to treatment, consent for treatment, and confidentiality are only some of the areas of litigation that bridge the judicial and mental health systems.

The right to treatment was first addressed in 1952 in civil commitment cases relating to sexual psychopaths. *Rouse* v. *Cameron* in 1966, based on arguments of cruel and unusual treatment and the right to due process, found that people judged criminally insane had the right to treatment (20). Since the early cases did not define criteria for treatment, but merely stated that some effort was required, there was little immediate impact. A decision by Judge Johnson of Alabama in 1972, based on a class action suit (*Wyatt* v. *Stickney*) related to conditions in state hospitals, required that right to treatment be enforced and implemented (21). Various courts have subsequently specified minimum standards for treatment.

Other cases have addressed the patient's right to the least restrictive environment for treatment. Donaldson, a patient in a Florida hospital for 14 years, sued for damages and demanded his release. The Supreme Court, in *Donaldson* v. *O'Connor,* ruled that patients cannot be confined in institutions against their will if they are not dangerous to society and themselves and have the necessary support to survive outside (22,23). A similar case went one step further when a federal court ordered the District of Columbia to create adequate facilities so that patients capable of treatment in a less restrictive community-based environment could be released from the hospital.

The right not to be treated raises often conflicting interests between the society, the therapist, and the patient. The implications of behavior control through the use of behavior therapies, drug therapy, and psychosurgery create problems that have been addressed by the judicial system and by mental health professionals. State laws on involuntary treatment acts determine when a person can be involuntarily committed and use criteria such as dangerousness to self and to others. The term *gravely disabled,* used in some state statutes for involuntary commitment, has not been clearly defined. Many people argue that dangerousness as a sole criterion for involuntary hospitalization deprives many mentally ill people of urgently needed protection and treatment. Relying solely on the gravely disabled criterion often means that a person is not hospitalized unless he or she faces imminent danger from starvation or exposure. People in less extreme circumstances may need treatment but cannot be committed as gravely disabled. However, the trend in mental health law regarding involuntary treatment seems to be moving away from the very narrow definitions of gravely disabled. Involuntary treatment laws in many states are being rewritten in ways that give communities, families, and professionals greater discretion in addressing the needs and determining the best interests of patients. In the past, many definitions of gravely disabled, although quite precise in their adherence to due process rights, were impossible to deal with when attempts were made by families, professionals, and others to secure treatment that was in the best interest of the mentally ill individual.

Conclusions

Our society is slowly working toward a better understanding of the nature of mental health. Much of what is currently known and believed is predicated on a mixture of fact and untested theory. Despite monumental efforts to incorporate the current knowledge and beliefs about the biologic, sociologic, and environmental factors in mental illness, even the Community Mental Health Centers, touted as a giant step away from the medical model and psychoanalytic practices, continue to adhere to the more traditional modes, varied only by the provider of therapies. The mental health system is working vigorously to catch up with current knowledge and philosophy, but its efforts are warped by a confusing mixture of funding sources and mandates dictated more by special interests and budgetary concerns than by the efficacy of therapeutic practices.

Many people who seek services cannot pay for them, and even those who can afford to pay may not find comprehensive services in private psychiatric offices or facilities. Public services are structured by the agencies that pay for them and may not recognize the problems of those who might seek services. Finally, in the current mental health system, where it is not clear who should be doing what to whom, there is little documented evidence as to which providers are better able to provide what services. With such a muddled and complex system, it is not surprising that many potential users become confused and either seek inappropriate services or none at all.

Despite the many problems that exist in the system, mental health professionals, citizen advocates, and consumers continue to labor toward better and more stable funding, better and more services, and less stigma for mental illness. Custodial treatment still exists. Many people do go unserved or inappropriately treated. But the problems of the mentally ill continue to receive attention and concern, and the mental health system continues to gain credence and legitimacy within the larger health care system.

REFERENCES

1. Levine M: *The History and Politics of Community Mental Health.* Oxford, Oxford University Press, 1981.
2. Weiner DB: The apprenticeship of Philippe Pinel: A new document, "Observations of Citizen Pussin on the Insane." *Psychiatry* 1979; 136:1128–1134.
3. Shore JH, Kinzie JD, Hampson JD, et al: Psychiatric epidemiology of an Indian village. *Psychiatry* 1973; 36:70–81.
4. *Diagnostic and Statistics Manual.* Washington, DC, American Psychiatric Association, Taskforce on Nomenclature Statistics, 1978.
5. President's Commission on Mental Health: *Final Report,* vol II, *Task Panel Reports.* US Government Printing Office, 1978.
6. Eaton W, Regier D, Locke B, et al: The epidemiologic catchment area program of the National Institute of Mental Health. *Public Health Rep* 1981; 96:319–325.
7. Novack A, Bromet E, Neill T, et al: Children's mental health services in an inner city neighborhood; 1. A 3-year epidemiological study. *Am J Public Health* 1975; 65:133–138.
8. Heiman E, Kahn M: Mental health patterns in a barrio health center. *Int J Soc Psychiatry* 1975; 21:197–202.
9. Mayo J: The significance of sociocultural variables in the psychiatric treatment of black outpatients. *Comp Psychiatry* 1974; 15:471–482.
10. Cole J, Pilisuk M: Differences in the provision of mental health service by race. *Am J Orthopsychiatry* 1976; 46:510–525.
11. Rosen B: Mental health and the poor: Have the gaps between the poor and "nonpoor" narrowed in the last decade? *Med Care* 1977; 15:647–661.
12. Rumer R: Community mental health centers: politics and therapy. *J Health Politics, Policy, Law* 1978; 3:531–558.
13. Schwartz DA: Community mental health in 1972, an assessment, in Barten HH, Bellak L (eds): *Progress in Community Mental Health,* New York, Grune and Stratton, 1972, vol II, pp 3–34.
14. Letter from M. Brewster Smith, PhD, President and Officer of the American Psychological Association, to Max Clelland, Administrator, Veterans Administration, Washington, DC, October 18, 1978.

15. Spoerl OH: Treatment patterns in prepaid psychiatric care. *Am J Psychiatry* 1974; 131:56–59.

16. Schiedemandel P: Utilization of psychiatric services. *Psychiatric Ann* 1974; 4:58–74.

17. Pemburton A, Witlock F, Wilson P: Knowledge about where to find help: A preliminary analysis. *Soc Sci Med* 1975; 9:433–439.

18. Crawford CD, Leadley S: Interagency collaboration for planning and delivery of health care. *Fam Community Health* 1979; 2:321–324.

19. Redlich F, Kellert S: Trends in American mental health. *Am J Psychiatry* 1978; 135:22–28.

20. *Rouse v Cameron*, 373 F2d 451 (DC Cir 1966).

21. *Wyatt v Stickney*, 344 F Supp 383 (MD Ala 1972).

22. *Donaldson v O'Connor*, 493 F2d 507 (Stu Cir 1974).

23. *O'Connor v Donaldson*, 43 USLW 4929 (1975).

PART FOUR

Resources for Health Services

CHAPTER 9

Technological Resources for Health

Robert F. Rushmer

During the past 30 years, revolutionary changes have involved virtually every aspect of health services in this country. Many adaptations have been discussed in earlier chapters of this book. Some of the most dramatic changes involve new technological resources that are now available to detect and treat disease. These changes and their implications are the subject of this chapter, which reviews the historical developments presaging modern technological achievements, their contributions to health care, and the unpredicted consequences and complications resulting from their applications.

The most comprehensive basic medical research enterprise in the world has engaged the attention of faculties in schools of medicine, public health, dentistry, nursing, and allied fields. Sophisticated sensors and analytical techniques have been developed to provide objective and quantitative information. The functional characteristics of various organ systems can be assessed in health and disease with greater precision and more detail than could have been conceived of even a few decades ago. Some of the basic research techniques have been converted into expanding arrays of diagnostic equipment, many of which are semiautomated, to provide information regarding the chemical and cellular composition of blood in remarkable detail. Microstructure of tissues and cellular components is revealed in amazing detail by the enormous magnification provided by electron microscopy. The size, shape, movement, and function of many internal organs are revealed by images produced by various forms of energy probes without pain, hazard, or disturbance to patients. Continuous measurement and display of vital functions can now be used to monitor the condition of patients in intensive care and during and after surgery or injury. Life support systems now permit surgeons to invade virtually any organ of the body to remove, repair, reconstruct, or replace components that have been distorted or destroyed by disease processes. Engineering technologies have been successfully employed to provide functional substitutes and supplements to many of the most important bodily functions.

The traditional family physician conducting medical practice out of a little

Supported in part by NIH Grant LM00010-01 from the National Library of Medicine.

black bag has been largely replaced by the highly trained specialists and new health professionals required to use effectively the increasingly complex equipment available for management of diseases of the various organ systems. Hospitals have assumed expanded roles as the institutions specifically designed and organized for ready access by patients and physicians to the many and varied health services that are the essence of modern medicine and surgery. The government has become increasingly involved in the details of health care, not only in supporting research but also in ensuring the safety and effectiveness of new devices (e.g., the Food and Drug Administration) and in providing financial support of health services for the military, veterans, the aged, the poor, and potentially the entire population under comprehensive national health insurance.

HISTORICAL HERITAGE OF HEALTH TECHNOLOGIES

At the beginning of this century, medical science was struggling for professional respectability, and rightly so. The methods of treatment of most medical problems were largely ineffectual, with remarkably few exceptions (i.e., surgical removal or repair and certain effective drugs, minerals, and hormones). Otherwise, home remedies were virtually as effective as the ministrations of physicians. Medical schools were much more numerous than they are today. Most of them were diploma mills, and even the best of them had little research activity. Basic medical research was heavily oriented toward subjective descriptions of structure, function, and taxonomy. The mechanisms of function and control were generally estimated on the basis of temporal relationships observed or recorded with crude mechanical devices and recording techniques. Quantitative measurements and dynamic analysis of functional relationships were extremely primitive, far outdistanced by the progress of 300 years in mathematics, chemistry, and physics. Most of the devices proposed and employed for diagnosis or treatment were outright fakes employed by charlatans. It has been estimated that at the turn of the century New York City contained some 20,000 quacks and only about 6,000 "regular" medical practitioners (1). The amazing variety of charms, amulets, and pseudoscientific gadgets with which health hucksters of the day engaged the gullible public defies imagination. The amazing but tragic diversity of devices "guaranteed" to cure long lists of unrelated ailments included impressive names such as Magneto Electric Device, Micro-dynamometer, Spectrochrome, Perkin's Patent Metallic Tractors, and Orgone Energy Accumulator. These devices were widely and persuasively advertised in newspapers, magazines, and even in the Sears Roebuck catalogue (2).

A full-scale campaign was waged for many years against these excesses by Morris Fishbein, editor of the *Journal of the American Medical Association* (3). Reticence by modern medicine to adopt new technologies may stem in part from this colorful but shameful period.

The nation's basic medical research capacity became established with the medical school reforms following the Flexner Report of 1910, which critically assessed medical education in the United States (4). These changes formed the necessary foundation for both fundamental and clinical research in medical schools, but the modern era of biomedical research was delayed until the period after World War II.

The Surge Toward Scientific Medicine

The national commitment to large-scale biomedical research and development did not originate from the medical community but instead was initiated by persuasive and persistent pressure by concerned citizens. This fascinating saga was detailed by Stephen Strickland (5).

The story begins with Matthew M. Nealey, senator from West Virginia. In May 1928, Senator Nealey made an impassioned speech to the Senate comparing cancer in its brutality to the guillotine and introduced legislation authorizing the National Academy of Sciences to investigate cancer and report to Congress on what the federal government could do to assist in coordinating cancer research, "conquering this most mysterious and destructive disease." Mary Lasker and her husband Albert, an advertising executive, were responsible for organizing an extremely effective "lay lobby" engaged in actively mobilizing the interest and support of key congressmen with whom they were acquainted. With patience and persuasion, the active support of powerful people such as Senator Claude Pepper of Florida was attained. Public opinion was aroused by extensive use of press releases to newspapers and other communication channels. After extensive efforts, the Ransdel Act was signed into law in 1930 to establish a National Institute of Health (NIH) and to erect additional buildings to house research activity as a Public Health Service. Dr. Roller E. Deider, director of the original Institutes of Health, is reported to have indicated to the Appropriations Subcommittee of the House of Representatives that the NIH would not be able to use any money beyond the $1.75 million requested, and that the NIH leadership wanted to stay within that figure (5).

Since World War II, the NIH and the biomedical research enterprise of this country have soared to meteoric heights, both in scope and in expenditures. The enormous influence exerted by the lay lobbies and the voluntary health agencies (i.e., the American Cancer Society, the American Heart Association, and many others) have tended to place cancer and heart disease before the public as principal targets for both medical research and the development of new and sophisticated technologies. The technical triumph of creating the atom bomb in a few short years by the Manhattan Project gave the mistaken impression that scientists could solve virtually any problem if provided with sufficient funds. This impression was reinforced by the rapid and successful series of dramatic moon landings by the National Aeronautics and Space Administration. The fundamental knowledge required for these impressive accomplishments was well established in advance and required only the solution of complex technical problems for which technologies were clearly attainable. There was widespread confidence in most quarters that by appropriating enough money for scientific research and development, virtually any problem could be solved.

The targets selected as highest priority were cancer and heart disease, based on the perception that they are the great killers. Other most favored health problems were addressed in sequence as the various categorical Institutes of Health were established. There is little evidence that the principal participants gave serious consideration to the question of whether the existing basic knowledge was an adequate foundation for the launching of major, definitive research programs to conquer cancer, cure heart disease, or overcome other diseases. Many persistent problems have resisted the development of definitive therapy because their ultimate causes remain mysterious. It is difficult to devise a cure for a problem with an unknown cause. To place this consideration in perspective, if President John F. Kennedy had responded to the challenge of Sputnik by a declaration that America would *overcome gravity* instead of deciding to send a man to the moon, the scientific community would have failed to achieve its goal. A great deal is known about gravity and its effects, but very little is known about its cause. An antigravity device cannot even be conceived at present because of a lack of knowledge of basic mechanisms. A corresponding situation pertains to the problems of most chronic diseases, conditions that persist as the most common hazards to the aging populations of modern societies, as discussed in Chapters 1 and 2.

There are several theories regarding the causes of cancer, which include radiation, mutations, carcinogenic materials, viruses, and others. Similarly, there are several competing theories about the origins of the abnormal swellings in blood vessels known as *atherosclerosis*. However, the very existence of many conflicting theories is a sure sign that the actual cause is unknown. The same arguments can be advanced regarding the ultimate causes of chronic diseases of the lung, the kidney, the joints, and many other organs. For lack of specific causative targets, there is currently a major preoccupation with peripheral (i.e., risk) factors. For example, there is little doubt that smoking is a contributing factor to both lung cancer and heart disease, but it is equally obvious that smoking is not the direct cause, because these diseases occur in people who do not smoke. With this historical perspective in mind, it is easier to understand and appreciate the factors responsible for the present priorities for research and development of medical techniques and technologies.

Factors Favoring Health-Related Research

Immediately after World War II, science and technology stood high in national esteem. The magnitude of the health problems of the country had been vividly exposed by the fact that some 30% of draftees were rejected for health-related reasons. There was widespread concern that a postwar depression might ensue. Programs to bolster the economy were sought, and health became an important one. Many counties in the country were lacking health services, and the importance of health as a human right emerged, along with other social reform movements. Legislation in support of research and development for health rapidly became one of the most popular political issues of the period. The stage was set for a rapid buildup of the nation's health-related research capacity, centered for the most part in the various medical schools throughout the country.

The Basic Medical Research Enterprise

Dr. James Shannon was appointed director of the National Institutes of Health during the crucial period between August 1955 and September 1968, the "golden age" of NIH. With the wholehearted support of the leadership in both the House of Representatives and Senate, the annual budgets for NIH exploded at an unprecedented rate. Indeed, appropriations for NIH exceeded the administrative requests in all but 4 years during a span of about 15 years. Dr. Shannon was perceptive enough to realize that the level of biomedical knowledge with regard to function, control, and response to diseases by the various organ systems was not substantial enough to serve as the foundation for a broad attack on the major diseases affecting the population. He convinced his backers in Congress and many of his scientific colleagues of the absolute necessity for mounting major programs in fundamental research. As a consequence, large and growing projects and programs in basic medical research rapidly emerged in medical schools in both basic medical science departments (e.g., anatomy, biochemistry, physiology) and clinical departments. In a few short years, the United States could justifiably boast of having the most comprehensive and advanced biomedical research enterprise in the world.

Initial Success Stories

During the immediate postwar period, technical developments of great importance appeared to confirm the exalted expectations of medical research. The sulfa drugs and antibiotics emerged just before and during the war, and quickly demonstrated their enormous effectiveness in combating many different types of infections. Rheumatic fever, a common and dreaded cause of heart disease in children, came under control through prophylactic use of these antibiotics. Improved life support systems that sustained respiratory and circulatory function during chest surgery provided opportunities to alleviate surgically or to correct a wide variety of congenital and acquired defects in the valves and walls of the heart chambers. As these surgical techniques became perfected, the need for more definite and quantitative diagnostic techniques emerged. For this purpose, techniques involving cardiac catheterization were developed for measuring the pressures, oxygen content, and dye concentration in blood by inserting long hollow tubes through veins (or arteries) into the chambers of the heart. A surge of progress resulted in the rapid accumulation of knowledge regarding the function of the heart and lungs in health and disease. The anatomic location and severity of the defects were elucidated by shadows cast on x-ray plates by radiopaque dyes coursing through the channels and chambers of the heart and circulation (angiocardiography).

Many of the conditions that had previously been regarded as degenerative changes due to aging were reconsidered and classified as diseases for which cures might reasonably be sought. For example, the association of high levels of fatty materials in the blood with the development of atherosclerosis caused this condition to be regarded for the first time as a metabolic disease that might be treatable, just as diabetes or other metabolic diseases could be managed. A similar change in attitude occurred with respect to other chronic diseases such as arthritis and cancer. A major search for chemical agents capable of destroying cancer cells while sparing normal cells was launched by generous funding of a massive cancer chemotherapy program. The rich rewards originally expected to result from medical research appeared to be forthcoming.

By 1960, the NIH had received a half-billion dollar budget and spent over half of it on more than 11,500 projects devoted to a wide variety of research endeavors. About 90% of all federally supported projects were initiated in the nation's universities and medical schools. The benevolent extravagance of Congress had produced such reckless expansion of the biomedical research enterprise that few were surprised when Congressman Lawrence H. Fountain, chairman of the Intergovernmental Relations Subcommittee of the House Government Operations Committee, and his committee began to discover evidence of weaknesses in the methods used to award, monitor, and account for these vast sums (5). The inevitable criticisms and concerns of critical congressmen grew and gradually contributed to mounting pressure for results. The momentum favoring continued research and development persisted for some years despite the growing criticism. Total federal expenditures for health research mounted from $550 million in 1960 to more than $3 billion in 1974, as indicated in Table 9-1. The distribution of these funds among the various agencies of government has strongly favored the National Institutes of Health as displayed in Figure 9-1. However, despite continued growth in dollar amounts, the appropriations for NIH reached a plateau in the mid-1960s when corrections are applied to account for inflation.

Pressures for Payoff

Along with continued financial support of research, there developed a growing and urgent expectation of tangible health benefits from the decades of generous support of biomedical research. Despite a veritable deluge of new and important basic information regarding the structure, function, and control of organs and their responses to disease, the primary targets, the great killers, were not succumbing to the onslaught of research as rapidly as expected. Indeed, certain kinds of cancer, heart disease, chronic lung disease, and various resistant infections were gaining in prevalence.

In response to the mounting pressures for payoff, three main trends emerged more or less simultaneously. First, risk factors were explored by large-scale epidemiological studies designed to seek clues to the causes of major diseases. For example, the contributions of smoking, diet, and lack of exercise became the targets for major campaigns exhorting the public to promote their own health by individual health maintenance. With attention now concentrated on the individual's propensity for forming unhealthy habits, the responsibility for relatively slow progress in conquering killers was subtly shifted from the medical community to the public. Second, the rapid development of sophisticated technologies for basic and clinical research was converted into a growing array of diagnostic methods—a "diagnostic imperative." Third, substitutes and supplements for the function of various organs were developed to "treat" chronic disabilities lacking effective or definitive therapy.

The technological developments in health care were greatly influenced in this direction by the latter two trends. Intensive campaigns against smoking, drinking, and dietary indiscretions have affected behavior to varying degrees. The medical research community has been exposed to powerful pressures to expand greatly the diagnostic capability and to develop technical substitutes or supplements for various organ functions.

DEVELOPMENT OF DIAGNOSTIC TECHNOLOGIES

At the turn of the century, physicians were still highly dependent upon their own subjective senses for gathering diagnostic data. They were aided by the newly developed x-ray machines, the electrocardiogram, and a few laboratory tests on blood and urine. During the first half of this century, technical progress was remarkably slow. There appeared to be far more technical progress in the appliances added to the average kitchen than those in the typical doctor's office. Many modern diagnostic devices have been developed by modifying and refining research tools originally intended for basic medical research.

TABLE 9-1. The Growth in Expenditures for Health Related Research and Development, 1960–1980

Source of Funds		Expenditures in Millions of Dollars							
	1960	1962	1964	1966	1968	1970	1974	1980
Total	$932	$1,372	$1,730	$2,147	$2,600	$2,856	$4,452	$7,891
Government	558	901	1,180	1,471	1,754	1,868	3,038	5,178
Federal	448	782	1,049	1,316	1,582	1,667	2,754	4,723
State and local	110	119	131	155	172	201	284	455
Industry	253	336	400	510	661	795	1,187	2,391
Private nonprofit	121	135	150	166	185	193	227	322
Foundations	40	40	43	44	49	47	54	—
Voluntary health agencies	36	38	42	47	57	61	84	—
Other	45	57	65	75	79	85	89	—

SOURCE: National Institutes of Health: Basic data relating to the National Institutes of Health, 1976; US Dept of Health and Human Services: *Health, United States, 1981.* Government Printing Office, 1982.

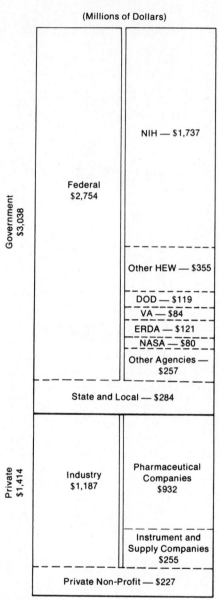

(Millions of Dollars)

Figure 9-1. Distribution of biomedical research and development funds by source of expenditures, United States, 1974.

SOURCE: *Opportunities for Assessment.* Office of Technology Assessment, US Congress, 1976.

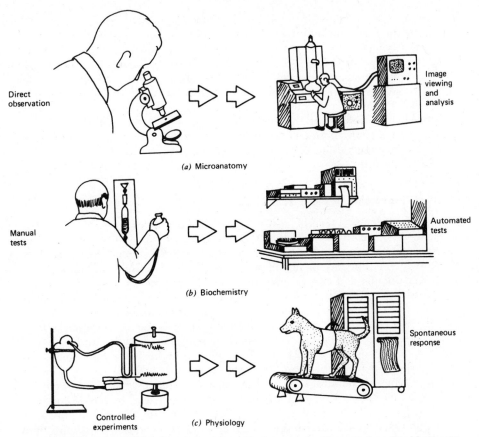

Figure 9-2. Changing technologies for biomedical research. *Note:* Before World War II, biomedical research was generally conducted using relatively primitive tools for observation and measurement. Since then, technologies have become increasingly sophisticated, with such commercially available equipment as electron microscopes, elegant and sometimes automated chemical analyses, and new sensors capable of continuously monitoring the performance of internal organs in comprehensive and quantitative scales.

Basic Medical Research Technologies

The traditional approaches to basic medical research were leisurely and scholarly, largely dependent upon subjective observations leading to descriptions, classifications, and concepts of functional cause and effect based mainly on time relationships. Structure was investigated by microscopy, composition by manual chemical analysis, and function by relatively crude recordings using mechanical levers and smoked drums (Fig. 9-2).

Revolutionary changes occurred after World War II. The explosive expansion of basic medical research required whole new arrays of tools and analytical techniques. Quantum jumps in magnification were attained by means of electron microscopes, ultimately coupled with sophisticated technologies for image analysis. The diversity, accuracy, and speed of chemical analyses were all enormously enhanced by spectrophotometers, ultracentrifuges, chromatographs, and fluorescence techniques. A variety of new sensors were developed to provide accurate information regarding the mechanical function of internal organs. For example, tiny devices for continuously measuring the changing pressures, dimensions, and blood flow in the heart and major blood vessels could be implanted to investigate functions in healthy, active animals under both spontaneous and experimentally induced conditions (6). Such techniques provided comprehensive analyses of the function of this hydraulic system in many of the same terms engineers employ for analyzing the performance of mechanical systems. The few examples shown in Figure 9-2 are representative of an enormous expansion of the basic medical research capacity, a major advance toward the "science" of medicine, which had progressed so slowly in earlier centuries.

Clinical Conversion of Basic Technologies

The newly developed tools of basic research were readily converted into diagnostic devices. They greatly expanded the diagnostic capacity of clinical medicine and at the same time represented tangible rewards for research support. For example, the electron microscope has opened new vistas in the study of subcellular elements in both fundamental and clinical investigations of virus infestations, cancer, genetic disturbances, and many other central issues. The growing number of laboratory tests for the chemical and cellular composition of blood, body fluids, and tissue samples has completely transformed laboratory procedures. Automation of testing sequences allows batch processing of small samples to provide multiple simultaneous test results (as many as 24 tests from single samples). Today, larger hospital laboratories provide more than 300 tests, in contrast to only one or two dozen different types of chemical tests 30 years ago. The unit cost for each test has been greatly reduced, but the volume has increased enormously. The physical measurements of pressure, electrical activity, and other characteristics of vital organs are now widely used for diagnosis and for monitoring the condition of patients during intensive care (e.g., during and after surgery or in life-threatening situations).

Diagnostic testing technologies can be conveniently grouped into three categories (Fig. 9-3). The analysis of samples (e.g., blood, body fluids, and tissues) has been expanded and speeded by automation, particularly in testing their chemical composition. Spectroscopy, chromatography, flame photometry, and other techniques commonly employed in academic and industrial applications have proved to be extremely valuable for clinical diagnosis. In addition, the number and types of blood cells are routinely tallied semiautomatically. Pathologic changes in cells and tissues are accentuated by special staining and microscopic techniques. The use of automation in processing samples for the study of tissues and bacteria has been much slower and less effective than the use of automation in chemical analysis, where great strides have been taken.

Intrinsic Energy Sources

The traditional methods of clinical diagnosis have always relied heavily on detecting and assessing changes in energy sources produced within the body. For example, excitable tissues produce recordable electrical potentials as a by-product of their functional activity. These potentials can be routinely recorded from the brain (electroencephalography), heart (electrocardiography), and muscles (myography). Similarly, changes in pressures within the fluid-filled spaces of the body can be

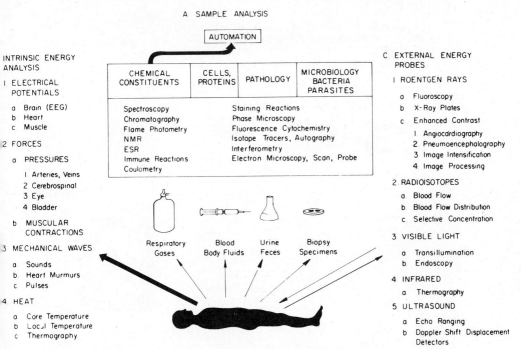

Figure 9-3. Three primary categories of diagnostic technologies currently available. *Notes:* (A) The chemical and cellular constituents of blood and body fluids can now be characterized by a large and growing selection of procedures, many of which have been automated to provide multiple, simultaneous values from a single small sample. Techniques for eliciting information from other samples of fluids and tissues involve histologic examination with various types of staining procedures and culturing techniques for identifying microorganisms. (B) Traditional components of the physical examination include subjective observations of intrinsic energy sources such as sounds, pulses, and temperature. Electronic devices supplement subjective senses by recording such items as electrical potentials, pressures, sounds, and temperature. (C) External energy probes elicit valuable information regarding the size, shape, location, movement, and function of internal organs by directing beams of energy into the body and analyzing the energy coming out. The versatility of diagnostic x-rays is generally known. These rays are being extended by means of other wave energies such as guided light, infrared light, ultrasound, and atomic energies.
SOURCE: Reprinted by permission from Rushmer RF: *Cardiovascular Dynamics*, ed 4. Philadelphia, WB Saunders Co, 1976.

recorded from arteries, veins, heart chambers, the spinal canal, the eye, the bladder, and elsewhere. Mechanical waves are produced by the heart (pulses and heart sounds) and have attracted physicians' attention for many centuries. The heat produced by the metabolic activity and its regulation are reflected in body temperature. These traditional sources of information are still widely employed and the technologies have been refined, but not greatly advanced.

External Energy Probes

Highly significant progress in diagnostic technologies has resulted from the many and varied applications of energy beams in probing the structure and function of

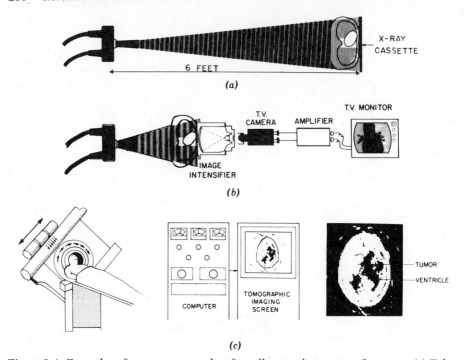

Figure 9-4. Examples of x-ray energy probes for collecting diagnostic information. (a) Tele-roentgenography, (b) image intensifier, (c) computerized axial tomography.
SOURCE: Reprinted by permission from Rushmer RF: *Cardiovascular Dynamics*, ed 4, Philadelphia, WB Saunders Co, 1976.

internal organs. The development of advanced optics and fiberoptics has provided long, flexible light guides for direct vision of the inner walls of virtually all hollow organs of the body (e.g., bronchi, stomach, bowel, bladder, uterus, and abdominal cavity). Light will penetrate the tissues of the body, but it is so badly scattered that the eye cannot observe internal organs through the skin. The interactions between different wave bands of energy and tissues have provided a whole new array of methods for extending the human senses beyond the normal range. For example, x-rays penetrate the body tissues with much less scattering than light and are absorbed to varying degrees by tissues such as lungs or bones. The images on fluorescent screens or x-ray plates provide valuable information regarding the size, shape, position, and displacement of many internal organs (Fig. 9-4).

The enormous potential of x-rays as diagnostic probes is being realized as a prototype for developments using other promising wave energies. By inserting or injecting appropriate radiopaque substances, the functional characteristics of certain organs can be explored. For example, fluid mixtures containing barium can be observed traversing the stomach and intestines. Certain functions of the kidneys and liver can be observed on sequential x-ray films after injection of appropriate materials into the bloodstream as they become concentrated in the gallbladder or urinary passages. By injecting radiopaque materials into the bloodstream, the distribution of blood in various organs can be visualized. High-speed computers can derive the shapes of some organs in three dimensions from simultaneous exposures in two planes. Monochromatic x-ray beams are a potentially useful analytical tool for painlessly exploring the composition of tissues (e.g., the iodine content of the thyroid gland or constituents of bone).

Computerized Axial Tomography (CAT) Scanners

Tomography is a term applied to the development of x-ray images of various planes in the body by specialized techniques. For example, an x-ray tube programmed to move in one direction while the x-ray plate is moved in the opposite direction will produce an image in a single plane that effectively remains stationary and un-blurred by the movement. The application of high-speed computers to this rela-tively simple mechanical process has produced costly but versatile instruments that have attracted the attention of physicians and the public alike. It has been recog-nized since 1917 that a two-dimensional image can be reconstructed from a large set of individual projections. Using a very narrow beam of x-rays penetrating the body from many different angles and positions, an enormous amount of data can be collected and processed to reconstruct an image of a plane transecting the body perpendicular to its long axis (7). This process provides an infinite number of views of the body that cannot be obtained using directly penetrating beams in the tradi-tional manner. The process is illustrated schematically in Figure 9-4. An x-ray tube is mounted on one side of a large housing, and a sensitive x-ray detector is posi-tioned on the opposite side and coupled to the x-ray tube so that they move to-gether. The tube and detector scan steadily back and forth across the portion of the body positioned within the circular orifice. The intensity of the x-rays that reach the detector is recorded at each of 160 positions along each scan. The housing then rotates 1 degree, and another series of scans ensues. The process is repeated 180 times to produce 28,000 values for x-ray intensities of beams penetrating from all these positions and angles. They are stored and analyzed in the computer and reproduced as an image of some 6,400 to 25,000 tiny areas (pixels) in the plane of the scan. Very subtle differences in x-ray absorption are recorded to delineate both normal and pathologic structures with different radio intensity. The original de-vices were designed for scanning the brain, but rapid progress has led to equipment for producing images of virtually any transverse plane of the body with increasing speed and definition. The many useful applications of x-rays represent prototypes for future developments in a number of other forms of wave energy (8). Recent developments in clinical use of Nuclear Magnetic Resonance (NMR) are especially exciting (9).

Diagnostic Ultrasound

The normal hearing range extends to only about 20,000 Hz (cycles per second). Very high frequency sounds can be readily generated by electric pulsations of certain types of ceramic crystals at frequencies in excess of 1 mHz (1 million cycles per second). Relatively narrow beams of such ultrasound have proved extremely useful in detecting the location and distance of ships and underwater objects by a device commonly known as *sonar*. Such beams penetrate the tissues with nearly the same ease as water and are absorbed and scattered by tissues to different degrees than are x-rays. Thus, ultrasound can be employed to extract entirely different information regarding the internal organs from that revealed by x-ray techniques. A common example is the application of sonar techniques to measure the time re-quired for pulses to traverse the brain substance and be reflected from a midline

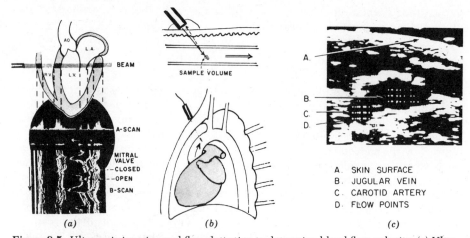

Figure 9-5. Ultrasonic imaging and flow detection to determine blood flow velocity. (a) Ultrasonic scans (A and B), (b) pulsed Doppler, (c) Duplex scan.
SOURCE: Reprinted by permission from Rushmer RF: *Cardiovascular Dynamics*, ed 4. Philadelphia, WB Saunders Co, 1976.

structure and the far side of the skull. A displacement of a midline structure of the brain may indicate a developing brain tumor.

Ultrasonic images can be derived by scanning techniques corresponding to those described above for x-rays. By moving the source and receiver of ultrasound through various positions and angles, an image of internal organs can be effectively produced on the surface of a television-like screen. Detailed transverse images can now be obtained of the brain, eye, abdomen, uterus, and other organs. The process promises to be rendered more effective and faster by current developments in arrays of ultrasound transducers and receivers coupled to high-speed computers to improve both resolution and efficiency.

Ultrasound has unusual and valuable backscattering (reflecting) properties that provide extremely valuable information. For example, a beam of ultrasound traversing the heart (Fig. 9-5) is backscattered from the walls of the chambers and from the valve leaflets. The movements of these various internal structures of the heart can be continuously observed on the face of an oscilloscope (A scan) or recorded on moving paper (B scan) for future analysis. Abnormal positions or movements of the various structures of the heart can be detected by such mechanisms. Ultrasound is also backscattered from blood cells, providing a means of registering changes in blood flow velocity by the Doppler shift principle, the physical mechanism that causes a change in the pitch of a whistle on a moving train as it passes by. The changing velocity of blood ejected from the heart can be continuously indicated by placing an ultrasonic probe at a strategic location just above the sternum, or breastbone (Fig. 9-5).

A combination of ultrasonic imaging and flow detection provides a means of obtaining information on blood flow velocity directly on the corresponding location in the body, as indicated in Figure 9-5. It is even possible to produce an image of the places where blood is flowing faster than some predetermined rate when this information is of interest. The many and varied applications of diagnostic ultrasound are being increasingly exploited in clinical laboratories, providing a whole new spectrum of clinically useful information.

Radioisotopes

The energy emitted by radioisotopes contributes additional information of value to the diagnosis of certain ailments. Injected intravenously, certain isotopes accumulate selectively in specific organs (e.g., iodine in the thyroid) as an indicator of function. The distribution of concentrations can be employed to indicate the blood flow in various internal organs. Arrays of isotope sensors (gamma cameras) can produce images illustrating the geometric distribution of isotopes in specific locations or organs and can be interpreted to indicate the position of blocked blood vessels in the lung or heart.

Thermography

Infrared cameras commonly employed to display geographic characteristics of the ground from high-flying aircraft or satellites can also be used to record the temperature distribution over the surface of the body. Such thermographs have excited some enthusiasm as a means of detecting pathologic processes (cancer or infection) under the surface of the skin. The expected promise of thermography has not yet been fulfilled.

Other forms of energy are also potentially useful as diagnostic probes. For example, microwaves may have value in exploring changes in the air-containing portions of the lung under various conditions.

This brief survey of the rapidly developing fields of diagnostic energies indicates the dramatic new ways in which more objective and quantitative information can be elicited using increasingly sophisticated equipment. The enthusiasm with which these new technologies are adopted should be tempered by important economic considerations.

Effects of Energy Probes on Health Care Costs

The practice of scientific medicine necessarily entails the accurate identification of the disease or disabilities of each patient. The diagnostic wave energy techniques described above all have the common attribute of deriving large quantities of potentially relevant information with minimal disturbance, discomfort, or hazard to the patient. CAT scanning has attained a very high level of sophistication that has greatly increased the versatility and definition of its applications. The potential for providing additional information from the other wave energies is as great as or greater than that of x-rays. Thus, the economic impact of CAT scanning can be used as a prototype to explore the potential economic impact of the large-scale commercial development of new technologies.

CAT scanners have experienced rapid technological change, with the development of three generations of models since the early 1970s. The enthusiasm with which the equipment was adopted produced a demand that outran the supply. With each new generation, the older versions became obsolete. A report by the Institute of Medicine indicated that purchase prices and installation charges range from $300,000 to $700,000 and annual operating costs range from $259,000 to $371,000, averaging about $285,000 (8). These high costs can be amortized only through high volume use of the equipment (i.e., 2,500 patient examinations per year as a minimum). The enthusiasm with which hospitals acted obtain this equipment exceeded reasonable bounds, so restraints are being considered or imposed by health planning agencies. Since the clinical effectiveness of these devices is not yet fully established, the uninhibited demand for them is decidedly premature. Furthermore, there is a growing conviction that the CAT scanner is being used primarily as an "add on" to supplement the traditional diagnostic procedures; therefore, its favorable properties are not being effectively used to reduce the need for other traditional tests.

The estimated increase in health costs of $1 billion per year due to the expansion of CAT scanning is serious enough. Exactly the same arguments can be advanced for correspondingly costly and sophisticated machinery employing other diagnostic wave energies such as ultrasound and NMR. They provide types of information entirely different from x-rays (9).

Expanding Electronics Industry

The development of sophisticated diagnostic equipment has spurred the growth of a huge medical electronics industry. This industry began at the turn of the century with electrocardiographs and x-ray systems, but the major advances occurred only after 1950 with the advent of large-scale cardiac monitoring, cardiac catheterization, scintillation (gamma) cameras, medical computers, and other complicated equipment (Fig. 9-6). The domestic market for diagnostic, therapeutic, and monitoring medical electronic equipment reached $840 million in 1974 and was estimated to exceed $1.4 billion in 1979. The growing ability to obtain ever more comprehensive and reliable information for purposes of diagnosis is generally regarded as a technical triumph of unquestioned value to the profession and society as a whole. However, consideration must be given to the price of progress in terms of two central issues. First, the ability to gather clinical data has proceeded so rapidly that it has outdistanced the ability to treat many of the conditions that can now be recognized

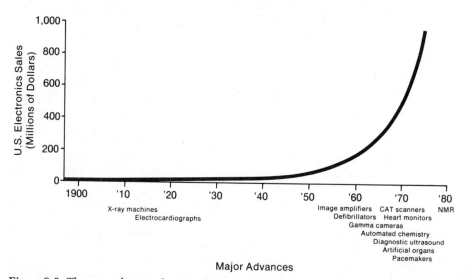

Figure 9-6. The expanding production of electronics for application in medicine. *Note:* The meteoric rise in expenditures for medical electronics began in the late 1940s and now exceeds $1 billion annually. Many of the technical developments that contributed to this industrial expansion are indicated at the bottom of the graph.

with confidence. Second, diagnostic technologies have added greatly to the soaring costs of health care, due in part to pervasive pressures toward overuse and inadequate incentives for restraint on the part of either the physician or the patient.

There is a growing awareness that semiautomatic or routine applications of diagnostic testing may yield little information or even provide unwarranted reassurance. For example, an x-ray film of the skull is virtually routine in the case of head injury, without much regard for severity. Evaluation has revealed that there are only relatively minor benefits to the patient compared to the rather large expenditure involved. Yet both patient and physician may feel uneasy at the thought of dispensing with this semiautomatic ritual.

THE BASIS FOR BENEVOLENT EXTRAVAGANCE (DIAGNOSTIC IMPERATIVE)

The technical revolution in health care has resulted in an enormous increase in the array of alternatives available to the physician for both diagnosis and management of diseases. At midcentury, the average hospital laboratory routinely performed one or two dozen tests on blood, body fluids, or other samples obtained from the body. Today, automated sequences can rapidly and precisely perform 12 to 20 different tests on a single small sample. The number of clinical laboratory tests is approximately 600 and continues to increase. Modern physicians have a new role as professional purchasing agents for their patients, selecting the appropriate choices for each patient from an enormous array of diagnostic and therapeutic options. Because of long tradition and practical considerations, these choices are heavily biased toward thoroughness and the comprehensive use of available resources. Medical education occurs in an environment provided by highly trained specialists strongly inclined toward research and inclusive studies at the cutting edge of science. The public and professional peers also expect that all the necessary steps will be taken in the best interests of the patient. The standards of practice in the community and the legal liability of health professionals represent risks from using restraint to the point of "cutting corners." The natural inclination of all concerned to use fully the resources commonly regarded as necessary is reinforced by the many mechanisms for defraying costs by insurance or subsidies that eliminate some or most of the out-of-pocket costs at the time of the encounter.

The Medical Uncertainty Principle

The manifestations of diseases are variable and often unpredictable in different individuals. This fact has led Aaron Wildavsky to state that medical management is open-ended (10). No matter how thorough a physician's diagnostic or therapeutic management may be, there is always at least one more test or one more treatment that can be justifiably ordered in the best interests of the patient's health and welfare.

One obvious consequence is a widespread difference in the strategies of different physicians with reference to the completeness or thoroughness of their diagnostic and therapeutic efforts. In one study, variation in the use of laboratories ranged up to 17-fold among 33 faculty internists caring for a homogeneous population at a university clinic (11) (variation in the use of prescribed drugs was 400%). If it costs $1,000 to attain 90% confidence or certainty of a diagnosis, it will require many times that amount to reach 95 or 97% confidence that the diagnosis is accurate or that the treatment has been maximally effective. There is little prospect for achieving major cost containment so long as the patient, physician, hospital, and third-party funding sources all desire to reduce risk or uncertainty to a minimum. In addition, conservative use of resources provides no rewards but instead risk patient dissatisfaction or loss of professional status.

The ready availability of diagnostic test procedures has naturally encouraged their use in monitoring the course of disease processes and attempting to detect ailments at the earliest possible moment. There is a widespread conviction that physicians are more likely to order routinely more laboratory tests than are strictly necessary for assessing a recovery process. Similarly, there are both theoretical and practical reasons to suspect that periodic health examinations for early detection of ailments are costly in relation to the benefits attained.

Early Detection of Asymptomatic Disease

Prevention maintenance is a concept of proven effectiveness in the maintenance of complicated machinery in industry. It is also an attractive idea when applied to the human body. There is an implicit assumption that the early recognition of a malfunction before it becomes serious or even manifest would allow corrective steps to be taken before more serious damage had occurred. In the case of machinery, a defective or failing part can be replaced if it is discovered at an appropriate time. However, the success of early recognition of subclinical malfunctions in the human body is dependent upon the ability to take corrective action. There are several categories of disease and disability that do not lend themselves to this concept. For example, acute, self-limited diseases cannot readily be diagnosed before they occur. If they are self-limited, management has little effect. On the other hand, serious illnesses for which therapy is ineffective are not significantly influenced by early recognition.

The Annual Checkup.   For many years, doctors have followed the lead of the dental profession in recommending an annual or periodic checkup. The periodic health examination of persons without symptoms, a symbolic cornerstone of modern medical practice, is now undergoing rather critical consideration. The principal components of a periodic checkup are an interim history, followed by a physical examination and usually by selected laboratory tests. There can be little doubt that periodic contact with a personal physician helps to improve rapport and cement relationships, but there are nagging questions regarding the overall effectiveness of the ritual. There are few useful guidelines for selecting laboratory tests that are appropriate for a healthy person during periodic checkups.

Doctors' Dilemmas.   The question arises, "how can a physician select tests that are potentially relevant, from among 600 or more options, without the guiding signs or symptoms that would make the selection more logical?" The common compromise is a sequence of laboratory tests, varying in number and complexity, depending on the personal preferences of the physician. The problem does not end with the initial selection of screening procedures because tests beget more tests. For example, if a physician orders a profile of 12 tests and considers the range of normal to be at the 95% confidence level, one can predict statistically that 54% of a healthy

**TABLE 9-2. Targets for Appropriate Preclinical
Detection of Disease**

Stage in Life	Targets for Selective Screening
The fetus and first year of life	Rhesus incompatibility with mother Phenylketonuria Congenital dislocation of hip Some congenital heart defects
Preschool age	Hearing abnormalities Amblyopia
Childhood and adolescence	Smoking Congenital heart defects
Adulthood	Smoking Breast cancer Cancer of the cervix Cancer of the colon and rectum Hypertension Bacteriuria in pregnancy
The aged	Hypertension Conditions and states amenable to rehabilitative intervention where the goal is not cure or extension of life but improvement of quality of life

SOURCE: Spitzer WO, Brown B: Unanswered questions about the periodic health examination. *Ann Intern Med* 1975; 83:257–263.

population will have at least one value outside the range of normal (12). When the reports of the tests contain abnormal values, the physician is in a quandary. He or she is duty bound to determine whether or not those measurements that fall outside the normal range are false positive or are actual indications of disease. This determination requires a further round of examinations and more tests. Follow-up studies of patients with such doubtful test results on routine examinations have demonstrated that as many as 70% had results that were normal on repeat examinations.

The World Health Organization is heavily involved in searching for diseases among large populations of apparently healthy people under various conditions. A series of restrictive requirements has been reviewed by Sackett (13). These limitations preclude screening of healthy people except for a few exceptional circumstances. For example, Walter Spitzer and Bruce Brown (14) carefully analyzed the conditions for which screening would be justified for healthy populations and developed a list that is surprisingly short (Table 9-2).

Dangers of Drugs

It is normally assumed, with some justification, that modern methods of diagnosis and treatment carry only a negligible risk. While it is true that complications rarely occur as a result of diagnosis and treatment, the hazards are not negligible. It is important to recognize that any drug capable of producing a functional change in the body is a potential poison if administered in sufficiently high doses. Even aspirin, which has been given with impunity for generations, is not without potential hazard. It has been reported that at least 10% of all the adverse drug reactions recorded in American hospitals are caused by aspirin. In fact, one out of every 500 people who take the drug experience undesirable side effects such as skin rashes, asthma, or gastrointestinal bleeding. This is a widespread international problem. There are two major types of dangers from drugs. One is the unusual sensitivity of individuals to a particular type of medication, and the other is the complicated interaction of drugs that may enormously enhance their potentially toxic effects when given in combination.

Drug Interactions.   At the present time, the American public ingests drugs at a frightening rate. It is exceedingly difficult for the average physician to be certain what drugs a particular patient may be taking on his or her own, which might seriously interact with the drug being prescribed. It has been proposed seriously that the side effects of drugs should be listed in such a way that both the physician and the patient would be aware of them.

Delayed Complications.   There are certain drugs that have no obvious effects at the time of administration but trigger problems later on in subsequent generations. The thalidomide experience (1960–1963) was a case in point, creating a great tragedy by producing deformed children. Even more subtle was the experience of those individuals whose mothers received stilbestrol preparations 2 decades ago to prevent premature delivery. It has now been fully documented that the female children of these women are developing precancerous cells in their vaginal tracts at an alarming rate. There was no reason to consider this possibility at the time the drug was being administered.

An even more striking event occurred in the more distant past. Everyone assumes that oxygen is an innocuous material; in fact, it is vital and life-giving. However, an epidemic of blindness occurred among premature infants in the 1950s because physicians, in attempting to help premature babies survive, placed them in an environment containing very high concentrations of oxygen. A greatly increased incidence of blindness in premature babies resulted and for several years appeared to be a mysterious epidemic of unknown origin. It was finally established by controlled studies that administration of oxygen-rich mixtures to premature babies was responsible for degenerative changes in the eyes, resulting in blindness. Such painful lessons from the past indicate the importance of using care and judgment in the development, acceptance, and widespread use of new techniques and technologies, no matter how innocuous they may seem.

MONITORING METHODS

Techniques for continuously displaying the electrocardiogram, arterial pressures, and other vital signs have been incorporated into equipment for monitoring the conditions of patients requiring intensive care. Such equipment is now widely used during and after high risk surgical operations (e.g., intracardiac surgery). Similar systems are also employed in the care of patients after heart attacks in the familiar coronary care units. Such sophisticated facilities, involving continuous surveillance by highly trained personnel, have been enthusiastically incorporated into hospitals of virtually all sizes. There is now an oversupply of coronary care beds, and experience has demonstrated that the quality of care tends to diminish in underused facilities. Cooperative activities in sophisticated settings require an unremitting and continuous flow of patients to maintain optimal performance. The supply of coronary care units in Massachusetts was evaluated using definitive criteria such as a maximum of 30 minutes' travel time and a 95% chance of obtaining a bed in the geographically closest unit (15). It was estimated that the 94 coronary care units in the state, with 446 beds, could be effectively reduced to 39 units and only 336 beds with both dollar savings and improved performance.

EMERGENCY MEDICAL SERVICES

The Emergency Medical Services Systems Act of 1972 provided aid to states and localities to establish coordinated, cost effective, areawide emergency medical service systems. This act was a response to the established fact that the most common hazards to life and health between the ages of 1 and 35 years are due to injuries from accidental or intentional violence. In recent years, an enviable record of performance has been achieved by dedicated emergency medical technicians, appropriately trained and using modern equipment. Specifically, many metropolitan areas are served by integrated systems of mobile units capable of responding rapidly to the types of emergencies that can beset citizens in modern society. The developing communication-transportation networks have attained the present level of performance by combining highly concentrated special training with appropriate equipment. For example, the successful management of acute heart attacks is heavily dependent upon having sophisticated portable defibrillation equipment incorporating methods for monitoring heart rhythms. In addition, respiratory assist devices, appropriate selection of drugs, and effective communication with physicians in emergency centers all combine to provide a very successful application of technology. Indeed, most doctors concede that patients are probably more effectively treated by experienced emergency medical technicians for heart attacks, drowning, traffic accidents, physical violence, or other similar hazards than by physicians. Very few physicians have such broad and concentrated experience with these particular threats to life and health.

In some communities, large proportions of the population have received training in cardiopulmonary resuscitation (CPR) for immediate life support during the critical minutes after a heart attack. For example, heart attack victims are probably better off in Seattle, where the CPR training extends to more than 20% of the population, than in many other cities. The success of civilian support is again highly dependent upon the backup of appropriately equipped emergency personnel, but it represents a vivid example of a growing trend toward public participation in health care for serious illness. Another prime example is the home care of patients with chronic kidney failure by means of sophisticated dialysis machines.

THERAPEUTIC TECHNOLOGIES

The application of engineering to clinical care has produced some spectacular achievements that are widely recognized by the public as a result of extensive coverage by the mass media. Increasingly sophisticated technologies embodied in the artificial heart-lung machines support open heart surgery. Credible visions of bionic human beings have been produced by implantable heart pacemakers, artificial kidneys, powered prostheses for amputees, and the prospects of an implantable artificial heart. These notable achievements have tended to obscure the rather disappointing rate of progress toward the control, cure, or prevention of many of the most important health hazards and disease states that Americans must confront.

Advances in therapeutic capability from symptomatic management through various steps toward cure, prevention, and elimination of diseases are illustrated schematically in Figure 9-7. The length of the arrow indicates the extent of progress, and the thickness indicates the current prevalence of the various ailments.

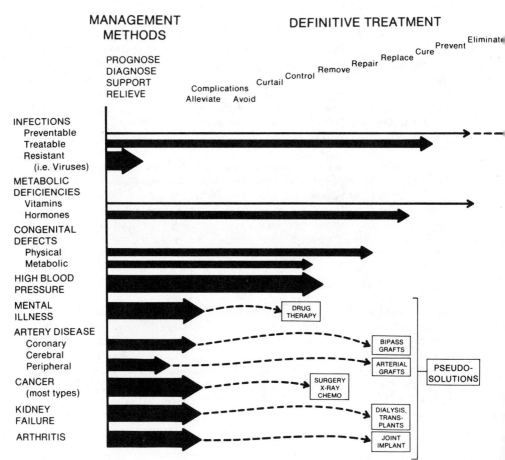

Figure 9-7. Advances in medical technology. *Note:* Progress in providing effective therapy differs widely for different conditions. For example, prevention, cure, and control have been attained for many infections. Many congenital malformations can be corrected by surgery, and high blood pressure can be effectively controlled. For conditions lacking definitive therapy, sophisticated technologies have been developed to replace or supplement the structure and function of affected organs. These technical triumphs should be regarded as pseudosolutions of value to current patients but not really directed toward the underlying causes and cures that must ultimately be developed for the benefit of future generations.

Great strides have been taken toward the control, cure, or even elimination of many infectious diseases that formerly attained epidemic proportions (e.g., cholera, plague, smallpox, typhoid fever, malaria). Many infections persist to plague the public, particularly viruses responsible for colds, influenza, hepatitis, gonorrhea, and other resistant organisms. These are now the most common infections, and progress toward their elimination is relatively limited, as indicated in Figure 9-7.

Advances in nutrition and endocrinology have gone far toward the prevention of vitamin deficiencies (e.g., ricketts, scurvy, beri-beri) and other deficiency diseases. The notable achievements in surgical correction of congenital heart disease have converted many impending tragic deaths into prospects of normal life spans. The development of drugs and procedures for controlling blood pressure has undoubtedly reduced the immediate threat of this condition, but it is uncertain whether the control of hypertension avoids the underlying processes leading to changes in arterial walls.

The most prevalent killer disease is atherosclerosis, or "hardening of the arteries," which is the uncontested leading cause of death. The current campaigns against excess consumption of fat and cigarettes obscures the fact that these are only peripheral factors and the direct causes of the thickening of arterial walls remain controversial and mysterious. During the past 30 years, a whole series of surgical operations has been touted in succession as means of providing an increased blood supply to the heart muscle when the coronary arteries are obstructed. These include methods of producing scar tissue on the surface of the heart by sprinkling talcum powder, roughening the heart surface with sandpaper, and inserting the cut ends of the arteries into the wall of the heart. Although none of these procedures has physiologic validity, their advocates initially claimed high rates of success. They have now fallen into disuse and have been replaced by a much more logical approach, the coronary bypass operation.

Bypass procedures use techniques of delicate vascular surgery that now permit skilled surgeons to install an accessory channel from the aorta (the main artery emerging from the heart) to a point beyond an obstruction, with widely reported success in relieving chest pain. There is little doubt that this operation relieves the chest pain in many patients, but the overall effectiveness in prolonging useful life is still under critical evaluation by controlled studies. Even before these studies have been completed, the coronary bypass operation has become one of the most common operations in this country (some 70,000 in 1977, at an average cost of $12,000 each). The unbridled enthusiasm for this surgical approach has been dampened for conservative physicians, but the advocacy of the surgical advocates remains intense. A provocative evaluation of this situation has been presented by Thomas Preston (16). It is interesting to note the widely varied rates of performance of the operation in different parts of the world (Table 9-3).

Critical evaluation of the outcome of coronary bypass surgery has indicated 1) excessive zeal exhibited by the most vigorous proponents of the operation and 2) persistent doubts regarding outcomes of surgery with respect to the potential for extending life as well as relieving the chest pain that is such a serious problem for many patients. The controversy regarding the long term outcome discloses a fundamental weakness in current approaches to assessment of modern medical technologies. The data in support of the beneficial effects of the operation are being assembled by a select few of the leading surgeons in the most prestigious institutions, which are the most fully equipped and staffed in the country. It seems optimistic in the extreme to extrapolate these data to the wide variety of professional personnel and institutions across the country.

TABLE 9-3. Coronary Bypass Surgery Rates in Selected
Locations

Location	Rate (Operations/ 100,000 Population)
Sweden, England, Finland	2[a]
Prepaid plans in the United States	4[a]
Average for the United States	28[a]
Western Washington State	45[b]
Eastern Washington State	90[b]
Spokane, Washington	116[b]

[a]From Preston T: *Coronary Artery Surgery: A Critical Review.*
New York, Raven Press, 1977.

[b]From *Guidelines for Heart Surgery Programs.* Seattle, Washington State Medical Association, 1977.

Pacemakers for the heart represent another major technical advance. The heart is provided with a built-in electrical ignition system that initiates each heartbeat in a regular fashion. When the conduction system of the heart is interrupted by disease, the heart rate may become dangerously low. An artificial ignition system can now be installed under the skin with wires leading to the heart muscle to maintain the heart rate at appropriate levels. The need to replace these devices after 2 or 3 years is being alleviated by the development of nuclear-powered devices with a much longer life expectancy. While the coronary bypass operation represents the installation of a structural element, an accessory blood channel, the pacemaker represents an electromechanical substitute for a vital function.

Another functional supplement or substitute is the artificial kidney, a major technical achievement. In earlier days, patients whose kidney function became insufficient to clear the blood of wastes were doomed to death. During World War II an artificial kidney was developed by Wilem Kolff from a used washing machine that was capable of sustaining life for a few days or weeks in patients with temporary kidney failure. Advances in biomaterials provided the essential tubing that could shunt blood from an artery to a vein outside the body and provide access to the circulation so that the blood could be cleansed of wastes for months, years, or even indefinitely. Applications of engineering technologies have provided a steady series of improvements in artificial kidney design. The dialysis machines are now so reliable that patients and their families can perform the necessary meticulous processes of this potentially life-threatening treatment several times a week at home after an intensive training period of only about 3 weeks. Current research and development efforts have attained miniaturization to the point where the dialysis devices may become portable, perhaps the size of a thermos bottle.

Structural Substitutes

The various tissues of the body have characteristics that are extremely difficult to duplicate. For example, the search for a substitute for skin to replace this vital covering when lost through damage, disease, or destruction (e.g., burns) has not yielded material that even approximates its protective properties. Surgeons in burn centers are still dependent largely on sources of mammalian skin from humans (or pigs). In other instances, substantial progress can be recognized. The problem is not new since artificial teeth have been known since antiquity. Arthritis is an extremely common disease resulting in destruction of joint surfaces that can render movement excruciatingly painful. The development of artificial joints has provided an alternative to this kind of suffering. Indeed, the installation of these artificial bone-joint combinations has become one of the most common orthopedic procedures at present.

Newly developed materials are now becoming widely used for a variety of purposes, including artificial heart valves and artificial ducts or channels that substitute for the esophagus, bile ducts, and arteries. Structural elements include bone implants, cartilage replacements (ear, nose, or joint) artificial tendons, and cosmetic implants to improve external appearance.

Artificial extremities of widely varying complexity have been developed for amputees. Sophisticated controlled and powered hands and arms are fully developed but have not been widely accepted because of a preference for the rather simple mechanical versions that remain dominant in present use.

Pseudosolutions

The functional and structural supplements and substitutes mentioned above are identified as "pseudosolutions" in Figure 9-7 because they appear to represent attractive solutions to complications of diseases but do not deal with the underlying disease process. Excessive enthusiasm over successful relief of symptoms by means of structural and functional substitutes can divert essential attention and resources from the more important tasks of identifying the underlying causes of these diseases and disabilities, which could lead to ultimate prevention and cure in the future. Considerations applicable to most of these technologies can be illustrated by a specific example.

The dialysis machines that support the lives of patients with inadequate kidney function are recognized as technical triumphs of vital importance to the patients who are dependent upon them. Congress has included financing for patients requiring dialysis under Medicare to cover costs too great for most individuals to sustain. In 1976, this program provided care for 21,500 eligible patients at a cost of $448 million. The cost is expected to reach $1 billion by 1984 and perhaps $1.7 billion by 1990, covering some 70,000 patients (17). There is no question of withdrawing this kind of support from patients who would die without it. However, it seems desirable to query what alternatives are being neglected because of this large allocation of funds for the benefit of a relatively small number of patients. For example, kidney transplants are recognized as preferable to continued enslavement to dialysis machines. The common rejection of kidney transplants can be avoided only by greater understanding of the underlying immune reactions. Our policymakers must carefully consider whether the huge expenditures for dialysis are diverting efforts away from solving the immune reaction problem or developing a basic understanding of kidney disease processes. The potential benefits of the much preferred treatment, cure, or prevention of kidney disease for future generations could be sacrificed in exchange for limited benefits for a relatively small number of patients today. These considerations apply to all of the present pseudosolutions but are perhaps best exemplified by the artificial heart.

Totally Implantable Mechanical Heart

The concept of substituting an artificial pumping device for the heart appeared realizable in 1939, when John Gibbon succeeded in keeping cats alive for nearly 3 hours with a mechanical apparatus that substituted for both the heart and lungs. The life support systems that opened the thorax and the heart chambers to surgical repair and reconstruction were the direct result. By the late 1950s, heart assist devices had reached a stage that encouraged some investigators to push for a totally implantable heart. Congress earmarked appropriations for such a development in 1965. Most of the technologies, essential materials, and successful implantable pump systems have been developed. Animals have been kept alive for weeks with implanted pumps and external power sources. Methods of meeting the power requirements remain elusive. The original projections were for the manufacture of sufficient devices to serve extremely large numbers of patients (as many as 200,000 per year). Growing concerns over the ultimate consequences of technical success stimulated the convening of a special interdisciplinary panel to consider the personal, social, and cultural implications of successful development of such hearts (18). This survey constituted one of the first and foremost assessments of the overall impact of technologies in the field of health care.

TECHNOLOGY ASSESSMENT: A NEW NEED

Most of the pressing problems of modern society can be traced to unpredicted consequences of technological triumphs (e.g., population explosion, urbanization, pollution). This realization has prompted a growing interest in developing techniques for evaluating, in advance, the potential and probable impacts of new technologies while their development is still in progress.

There is growing interest in the problem of assessing the effectiveness of procedures in affecting the course of illness in relation to their costs. The significance of a single source of information in a diagnostic pattern or the contribution of a particular therapy to favorable outcomes has proved to be extremely difficult to evaluate, primarily due to deficient criteria. The problem of evaluating the cost-benefit relationship is even more difficult when the concept is extended beyond the immediate effects on individual patients to encompass the psychosocial, economic, and political impact of technologies on local or national scales. A notable example is the obvious impact of providing artificial kidneys to 60,000 patients at a cost of more than $1.5 billion on the nation as a whole, in addition to the interpersonal relationships within families and the legal, ethical, and philosophical implications for our society. Such considerations also apply, in varying degrees, to the many other incremental additions to health technologies that have bloomed with breathtaking speed to revolutionize the principles and practices of health care in 3 short decades. Since these changes are continuing, it is increasingly necessary to consider carefully their portents for the future.

FUTURE FORECASTS

Health care technologies have induced revolutionary changes in the practice of medicine and surgery during the past 25 years. The original emphasis on basic medical research during the golden age of NIH has been reduced and diverted toward more tangible health benefits by pressures for short term payoffs by the public and their representatives in Congress. Both attention and resources need to be restored for the elucidation of the fundamental causes of the most common and critical diseases as the essential ingredient for more definitive diagnosis of and therapy for persistent health problems.

Greatly expanded research is needed in such critical areas as virology, immunology, genetics, and related subjects that are fundamental to many of the diseases affecting humanity (e.g., cancer, atherosclerosis, arthritis, and allergies). In addition, the mechanisms that are directly involved in the production of specific lesions need to be explored in depth before definitive diagnosis and therapy can be developed to optimal levels. Diagnostic equipment has greatly expanded in diversity, objectivity, and relevance. Ideally, a definitive diagnostic test can indicate the nature and severity of an ailment from a single quantitative value. Some of the infectious diseases can be diagnosed with this degree of certainty and, in general, their causes are known. Despite enormous progress in both basic and clinical medicine, the causes of most other common persistent disease problems remain uncertain. Continued commitment to basic medical research should progressively elucidate the causes of a growing list of diseases, creating opportunities for definitive and quantitative diagnoses. Continued pressures for payoffs will ensure that the fruits of basic research technologies will be promptly converted into diagnostic methods.

The current tendency to develop extremely costly substitutes for definitive therapy, technical pseudosolutions, is likely to continue at the peril of the economic stability of the country. The need for multidisciplinary evaluation of the ultimate impact of health technologies is just now becoming more widely apparent. Technology assessment is a concept whose time has come, perhaps too late to avoid the mistakes of the past but absolutely essential to avoid even worse problems in the future.

The impact of health care technology has affected all components of the health services system and the public's relation to it. Health care professionals have become increasingly dependent upon these technologies and have assumed the role of professional purchasing agent for the patient in selecting appropriate health services. One consequence has been the progressive specialization of physicians and other professionals. A corresponding decrease in the number of general practitioners has depleted the ranks of primary care physicians. The sophistication of health technologies has increased the dependence of patients on the health professionals to the point where they become helpless in treating even trivial health problems. The average citizen must become more responsible for health maintenance and for the management of the most common self-limited ailments through aided self-care. The well established technologies of communication and transportation must be mobilized into readily accessible networks by which the citizen can assume these responsibilities with confidence and with appropriate protection against complications.

There is growing evidence that health technologies have been developed too far, too fast, and with exuberant enthusiasm by health professionals. The outcome for the public in terms of their actual health status has been recognized in the improved management of life-threatening ailments. However, the common malfunctions and chronic complaints that reduce the quality of life for many people have gone essentially unchallenged. A realignment of priorities seems timely to support the health status of the productive population between 16 and 55 years of age, even if this requires a reduction in the resources devoted to prolonging life and postponing death in the aging population. The process of technology assessment must be developed and progressively refined to permit such crucial evaluation of current and future priorities. The single most important requirement for effective technology assessment is the broad consideration of interdisciplinary impacts on the social, economic, legal, and political aspects of modern society.

The need for long-range health planning on a national scale has been recognized for years. The excessive duplication of costly technologies is one of the most pressing problems to be resolved. The crucial first step, the development of national health goals, policies, strategies, and criteria for evaluation, has not been taken. However, there is awakening interest in these needs, as evidenced by requirements written into legislation.

The ramifications of these issues are vast. They fundamentally affect every facility and service discussed in the previous chapters of this book. They are also driving forces that are strongly influencing the quantity and form of the resources devoted to health care and the means by which our nation controls those resources.

REFERENCES

1. Maple E: *Magic, Medicine and Quackery*. London, Robert Hale, 1968.
2. Ray C: *Medical Engineering*. Chicago, Year Book Medical Publishers, Inc, 1975.
3. Fishbein M: *Fads and Quackery in Healing*. New York, Covici, Friede, Publishers, 1932.
4. Duffy J: *The Healers; The Rise of the Medical Establishment*. New York, McGraw-Hill Book Co, 1976.
5. Strickland SP: *Politics, Science, and Dread Disease; A Short History of the United States Medical Research Policy*. Cambridge, Mass, Harvard University Press, 1972.
6. Rushmer RF: *Cardiovascular Dynamics*, ed 4. Philadelphia, WB Saunders Co, 1976.
7. Gordon R, Herman GT, Johnson SA: Image reconstruction from projections. *Sci Am* 1975; 233(4):56–71.
8. Institute of Medicine: *Computed Tomographic Scanning: A Policy Statement*. Washington, DC, National Academy of Science, 1977.
9. American Hospital Association: *NMR: Nuclear Magnetic Resonance*. Guideline Report, Hospital Technical Series. Chicago, AHA, 2:8, March, 1983.
10. Wildavsky A: Doing better and feeling worse: Political anthology of health policy, in Knowles J (ed): *Doing Better and Feeling Worse: Political Anthology of Health Policy*. New York, WW Norton and Co, 1977.
11. Steven S, Kenders K, Cooper J, et al: Use of laboratory tests and pharmaceuticals: Variation among physicians and effect of cost audit on subsequent use. *JAMA* 1973; 225:969–973.
12. Richard R: The probability of abnormal 12-channel results in normal people. *Minn Med* 1972; 55:944.
13. Sackett DL: Laboratory screening: A critique. *Fed Proc* 1975; 34:2157–2161.
14. Spitzer W, Brown B: Unanswered questions about the periodic health examination. *Ann Intern Med* 1975; 83:257–263.
15. Bloom BS, Peterson OL: Patient needs and medical-care planning: The coronary-care unit is a model. *N Engl J Med* 1974; 290:1171–1177.
16. Preston T: *Coronary Artery Surgery: A Critical Review*. New York, Raven Press, 1977.
17. Congress: *Development of Medical Technology: Opportunities for Assessment*. Office of Technology Assessment, 1976.
18. National Heart and Lung Institute: *The Totally Implantable Heart*. Report of the Artificial Heart Assessment Panel, National Institutes of Health; Department of Health, Education, and Welfare, 1973.

CHAPTER 10

Health Care Personnel

Ira Moscovice

Health care personnel play an important role in the provision of services to meet the health needs of the population. This chapter highlights recent health care personnel trends and discusses issues of provider supply, education/training, distribution, specialization, and the role of the federal government in the production of health care personnel.

At the outset, it is important to recognize that health care personnel are only one of a larger group of interrelated and interdependent components that together comprise the *health care system,* defined as the formal linkage of a variety of resources that facilitate the delivery of a full range of health services appropriate for a defined population and/or service area (1). Important components of a health care system, as discussed in this book, include personnel (physicians, dentists, nurses, and support staff), physical facilities such as hospitals and nursing homes, medical technology, equipment and supplies, transportation and communication resources, and public and private reimbursement mechanisms (2).

The U.S. health care system is large, complex, and often fragmented, as noted in Chapter 1. Various chapters in this book have described the important trends concerning other health system components. This chapter will demonstrate the reliance of health care personnel and other components of the system on each other and on external pressures including technology, regulation, economic growth, aging of the population, and urbanization.

EMPLOYMENT TRENDS IN THE HEALTH CARE INDUSTRY

The twentieth century has witnessed a dramatic growth in the number and types of personnel employed in the health care industry. Table 10-1 shows the rapid gains in health sector employment in the United States, starting with a pool of fewer than

TABLE 10-1. The Health Sector as a Proportion of All Employed Persons, by Decade: 1910–1980

	1910	1920	1930	1940	1950	1960	1970	1980
Employment in health sector (1,000s)[a]	479	624	859	972	1,394	1,966	3,130	5,030
Total number of persons employed (1,000s)[b]	38,167	41,614	48,829	44,888	56,225	64,639	78,627	97,270
Health sector as a proportion of all occupations	1.3%	1.5%	1.8%	2.2%	2.5%	3.0%	4.0%	5.2%
Total U.S. population (1,000,000s)	92.4	106.5	123.1	132.6	152.3	180.7	205.1	227.7
Rate of health personnel per 100,000 population	518	586	698	733	915	1,088	1,428	2,209

SOURCE: Adapted from Mick, S. Table 7, Understanding the problems of human resources in health, 1925–77: Recommendations from the CCMC and current realities, paper prepared for a conference at Georgetown University, May 1977.

[a]These figures do not include secretarial and office workers, craftsmen, laborers, and other personnel such as cooks, janitors, and so on who work in supporting roles in the health care industry.

[b]Figures for 1980 include employed persons 16 years of age and over; figures from 1940 to 1970 include employed persons 14 years of age and over; earlier data are based on persons 10 years of age and over.

500,000 employees in 1910 and growing to more than 5 million by 1980. These figures include primarily those individuals with training and skills unique to the health care industry and exclude clerical staff, craftsmen, laborers, and others who have supporting roles in the delivery of health services. It has been estimated that almost one-third of all health sector employees fall into this supporting category (3). The importance of these approximately 1.5 million nonclinical workers should not be overlooked.

The health care industry is the largest single employer of all the industries monitored by the Department of Labor (4). It has maintained a steadily increasing proportion of all persons employed, and currently includes 5.2% of the U.S. labor force. Thus, employment in the health sector has outpaced overall employment in our economy as well as total population growth. This growth is accentuated by the fourfold increase in the rate of health care personnel per 100,000 population, from a low of 518 in 1910 to a high of 2,209 in 1980 (Table 10-1).

More extraordinary than the increased supply of health care personnel has been the emergence of a wide variety of new categories of personnel, including physicians' assistants (PAs), nurse practitioners (NPs), dental hygienists, and laboratory technicians, nursing aides, orderlies and attendants, home health aides, occupational and physical therapists, medical records personnel, radiologic technicians, dieticians and nutritionists, social workers, and the like. The Department of Labor currently recognizes almost 700 different job categories in the health industry (4). The most rapid growth in the supply of health care personnel has occurred in these recently developed categories (Table 10-2).

The traditional health care occupations of physicians, dentists, registered nurses, pharmacists, and optometrists generally have experienced dramatic declines in their relative proportion of all health care personnel as compared to the marked increase in recent decades in the supply of medical, nursing, and dental allied health personnel. One exception is registered nurses, who continue to comprise the largest single group of health care personnel. By 1980, more than two-thirds of all personnel employed in the health care industry were in nontraditional allied health or support services positions (5).

The primary reasons for the increased supply and wide variety of health care personnel in the twentieth century are the interrelated forces of technological growth, specialization, and the emergence of the hospital as the central focus of the health care system. The hospital became the setting where new technology could be implemented and where medical, nursing, and other health professional students could be educated. The technological revolution has led to the increased use of hospitals, with a corresponding concentration there of health care personnel. Almost 60% of all health care personnel work in hospitals today (6).

Technological innovation has also led to increased specialization of health care personnel, primarily during the last 30 years. This specialization has resulted in the formation of new categories of health care providers within the traditional professions (e.g., pediatric nephrologists and gastroenterologists in medicine, periodontists in dentistry) and the advent of new types of allied health professionals (e.g., occupational therapists, radiologic technicians, speech pathologists).

These health care personnel trends will be discussed in greater detail by focusing on three of the more traditional groups of professionals—physicians, dentists, and nurses—and two of the recently developed categories of personnel—physicians' assistants and nurse practitioners.

TABLE 10-2. Employment in Selected Occupations in the Health Field, United States, 1950–1980

	1950	1960	1970	1975	1950–1975 (Percent Increase)	1980
Physicians (MDs)	209,000	247,300	311,200	364,500	74	432,400
Dentists	79,200	91,100	102,200	112,000	41	126,200
Registered nurses	316,200	527,000	750,000	961,000	204	1,235,200
Optometrists	14,800	16,100	18,400	19,900	34	22,300
Pharmacists	89,200	92,700	109,600	122,500	37	144,200
Dental hygienists	7,000	12,500	16,000	23,500	235	NA[a]
Dental assistants	55,200	82,500	92,500	120,000	118	NA
Licensed practical nurses	146,000	245,000	400,000	477,000	226	NA
Occupational therapists	2,000	8,000	12,800	13,700	585	NA
Physical therapists	4,600	9,000	24,000	26,100	467	NA
Social Workers	6,200	11,900	29,800	40,000	545	NA

SOURCE: Torrens P, Lewis C, Health care personnel, in Williams S, Torrens P (eds): *Introduction to Health Services*, New York, John Wiley & Sons, Inc, 1980, Table 9-1, and *Third Report to the President and Congress on the Status of Health Professions Personnel in the United States*, US Dept of Health and Human Services, publication No. (HRA) 82-2. Governmental Printing Office, January 1982.

[a]NA = not available.

THE EXPANDING SUPPLY OF PHYSICIANS

Shortage or Surplus?

The number of physicians in the United States has increased rapidly in the last 15 years, with nearly 450,000 active physicians practicing in 1980 (Table 10-3). Since 1965, there has been a 55% increase in the supply of physicians, resulting in an average of approximately one physician per 500 population in 1980. The increase in physician supply has been primarily due to two important trends—the rapid increase in the number of graduates from medical schools since 1965 and the substantial immigration of foreign-trained physicians into the United States (7).

Table 10-4 shows the substantial increase in both the number of medical schools and the number of enrolled medical students over the past 2 decades. By 1980, the yearly number of graduates from medical schools had doubled in just 15 years. This increase can be directly attributed to the massive federal outlays for training, research, and construction since the early 1960s. By the early 1970s, 40 to 50% of medical school support came from federal sources (8).

The second important factor in the rapidly increasing supply of physicians has been the influx of foreign medical graduates (FMGs) into the United States. By the mid-1960s, favorable immigration policies for physicians had encouraged this movement. By the early 1970s, FMGs accounted for more than 40% of new physician licentiates, 30% of filled residency positions, and 20% of active physicians in the United States (Table 10-5). One-third of the growth in the supply of physicians in the past decade has been due to increases in the number of physicians trained outside the United States (9).

Table 10-5 indicates that the vast majority of the increase in FMG supply occurred before 1976. That year marked the passage of PL 94-484 (the Health Professions Education Assistance Act of 1976), which stated, "there is no further need for affording preference to alien physicians and surgeons in admission to the United States under the Immigration and Nationality Act." The enactment of PL 94-484 has noticeably limited the emigration of FMGs to the United States. Further growth in the number of U.S. physicians will not be influenced as much as it has been in the past by the influx of FMGs.

In summary, there has been a marked increase in the supply of U.S. physicians in the last 2 decades due to an increased number of medical school graduates and the immigration of FMGs. An obvious question is, why was it necessary to use this dual strategy for increasing the physician supply? The answer is twofold: First, before the 1970s, policymakers strongly believed that there was a serious shortage of physicians in the United States, with several studies estimating the shortage in 1975 to be in the range of 10,000 to 50,000 (10). Second, our country has not had a coordinated physician personnel policy; undergraduate and graduate medical education systems have operated independently of each other (7). Historically, the students graduating from U.S. medical schools have filled only two-thirds of the available residency positions, leaving the less desirable positions (e.g., those in inner city and county hospitals, health departments, nursing homes, and underserved areas) for FMGs. FMGs have helped to staff U.S. hospitals and have been more willing than U.S. medical school graduates to practice in relatively unpopular geographic and/or specialty areas.

It is not surprising, then, that the twofold strategy for increasing the physician supply more than met the perceived physician shortages of the 1960s and early

TABLE 10-3. Number of Active Physicians: 1965, 1970, 1975, 1980

Health Occupation	1965		1970		1975		1980		Percent Increase, 1965–1980
	Number	Personnel per 100,000 Population	Number	Personnel per 100,000 Population	Number	Personnel per 100,000 Population	Number	Personnel per 100,000 Population	
Physicians	288,700	145.5	323,200	154.5	377,400	176.8	449,500	202.3	55.7
MDs	277,600	139.9	311,200	148.7	363,300	170.2	432,400	194.6	55.8
DOs	11,100	5.7	12,000	6.0	14,100	6.6	17,100	7.7	54.1

SOURCE: *Third Report to the President and Congress on the Status of Health Professions Personnel in the United States*, US Dept of Health and Human Services publication No. (HRA) 82-2. Government Printing Office, January 1982.

TABLE 10-4. Number of Medical Schools, Students, and Graduates: Selected Academic Years 1950–1951 Through 1979–1980[a]

Academic Year	Number of Schools	Number of Students		Number of Graduates
		Total	First Year	
1950–51	79	26,186	7,177	6,135
1955–56	82	28,639	7,686	6,845
1960–61	86	30,288	8,298	6,994
1961–62	87	31,078	8,483	7,168
1962–63	87	31,491	8,642	7,264
1963–64	87	32,001	8,772	7,336
1964–65	88	32,428	8,856	7,409
1965–66	88	32,835	8,759	7,574
1966–67	89	33,423	8,964	7,743
1967–68	94	34,538	9,479	7,973
1968–69	99	35,833	9,863	8,059
1969–70	101	37,669	10,401	8,367
1970–71	103	40,487	11,348	8,974
1971–72	108	43,650	12,361	9,551
1972–73	112	47,546	13,726	10,391
1973–74	114	50,886	14,185	11,613
1974–75	114	54,074	14,963	12,714
1975–76	114	56,244	15,351	13,561
1976–77	116	58,266	15,667	13,607
1977–78	122	60,456	16,134	14,393
1978–79	125	62,754	16,620	14,966
1979–80	126	64,195	17,014	15,135

SOURCE: *Third Report to the President and Congress on the Status of Health Professions Personnel in the United States*, US Dept of Health and Human Services publication No. (HRA) 82-2. Government Printing Office, January 1982.

[a]Includes schools of basic medical sciences.

1970s. The final report of the Graduate Medical Education National Advisory Committee (GMENAC) estimates there will be a surplus of 70,000 physicians by 1990 (11). How the federal government reacts to this perceived surplus will influence physician supply in the remaining decades of this century.

Trends in Specialty Distribution

The significant increase in the supply of physicians described above has led to major concerns about the specialty and geographic distribution of physicians. Simply increasing the supply of physicians did not guarantee that necessary medical services would be readily available to the general population. Of particular interest was the availability of primary care—the entry level into the health care system where basic medical services are provided. Primary care includes the diagnosis and treatment of common illnesses and diseases, preventive services, home care ser-

TABLE 10-5. Foreign Medical Graduates (FMGs) as a Percent of New Licentiates, Filled Residencies, and Number of New Entry FMG Aliens, United States, Selected Years

Year	FMGs as a Percent of New Licentiates	FMGs as a Percent of Total Filled Residencies	Total New FMG Entries to the United States	U.S. Medical Graduates
1966	18.5	30	6,628	7,574
1967	22.9	32	8,115	7,743
1968	22.4	32	8,405	7,973
1969	23.1	33	6,939	8,059
1970	27.3	33	7,630	8,367
1971	35.2	32	7,879	8,974
1972	46.0	32	7,024	9,551
1973	44.4	30	8,123	10,391
1974	40.0	29	8,352	11,588
1975	35.0	26	7,316	12,714
1976	36.0	24	7,514	13,561
1977	32.2	18	6,681	13,607
1978	23.6	16	3,467	14,393

SOURCE: *Third Report to the President and Congress on the Status of Health Professions Personnel in the United States,* US Dept of Health and Human Services publication No. (HRA) 82-2. Government Printing Office, January 1982.

vices, and uncomplicated minor surgery and emergency care, as discussed in Chapter 5.

The increased supply of physicians has not resulted in major changes in the proportion of physicians in the primary care specialties—general practice, family practice, general internal medicine, and general pediatrics (Table 10-6). Within the primary care specialties, the number of family practitioners, internists, and pediatricians grew faster than the overall physician supply in the 1970s. However, these gains were offset by the declining number of general practitioners due to death or retirement.

The strong growth in surgical specialties that characterized the specialty distribution up to 1970 ceased in the following years. This trend, as well as the introduction and growth of family practice in the 1970s and the increased emphasis on training in internal medicine, are shown in Table 10-7. These data reflect the efforts of PL 94-484 to increase support for primary care residencies and decrease support for surgical residencies (9).

Despite these efforts, only 40% of physicians are currently in primary care specialties providing basic medical services, and almost 30% are surgeons. The final report of the GMENAC projects significant surpluses of surgical and medical specialties, with a near balance of supply and demand for primary care specialties in 1990 (Table 10-8).

The real goal of any physician supply policy should be to provide appropriate medical services that are readily accessible to the general population. Knowledge of the physician specialty distribution does not provide information on physician productivity, practice case mix, or the scope of services provided. The recent controversy over the extent of primary care provided by specialists and specialty care

TABLE 10-6. Number of Active Physicians (MDs) and Percentage Distribution by Specialty Groups

Specialty	1963		1968		1976		1980[b]		1990[b]	
	Number	Percent	Number	Percent	Number	Percent	Number	Percent	Number	Percent
All specialties	261,728	100.0	296,312	100.0	348,443	100.0	430,150	100.0	566,930	100.0
Primary care specialties[a]	110,071	42.1	116,760	39.4	135,881	39.0	166,790	38.8	239,830	42.3
Other medical specialties	12,291	4.7	15,762	5.3	18,955	5.4	26,580	6.2	41,080	7.2
Surgical specialties	67,745	25.8	81,820	27.6	98,667	28.3	113,200	26.3	129,610	22.9
All other specialties	71,621	27.4	81,970	27.7	94,940	27.3	123,580	28.4	156,410	27.6

SOURCE: Rosenblatt R, Moscovice I: *Rural Health Care*. New York, John Wiley & Sons, Inc, 1982, Table 4.2.

[a]Includes general practice, family practice, general internal medicine, and general pediatrics.
[b]Projections.

TABLE 10-7. Trend Data on Number and Percent Distribution by Specialty of First-Year Residents, 1960, 1968, 1974, 1976, 1978, and 1979

Total Number and Percent Distribution of First-Year Residents

Specialty	1960		1968		1974		1976		1978		1979	
	Number	*Percent*	*Number*	*Percent*	*Number*	*Percent*	*Number*	*Percent*	*Number*	*Percent*	*Number*	*Percent*
All specialties	11,080	100.0	12,864	100.0	18,834	100.0	19,831	100.0	22,291	100.0	22,477	100.0
Primary care specialties	3,443	31.1	3,796	29.4	7,724	41.0	9,432	47.5	11,070	49.7	11,107	49.4
General practice	364	3.3	258	2.0	162	0.9	196	1.0	—	—	—	—
Family practice	—	—	—	—	1,199	6.3	1,828	9.2	2,296	10.3	2,347	10.4
Internal medicine	2,193	19.8	2,589	20.1	4,533	24.2	5,522	27.9	6,704	30.1	6,729	29.9
Pediatrics	886	7.9	949	7.3	1,810	9.6	1,886	9.5	2,070	9.3	2,031	9.0
Surgical specialties	4,274	38.6	4,754	37.0	5,852	31.0	5,653	28.5	6,222	27.9	6,343	28.2
General surgery	2,122	19.1	2,394	18.6	2,639	14.0	2,575	13.0	2,730	12.2	2,817	12.5
Neurologic surgery	101	0.9	119	0.9	129	0.7	121	0.6	121	0.5	127	0.6
Obstetrics and gynecology	917	8.3	759	5.9	1,030	5.5	1,065	5.4	1,218	5.5	1,244	5.5
Ophthalmology	288	2.6	418	3.2	504	2.7	455	2.3	523	2.3	505	2.2
Orthopedic surgery	353	3.3	403	3.1	609	3.2	563	2.8	684	3.1	684	3.0
Otolaryngology	153	1.4	206	1.6	270	1.4	239	1.2	270	1.2	293	1.3
Plastic surgery	47	0.4	90	0.7	184	0.9	184	1.0	200	0.9	202	0.9
Thoracic surgery	89	0.8	137	1.1	147	0.8	142	0.7	144	0.6	134	0.6
Colon and rectal surgery	—	—	6	0.1	30	0.2	32	0.2	39	0.2	44	0.2
Urology	204	1.8	222	1.7	310	1.6	277	1.4	293	1.3	293	1.3

SOURCE: *Third Report to the President and Congress on the Status of Health Professions Personnel in the United States,* US Dept of Health and Human Services publication No. (HRA) 82-2. Government Printing Office, January 1982.

TABLE 10-8. Ratio of Projected Supply to Estimated Requirements, 1990

	Ratio (%)	Requirements	Surplus (Shortage)
Shortages			
Child psychiatry	45	9,000	(4,900)
Emergency medicine	70	13,500	(4,250)
Preventive medicine	75	7,300	(1,750)
General psychiatry	80	38,500	(8,000)
Near Balance			
Hematology/oncology-internal medicine	90	9,000	(700)
Dermatology	105	6,950	400
Gastroenterology-internal medicine	105	6,500	400
Osteopathic general practice	105	22,000	1,150
Family practice	105	61,300	3,100
General internal medicine	105	70,250	3,550
Otolaryngology	105	8,000	500
General pediatrics and subspecialties	115	36,400	4,950
Surpluses			
Urology	120	7,700	1,650
Orthopedic surgery	135	15,100	5,000
Ophthalmology	140	11,600	4,700
Thoracic surgery	140	2,050	850
Infectious diseases-internal medicine	145	2,250	1,000
Obstetrics gynecology	145	24,000	10,450
Plastic surgery	145	2,700	1,200
Allergy immunology-internal medicine	150	2,050	1,000
General surgery	150	23,500	11,800
Nephrology-internal medicine	175	2,750	2,100
Rheumatology-internal medicine	175	1,700	1,300
Cardiology-internal medicine	190	7,750	7,150
Endocrinology-internal medicine	190	2,050	1,800
Neurosurgery	190	2,650	2,450
Pulmonary-internal medicine	195	3,600	3,350
Estimated			
Physical medicine and rehabilitation	75	3,200	(800)
Anesthesiology	95	21,000	(1,550)
Nuclear medicine	N/A	4,000	N/A
Pathology	125	13,500	3,350
Radiology	155	18,000	9,800
Neurology	160	5,500	3,150

SOURCE: *Third Report to the President and Congress on the Status of Health Professions Personnel in the United States,* US Dept of Health and Human Services publication No. (HRA) 82-2. Government Printing Office, January 1982.

provided by primary care physicians highlights this point (12,13). Future needs for physicians cannot be based solely on knowledge of the number and types of physicians in our country.

Geographic Distribution of Physicians

One of the assumptions underlying federal health personnel policy in the 1960s and early 1970s was that a significant increase in the overall supply of physicians would both resolve the problem of a serious shortage and improve the geographic distribution of physicians. Clearly, there is no longer a shortage of physicians in the United States. Nevertheless, the chronic shortage of physicians in rural and inner city areas continues to persist (14).

With the output of physicians from medical schools outpacing the growth of the U.S. population, the population/physician ratio declined from one physician per 840 people in 1960 to one per 578 people in 1978 (Table 10-9). From 1960 to 1970, the vast majority of these physicians located in urban areas. However, the supply of physicians increased in both Standard Metropolitan Statistical Areas (SMSAs) and non-SMSAs in the 1970s. People living in SMSAs had a 22% decrease in the population/physician ratio while those living in non-SMSAs had an 18% decrease. Table 10-9, clearly shows the inverse relationship between physician supply and county size; larger counties have fewer people per physician.

The recent increase in physician supply has not been enjoyed by all counties. In 1978, 138 rural counties had no physicians at all, and counties with the smallest populations have gained few new physicians (14). Also of note are the small gains in the population/physician ratio in the largest metropolitan areas (>5 million population) in recent years. These areas appear to be reaching a saturation point (9).

The impact of specialization on the geographic distribution of physicians is not surprising. Until recently, general practitioners were the majority of physicians in rural areas. The supply of general practitioners has since dwindled, to be replaced in the late 1970s and early 1980s by recently trained family practitioners and other specialists. Table 10-10 shows the geographic distribution of recent family practitioners and other medical graduates. In 1975, general and family practitioners under 35 years of age located in non-SMSAs more frequently than their specialist counterparts. This trend has increased even further, with more than one-third of recent family practitioner graduates locating in nonmetropolitan areas (9). Family practitioners will undoubtedly be the core of the future rural physician supply.

As mentioned earlier, large metropolitan areas are rapidly becoming physician-saturated. Policymakers have traditionally assumed that physicians, particularly specialists, would not locate in rural areas as their supply increased. These views have been recently challenged by research that concluded that economic or market forces have caused major changes in the distribution of board-certified specialists (15). By 1977, communities with more than 20,000 residents often had board-certified specialists. Board-certified specialists who are moving to nonmetropolitan areas appear to be settling in regional centers that already have a sufficient number of physicians (2). Thus, those areas in greatest need of physicians (counties with populations under 25,000) still have great difficulty in attracting family practitioners or specialists.

Physicians have been reluctant to locate in rural areas for such reasons as lack of adequate medical facilities, professional isolation, limited support services, inadequate organizational frameworks including lack of group practices, excessive

TABLE 10-9. Population/Physician Ratios by SMSA and County Size, 1950–1978

SMSA or County Size Classification[a]	Population/Physician Ratio							% Decrease, 1976–1978
	1950	1960	1970	1972	1974	1976	1978	
U.S. total	845	840	728	687	658	617	578	6.3
SMSA total	707	721	622	584	558	522	489	6.3
>5,000,000	511	551	458	433	414	395	380	3.8
1,000,000–5,000,000	676	680	585	545	521	486	454	6.6
500,000–1,000,000	823	803	708	658	620	571	531	7.0
50,000–500,000	935	943	835	788	747	694	636	8.4
Non-SMSA total	1,412	1,443	1,416	1,378	1,328	1,250	1,165	6.8
>50,000	997	973	850	815	768	711	656	7.7
Potential SMSAs[b]	1,240	1,240	1,143	1,098	1,041	983	910	7.4
25,000–50,000	1,409	1,448	1,470	1,439	1,398	1,304	1,210	7.2
10,000–25,000	1,617	1,765	1,962	1,967	1,933	1,854	1,763	4.9
<10,000	1,802	1,994	2,352	2,333	2,452	2,324	2,260	2.8

SOURCE: Fruen M, Cantwell J: Geographic distribution of physicians: Past trends and future influences, Table 1. *Inquiry* 1982; 19:44–50.

[a]Classified on the basis of 1978 population estimates.

[b]Potential SMSAs are counties that do not meet all the requirements to be designated SMSAs but are considered "prime candidates to achieve SMSA status in the near future."

TABLE 10-10. Percent Distribution of Recent Family Practice and Other Medical Graduates to Counties Grouped by Urban Classification

	All Counties	Metropolitan[a]	Nonmetropolitan Urban[b]	Rural Large Town[c]	Rural Small Town[d]
1977–1979 graduates, 1979 data					
Family practitioners	100.0	64.6	26.7	1.6	7.2
1975 data: MDs under age 35					
All physicians	100.0	92.6	6.4	.2	.8
All primary care MDs					
General/family practice	100.0	78.1	16.2	.8	5.0
Internal medicine	100.0	95.3	4.2	.2	.3
Pediatrics	100.0	94.2	5.2	.2	.4
Other medical specialties	100.0	95.1	4.7	.1	.1
General surgery	100.0	94.9	4.4	.2	.5
Obstetrics-gynecology	100.0	94.1	5.4	.3	.2
Other surgical specialties	100.0	91.9	7.7	.1	.2
Other specialties	100.0	93.8	5.6	.1	.1

SOURCE: *Third Report to the President and Congress on the Status of Health Professions Personnel in the United States*, US Dept of Health and Human Services publication No. (HRA) 82-2. Government Printing Office, January 1982.

[a]Counties defined as part of a Standard Metropolitan Statistical Area in 1976.

[b]Non-metropolitan counties with no more than 25% urban population in 1970.

[c]Counties with a town of at least 5,000 persons in 1970.

[d]Counties with a town of less than 5,000 persons in 1970.

workloads and time demands, economic disincentives, lack of social, cultural, and educational opportunities, and spouse influence (16). Efforts to improve the distribution of physicians have tried to address these factors.

Federal efforts to improve the distribution of physicians have included loan forgiveness, the National Health Service Corps, Area Health Education Centers, and extensive support for the development of family practice training programs. The National Health Services Corps (NHSC) is different from earlier institutions used to improve physician distribution. The NHSC directly employs and places physicians in underserved areas (16). This program grew rapidly in the 1970s and became a centerpiece of federal intervention in health care delivery. The NHSC became the staffing mechanism for other federal health projects in underserved areas, and more than 1,000 NHSC sites with more than 2,000 assignees have been developed. The NHSC has also administered a large scholarship program that paid educational expenses and living allowances for medical students in return for service in an underserved area upon graduation. However, changes in administrative policy, political pressures, and the difficulties of managing a large and diverse program have disrupted the operation of the NHSC (17). The future of the NHSC is currently in doubt due to the Reagan administration's efforts to contain federal health care costs.

Area Health Education Centers (AHEC) are another federal effort to improve the distribution of physicians and other health providers in rural areas by decentralizing their educational training opportunities and linking rural health providers and facilities with large urban health centers (18). Urban educational resources became available to rural physicians to meet local personnel needs, extend local clinical training opportunities, and improve continuing education for local providers. In 1982, 18 AHECs were attempting to decrease the isolation of rural health care providers.

Other efforts to improve physician distribution include the attempts of Officers of Rural Health in states such as North Carolina, Colorado, Wyoming, and Nevada to increase the recruitment and retention of health care providers in rural areas, and cooperative ventures of consortiums of states to decentralize medical education programs and coordinate the placement of graduates (16). Examples of cooperative programs include the WAMI program (Washington, Alaska, Montana, and Idaho) and WICHE (Western Interstate Commission for Higher Education (19). Finally, private foundations have also supported the development of innovations in rural health delivery systems. Recent efforts have included the Rural Practice Project sponsored by the Robert Wood Johnson Foundation and the Innovations in Ambulatory Primary Care program sponsored by the W.K. Kellogg Foundation (20,21).

Despite the variety of approaches that have attempted to alter the urban/rural location of physicians, maldistribution persists. Recent studies implying that market forces have altered the distribution of board-certified specialists are preliminary at best. Many rural communities still find it difficult to recruit and retain physicians. Those communities with the greatest need continue to have the biggest problems in attracting physicians.

Developing policies to alter the physician distribution requires knowledge of which areas are underserved, plus the reasons for this problem and the amount and type of resources necessary to address it (22). The limited impact of previous attempts suggests that broader policy options should be considered. The possibilities include changing reimbursement systems or offering tax incentives to provide a financial reward for physicians practicing in underserved areas; modifying the medical school admissions process to place emphasis on applicants interested in primary care practice; or changing the undergraduate and graduate medical education system to ensure that the curriculum, counseling, clinical setting, and role models presented to medical students are related to the needs of society (14).

Physician maldistribution persists in the United States. Inefficient policies that continue to produce an excess of specialists in return for a small number of primary care physicians who locate in rural areas need to be carefully examined. Future federal and state policies that influence the training and reimbursement of physicians should be compatible with goals for improved physician distribution.

The Medical Education Pipeline

The 1970s were a period of change for both undergraduate and graduate medical education. The stereotype of the typical medical student—a white urban male who will eventually practice a medical or surgical subspecialty in a large urban setting—started to change.

On the undergraduate level, medical school class size increased by more than 50%, with the 1980–1981 entrance class totalling more than 17,000 students (23). The number of applicants to medical school, however, has declined approximately 15% from its peak in the mid-1970s and has remained relatively constant for the past few years. This decline has been caused by the reduced number of reapplicants; the skyrocketing costs of medical school tuition, which averages well over $10,000 annually in private schools and approaches $20,000 per year in several schools; and recent cutbacks in federal grants and loans for medical students.

The undergraduate medical curriculum remains broad-based, with the first 2 years consisting of lectures and laboratory work in the basic sciences, followed by 2 years of work in the clinical sciences through seminars and work in hospital wards and clinics. The role models and values in most medical schools continue to emphasize acute care for hospitalized patients (24). However, the professional socialization of the medical student has shown signs of changing, with increased emphasis on preceptorships in primary care settings and shifts in the focus of a growing number of medical school faculty from research to service. The latter has occurred due to recent changes in the distribution of medical school funding that have resulted in a deemphasis of federal support and greater reliance on state and local support as well as revenues from faculty practice income (9).

Another important issue affecting the medical education system has been the small number of women and minority students in medical schools. Concerted efforts have been made in the past decade to increase their enrollment, resulting in a sizeable increase over the decade from 11 to 28% of female first-year medical students and a moderate increase from 9% to 13% of minority first-year students (Tables 10-11 and 10-12). The proportion of minority medical students has stabilized over the last 5 years, but the proportion of black medical first-year students has recently declined. There are several factors for this decline, including increased tuition, reduced availability of scholarships, and the aftermath of legal challenges to affirmative action efforts (25).

The graduate medical education pipeline has also undergone major changes in the past decade. The number of residency positions increased by 75% to more than 22,000 by the end of the decade, with the percentage of filled positions increasing to over 90% (9). The increase in fill rate was due to an increased demand for first-year

TABLE 10-11. First-Year Students in Medical Schools, by Sex: Academic Years 1970–1971 Through 1979–1980

Academic Year	All First-Year Students	Male Students	Female Students	Percent Female of First-Year Students
1970–71	11,348	10,092	1,256	11.1
1971–72	12,361	10,668	1,693	13.7
1972–73	13,726	11,411	2,315	16.9
1973–74	14,185	11,442	2,743	19.6
1974–75	14,963	11,703	3,260	22.3
1975–76	15,351	11,695	3,656	23.8
1976–77	15,667	11,791	3,876	24.7
1977–78	16,134	11,985	4,149	25.7
1978–79	16,620	12,436	4,184	25.2
1979–80	17,014	12,266	4,748	27.9

SOURCE: *Third Report to the President and Congress on the Status of Health Professions in the United States,* US Dept of Health and Human Services publication No. (HRA) 82-2. Government Printing Office, January 1982.

residency positions by graduates of U.S. medical schools. In fact, the proportion of residencies filled by FMGs significantly decreased in the 1970s (Table 10-5).

The specialty distribution of residencies also changed dramatically in the 1970s, with greater emphasis being placed on primary care specialties (Table 10-7). By the end of the decade, almost one-half of all first-year residency positions were in the primary care specialties of family practice, internal medicine, and pediatrics. The growth in these specialties has stabilized since 1976 and will not increase further unless stimulated by new federal and state policies (26).

In the past decade, policymakers have recognized the strong interdependence of medical training and overall physician personnel policies. Earlier federal legislation (Health Professions Education Assistance Acts—HPEA—of 1963, 1965, 1968, and 1971) generally focused on increasing the size of medical school classes by funding the construction and operation of medical schools. Only recently have policymakers viewed the residency as a powerful influence on physician personnel policy.

In 1976, PL 94-484 attempted to address directly the geographic and specialty maldistribution of physicians as well as the country's excessive reliance on FMGs. The HPEA Act of 1976 tied the receipt of federal funds to the distribution of available residency slots in medical schools.

It should be noted that the federal goal of having 50% of first-year residencies in primary care specialties by 1979 was already satisfied in 1976, just before the implementation of the legislation (27). A shortcoming of PL 94-484 was the failure to consider switching into internal medicine and pediatrics subspecialties by first-year general internal medicine and general pediatric residents. PL 94-484 also affected residency positions by curtailing the inflow of FMGs into the United States through changes in immigration laws. The HPEA Act of 1976 has focused attention on the importance of the number and type of available residency positions. State governments have followed suit by starting to link their support of public and

TABLE 10-12. Minority Students in First Year of Medical School: Academic Years 1970–1971 Through 1979–1980[a]

Academic Year	All First-Year Students	Racial/Ethnic Category						Total Minority	Percent Minority of First-Year Students
		Black	Hispanic	Oriental	American Indian	Other Minority[b]			
1970–71	11,255	697	100	190	11	—		998	8.9
1971–72	12,258	882	158	217	23	—		1,280	10.4
1972–73	13,614	957	181	231	34	34		1,437	10.6
1973–74	13,898	1,027	230	259	44	71		1,631	11.7
1974–75	14,845	1,106	296	275	71	91		1,839	12.4
1975–76	15,216	1,036	336	282	60	73		1,787	11.7
1976–77	15,524	1,040	379	348	43	81		1,891	12.2
1977–78	16,134	959	609	418	46	—		2,032	12.6
1978–79	16,620	922	627	470	43	—		2,062	12.9
1979–80	17,014	960	766	512	55	—		2,293	13.5

SOURCE: *Third Report to the President and Congress on the Status of Health Professions in the United States*, US Dept of Health and Human Services publication No. (HRA) 82-2. Government Printing Office, January 1982.

[a]Excludes students at the University of Puerto Rico for academic years 1970–1971 through 1976–1977.

[b]Data were not provided for the category "Other minority" for certain years. Where such data are provided, they include a number of persons now counted under "Hispanic."

322

private medical schools to increases in the proportion of primary care residency slots.

The increased interest in the distribution of residency slots has heightened awareness of the strong relationship between community hospitals and neighboring medical schools. It is unclear exactly how much control medical schools have over the number and type of residencies offered. Community hospitals have become exceedingly dependent on residents to meet their staffing needs. Most of the costs (stipends for residents, teaching and support costs, cost of additional tests) of graduate medical education have been primarily supported by reimbursement for medical services provided by residents. This dual relationship demonstrates the influence that teaching hospitals can have on residency training.

In summary, graduate and undergraduate medical education has changed in the past decade. More structural changes can be expected in the 1980s as federal and state governments continue to pick up a sizeable share of medical education costs. The final report of the GMENAC recommends decreasing the size of medical school classes by 10% in 1984; no longer using capitation payments merely to influence specialty choice; and selectively using special-purpose grants to accomplish specific goals such as continued growth for family medicine and general medicine programs, support for primary care preceptorships, and renovation and construction of improved ambulatory training facilities.

Federal and state decision makers must continue their efforts to develop effective policies that influence physician training. In the current period of physician oversupply, federal and state policies will directly influence the ability to improve the geographic and specialty distribution of physicians in the United States.

DENTISTRY: A PROFESSION IN TRANSITION

By 1980, there were more than 121 thousand active dentists practicing in the United States. Although the supply of dentists has increased during the past decade, the ratio of active dentists to population has increased only slightly from 47.1 per 100,000 population in 1970 to 54.7 per 100,000 population in 1980 (Table 10-13). As in medicine, the increases that have occurred can be attributed to federal legislation passed in the 1960s and early 1970s that directly attempted to remedy a perceived shortage of dentists. This legislation resulted in increases in the number of dental schools from 47 to 60 in the past 2 decades and an increase in the number of first-year dental students from 3,600 to more than 6,000 in the same period (Table 10-14).

Some of the recent trends that have affected medical schools have also influenced dental schools. The percentage of female first-year students in dental schools increased significantly in the past decade, with one-fifth of current dental school students being female (9). The proportion of minority first-year dental students increased slightly over the same period, from 9% in 1970 to 13% by 1980 (9). Dental schools have started to deemphasize their support from federal sources and have increased their state support, dental clinic revenues, and fees from tuition. Another important recent trend has been the sizeable decrease in the number of applicants to dental schools. During the period 1975–1979, the number of dental school applicants decreased by almost one-third (from 15,734 to 10,520), resulting in an increase in the acceptance rate of dental school applicants from 37% to 58% during the same period (9).

TABLE 10-13. Total and Active Dentists and Dentist/Population Ratios: Selected Years, December 31, 1950–1980

Year	Number of Dentists[a]		Total Population (Thousands)	Dentists per 100,000 Population		Active Civilian Dentists[b]	Civilian Population (Thousands)	Active Civilian Dentists per 100,000 Civilian Population
	Total	Active		Total	Active			
1950	89,730	79,190	153,622	58.4	51.5	75,310	151,238	49.8
1955	97,960	84,370	167,513	58.5	50.4	78,270	164,597	47.6
1960	105,200	90,120	182,287	57.7	49.4	84,500	179,742	47.0
1965	112,450	95,990	195,539	57.5	49.0	89,640	192,633	46.5
1970	116,250	102,220	206,076	56.4	49.6	95,680	203,109	47.1
1975	126,590	112,020	214,446	59.0	52.2	106,740	212,308	50.3
1976	129,660	115,000	216,022	60.0	53.2	110,000	213,889	51.4
1977	132,670	117,890	217,739	60.9	54.1	112,720	215,620	52.0
1978	135,500	120,620	219,484	61.7	55.0	115,450	217,389	53.1
1979	138,450	123,500	221,195	62.6	55.8	118,330	219,100	54.0
1980	141,280	126,240	223,870	63.1	56.4	121,240	221,725	54.7

SOURCE: *Third Report to the President and Congress on the Status of Health Professions in the United States*, US Dept of Health and Human Services publication No. (HRA) 82-2. Government Printing Office, January 1982.

[a] Includes dentists in federal service.

[b] Dentists in the Veterans Administration and U.S. Public Health Service are counted as civilian dentists.

TABLE 10-14. Number of Dental Schools, Students, and Graduates: Selected Academic Years 1950–1951 Through 1980–1981

Academic Year	Number of Schools	Number of Students		Number of Graduates
		Total	First Year	
1950–51	42	11,891	3,226	2,830
1955–56	43	12,730	3,445	3,038
1960–61	47	13,580	3,616	3,290
1961–62	47	13,513	3,605	3,207
1962–63	48	13,576	3,680	3,233
1963–64	48	13,691	3,770	3,213
1964–65	49	13,876	3,836	3,181
1965–66	49	14,020	3,806	3,198
1966–67	49	14,421	3,942	3,360
1967–68	50	14,955	4,200	3,457
1968–69	52	15,408	4,203	3,433
1969–70	53	16,008	4,355	3,749
1970–71	53	16,553	4,565	3,775
1971–72	52	17,305	4,745	3,961
1972–73	56	18,376	5,337	4,230
1973–74	58	19,369	5,445	4,515
1974–75	58	20,146	5,617	4,969
1975–76	59	20,767	5,763	5,336
1976–77	59	21,013	5,935	5,177
1977–78	59	21,510	5,954	5,324
1978–79	60	22,179	6,301[a]	5,424
1979–80	60	22,482	6,132	5,256
1980–81	60	22,842	6,030	—[b]

SOURCE: *Third Report to the President and Congress on the Status of Health Professions Personnel in the United States,* US Dept of Health and Human Services publication No. (HRA) 82-2. Government Printing Office, January 1982.

[a]New York University enrolled 408 first-year students in 1978–1979, nearly twice as many as the 212 enrolled in 1979–1980. This was done so that a graduating class would not be lost when the university returned to a 4-year program from the earlier 3-year program. Considering this change, the apparent drop in first-year enrollments in 1979–1980 is significant since, had the university not doubled its enrollment, the number of first-year students in 1978–1979 would have been 6,097.

[b]Data are not available at this time.

Unlike their physician counterparts, dentists typically work in solo private general dental practices. The 1979 Survey of Dental Practice by the American Dental Association estimates that 73% of all dentists practice alone, with another 17% having a single colleague as a partner (28). Only one of every seven dentists are specialists, and the number of specialists has remained relatively stable over the past 5 years. Orthodontists comprise about two-fifths of all dental specialists, with oral surgeons totaling an additional one-fourth of the specialist population (Table 10-15).

There is significant variation in the distribution of dentists across regions of the

TABLE 10-15. Number of Active Dental Specialists by Specialty: December 31, 1980

| | All Dental Specialists | |
Type of Specialist	Number	Percent Distribution
All specialists	17,160	100.0
Orthodontists	6,563	38.2
Oral surgeons	3,960	23.1
Periodontists	2,242	13.1
Pedodontists	2,063	12.0
Endodontists	1,174	6.8
Prosthodontists	949	5.6
Public health dentists	110	0.6
Oral pathologists	99	0.6

SOURCE: *Third Report to the President and Congress on the Status of Health Professions Personnel in the United States,* US Dept of Health and Human Services publication No. (HRA) 82-2. Government Printing Office, January 1982.

United States and metropolitan/nonmetropolitan areas (Table 10-16). This variation is caused by the same factors that have led to physician maldistribution, as well as by the lack of reciprocity in the licensing of dentists across states. More than half of all dentists practice in the state where they trained, yet 18 states do not have a school of dentistry (9). The northeastern and western portions of the country have the highest dentist/population ratios, and the South, with its increased rural area, has the lowest ratio. Metropolitan areas have 60 dentists per 100,000 population compared to 37 per 100,000 in nonmetropolitan areas. These figures do not reveal the even larger supply of dentists practicing in the biggest metropolitan areas and nonmetropolitan areas with large cities. Thus, the smallest, poorest rural communities continue to have the greatest need for dentists. The likelihood of improving this situation in the near future is not good, as previous efforts to broaden the distribution of dentists have generally been ineffective (16).

Auxiliary Personnel

The practice of dentistry has undergone major technological and organizational changes in the past 2 decades. Of particular importance has been the increased use of dental auxiliary personnel. The three major types of dental auxiliaries are dental hygienists, dental assistants, and dental laboratory technicians. Dental hygienists provide oral prophylaxis services and dental health education and are the only group of dental auxiliaries that is licensed. Dental assistants have generally supported the dentist at chairside and have had the opportunity in some states to perform expanded functions under the supervision of the dentist. Dental laboratory technicians make oral appliances following the written prescription of a dentist.

In 1978, nearly all dentists had at least one auxiliary, with more than half of all dentists employing hygienists (Table 10-17). The government has supported the training of approximately 10,000 expanded-function dental auxiliaries (dental hygienists or dental assistants who receive additional education and training that enables them to perform a broader range of clinical functions), as well as the training of dental students to help improve their administrative and organizational skills

TABLE 10-16. Dentist/Population Ratios According to Geographic Region and Location: United States, 1979

Geographic Region	All Areas	Metropolitan Areas			Nonmetropolitan Counties		
			Population			Size of Central Cities	
		Total	1 Million or More	Less Than 1 Million	Total	10,000 or More	Less Than 10,000
				Number of active civilian dentists per 100,000 population			
United States	54.2	60.4	65.7	53.9	37.4	44.1	30.9
Northeast	66.3	69.9	76.2	59.8	46.2	47.4	43.3
New England	66.3	70.2	80.8	65.0	50.7	50.3	51.6
Middle Atlantic	66.3	69.7	75.6	56.2	43.9	45.9	38.7
North Central	51.7	56.6	60.6	50.8	40.5	46.9	35.0
East North Central	51.5	55.4	59.9	48.8	38.5	42.5	33.9
West North Central	52.2	61.1	63.5	57.6	42.7	53.9	36.0
South	43.5	51.4	55.5	49.1	29.3	36.6	23.7
South Atlantic	46.6	54.3	59.5	50.3	31.6	39.0	25.3
East South Central	40.2	52.2	41.3	52.6	27.3	36.7	21.5
West South Central	40.9	46.7	49.3	45.0	27.5	32.5	23.8
West	61.5	65.1	67.7	60.5	47.3	51.3	40.4
Mountain	54.2	61.2	65.1	59.7	43.3	49.4	37.1
Pacific	64.0	66.0	67.9	60.7	50.9	52.3	46.5

SOURCE: *Health United States, 1981.* Hyattsville, MD, US Dept of Health and Human Services, Public Health Service, December 1981.

TABLE 10-17. Percent of Independent Dentists Who Employ Auxiliaries: Selected Years, 1958–1978

	Percent of Dentists Who Employ Auxiliaries		
Year	*Dental Hygienists*	*Dental Assistants*	*All Types of Auxiliaries*[a]
1958	14.0	75.5	81.8
1964	20.2	82.4	89.9
1970	30.8	85.6	89.9
1972	36.9	90.2	93.6
1974	41.3	92.5	96.1
1976	47.0	86.7	94.5
1978	52.8	90.3	95.0

SOURCE: *Third Report to the President and Congress on the Status of Health Professions Personnel in the United States,* US Dept of Health and Human Services publication No. (HRA) 82-2. Government Printing Office, January 1982.

[a]Includes dental laboratory technicians and secretary-receptionists, as well as dental hygienists and dental assistants, who are employed full- or part-time.

in managing multiple auxiliary team practices (29). Support for the auxiliary concept has largely been due to an observed increase in productivity of dental practices that employ auxiliaries. Solo general practice dentists without auxiliaries averaged 42 visits per week in 1979; productivity monotonically increased with the number of auxiliaries employed, with 103 visits per week for those dentists employing four or more auxiliaries (28).

The dental profession is in transition. There has been a relative increase in the supply of dental services in recent years, resulting in a potential surplus of dentists before the end of the current decade unless there is a significant decrease in dental school enrollments (9). The role of the expanded-function dental auxiliary is unclear given this potential surplus and the depressed state of the economy. The demand for dental care is particularly sensitive to economic conditions, despite the significant growth in third-party payment for dental services (almost one-third of the U.S. population had some form of dental insurance coverage in 1979) (30). The substantial gains made in the prevention of dental disease through community water supply fluoridation will tend to reduce the demand for dental services in the future. All of these factors support the hypothesis that dental practice will be increasingly competitive in the 1980s. The impact of this increased competition on the price of dental care, the distribution of dentists, and the diffusion of innovations, such as the use of expanded-function dental auxiliaries, will shape the practice of dentistry in the coming years.

NURSING: SHORTAGES
AND FUTURE ROLE CHANGES

The Paradox of Increased Supply But Continued Shortage

Registered nurses are the largest group of licensed health care professionals in the United States. The supply of nurses increased from 316,000 in 1950 to 1,235,000 in 1980, resulting in a twofold increase in the nurse/population ratio during the same period. The supply of nurses has grown at a rate twice that of the population for the period 1950–1980 (31). The yearly number of nursing graduates has also doubled from 35,000 in 1966 to 70,000 in 1976 (32).

Table 10-18 presents a profile of the registered nurse supply from two surveys in 1977 and 1980 that were sponsored by the federal Bureau of Health Professions. The surveys indicate a 15% increase in the total registered nurse supply, with a 24% increase in the number employed in nursing. Despite these increases, almost one-fourth of nurses are not currently employed in nursing positions.

Most nurses are women; almost three-fourths are married, and only 7% are minorities. The most salient change highlighted by Table 10-18 is the shifting educational pattern of registered nurses, with increased emphasis on a 4-year baccalaureate degree and continued significant reductions in hospital-based diploma school graduates. The potential impact of nursing education trends on the future supply of registered nurses will be discussed in greater detail below.

Another important aspect of the supply of nurses has been the changing distribution of nursing personnel (Table 10-19). From 1950 to 1970, registered nurses steadily declined as a proportion of total nursing personnel. This trend changed in the 1970s, when the supply of registered nurses dramatically increased. It has been hypothesized that these changes indicate a reversal of the substitution of lower-salaried nursing personnel for registered nurses in institutions (33). Hospitals and nursing homes currently employ almost three-fourths of all registered nurses. The proportion of registered nurses increased as the total supply of registered nurses grew in the 1970s and as the wage differential between registered nurses and licensed practical nurses decreased.

Despite the overall gains in registered nurse supply, for many years the shortage of nurses seemed to get worse (31). Understanding the causes for the imbalance between the supply and demand is not easy. Some have pointed to the large number of inactive nurses as the main reason for the perceived shortage. However, Table 10-18 shows that the proportion of nurses actively employed increased from 70% in 1977 to 76% in 1980.

Although a 24% inactive rate may seem high, the labor force participation of nurses is similar to that of women in comparable professions. Personal characteristics and the role of women in society appear to be as important as job characteristics in influencing nurses to work (2). Only 8% of unemployed nurses are actively seeking nursing employment; the vast majority of unemployed nurses are over 50 years of age or married with children at home (34). One job characteristic that appears to influence the nurse employment rate is salary. Nurses are not paid well relative to their training and responsibilities, and the nurse shortage has been termed a shortage at a price due to lagging salaries (33).

Approximately one-third of employed nurses work part-time (31). The majority of part-time nurses are married with children at home. The proportion of nurses working part-time remained constant from 1977 to 1980. Although concern has also been focused on nursing attrition due to burnout and/or poor working conditions, recent surveys indicate only a small increase in the number of nurses working in other professions (31). Thus, the possible shortage of nurses cannot be attributed to increases in the number of part-time workers or attrition from the profession.

The reason for the perceived shortage of nurses is not clear. The most likely explanation appears to be increased demand for nursing services from several sectors of the health care system—acute hospital-based care, long term care for the growing number of chronically ill people, home-based care, and preventive care.

TABLE 10-18. Statistical Profile of Registered Nurses, September 1977 and November 1980[a]

Characteristic	Total Registered Nurses		Total Employed in Nursing		Total Not Employed in Nursing	
	1977	1980	1977	1980	1977	1980
Total number	1,401,633	1,615,846	978,234	1,235,152	423,400	379,712
Median age	39.8	38.4	37.7	36.3	46.1	47.1
Percentage male	1.9	2.7	2.1	3.0	1.4	1.6
Percentage minority	6.2	7.0	7.5	8.2	3.5	3.4
Percentage married	72.4	70.8	68.9	68.1	80.5	79.8
Percentage married with children at home	45.7	47.5	43.8	46.3	50.1	51.6
Percentage whose basic nursing education was:						
Diploma	74.8	63.4	71.4	59.6	82.6	75.7
Associate degree	11.3	18.5	13.7	21.2	5.8	9.7
Baccalaureate or higher degree	13.7	17.3	14.6	18.5	11.4	13.6
Percentage whose highest nursing related education was:						
Diploma	67.0	54.6	63.4	50.9	75.1	66.4
Associate degree	11.3	17.7	13.5	20.0	6.0	10.1
Baccalaureate	17.5	22.1	18.5	23.2	15.4	18.4
Masters or doctorate	4.1	5.1	4.4	5.3	3.3	4.4

SOURCE: Levine E, Moses E: Registered nurses today: A statistical profile, in Aiken L (ed): *Nursing in the 1980's: Crises, Opportunities, Challenges,* (L. Aiken, ed.) Philadelphia, JP Lippincott, 1982, Table 26.1.

[a]Percentages included on this table are derived from the segment of the total population indicating the particular characteristic being studied.

TABLE 10-19. Percent Distribution of Active Nursing Personnel by
Type of Personnel, Selected Years, 1950–1976

	1950	1960	1970	1976
Registered nurse	51%	46%	37%	39%
Licensed practical nurse	19%	19%	20%	20%
Nursing aides, orderlies, attendents	30%	35%	43%	41%

SOURCE: Adapted from Donabedian A, Axelrod S, Wyszewianski L: *Medical Care Chartbook*. Washington, DC, AUPHA Press, 1980, Chart E-50.

The demand for nursing services should continue to grow. Less attractive hospitals will continue to have nursing vacancies on evening shifts and in their intensive care and coronary care units. The expected growth in the supply of nurses will not be able to meet all the demand for nursing services in the future. To achieve an improved balance between the supply and demand for nursing services, institutional and other employers must become more sensitive to the special needs of working women.

Like many other health care professionals, nurses are not distributed evenly throughout the United States. The maldistribution appears to be due to the geographic immobility of women who are married and second wage earners in a family, as well as the inability of rural and inner city hospitals to offer an adequate range of incentives (e.g., flexible hours, increased salaries, and fringe benefits) to attract nurses (2).

Rural institutions have found that urban-based education and training programs are often not relevant to rural needs. Rural hospitals must frequently hire recent nursing graduates with limited skills and often resort to depending on pool nurses from temporary employment agencies (2). This problem is of particular concern due to the increased responsibilities and range of skills required of rural nurses. In the near future, rural providers are not likely to improve their chances of attracting well-trained nurses with a broad range of skills.

Nursing Education and Role Changes

The federal government provided $1.5 billion for nursing education during the period 1965–1981. This support, as well as market forces, helped to increase the number of nursing graduates entering the profession in the 1970s. Table 10-20 shows the twofold increase in the number of admissions to registered nursing programs over the past 2 decades. Of particular interest is the shift that has occurred in the control of nursing education from the hospital to nursing educators in colleges and universities.

There are three forms of training that lead to licensure as a registered nurse: 3-year diploma programs that are hospital based, 2-year associate degree programs that are generally community college based, and 4-year baccalaureate nursing programs in universities or 4-year colleges. In 1960, 83% of all nursing graduates were trained in hospitals; in 1980, 83% were trained in colleges and universities (35). The number of graduates from diploma programs has decreased rapidly since 1965 as baccalaureate and associate programs have grown.

TABLE 10-20. Admissions to Schools Offering Initial Programs in Registered Nursing by Type of Program, 1959–1979[a]

| | Registered Nursing Programs | | | |
Year	Bacca-laureate	Diploma	Asso-ciate Degree	Total
Calendar year				
1952	5,402	37,140	—	42,542
1953	5,771	38,947	609	43,327
1954	6,083	38,106	741	44,930
1955	6,985	38,884	629	46,498
Academic year				
1955–56	6,887	37,763	559	45,209
1956–57	7,106	37,571	578	45,255
1957–58	6,866	36,402	953	44,221
1958–59	7,275	37,722	1,266	46,263
1959–60	7,555	40,013	1,598	49,166
1960–61	8,700	38,702	2,085	49,487
1961–62	9,044	38,257	2,504	49,805
1962–63	9,597	36,434	3,490	49,521
1963–64	10,270	37,936	4,461	52,667
1964–65	11,835	39,609	6,160	57,604
1965–66	13,159	38,904	8,638	60,701
1966–67	14,070	33,283	11,347	58,700
1967–68	14,891	31,268	14,870	61,389
1968–69	15,983	29,267	18,907	64,157
1969–70	19,048	30,718	25,583	75,349
1970–71	20,413	28,980	29,889	79,282
1971–72	27,357	29,801	36,996	94,154
1972–73	30,478	29,848	44,387	104,713
1973–74	32,672	26,943	48,595	108,210
1974–75	35,192	24,696	50,180	110,068
1975–76	36,656	23,622	53,033	113,311
1976–77	36,947	22,243	54,289	113,479
1977–78	37,664	20,611	53,653	111,928
1978–79	36,087	18,499	54,131	108,717

SOURCE: *The Recurrent Shortage of Registered Nurses,* US Dept of Health and Human Services publication No. (HR) 81-23. Bureau of Health Professions, September 1981.

[a]Registered nursing programs include 49 states and the District of Columbia for all years, Puerto Rico beginning 1953, Virgin Islands beginning 1965, Guam beginning 1966, and Alaska beginning 1978.

Leading nurse educators have recently proposed that a baccalaureate degree be required for licensure as a registered nurse (36). The 1985 New York State Nursing Association's proposal (1985 NYSNA) attempts to create a distinction between professional nurses with baccalaureate degrees and nurse technicians with associate degrees; diploma school graduates and licensed practical nurses would no longer be relevant (37). The legislative response to this controversial proposal has been poor to date. A synthesis of the potential problems associated with the proposal suggests that it would result in increased costs and length of nurse training and restricted access to the nursing profession, and would exacerbate the nursing shortage in many areas of the United States (38). The burden of proof remains with the proponents of the 1985 NYSNA proposal to show that these problems would be offset by the improved quality of care provided by university-trained registered nurses. Nurse training has changed dramatically in recent years, with the potential for even greater change in the future. The decisions made concerning the 1985 NYSNA proposal will have important implications for the future supply of registered nurses.

The nursing profession is attempting to change its role in the health care system. The leaders of the profession have called for an expansion of the independent role of the nurse within the hospital and the creation of new professional roles outside the hospital (35). Hospitals continue to employ approximately two-thirds of all nurses and will remain their major employer due to continued technological advances and increased insurance coverage for the general population. Nurses are seeking to clarify their relationship to physicians, particularly within the context of clinical decision making in the hospital (35). They are developing new delivery modes, such as primary nursing, in which the nurse assumes direct responsibility for comprehensive care for a group of patients over a given time period.

A variety of new roles has emerged for the registered nurse. Included are positions such as clinical nurse specialist, nurse practitioner, nurse anesthetist, and nurse clinician. These positions involve employment in new ambulatory care settings (Health Maintenance Organizations, ambulatory surgery centers), nursing homes, and home care programs providing care for the elderly and others with chronic illnesses, as well as positions in hospitals.

Nursing professions want to control their future. They are trying to shed the traditional stereotype of the nurse as an underpaid female hospital laborer. In the process, considerable controversy has been created both inside and outside the profession. Associate degree and diploma graduates want to continue to function in viable roles within the nursing profession. Institutions desire to employ combinations of nursing personnel suitable for their particular environments. These forces, as well as the current restrictive interpretation of state nurse practice acts, suggest that there will be no easy solutions to changing, and hopefully strengthening, the future relationships of nurses, physicians, and health care institutions.

NEW CATEGORIES OF HEALTH CARE PERSONNEL: PHYSICIAN ASSISTANTS AND NURSE PRACTITIONERS

The perceived shortage of physicians in the mid-1960s led to the development of two new types of health care providers—physician assistants (PAs) and nurse practitioners (NPs). The first PA training program was established at Duke University in 1966; the initial NP program was started at the University of Colorado in 1965.

PAs are persons qualified by academic and practical training to provide patient services under the direction and supervision of a licensed physician who is responsible for the performance of the PA (39). PAs are able to diagnose, manage, and treat common illnesses, provide preventive services, and respond appropriately to common emergency care situations. The typical PA training program consists of 2 years of didactic study followed by clinical training. However, training programs vary widely in terms of admission requirements, curriculum, and site of educational training. There are currently 51 programs training PAs in the United States.

NPs are registered nurses who have completed formal programs of study preparing them for expanded roles and responsibilities (40). These expanded roles include obtaining comprehensive health histories, assessing health status, performing physical examinations, formulating and managing a care regimen for acute and chronically ill patients, teaching, and counseling (41). There are a range of training programs for different types of NPs, including pediatric, nurse midwife, family, adult, psychiatric, and geriatric programs. Slightly more than half of the more than 200 NP training programs are certificate programs that generally last for 8 to 12 months; the remainder are master's programs lasting from 1 to 2 years.

GMENAC estimates that approximately 16,000 NPs graduated from formal training programs by the end of 1979, and more than 2,000 new NPs are expected to graduate each year (40). The Association of Physician Assistant Programs estimates a PA supply of 11,000 at the beginning of 1980, with approximately 8,800 active (40). The PA totals include formal PA training program graduates and others who have passed the PA certifying examination. Currently, 1,500 new PAs graduate from PA training programs every year.

Almost three-fourths of PAs work in primary care specialties, with the majority in family practice (9). Surgical specialties accounted for 12% of all PAs, with general surgery and orthopedic surgery having the largest number. PAs have located in nonurban areas more frequently than physicians or the general population (16). Many PA programs were designed to train assistants to rural physicians and have succeeded in placing graduates in rural areas.

Several estimates are available on the specialty distribution of NPs. GMENAC estimates that 30% are family NPs, 25% are pediatric NPs, 20% are adult NPs, 10% are maternity NPs, 10% are midwives, and 5% are other types. NP graduates have been more likely than PAs to locate in urban areas. Research suggests that the structure of training programs is an important factor affecting the geographic distributions of NPs and PAs (40).

There are important differences in the perceived roles of PAs and NPs (42). PAs are viewed by the medical profession as physician extenders who can perform many of the usual functions completed by physicians. Nurses view the NP as a registered nurse in an expanded role. The expanded role includes greater supervision of and responsibility for primary patient care, with extra emphasis on the traditional nursing values of prevention and counseling. Despite these differences in perceived roles and in education and training requirements, PAs and NPs appear to be similar in many of their performance characteristics.

Several issues related to the performance of NPs and PAs are generally agreed upon as resolved. The research literature provides sufficient evidence that NPs and PAs are well accepted by patients, provide similar quality of care as physicians for basic health care problems, increase the availability and accessibility of health services, increase physician productivity in small primary care practices by up to 50%, and are generally cost effective from an employer's perspective (25,42–44). The individual effectiveness of a PA or NP is strongly related to environmental characteristics of the practice, including size, organizational structure, and location, as well as the physician's work style and willingness to delegate responsibility to the PA or NP (25).

Issues in PA and NP Use

Major issues that need to be resolved before PAs and NPs can be used fully are legal restrictions to practice, reimbursement policies, and relationships with physicians. The legal status of PAs and NPs is uncertain and varies considerably across states. Some states permit considerable delegation of tasks and responsibilities to the PA, including drug prescriptions with physician countersigns within 24 hours. New Jersey prohibits PAs from being employed in nonfederal facilities, and three states have no PA practice legislation (9). State legislation governing expanded medical delegation has been unduly restrictive with respect to the scope of practice of qualified nonphysicians (45).

Laws and regulations governing the expanded role of the nurse are changing rapidly but inconsistently. Although the majority of states have altered their nurse practice acts to facilitate expanded roles, the constraints on the scope of practice of NPs varies from state to state. For example, independent diagnosis, treatment, and prescription are prohibited for NPs in Wyoming but not in Colorado (2). Although the restrictions appear to be fewer for NPs than for PAs, changes in legal authority must take place before NPs will be able to practice independently. The nonphysician health care provider technical panel of GMENAC recommends that state laws and regulations should not require physician supervision of NPs and PAs beyond that needed to assure quality of care (40).

Third-party reimbursement imposes a major constraint on the use of PAs and NPs. Current policies almost always link the reimbursement of PAs and NPs directly to the employing physician or institution. Most insurers do not recognize PAs and NPs as legitimate providers of medical care. Private fee-for-service physician practices or other ambulatory settings have had difficulties in securing reimbursement for nonphysician services. However, institutions such as hospitals can include PA or NP compensation as part of their "reasonable cost" basis for reimbursement purposes (40).

To date, there has been little success in improving reimbursement for services provided by PAs and NPs. The implementation of the Rural Health Clinic Services Act of 1977 (PL 95-210) highlights the problems involved in attempting to change reimbursement policies. This act amends Titles XVIII and XIX of the Social Security Act to allow Medicare and Medicaid reimbursement to certified rural clinics staffed by PAs and NPs. Only a small number of clinics are participating in the program due to the complexities of the reimbursement formula, excessive paperwork, and inadequate patient load to make certification worthwhile (16). Many states have not promoted the program due to the reduction in their Medicaid budgets.

Reimbursement problems may be even greater than legal restrictions. Policymakers must carefully review inconsistent federal policies that fund the training of PAs and NPs but then deny reimbursement for the services they provide.

A third area of concern is future relationships of PAs and NPs with physicians.

In the past, physicians have shown reasonable acceptance of these personnel (42). The current perceived surplus of physicians could result in reduced employment opportunities for PAs and NPs. Nonphysician health providers may be forced to compete with new physician graduates for available jobs.

Delegation of tasks and responsibilities is an important issue for physicians who decide to employ PAs and NPs. The substitutability of PAs and NPs for physicians depends upon the volume and types of services delegated. PAs and NPs are cost effective only if they are used appropriately by their employers, whether physicians or institutions.

The future of NPs and PAs is uncertain. Past employment of these providers was motivated by the shortage and geographic maldistribution of physicians. The shortage has now turned into a surplus, and physicians have started to locate in previously underserved areas. These trends may cause problems for future employment of NPs and PAs, who will need to adapt to the changing health care environment. Emerging roles for NPs and PAs include providing primary care to underserved areas and populations, such as the elderly and the mentally ill, providing preventive care, and providing specialty services in hospitals in lieu of house staff (25). Resolution of problems regarding legal restrictions, reimbursement policies, and relationships with physicians will undoubtedly influence the ability of NPs and PAs to meet these new challenges. NPs and PAs will thrive in the future only if they are cost effective from both an employer's and a social policy perspective.

FUTURE ISSUES FOR HEALTH CARE PERSONNEL

This chapter has summarized recent trends in health care personnel supply. Federal and state support has resulted in large increases in the number of graduates from health professions schools. The significant increase in the supply of health personnel has guaranteed a future surplus of many types of health care professionals.

The federal and state investment in health care personnel has improved access to health services, helped health professions schools remain fiscally viable, and increased opportunities for careers in the health professions for women and minorities (46). Federal and state support for health professional training programs is likely to be reduced in the future. Budgetary pressures will cause a reallocation of funds that are targeted for health professions programs to other portions of federal and state budgets. It will be important to monitor the impact of future cutbacks on enrollments in health professions schools.

The health care system has exhibited an extraordinary capacity to expand. Federal and state decision makers have focused their efforts on constraining, or at least stabilizing, overall health care expenditures. Approaches that could be used to help contain expenditures range from fostering competition between health care providers to improve the efficiency of service delivery, to using the reimbursement mechanism to influence provider behavior, to limiting the supply of health care professionals.

Health care cost containment strategies need to be developed in concert with health care personnel policies. The health care system offers strong resistance to fiscal cutbacks. Major system changes—competition between health providers, alterations in reimbursement policies, and the like—can best be implemented if constraints on the flexible use of health personnel are reduced. Alternatives to the existing methods of training, licensing, regulating, and reimbursing health personnel should be seriously considered.

The surplus of personnel has been identified as one of the factors that have led to increased health care expenditures. Future health care personnel policies, at both the federal and state levels, will need to be targeted to meet specific goals. Modifications in the number and types of health professionals that are trained must be considered in light of the current focus on cost containment.

Efforts to contain health care costs will not be successful unless the practice behavior of current and future health care professionals can be modified. Further changes in the number and types of health professionals that are trained should take into account the behavioral modifications that are desired. These are the challenges facing decision makers and educators concerned with future health care personnel policies in the United States.

REFERENCES

1. *Health Care Delivery in Rural Areas.* Chicago, American Medical Association, 1976.

2. Moscovice I, Rosenblatt R: *The Viability of the Rural Hospital.* Boulder, Colo, Western Interstate Commission for Higher Education, 1982.

3. Sorkin A: *Health Manpower.* Cambridge, Mass, Lexington Books, 1977.

4. Torrens P, Lewis C: Health care personnel, in Williams S, Torrens P (eds), *Introduction to Health Services.* New York, John Wiley & Sons Inc, 1980.

5. US Bureau of the Census: *Statistical Abstract of the United States.* US Government Printing Office, 1981.

6. *Health, United States, 1981,* publication No. (PHS) 82-1232. Hyattsville, Md, US Dept of Health and Human Services, 1981.

7. Stevens R: The muddle over medical manpower. *Prism* 1975; 3:10–63.

8. Reinhardt U: *Physician Productivity and the Demand for Health Manpower.* Cambridge, Mass, Ballinger Publishing Co, 1975.

9. *Third Report to the President and the Congress on the Status of Health Professions Personnel in the United States,* publication No. (HRA) 82-2. US Dept of Health and Human Services, 1982.

10. Hansen W: An appraisal of physician manpower projections. *Inquiry* 1970; 7:102–114.

11. *Report of the Graduate Medical Education Advisory Committee to the Secretary, DHHS,* vol 1: *GMENAC Summary Report,* publication No. (HRA) 81-653. US Dept of Health and Human Services, 1980.

12. Aiken L, Lewis C, Craig J, et al: The contribution of specialists to the delivery of primary care. *N Engl J Med* 1979; 300:1363–1370.

13. Rosenblatt R, Cherkin D, Schneeweiss R: The structure and content of family practice: Current status and future trends. *J Family Pract* 1982; 15:681–723.

14. Fruen M, Cantwell J: Geographic distribution of physicians: Past trends and future influences. *Inquiry* 1982; 19:44–50.

15. Schwartz W, Newhouse J, Bennett B, et al: The changing geographic distribution of board-certified physicians. *N Engl J Med* 1980; 303:1032–1037.

16. Rosenblatt R, Moscovice I: *Rural Health Care.* New York, John Wiley & Sons Inc, 1982.

17. Rosenblatt R, Moscovice I: The National Health Service Corps: Rapid growth and uncertain future. *Milbank Mem Fund Q* 1980; 58:282–309.

18. Gessert C, Smith D: The national AHEC program: Review of its progress and considera-
    tion for the 1980's. *Public Health Rep* 1981; 96:116–120.

19. Schwartz R: Regional medical education: The WAMI program, in Purcell E (ed): *Recent
    Trends in Medical Education.* New York, Josiah Macy Jr. Foundation, 1976.

20. Moscovice I, Rosenblatt R: Rural health care delivery amidst federal retrenchment: Les-
    sons from the Robert Wood Johnson Foundation's Rural Practice Project. *Am J Public
    Health* 1982; 72:1380–1385.

21. *1977 Annual Report.* Battle Creek, Mich, WK Kellog Foundation, 1977.

22. Hadley J: Alternative methods of evaluating health manpower distribution. *Med Care*
    1979; 17:1054–1060.

23. Ginzburg E, Brann E, Hiestand D, et al: The expanding physician supply and health
    policy: The clouded outlook. *Milbank Mem Fund Q* 1981; 59:508–541.

24. *Report of GMENAC to the Secretary, DHHS:* Vol 5: *Educational Environment Technical
    Panel,* publication No. (HRA) 81-655. US Dept of Health and Human Services, 1980.

25. Scheffler R, Yoder S, Weisfeld, N, et al: Physicians and new health practitioners: Issues
    for the 1980's. *Inquiry* 1979; 16:195–229.

26. Steinwachs D, Levine D, Elzinga J, et al: Changing patterns of graduate medical educa-
    tion. *N Engl J Med* 1982; 306:10–14.

27. Jacoby I: Graduate medical education: Its impact on specialty distribution. *JAMA* 1981;
    245:1046–1051.

28. *The 1979 Survey of Dental Practice.* Chicago, American Dental Association, 1980.

29. Machlin S: Dental manpower, in *Health, United States, 1981,* publication No. (PHS) 82-
    1232. US Dept of Health and Human Services, 1981.

30. *Sourcebook of Health Insurance Data: 1981–1982.* Washington, DC, Health Insurance
    Association of America, 1982.

31. Levine E, Moses E: Registered nurses today: A statistical profile, in Aiken L (ed): *Nurs-
    ing in the 1980's: Crises, Opportunities, Challenges.* Philadelphia, JP Lippincott Co,
    1982.

32. Fagin C: The shortage of nurses in the United States. *J Public Health Policy* 1980; 1:293–
    311.

33. *The Recurrent Shortage of Registered Nurses,* US Dept of Health and Human Services
    publication No. (HRA) 81-23. Bureau of Health Professions, 1981.

34. Moses E: *The Registered Nurse Population: An Overview,* report No. 82-5. Hyattsville,
    Md, Bureau of Health Professions, US Dept of Health and Human Services, 1981.

35. Aiken L: The impact of federal health policy on nurses, in Aiken L (ed): *Nursing in the
    1980's: Crises, Opportunities, Challenges.* Philadelphia, JP Lippincott Co, 1982.

36. Fagin C, McClure, M, Schlotfeldt, R: Can we bring order out of the chaos of nursing
    education? *Am J Nurs* 1976; 76:98–107.

37. *Resolution on Entry Into Professional Practice.* New York, New York Nurses Association,
    1974.

38. Dolan A: The New York State Nurses Association 1985 Proposal: Who needs it? *J Health
    Polit Policy, Law* 1979; 2:508–531.

39. *Physician Assistants: Education, Accreditation, and Consumer Acceptance.* Chicago,
    American Medical Association, 1975.

40. *Report of GMENAC to the Secretary, DHHS:* Vol 6: *Nonphysician Health Care Provider
    Technical Panel,* publication No. (HRA) 81-656. US Dept of Health and Human Services,
    1980.

41. Abdellah F: The nurse practitioner 17 years later: Present and emerging issues. *Inquiry*
    1982; 19:105–116.

42. Kane R, Wilson W: The new health practitioner—the past as prologue. *West J Med* 1977; 127:254–261.

43. Record J, McCally M, Schweitzer S, et al: New health professions after a decade and a half: Delegation, productivity and costs in primary care. *J Health Polit Policy, Law* 1980; 5:470–497.

44. Lawrence D: The impact of physician assistants and nurse practitioners on health care access, costs, and quality. *Health Med Care Serv Rev* 1978; 1:1–12.

45. Kissam P: Physician's assistants and nurse practitioner laws: A study of health law reform. *Kansas Law Rev* 1975; 24:1–65.

46. Ginzburg E: Investments in health manpower: A possible alternative, in MacLeod G, Redman R (eds): *Health Care Capital: Competition and Control.* Cambridge, Mass, Ballinger Publishing Co, 1978.

CHAPTER 11

Financing
Health Services

William C. Richardson

Financing of health services cannot be considered independently from the various other dimensions of the system that are presented in this book. For example, human resource development, medical care technology, health services use, and institutional arrangements all are affected by, and in turn affect, the economic aspects of the system. The purpose of this chapter is to describe and analyze health services financing from four perspectives: health service expenditures and trends in health care costs, financial arrangements and economic relationships in the health care market, organizations or institutions financing health services, and major financial issues and alternatives for the future.

HEALTH CARE EXPENDITURES

Distribution and Sources

The United States spent $1,365 per person for all health services during 1982 (1). This total national expenditure of $322 billion included money spent for hospital care, physicians' services, dentists' services, drugs, nursing home care, other personal health care, construction of hospital facilities, government-funded research, and the cost of administering health insurance plans. By far the largest category of expenditure was for hospital care, which accounted for 42% of all health expenditures (Table 11-1). About four out of every five dollars spent for these services go to community hospitals. Community hospital expenditures are divided between inpatient services and outpatient services in a ratio of approximately 9:1.

The second largest category of expenditures is for physicians' services (2). Just under one-fifth (19.2%) of the dollars spent went to physicians. The professional services of dentists (6.0%), drugs (6.9%), nursing home care (8.5%), and other personal health care (6.3%) were of approximately equal magnitude. Somewhat more than one-half of the drug expenditures are accounted for by prescription drugs. Only 2.7% of total expenditures were devoted to traditional public health activities.

TABLE 11-1. National Health
Expenditures by Type of Care, United
States, Fiscal Year 1982

Type of Care	Percentage
Hospital care	42.0
Physicians' services	19.2
Dentists' services	6.0
Drugs and drug sundries	6.9
Nursing home care	8.5
Other personal health care	6.3
Other health spending	11.1
Total	100.0

SOURCE: Gibson RM, Waldo DR, Levit KR: National Health Expenditures, 1982. *Health Care Financing Rev*, Fall, 1983.

This proportion declined from a level of 3.1% in 1975, primarily as a result of more rapid increases in nonpublic health expenditures.

The expenditure of $322 billion (10.5% of the gross national product), or $1,365 per person, is substantial by any standard. The distribution of expenditures across sources of financing, however, reflects the diffusion of these expenditures in such a manner as to lessen their visibility in the society and, usually, their obvious impact on individual families. Approximately 89% of total national health expenditures are accounted for by the cost of personal health care. Only 32% of personal health care costs were paid for directly by individuals or families in 1982. An additional amount, representing various insurance premium payments paid for directly by individuals or families, results in a total of approximately 40% of personal health care costs that are "out-of-pocket" expenses paid directly by consumers.

So as not to double count, consider only the 32% in direct payments to providers. Of the other 68% of payments for personal health care in 1982, 29% was financed through the federal government, 11% by state and local governments, 1% by charity and private industry, and the remaining 27% of personal health care expenditures was paid as a result of private health insurance benefits.

The dispersion of sources of health care financing is particularly pertinent in light of the uneven distribution of health care costs across the population. For example, in 1974 slightly over 1% of the population accounted for approximately 20% of national health care expenditures, or an average of $8,600 per capita (3).

Because of the high proportion of expenses paid through governmental programs and voluntary health insurance, generally referred to as third parties, patient care decision making in any particular illness is more likely to be influenced by the existence or availability of sophisticated medical resources than by the costs entailed. On the other hand, as discussed further later in this chapter, the societal implications of both the uneven distribution of catastrophic illness expenses and their magnitude are very consequential.

Recent advances in medical technology (Chapter 9), including expensive equipment and large numbers of highly trained personnel, while important, account for only one-half of the expenditures of the so-called catastrophic population. The other half represent the 1.2 million catastrophically ill individuals who are patients in long term care institutions. As Birbaum points out, "[these] are persons

TABLE 11-2. National Health Expenditures as Percent of GNP, United States, Selected Fiscal Years 1950–1982

Fiscal Year	Percent of GNP
1950	4.6
1960	5.2
1965	6.0
1970	7.5
1975	8.6
1982	10.5

SOURCES: Gibson RM: National health expenditures, 1978. *Health Care Financing Rev,* Summer 1979, p 3. Gibson RM, Waldo DR, Levit KR: National health expenditures, 1982. *Health Care Financing Rev* Fall, 1983.

for whose conditions there are no technological remedies yet who are no longer able to care for themselves. Thus, the levels of technology and know-how polarize catastrophic expenses. To a significant extent, catastrophic illness is a result of an absence of technology" (3).

Trends in Health Care Expenditures

Between 1950 and 1982, per capita health care expenditures in the United States have increased more than 10-fold. As presented in Table 11-2, the nation was devoting twice as large a proportion of the GNP to health services in 1982 as in 1950 (10.5% versus 4.6%). During that same period, there was a dramatic shift in the sources of funds from the private to the public sector. For example, in 1950 and continuing until 1966, between 25 and 26% of national health expenditures were financed through governmental agencies. With the enactment of Titles XVIII and XIX of the Social Security Act (Medicare and Medicaid), the government share began to increase. This increase was dramatic in 1967 and 1968, and has since been more gradual. Estimates for 1975 through 1982 indicate a fairly stable proportion of expenditures financed through government, ranging between 42 and 43% of the total.

It is obvious from the increasing proportion of the GNP accounted for by health care expenditures that the rate of growth in this industry has been substantially higher than for the economy as a whole. The increases in total expenditures can be attributed to three principal factors: growth in the population, changes in the quantity and nature of the services consumed, and price inflation. With respect to the second factor, for example, and as noted in Chapter 3, there have been increases in the rate of hospital admissions per 1,000 population and in the number of doctor visits per person. There have also been increases in the numbers of tests and procedures performed, and, more generally, an increased intensity of medical care technology used in treating various conditions. The population growth factor has always been the smallest component of expenditure increases for health services. Further, over the years it has declined, accounting for one-fifth of the rise in total expenditures in 1950 compared to one-twentieth of the increase in expenditures in the late 1970s.

From 1950 through the 1970s, a more important factor in expenditure increases has been the change in the nature of the services provided. By the early 1970s, this element accounted for at least half of each year's increase. Furthermore, this factor may be understated relative to price increases due to the way in which consumer prices are measured.

An important aspect of changes in the type or intensity of services is that changes in technology, on balance, tend to be cost-raising rather than cost-saving. Such an assertion says nothing about the cost effectiveness of new technology since the end result may reflect benefits that outweigh the increased cost, benefits that are less than the increased cost, or indeed, no benefits at all.

A study by Scitovsky and McCall (4) of the treatment for several common conditions and the changes in services and associated costs over a 20-year period illustrates the impact in the intensity factor. For example, there has been a steady increase in the average number of diagnostic laboratory tests per case over the 20-year period. Similar results are evident for other procedures such as x-ray films and electrocardiograms (EKGs). On the other hand, hospital lengths of stay declined quite consistently over the 20-year period, offsetting in some cases the increases in intensity. On balance, however, the changes in medical practice tended to be cost-raising rather than cost-saving. It is also not evident that there is a relationship between the decline in hospital lengths of stay and the increase in diagnostic and therapeutic procedures used. Thus, the latter may continue on into the future after the former has reached some apparently irreducible minimum.

Price increases, per se, have accounted for substantial increases in personal health expenditures in recent years. This fact is due in part to increased demand fostered by rising incomes and the greater prevalence of health insurance benefits, but also reflects a catchup phenomenon after the removal of controls under the Economic Stabilization Program of the early 1970s and subsequent higher rates of general inflation in the U.S. economy. Again, as is evident from the increasing proportion of the GNP accounted for by personal health care expenditures, resources devoted to this sector of the economy have outpaced most other items. Price increases are currently the dominant factor in rising expenditures and, as is evident from Table 11-3, have in most years been outpacing price increases for other major items, along with housing and fuel most recently (1, 4).

From the distribution of national health expenditures by type of service over time, it is evident that hospital care, including outpatient hospital services, has been accounting for an increasing share. For example, in 1929 hospital care was responsible for 18% of total expenditures, a figure that had increased to 31% by

TABLE 11-3. Consumer Price Increases, United States, Selected Years[a]

Consumer Price Index (CPI) Item	Percentage Increase for Year						
	1975	1976	1977	1979	1980	1981	1982
CPI, all items	9.1	5.7	6.5	8.5	12.3	12.7	9.5
Medical care services	12.6	10.0	9.9	8.8	10.1	10.8	11.4
Housing	10.8	6.2	7.0	10.9	15.6	15.9	10.9
Fuel, oil and coal	9.6	6.6	13.0	7.6	33.8	23.9	10.4
Apparel and upkeep	4.5	3.7	4.5	3.7	5.0	6.8	4.2

SOURCES: Gibson RM, Fisher CR: National health expenditures, fiscal year 1977. *Soc Secur Bull* 1978; 41(7):10; Waldo DR: *Health Care Financing Trends, Health Care Financing Adm* 1982; 2(5):13.

[a]The data for 1979–1982 are for the year ending in March.

1950, 33% by 1960, 37% by 1970, and stood at 42% for the year ending September 1981. On the other hand, the proportion of expenditures accounted for by physicians' services has been quite stable since 1950, declining slightly from 22.4% in that year to 19.2% in 1982. Most other categories of personal health care expenditures have declined as a proportion of the total, with drugs, eyeglasses, and appliances all accounting for substantially less. The other major category, in addition to hospital care, that has accounted for an increasing proportion of total expenditures is nursing home care. Nursing home costs, which are discussed in Chapter 7, increased from less than 1% of national health expenditures in 1940 to 8.5% of all expenditures in 1982.

As was noted earlier, health care expenses fall unevenly on the population. As would be expected from the discussion of factors affecting use in Chapter 3, age is a major determinant of hospital, nursing home, physician, and other health care expenses. If age 65 is considered as the lower limit for the elderly segment of the population, per capita expenditures for the elderly in 1976 ($1,522), for example, were three times higher than the per capita figure for younger persons. Further, the rate of increase in per capita expenditures for the elderly since the passage of Medicare has been greater than the rate of increase for the remainder of the population by approximately two percentage points (5). Somers points out that the cost experience of federal Medicare and Medicaid health financing programs has been so conspicuously unfavorable, with recent annual increases over 15%, as to have a major impact on other federal programs. She cited Medicare and Medicaid, for example, as being major factors in "the continued postponement of national health insurance for the entire population, [as well as] preventing the extension of benefits to desperately needed long-term care services for the elderly" (5).

The factors responsible for increases in health care expenditures for the elderly are somewhat different than for the remainder of the population. For example, population increases in this age category are far more substantial. In addition, women, who are heavier users of health services than men, are increasing as a proportion of the elderly population. Family social support also seems to be declining, with the result that society can expect "a growing proportion of elderly persons who will be living without the traditional support of either a legal spouse or children" (5). Finally, Somers notes that the use and type of health services, as a component accounting for the increase in expenditures, is also different from the rest of the population. Even with the implementation of Medicare in the mid-1960s, there was no increase in the average number of physician visits per day by the elderly during the following decade, nor was there an increase in the number of days of hospital care per 1,000 older persons. Increases in admission rates were more than offset by a decline in lengths of stay. On the other hand, the services provided within these broader categories of use have changed. For example, surgery rates for the elderly more than doubled over the decade after the implementation of Medicare, and there has been greater use of more complex, and therefore more expensive, medical procedures and other services.

FINANCIAL ARRANGEMENTS AND ECONOMIC RELATIONSHIPS

The health care market has long been recognized as a special case in terms of financial arrangements, economic relationships, and the formulation of public policy. This is not to say that the familiar concepts of economics such as supply and demand, production functions, and so forth are not applicable or useful in analyzing health care financing. Rather, it is an indication that the health care market is a complex one, involving as it does third-party financing (governmental programs and voluntary underwriting), employers who pay a majority of the premiums for their employees, physicians who both provide care and act as the patient's agent in obtaining care, not-for-profit hospitals, assorted regulatory agencies, and so forth. Thus, no simple model will help to explain or predict the behavior of the various participants, nor are there any simple solutions to the various problems found in the health care market.

Patient-Physician Relationships

This section considers financial and other relationships between patients and non-institutional providers. The physician is used as the example throughout the section since the physician is the most prevalent and traditional provider relating to the patient. However, numerous other providers including, for example, dentists and optometrists, have similar relationships with patients, and the discussion applies to them as well.

The patient generally initiates the medical care process, seeking to find out what is causing a physical or mental discomfort and what should be done about it or, less often, simply seeking reassurance or possibly an examination in the absence of symptoms (a general checkup). It is important to recognize that, faced with this initial contact, the physician has tremendous discretion in responding and tremendous control over the subsequent medical care process. Patients cannot order tests, prescribe drugs, or admit themselves to the hospital. The physician, on the other hand, while having substantial discretion within the bounds of professionally acceptable practice, may be limited by knowledge and availability of various services, local practice patterns, specialty orientation, and the professional referral network, including the hospital's medical staff organization (Chapter 6).

Financing is critical in determining the types of services available, the relative emphasis given to primary, secondary, and tertiary patient care, and the combinations of resources the physician uses to achieve various diagnostic or patient management objectives. The physician's role can be considered as consisting of three elements: entrepreneurial, technical, and professional. The entrepreneurial element includes choice of specialty, practice setting, and services to be provided directly by the practice. The technical element includes the physician's personal laying on of hands, and the professional element includes the critical role of acting as the patient's agent. These elements occur to varying degrees, depending on practice setting and the associated economic incentives. For the most part, however, the entrepreneurial element has been a major one, and the range of professionally acceptable options available to independent, fee-for-service physicians acting as the patient's agent has been substantial.

Before the advent of third-party insurance coverage for physicians' services, both the patient and the patient's agent, the physician, were necessarily concerned with the patient's ability and willingness to pay for various options. An analogous situation still exists today for the most part in dentistry, where patients have the choice of more or less expensive types of restoration.

Indeed, the practice of medicine in the days when the patient paid the bill was not unlike dentistry today in the sense that the general practitioner was responsible for delivering most of the services within the context of the practice setting. Medicine has changed, however, so that a great deal of the care that is rendered, particularly expensive care, is likely to be provided by a referral specialist or within an inpatient setting. In the entrepreneurial role, the physician has decided what services will be available within the practice, what patterns of referral will be established, and what other resources will be available (such as particular hospitals). The physician's technical role may be limited to a specialty or subspecialty. Factors associated with both the entrepreneurial and technical roles will impinge upon the decisions made within the context of the professional role where the physician serves as the patient's agent.

In combining resources to serve the needs of any particular patient, the physician may draw on the practice for providing ancillary services such as diagnostic tests, may refer to another physician, typically a specialist, or may hospitalize the patient. In understanding the financing of health services and the economic relationships that exist, it is not sufficient to consider only whether or not the patient has third-party coverage for these various options, although this is important. In addition, the costs to the physician, in the entrepreneurial sense of various choices, must be considered. A physician with a busy practice could manage only a limited number of very sick but potentially ambulatory patients if such management required instructing the family on how to care for the patient, being available for repeated consultation with the family when certain changes in the medical condition occurred, and arranging for the use of other professional services on an ambulatory basis. If, instead, the physician hospitalizes the patient, all of these costly functions are carried out by appropriately trained professionals within the institutional setting. The physician need only be available for daily rounds and occasional consultation, and has only to order procedures and consultations available within the hospital through a note in the medical record. The point of this discussion is that the physician can handle a larger and more complex patient load through increased use of the hospital. Thus, there are both professional and economic incentives to hospitalize; these incentives are especially strong since the physician does not have to pay for this service out of practice income either directly or indirectly because of the subsidization of hospitalization by third parties. This discussion assumes financing under a fee-for-service system, as well as an independent office practice. There are a number of mechanisms for reimbursing the physician, some of which introduce other types of incentives.

Physician Reimbursement

There are three principal mechanisms for paying for physicians' services. The first, which is the predominant method, is fee-for-service. Under this system, the physician is reimbursed for each procedure or service. Services can be small and discrete, such as a follow-up visit, a laboratory test, or the reading of an EKG; or they can be substantial and inclusive, such as a comprehensive fee for normal delivery or for a major surgical procedure, which would include prenatal or preoperative care, the procedure itself, and follow-up care. Relative value scales have been developed to reflect the relationship between procedures in terms of the time and skill required to provide services.

One problem with fee-for-service is the definition of a particular service and what is included in it. The more general issue, however, is the incentive inherent in the fee-for-service approach. The physician's income depends upon the volume of services provided and the price of those services. Obviously, more services result in a higher income, as would the provision of more complex and therefore expensive services. In particular, technical procedures tend to be weighted more heavily, given the amount of time it takes to perform them, than physician time when the physician is providing patient counseling, consulting, or a history and physical examination, as noted in Chapter 9.

A second mechanism for reimbursing physicians is capitation. Capitation involves paying the physician a fixed amount per person per unit of time without regard to the volume of services provided. Thus, a physician may agree to take responsibility for a group of patients, called a *panel*, for a month or a year, and would agree to provide to those patients whatever was necessary within a previously agreed range of services (for example, primary care). The capitation method assumes that the physician is qualified to provide the agreed upon services and will be available to do so. Since the physician's income is determined by the number of individuals in the panel, rather than the number of services provided, there is an incentive to maximize the number of patients in the panel and to minimize the number of services provided to each patient. This method assumes an organization serving as a third party (the National Health Service in England and Wales, for example). The third party can limit panel size, and can use various mechanisms to monitor the volume and mix of services being rendered. In addition, under such a system the patient would typically have a choice of physicians and the opportunity to switch should there be concern about underprovision of care or any other unattractive facet of the doctor's practice.

The third method for reimbursement of physicians is salary, or payment per unit of time. As in other sectors of the economy, salary is used only in organized settings where various other mechanisms are employed to assess or encourage the type of care given and the level of productivity.

Each of the three methods has been described in terms of compensation for the individual practitioner. Fee-for-service and capitation reimbursement can also be used for groups of physicians. For example, under the capitation method, a multispecialty group with broad responsibility for virtually all types of patient care can be paid on the basis of the number of persons enrolled with the group. The implicit incentives that apply to the individual practitioner can also be attributed to the group. However, payment of individual physicians by the group might be arranged on a salary or some other basis. Various related aspects of group practice are discussed further in Chapter 5.

Hospital Reimbursement Mechanisms

Next, let us consider hospitals and their relationships to both physicians and third parties. The community general hospital, which accounts for the largest segment of the resources used for inpatient care in the United States, is the focus of this discussion. Other types of hospitals are discussed further in Chapter 6.

Community hospitals offer a wide range of services, with the degree of technological complexity being largely a function of the composition of the hospital's medical staff. The typical hospital's objectives include providing as broad a range of services as can be supported by the community and to the largest feasible population. One way of achieving these objectives is through maximization of the quality of care as perceived by both physicians and prospective patients. Hospitals compete for patients indirectly by competing for physicians. Physicians, in turn, are attracted to hospitals by the status of members of the medical staff, the availability of those services needed in support of the physician's practice—in economic parlance, the production function—and the ease of access to hospital services for the physician's patients.

These characteristics are not remarkable in themselves. It is only when they are coupled with third-party reimbursement that the system strays from a self-correcting economic model. In 1975, 80% of consumer expenditures for hospital care were paid through voluntary hospital insurance. All third-party payments, including those by government, to all kinds of hospitals in the same year added up to 94.8% of total expenditures for hospitals (6). Although precise data are not readily available, it is estimated that third parties accounted for more than 90% of the revenue derived by community general hospitals. The effective price facing many patients at the time services are delivered is a small fraction of the price charged by the hospital for the service. The difference, of course, is financed through the various third-party mechanisms, both voluntary and governmental.

Like physicians, hospitals can be reimbursed through a variety of mechanisms. The first, which is analogous to fee-for-service, is reimbursement for specific services. A related method is reimbursement on a per-case basis. Hospitals can also be reimbursed using the capitation method, under which the institution receives a fixed amount for each enrolled patient. A fourth approach is to reimburse the hospital a proportion of its budget, with the shares for which various third parties are responsible being determined by the amount that their enrollees use the hospital in a given year. Finally, the hospital may be reimbursed on the basis of a day of care. That is, the third party pays an amount for each day that one of its enrollees is hospitalized.

With the exception of payment for specific services, all of these methods assume a formal relationship between the hospital and a third party, whether it be the state or federal government or a voluntary underwriter. Payment for specific services, on the other hand, is simply based on the hospital's charges. These charges may be inclusive, as for the daily service charge (for bed, board, and nursing services); or for the use of special facilities such as the operating room (usually on a per-minute basis after a minimum charge); or on an item-by-item basis, as for laboratory and radiology procedures. Increasingly, hospital charges are directly related to the unit cost of producing the service. Where they are not, some of the revenue generated from one source may possibly subsidize other services. In addition to cross-subsidization, financial requirements of the institution generally require that charges include an amount for future growth and development. Considering all methods of payment, operating margins, or the difference between revenues and expenses, for community hospitals have been approximately 3 to 4% in recent years.

In some states, the schedule of charges established by hospitals is subject to approval by a state rate commission. Almost by definition, charges are established on a prospective basis and are derived from the anticipated budget of the hospital. Rate review mechanisms, therefore, generally deal with the reasonableness of the proposed budget, including the projected cost of various services, the volume of use anticipated, and particularly the growth and development factor that arises from a projected positive operating margin.

Since each hospital charges for hundreds of different services, it is not feasible to determine the reasonableness of all charges. On the other hand, there are advantages to using charges for specific services as the basis for paying hospitals. First, it seems most equitable to determine the payment from each patient on the basis of those services actually used. This system is in contrast to approaches that will be described below, which tend to average payments across patients. Second, charges are a system well understood by the consumer since this is the approach used throughout the economy for most goods and services. Third, it is possible to introduce copayments, where the patient has responsibility for a fraction of the charge, into the insurance system for those services for which patient or physician cost consciousness is considered particularly important. Finally, if a uniform system of charges were developed, it would enhance the buyer's ability to compare hospitals on the basis of price, whether the buyer was a patient, a voluntary underwriter, or a government.

All community general hospitals use charges as one method of obtaining payment. Patients with commercial insurance coverage, some Blue Cross patients, and others who are responsible for part or all of their bill (e.g., for days that are not covered by a third party) are charged on this basis. By far the most important source of revenue to hospitals, however, has been the per diem system of reimbursement by which the hospital is paid for each day that a patient is in the hospital without regard to the particular service used. Most Blue Cross enrollees are in plans that have used per diem reimbursement for many years. When Medicare and Medicaid were adopted in the mid-1960s, these governmental programs adopted the Blue Cross approach to per diem hospital reimbursement. The trend for Blue Cross, however, is toward payment based on charges. In 1981, 59% of plan contracts, representing 40% of Blue Cross enrollees nationwide, had payment schedules based on full charges (42%) or a percentage of charges (17%) (7). Further, the Medicare program changed to per case reimbursement in 1983.

Per diem reimbursement as used by Blue Cross and government has been based on retrospectively determined costs. The approach is to determine the hospital's total cost of delivering patient care for a year, and then to divide this amount by the total number of patient days of care rendered by the hospital during the same period. The resulting cost per day (per diem) then becomes the amount to which the hospital is entitled for each day of care rendered to a particular third party's enrollees. For example, if a hospital's total costs were $35 million, and it had delivered 100,000 days of patient care in the course of the year, the resulting per diem costs would be $350. Thus, for each day that a Blue Cross or Medicare patient was in the hospital, the hospital could expect to receive this amount. In actual use, however, this method is far more complex.

Traditional per diem cost reimbursement, as noted above, is retrospective. The actual periodic payments to hospitals by third parties are generally based on some interim estimate of per diem costs, since these are not known until the end of the period. This payment may be calculated as a function of charges, the previous year's per diem costs plus a factor for inflation, or some similar approach. It is important to reemphasize, however, that after a year-end adjustment, the hospital will ultimately be paid its actual allowable per diem costs under this mechanism.

Two major issues that have accompanied per diem cost reimbursement over the years are the definition of allowable costs and equity between classes of patients. The issue of which hospital costs should be subject to per diem reimbursement has been debated for decades. Accommodations were reached between hospitals and Blue Cross plans in a number of areas. For example, when costs are incurred in nonpatient care areas where other sources of revenue are collected (e.g., gift shops and cafeterias), costs would be determined after deducting such revenue. In the patient care areas, teaching costs are considered allowable on the grounds that teaching improves the quality of patient care. Research costs, however, are generally not allowable because they may benefit patients ultimately but are not of direct benefit to a patient in the hospital at the time the research is conducted. Depreciation is allowed, usually on the historical cost basis. Bad debts are generally not allowed on the theory that cost reimbursement obviates bad debts for those patients subject to it. An exception is bad debts incurred in relation to deductibles and copayments associated with Medicare.

More generally, the Social Security Administration, in developing the regulations for implementation of the Medicare law, followed the traditional Blue Cross pattern by and large in determining reasonable costs. Notable exceptions were the policy followed with respect to equity among classes of patients and that part of hospitals' financial requirements needed for growth and development.

Hospital Reimbursement, Equity, and Hospital Growth

Blue Cross plans over the years have endeavored to enroll a broad cross section of the community; further, these plans historically have been in close alliance with hospitals. Thus, in developing cost reimbursement arrangements, Blue Cross assumed that its subscribers reflected the mix of all patients who were hospitalized. Consequently, Blue Cross reimbursed hospitals an average amount per day, without regard to the particular services, or their costs, employed on behalf of their subscribers.

The adaptation of per diem cost reimbursement under Medicare did not follow this line of reasoning. Because the program was originally intended only for those persons age 65 and over, certain costs were disallowed outright, such as for maternity and pediatrics. More consequentially, however, it was asserted by the Social Security Administration that because of the extended lengths of stay experienced by this population, the per diem cost for ancillary services, which tend to be concentrated in the earlier days of the hospital stay, should be lower on average than for those under age 65. Consequently, hospitals were reimbursed for ancillary service costs in proportion to the ratio of ancillary service charges for the elderly to ancillary service charges for those under age 65.

Hospitals argued that while ancillary service costs might be lower for the elderly on a per diem basis, nursing costs were higher. After several cost studies and some years, the Social Security Administration recognized the nursing differential. The point of this discussion is not to go into the details of cost reimbursement formulas, but rather to point out the difference between a per diem system that assumes that the patients of a particular third party are representative of all patients, versus one that recognizes in advance that its enrollees, or prospective patients, may be less expensive than average. Carried to its logical conclusion, the latter approach would result in reimbursement based on actual costs incurred by each patient, which is similar to a system based on charges that are directly related to units costs.

The issues of allowable costs and equity both come into play in considering the growth and development factor that is allowed hospitals. Blue Cross plans have typically included a plus factor in per diem reimbursement. This factor has ranged from 2 to 8% depending on the Blue Cross plan. The Social Security Administration included a 2% plus factor in its original formulation, but this charge was discontinued early in the Nixon administration. The plus factor is intended to recognize hospitals' financial requirements, and particularly the need for internally generated capital funds. On the other hand, it has been argued that the planning and development of community resources should not be tied to a particular hospital's ability to generate funds from depreciation, a plus factor, or a surplus from other sources. Some of the reservations that have been expressed about the growth and development factor relate more broadly to the incentives inherent in cost-plus reimbursement. In recent years, these concerns have led to a shift toward experimentation with prospective reimbursement.

Prospective Hospital Reimbursement

One approach to prospective rate setting has been discussed: reimbursement of hospitals on the basis of charges subject to prior approval. Such a system has been in operation in Indiana for more than 20 years under agreements between hospitals and Blue Cross. More recently, this approach has been adopted by several states using state rate commissions. The other major approach to prospective reimbursement is a modification of per diem cost reimbursement.

Prospective cost reimbursement differs from retrospective cost reimbursement in that the per diem amount is established before the beginning of a year (and thus before the hospital's actual costs are known), rather than being adjusted to reflect the actual costs incurred for the previous year. Under prospective per diem reimbursement, if a hospital's actual costs exceed its approved costs, the hospital would suffer a loss. Thus, there is an incentive for the hospital to keep its cost at or below the approved level. This situation is in sharp contrast to retrospective per diem cost reimbursement, under which the hospital receives payment for whatever costs it incurs, and therefore is not subject to a loss should costs be higher than anticipated. With a plus factor, the hospital may actually benefit from higher costs. This benefit would carry forward to future years since the hospital would be starting from a higher cost base.

Under prospective per diem cost reimbursement, however, the incentives for keeping costs below the approved level are weak. Even though the hospital may keep the difference between revenues derived from the prospectively approved per diem rate and the actual per diem costs, the institution has merely deferred expenditures to future years by carrying forward a surplus. In the process, the hospital risks obtaining a lower approved rate for future years by virtue of its lower base costs for the following period.

There are several approaches to establishing the prospective per diem rate. The two most common approaches, however, are based on a formula or on individual hospital-negotiated budgets. In the former, the rate-setting agency, whether it be a voluntary prepayment plan such as Blue Cross or a state rate setting authority, would establish a formula that provides the basis for determining the percentage increase in per diem costs that will be allowed for the following period. The starting point is generally the hospital's per diem cost for the preceding period, adjusted upward for input cost increases of various types including labor costs, services, supplies, and so forth. The overall increase would generally be subject to a ceiling established for each category of hospital. The categories might be based on hospital size, for example. With a strict exception policy, this approach seems to have the greatest potential for holding down the rate of increase in hospital costs. On the other hand, because it starts with the hospital's current per diem costs, it does not necessarily reward the more efficient hospital, and as noted above, there is some incentive to incur costs up to the allowed level. Further, since the unit of service is a day of care, there is an incentive for hospitals to place less pressure on the medical staff for reduced lengths of stay or, alternatively, to allow lengths of stay to increase somewhat in order to generate higher total revenues for the year. This tendency may offset savings that would otherwise accrue from a tight policy of allowable percentage increases in per diem costs. The rate-setting agency must also consider the financial viability of the institutions whose costs it is attempting to regulate.

The other extreme is the approach that considers each hospital's budget individually. It would probably be more difficult for a rate-setting agency to reduce the rate of increase in per diem costs under this system. Instead of a rather mechanistic formula under which few exceptions are allowed, the third party or state regulator must consider the particular circumstances and financial viability of each institution. Hospitals can make persuasive cases in terms of their financial requirements for the coming period, and these may be difficult to ignore or refute in the rate-setting process. The approach is also more difficult to administer since it involves individual consideration of large numbers of hospitals. On the other hand, this approach has the advantage of recognizing legitimate differences in hospitals, and particularly year-to-year changes in growth, case mix, and so forth. Standards are developed to determine the reasonableness of those elements of cost that comprise each hospital's projected budget. There is a tendency toward uniform measurement of hospital costs and services, and considerable effort is being directed toward grouping of hospitals, which may make the budget review process the more constructive approach in the long run.

The approaches to prospective rate setting described above are based on hospital costs. Some have argued that the connection between historical costs and prospective rates should be broken for purposes of establishing a cost containment strategy. An alternative approach would be to place limits on allowable increases in hospital revenue without regard to costs. The hospital would then have to manage its resources so as to operate within such revenue caps. The obvious drawback to this approach is its potentially arbitrary nature, especially if hospitals' operating situations are not considered. That is, for a reasonable system to be implemented, some account must be taken of the hospital's current and anticipated situation with respect to costs and volume of service. A cap on the percentage increase allowed for total revenues of an institution for a year, for example, would institutionalize existing differences between hospitals and not allow for the dynamic nature of hospital growth and development or, alternatively, of attrition.

Another approach is to regulate or determine the revenue that could be generated on a per-case basis, with differentiation across types of admissions by diagnostic category. The incentives in such a system are desirable in terms of cost containment behavior by hospitals with respect to both resource use and length of stay. However, this approach introduces incentives to increase admissions and to modify case mix.

The Social Security amendments enacted in 1983 included a change in Medicare reimbursement to a prospective per case payment system. The price per case now depends on the Diagnosis Related Group (DRG) into which the case falls. The amendments called for a phasing in of the DRG system over a four-year period. As the phase-in progresses, less weight is given to the individual hospital's actual cost-per-case and more weight is given to a national average price for each DRG.

The prospective payment system based on DRGs was not intended, at least initially, to reimburse all hospital costs. For example, capital expenses—depreciation, interest, and lease expenses—are paid on a cost basis, as are expenses of approved education programs. It is also recognized that some fraction of patients don't fit the diagnostic group to which the system assigns them. A provision is made for about five percent of socalled "outliers" for whom the hospital may request additional payment. Finally, provision is made for inflation using a hospital market basket approach and a plus factor for new technology.

In summary, hospital reimbursement as it has been developed over several decades has led to a heavy emphasis on cost-plus reimbursement, which in turn has enabled, and indeed encouraged, the diffusion of technology, the elaboration of hospital services, and an increase in the amenity level in most institutions. Since hospitals compete for physicians, and indirectly for patients, and seem to have as their objective to provide a wide range of services to the broadest possible segment of the community, it is not surprising that expenditures have increased. At the same time, attempts to deal with hospital financing through prospective rate setting are subject to many theoretical and practical difficulties. Some have argued that with economic incentives as strong as they are for hospitals to elaborate their services under the current arrangement, some more comprehensive set of incentives that tie together the interests of underwriters, physicians, and hospitals is the most feasible and desirable approach to containing health service costs. An emerging consensus, however, that prospective reimbursement is the most appropriate next step, at least for governmental reimbursement of hospitals, has led to adoption of this approach using the case or discharge as the unit of service. In the absence of fundamental changes in the health services system, the relationship between hospitals and governmental and voluntary insurers will continue to be of considerable importance.

Hospital and Nongovernmental Insurance Relationships

As will be discussed further below, voluntary health insurance underwriters have been very successful in enrolling a high proportion of employed persons and their dependents, with in-depth coverage of expensive episodes of illness, and in competing in an insurance market characterized by very sophisticated group coverage buyers or their brokers. Voluntary third parties have assumed the social responsibility of improving access to care by removing financial barriers for much of the population and by spreading the risk of high family health expenditures.

At the same time, commercial carriers and nonprofit prepayment plans such as Blue Cross have not played a major role in controlling the rise in hospital costs. No control function was originally intended by either the commercial carriers or Blue Cross, however, and under current arrangements little control is likely to exist in the absence of regulatory intervention. This situation is the result of the current relationships between underwriters and providers, existing incentives, and the historical development of these relationships.

There are two fundamental approaches to voluntary underwriting: indemnification and service benefits. Indemnification is the approach employed by commercial insurance companies for health insurance as well as a wide range of casualty coverages. With the indemnity approach, a contractual relationship is established between the company and the insured under which the insured agrees to pay a premium and the company, for its part, agrees to pay the insured a cash benefit in the event of a loss. For example, the insured may receive a certain dollar amount for each day of hospitalization as a result of an accident or covered illness, plus an additional amount equal to the charges for various ancillary services used during the stay in the hospital, up to some limit.

The service benefit approach, on the other hand, guarantees the insured individual, usually referred to as a *subscriber* or a *member*, services when needed in return for the premium, rather than a cash amount. For example, under a Blue Cross service benefit agreement the subscriber would be assured needed hospital services in the event of an accident or covered illness.

Under indemnity arrangements, the only contractual relationship is between the insurance company and the insured. With service benefits, the underwriter must have some way of arranging for the delivery of services in order to fulfill its contractual obligation to the subscriber. Thus, the third party with a service benefit must either contract for services or provide services directly. In the case of Blue Cross plans, the third party has agreements with member hospitals, usually including all community general hospitals in its service area. The hospitals agree to care for Blue Cross enrollees, accepting reimbursement as payment in full with the exception of copayments and exclusions, while the Blue Cross plan agrees to reimburse the hospital on an agreed-upon basis. Another example of a service benefit would be that provided by a Health Maintenance Organization that may own and operate its own hospital, may have a close affiliation with a community hospital, or may engage in contractual relationships with several hospitals.

The commercial underwriter's liability is limited to the dollar amount agreed to in the indemnity arrangement, and the patient is responsible for any additional amounts charged by the hospital. For these reasons and the absence of a contractual relationship between the insurance company and the institution, there is no reason to expect cost control behavior by insurance companies. Blue Cross plans might be in a better position to influence hospital costs, and several voluntary efforts have been undertaken. However, in many parts of the country there is a balance of power between Blue Cross plans and the hospitals since the Blue Cross plan must have hospital members to offer a service benefit, while the hospitals enjoy favorable reimbursement arrangements with Blue Cross. Although the relationship is weaker today than it once was, hospitals and Blue Cross plans in many areas view themselves as closely allied. At the same time, Blue Cross plans must compete in the insurance market and therefore feel the impact of hospital cost increases directly in establishing premiums for the following year. In many states, insurance commissioners have put pressure on Blue Cross at the time premium increases are up for approval, but in most cases these efforts have had little long term impact.

Another approach to the relationship between hospitals and third parties is to consider the market objectives of the third parties themselves. A common objective is the maximization of enrollments or market share, which is particularly true of nonprofit third parties such as Blue Cross. As hospital costs increase, the utility of having third-party coverage to protect against such costs also increases. Thus, rising hospital costs enable the third party to pursue its objective of increased enrollments and comprehensiveness of coverage, while at the same time supporting hospitals in their pursuit of greater quantity and quality of services. Thus, by financing hospital cost increases, Blue Cross increases the "potential negative impact on the consumers' wealth positions and thereby expands enrollments and coverage" (8:221). Also, to the degree that governmental programs such as Medicare reimburse hospitals for less than their full costs, these costs are likely to be passed on in the form of higher charges or reimbursement to those not covered by the governmental programs. This phenomenon is called *cost shifting*. The same insurance effect then results since the increased cost of hospitalization encourages additional insurance coverage because the expected loss to the prospective hospital patient is increased. These and other factors have been responsible for dramatic increases in insurance coverage for health services.

HEALTH INSURANCE COVERAGE IN THE UNITED STATES

In this section health care financing is considered from the consumer's perspective. What are the options available in terms of third-party insurance coverage from either private underwriters or government programs, how do they market or otherwise make coverage available, and what kinds of benefit structures are typical?

Development of Health Insurance Coverage

Third-party coverage for health care costs is a phenomenon largely of the last 40 years in this country. In 1940, for example, less than 10% of the population had coverage for inpatient care, and a negligible portion had coverage for any other type of health service. By 1979, almost four out of every five Americans under the age of 65 had private health insurance for inpatient services provided by both hospitals and physicians, 65% had some type of coverage for out-of-hospital physician visits, and the proportion with coverage for dental care was three out of 10 (Table 11-4) (9).

Virtually the entire population age 65 and over is covered under Medicare, with hospital benefits (Part A) protecting 98% and medical benefits covering 97% of the elderly. Further, more than three out of five persons over 65 have some form of private supplementary coverage, in addition to Medicare, for hospital services. An estimated 11% of the population under age 65 received benefits from the Medicaid program during 1976, and an additional 1% were covered under that portion of the Medicare program designed for the disabled under age 65. In contrast, census estimates (10) and a national survey supported by foundation sources (11) indicate that 12 to 13% of the U.S. population under age 65 have no insurance coverage at all.

In the early years of this century, it was not generally believed by those in the insurance industry that health care, particularly for illnesses, as distinct from accidents, was an insurable risk. To indemnify against a loss, the event causing the loss would ordinarily be expected to be clearly definable, undesirable from the point of view of the insured, and unpredictable on an individual basis but predictable, in the actuarial sense, for a group of individuals or for the entire population. Until the emergence of the twentieth-century hospital (Chapter 6), care for illness did not fit this definition. Although there were numerous experiments in the first quarter of this century to spread the risk of financial loss due to illness, there were no large scale efforts.

During the late 1920s, a comprehensive study of various facets of health care organization and financing under the aegis of the Committee on the Costs of Medical Care (12) demonstrated the degree to which a relatively small fraction of the population in any given year bore a substantial fraction of the costs of medical care. The hospital had emerged as the most appropriate setting for the treatment of serious illness for all socioeconomic classes, but had also resulted in substantial increases in health costs per episode of illness.

Rising health costs and the financial impact on families of the Great Depression led to the specter of potential debt for families with a member requiring hospitaliza-

TABLE 11-4. Estimates of Net Number of Different Persons Under Private Health Insurance Plans and Percent of Population Covered, by Age and Specified Type of Care, as of December 31, 1979

	All Ages		Under Age 65		Aged 65 and Over	
Type of Service	Number (in Thousands)	Percent of Civilian Population[a]	Number (in Thousands)	Percent of Civilian Population[b]	Number (in Thousands)	Percent of Civilian Population[c]
Hospital care	170,791	77.8	154,790	79.5	16,001	64.1
Physicians' services						
Surgical services	165,090	75.2	154,407	79.3	10,683	42.8
In-hospital visits	167,559	76.3	156,578	80.4	10,981	44.0
X-ray and laboratory						
examinations	166,374	75.8	155,774	80.0	10,600	42.4
Office and home visits	133,351	60.7	126,735	65.1	6,616	26.5
Dental care	60,269	27.4	58,747	30.2	1,522	6.1
Prescribed drugs						
(out-of-hospital)	131,237	59.8	126,865	65.2	4,372	17.5
Private-duty nursing	126,934	57.8	123,405	63.4	3,529	14.1
Visiting nurse service	161,082	73.3	152,671	78.4	8,411	33.7
Nursing-home care	97,632	44.4	85,698	44.0	11,934	47.8

SOURCE: Carroll, MS, Arnett RH: Private health insurance plans in 1978 and 1979: A review of coverage, enrollment, and financial experience. *Health Care Financing Rev* 1981; 3(1):55–87.

[a]Based on a Bureau of Census estimate of 219,625,000 as of January 1, 1980.

[b]Based on a Bureau of Census estimate of 194,648,000 as of January 1, 1980.

[c]Based on a Bureau of Census estimate of 24,977,000 as of January 1, 1980.

tion and very real financial difficulties for community general hospitals. These hospitals were increasingly dependent upon income generated from charges to private patients. The combination of a definable event such as medical or surgical inpatient treatment, the recognition of the need to spread financial risk across the community, and the need of institutions for a more reliable source of revenue led to hospital prepayment, which ultimately became the Blue Cross system. Blue Cross plans grew relatively slowly during the 1930s, although they were widely recognized as an important social movement.

The two objectives of providing a stronger financial base for community hospitals and spreading the risk of economic loss from hospitalization were viewed as being socially worthwhile. Also, the service benefit relationship between the third party and the hospital was markedly different from customary commercial indemnity insurance. As a result of these factors, special enabling legislation was passed in many states to encourage the development of Blue Cross on a nonprofit, tax-free basis, with exemption from the usual requirements of commercial insurance underwriters. Blue Shield plans, organized by the medical profession, also were developing during this period. However, the paid-in-full service benefit arrangement never took hold for physicians' coverage, with the exception of plans on the West Coast that were established to protect physicians and their patients from "contract practice," under which a particular physician or physician group would serve as the exclusive provider for an employer's workers.

During the 1940s and early 1950s, major growth occurred in both hospital coverage and inpatient medical-surgical coverage. Also during this period, the original social objectives of the Blue Cross system were undermined by the more conventional practices of commercial insurers.

Blue Cross plans originally spread the risk of loss across all segments of the community. This objective was accomplished by establishing a premium that was essentially the same regardless of the potential subscriber's degree of risk. The premium rate was the same whether an individual or a group of individuals was young and healthy or older and at greater risk. This approach was in sharp contrast to underwriting practices traditionally used by commercial carriers, who attempt to estimate the claims that will be experienced by a group and establish a premium rate accordingly. The common rate approach, used originally by Blue Cross, is referred to as *community rating* and the commercial insurance approach as *experience rating*.

As Blue Cross began to develop coverage for employee groups, and as this form of fringe benefit became increasingly popular during the 1940s, commercial insurance companies were able to penetrate the market by selectively offering equal or improved benefits for lower premiums by selling to groups that were of below-average risk. To the degree that more favorable groups obtained coverage from commercial underwriters, the remaining market was at greater risk and therefore the Blue Cross premium would necessarily be higher. As a consequence, Blue Cross plans eventually abandoned community rating, except in the case of small employers and individual coverage, and began to compete with commercial underwriters using experience rating. One consequence of this natural evolution of market forces was that neither Blue Cross and Blue Shield plans, nor commercial underwriters, were able to provide coverage in an economical fashion to two very important high-risk segments of the population: the aged, who were at high risk and had left the labor force, and the poor, who tended to be at higher risk and were typically not members of stable employee groups. This situation led to the passage of two federal programs, Medicare and Medicaid.

The competition for new enrollees between the prepayment plans (Blue Cross/ Blue Shield) and commercial underwriters was particularly vigorous during the 1940s and 1950s. A major impetus for the rapid growth of voluntary health insurance was its increasing popularity as a fringe benefit, with at least partial contributions by the employer. During World War II and the wage and price control years that followed, health insurance was recognized as a negotiable item under collective bargaining agreements and, furthermore, one that was exempt from controls. Thus, both industry and labor found it an attractive component of employee compensation.

Over the years, through collective bargaining or simply competition in the labor market, health insurance plans have changed in two respects. First, an increasing number of benefits have been added to plans, while existing benefits have been improved in the sense that the plan pays for a higher proportion of expenses incurred. Second, an increasing proportion of all employers pay part or all of the premium for their employees and, concomitantly, an increasing proportion of all premiums are paid for by employers. For example, of the almost 500 group health insurance plans for groups of 100 or more employees that took effect during the first 3 months of 1977, all but 6% were paid for entirely by the employers (39%) or involved contributions by both the employee and the employer (55%). It is estimated that more than 70% of all premium expenses for group insurance are paid for by employers.

In addition to group insurance available through Blue Cross/Blue Shield and commercial insurance companies, there is also coverage in the form of individual health insurance policies. These policies vary widely in the quality of the coverage and tend to be costly to administer. Further, since the individual who purchases a health insurance policy is not receiving coverage as a member of a group constituted for a purpose other than acquiring health insurance (employee group), which may be of lower than average risk, the claims experience for individual policy holders is usually less favorable. That is, an individual unable to obtain insurance through a group related to employment status or some other nonhealth-related status, such as being a student, would be more likely to apply for insurance if he or she anticipated illness. The same phenomenon may occur in the process of employment, but then the effect would be swamped or "averaged out" by the large number of people in an employed group.

Voluntary Health Insurance Plan Administration

Health insurance premiums vary tremendously, in large part because of the wide variations in benefit structure and in the composition of groups that buy the insurance. In addition, however, operating expenses (and profits) range from a relatively low proportion of the total premium to as much as one-half or more. Table 11-5 shows the operating expenses experienced by different categories of underwriters, and for commercial insurance companies by type of policy, for the years 1970, 1975, and 1980. These percentages have changed relatively little in recent years.

The operating expense of Blue Cross, (approximately 5% nationally), and of the independent plans have consistently been the lowest. By far the highest operating expense is associated with individual policies marketed by commercial insurance companies. While Blue Cross and the independent plans have much lower than average operating expenses, the reasons are somewhat different. What these organizations have in common is that they offer service benefits and therefore, as dis-

TABLE 11-5. Operating Expense as a Proportion of Premium
Income, 1970–1980

Type of Plan	1970	1975	1980
Blue Cross/Blue Shield, total[a]	7.2	7.4	7.4
Insurance companies, total	20.4	18.8	21.7
Group policies	12.8	12.7	16.3
Individual policies	46.6	46.1	43.7
Independent plans, total	7.7	7.5	NA[b]
Community	7.2	6.6	NA
Employer-employee-union	7.7	6.7	NA

SOURCE: Mueller MS: Private health insurance in 1975: Coverage, enrollment, and financial experience. *Soc Secur Bull* 1977; 40(6):18; Carroll MS:
Private health insurance plans in 1976: An evaluation. *Soc Secur Bull*
1978; 41(9):14; for 1980, private communication with Marjorie Smith Carroll, Office of Research, Demonstrations and Statistics, Health Care
Financing Administration.
[a]Data are adjusted for duplication.
[b]NA = not available.

cussed earlier, necessarily have a contractual relationship with providers. Thus, the
administrative expense associated with reimbursement is often lower. For example,
cost reimbursement under Blue Cross is administratively easier than reimbursement on the basis of itemized bills for a multitude of different providers. Similarly,
independent plans have well-established payment mechanisms developed for
member providers, some of which may be as straightforward to administer as paying
annual salaries.

Another important factor, however, involves the size of the average claim. It is
less expensive to administer a smaller number of large claims, as for hospital coverage, than a larger number of small claims, as for fee-for-service physician coverage.
Thus, Blue Cross, which primarily covers hospital services, has the lowest operating expense, while the independent plans, which tend to be more comprehensive
in coverage, have somewhat higher expenses as a proportion of the premium.

The group policies of insurance companies tend to have higher administrative
costs than Blue Cross/Blue Shield or the independent plans because they are
heterogeneous, organizationally have a wider range of providers to pay, do not have
established relationships with those providers, and offer more complex and often
more limited coverage. The individual policies sold by commercial insurance companies have operating expenses, and profits, that average 44 cents for every dollar of
premium collected.

In addition to the administrative costs associated with indemnity coverage,
commercial insurance companies have much higher selling and administrative expenses, including the cost of premium collections. In the group situation, health
insurance is offered through an employer, thus enabling the underwriter to reach a
relatively large number of subscribers through a single or master contract. In contrast, individual policies must be sold on a one-to-one basis. Further, the premiums
for group policies are usually collected by the union or employer and paid to the
insurance company in a lump sum. In contrast, insurance companies must collect
directly for the premiums on individual policies. Finally, keeping track of eligible
insureds is complicated in the individual policy case and is the responsibility of the
underwriter. By comparison, in the case of group policies, the employer advises

the underwriter, typically each month, of additions and deletions with respect to eligibility.

Benefit Structure of Health Insurance Plans

Plans may range from very limited individual coverage, such as indemnity of $60 per day for hospitalization as a result of an accident, to very comprehensive coverage, such as paid-in-full service benefits for all inpatient and outpatient services with few exclusions or limitations. The development of health insurance began with the identification of hospitalization as a definable and insurable risk. Medical-surgical benefits were the next to develop; these benefits usually included coverage for inpatient physician services, most notably surgeons' fees.

During the late 1950s, major medical insurance began to develop quite rapidly. This coverage paid for a wide range of medical services including hospital care, both inpatient and outpatient physician services, drugs, appliances, ambulance services, and so forth. Major medical insurance, however, included a deductible and coinsurance as well as an upper limit. The *deductible* is an amount to be paid by the insured before coverage takes effect. *Coinsurance* refers to a portion of the total expense that is expected to be borne by the insured. At present a common major medical policy would have a deductible of between $150 and $250, 20% coinsurance, and a maximum ranging from $100,000 to $250,000.

Basic hospital and medical-surgical coverage is often complemented by a major medical policy. Such a policy superimposed on a basic plan would generally have a much lower or possibly no deductible. Thus, the combination of plans would lead to payment in full for hospital confinements and physicians' services in the hospital, perhaps up to some limit under the basic plan, fairly substantial coverage for care in the hospital beyond such limits, and partial coverage for other medical services not included in the basic plan.

Another approach that has become increasingly prevalent in recent years is a comprehensive coverage that directly combines the basic and major medical plans. Under this benefit structure, most services are paid at 80 to 90% of reasonable charges after a fairly low deductible, such as $50 to $100 per year. Comprehensive plans often pay 100% after an out-of-pocket expense limit, such as $200 or $300 per year, has been reached by the insured. Certain types of benefits, such as psychiatric or dental coverages, may be subject to additional deductibles, coinsurance, or limits. For example, the psychiatric benefit may limit outpatient visits to a specified number of visits per year or to a dollar ceiling such as $1,000. At the same time, there may be a coinsurance of 50%. Similarly, dental care may be paid-in-full for preventive services up to two visits per year but have a 50% coinsurance feature for restorative care and limited provision for orthodontics.

The important point is that there are virtually an infinite variety of benefit packages. As noted earlier, the trend in recent years has been toward fuller coverage of traditional hospital and physician services, as well as the addition of new benefits. New benefits tend to be initiated with relatively conservative provisions, including coinsurance and limits. As experience accumulates, these benefits may then be broadened or deepened. A summary measure of the depth of coverage for various types of care is reflected in Table 11-6, which presents the proportion of consumer expenditures paid for through private insurance since 1950.

In 1950, only 12% of such expenditures were financed through private insurance. Almost all of the insurance payments were devoted to inpatient hospital and

TABLE 11-6. Proportion of Consumer Expenditures Met by Health Insurance, 1950–1979

Year	Total	Hospital Care	Physicians' Services	Prescribed Drugs	Dental Care (Out-of-Hospital)	Other Types of Care
1950	12.2	37.1	12.0	NA[a]	NA	NA
1960	27.8	64.7	30.0	NA	NA	5.0
1965	32.1	70.9	34.0	2.6	1.5	3.1
1970	37.5	78.2	42.9	4.1	5.4	4.9
1971	38.4	79.6	42.6	4.7	5.9	5.2
1972	38.1	75.8	45.0	4.9	6.2	5.3
1973	38.1	73.8	45.5	5.5	7.0	5.8
1974	40.2	76.2	49.4	6.1	8.1	6.1
1975	43.6	81.3	50.9	6.8	13.0	5.6
1976	45.2	81.3	52.7	8.0	17.7	5.6
1977	45.1	79.2	52.3	8.7	18.8	6.0
1978	45.4	80.4	50.7	9.2	20.4	6.1
1979	44.7	79.1	48.9	9.9	22.3	5.9

SOURCE: Carroll MS, Arnett RH: Private health insurance plans in 1978 and 1979: A review of coverage, enrollment, and financial experience. *Health Care Financing Rev*, 1981; 3(1):85.

[a]NA = not available.

physician services. Over the years the proportion of all consumer expenditures met by insurance has increased almost fourfold to 44.7% in 1979. Seventy-nine percent of consumer expenditures for hospital care were paid for through private insurance in 1979, while 49% of physician services and 22% of outpatient dental care were paid for through insurance. Outpatient prescribed drugs and all other types of care are still largely paid for out-of-pocket by consumers.

In 1979, Blue Cross/Blue Shield plans accounted for 39% of gross enrollments for the most basic insurance, hospital coverage (13). These were largely enrollments under group policies. This type of policy underwritten by commercial insurance companies accounted for another 34% of all enrollments, with individual policies underwritten by insurance companies yielding an additional 15%. The remaining 12% of enrollments for hospital insurance was accounted for by independent pre-paid group practice plans, individual practice associations, and employer and union plans. As their name implies, independent plans tend to be locally oriented, but some represent large systems, as for example the Kaiser-Permanente medical care system. Excluded from the insurance company figures are persons covered by self-insured and prepayment plans for which there is an administrative services arrangement with an insurance carrier, without the carrier being primarily at risk. Approximately 20 million persons are covered under such arrangements. They are included in the independent plan category.

Health Maintenance Organizations

In the early 1970s an umbrella label, *Health Maintenance Organization (HMO)*, was coined to characterize independent plans that offered service benefits for an enrolled population, covering hospital, physician, and related ancillary services. These plans offer service benefits, with the implied requirement that both hospital care and physician services be provided directly or on a contractual basis through the HMO.

The HMO has received considerable attention since federal legislation was passed in 1973 to promote this type of financing and organization through planning and operational grants and loans. About 200 such organizations exist in the United States in various stages of development with quite diverse characteristics. The federal legislation included complex and demanding requirements for these organizations if they were to become eligible for federal funding and mandatory inclusion in dual-choice health insurance offerings by employers. Under dual-choice, the employer must offer the employee more than one health insurance plan. Organizational aspects of HMOs are discussed in Chapter 5, and insurance considerations are presented here.

The ideals of community rating and comprehensive services, characteristics of some of the more successful earlier prepaid group practices or HMOs, put the newer organizations at a considerable disadvantage in the marketplace. Later amendments have made their promotion more feasible. At the same time, some states have passed legislation to protect developing HMOs and, in particular, to encourage their further development by requiring that employers include an HMO option in their fringe benefit offerings. What is it about the HMO that is so appealing from the public policy point of view?

Perhaps the major factor is that the HMO combines the insurance or underwriting function with the responsibility for delivering a broad range of health services. Thus, the underwriter (HMO) has to compete in the insurance market to be included as a benefit option for employees as the preferred employee choice among the alternatives offered, such as commercial insurance or Blue Cross/Blue Shield coverage. In addition, the plan must offer services that are professionally satisfactory and acceptable to patients. Thus, a central organization, the plan, has a strong incentive to offer services efficiently and in as cost effective a manner as possible so as to contain premium increases and expand benefits, both of which would attract enrollees in the dual-choice situation. The HMO, then, has been seen as an important model for encouraging natural regulation of the health care market through the usual forces of competition.

The better established HMOs, particularly prepaid group practice plans, have been operating successfully in various areas, largely on the West Coast and in New York City and Washington, D.C., since the 1940s. The development of these plans has been steady in their local geographic areas, and some, such as Kaiser-Permanente, have expanded into new geographic areas over the decades.

These prepaid group practice plans have been characterized by far more comprehensive benefits than the typical health insurance program. Comprehensive HMO coverage, including hospital and physician services for both the subscriber and dependents, typically without a deductible or coinsurance, has been a major attraction. The premium to cover this comprehensive benefit package has generally been higher than the premium associated with competing traditional health insurance programs. The total costs to the subscriber or member, however, must be considered in terms of premium payments combined with out-of-pocket expenses. On average, prepaid group practice is less expensive, for the same benefit package, than traditional underwriting using independent fee-for-service physicians and community hospitals.

A drawback to prepaid group practice enrollment is the required use of plan physicians, who themselves are grouped into area medical centers. Thus, an enrollee must find a physician within the group practice with whom family members are satisfied, and must have reasonable geographic access to health services if this type of HMO is to be attractive. The slow but steady growth of prepaid group practice over recent decades indicates that for many people the protection afforded by more comprehensive coverage at relatively less expense offsets limited choice of physician and lessened geographic availability.

Developments during the 1970s in financing health services, however, have raised some serious questions about the attractiveness of prepaid group practice in the future. As was noted earlier, there has been a tendency for a larger proportion of the premium, and often the entire premium, to be paid by employers and a tendency toward more comprehensive benefits to be offered by commercial insurance companies and Blue Cross/Blue Shield plans. These changes would appear to reduce the competitive advantage of prepaid group practice, since the latter arrangement still has inherent in it the organizational and geographic limitations, but is at a lesser advantage in terms of coverage and risk sharing. More recently, economic pressures have led to renewed interest by employers in cost-sharing arrangements such as deductibles and coinsurance. Thus, the incentives favoring more comprehensive HMO plans may again increase.

Employers and other purchasers of third-party coverage, such as governments, often benefit from the lower premium costs, given equal benefit structures, of prepaid group practice. But in the dual-choice situation, it is the subscriber or employee who makes the decision as to which plan to use. The issue then becomes one of who will benefit from the savings that accrue by selecting a prepaid group practice in contrast to a traditional insurance program.

An alternative form of HMO to the prepaid group practice is the individual practice association (IPA), in which contractual arrangements exist between the plan and individual physicians and multiple medical groups, who are at some financial risk in the event that the costs of services exceed premium income, but practice in their offices, widely dispersed throughout the community. The IPA arrangement offers a broader range of physicians who are more geographically accessible to an enrolled population, and thus may offset the drawbacks to prepaid group practice mentioned above. Such a plan can also use physicians already in practice and hospitals already operating in the community, rather than invest the substantial capital required to start a group practice, particularly one that ultimately operates its own hospital. Further, physicians can be reimbursed on a prorated fee-for-service basis, a method close to that to which they are already accustomed.

Yet another approach is the primary care network plan, sometimes also called the *case management* system. This system takes advantage of the gatekeeper role of the primary care physician by developing a contractual relationship with primary care physicians in the community, either on a fee-for-service or a capitation basis, to deliver their own services. These physicians then have the responsibility for handling referrals of enrollees to specialists and hospitals and of approving the charges for such care. Under this arrangement, reimbursement is withheld for care rendered by a specialist or in the hospital unless the patient was referred by the primary care physician. Ease of selection of a primary care physician depends, of course, upon the participating proportion and geographic dispersion of the primary care practitioners in the community.

A drawback of the IPA and network is that the plan or HMO has much less influence over the organization and method of physician practice than under the prepaid group arrangement. Such plans are more dependent upon the incentives built into the reimbursement agreement with physicians and sometimes hospitals. In contrast, the prepaid group can select physicians with practice styles consistent with the plan's operation, can organize facilities so as to encourage out-of-hospital management of illness, and can achieve the efficiencies inherent in combined ambulatory and inpatient delivery organizations.

To date, much of the experience with IPAs or primary care networks has been in settings in which they are competing with more traditional prepaid group practice, as well as with commercial insurance companies and Blue Cross/Blue Shield. Indeed, in some instances IPAs have been developed by physicians to meet the competitive threat of prepaid group practices moving into their area. Under these circumstances, it is difficult to judge how much influence specific economic incentives have on physician behavior in the sense of putting physicians at risk through reimbursement schemes, and how much of the savings that may accrue from the IPA arrangement are due to greater physician motivation and peer control. Nor is success assured. A number of plans started during the 1970s have failed in the marketplace.

Major Government-Financed Programs

As noted earlier, the development of private health insurance in this country, and particularly the evolution of experience rating of premiums under both commercial insurance plans and Blue Cross/Blue Shield, left two major segments of the population without access to adequate coverage. The first group, the elderly, tend to be out of the labor force and therefore not eligible for group coverage, experience a substantial drop in income and typically a deteriorating wealth position, and are at increasing risk of major illness and therefore financial loss. The poor are also at greater risk of illness and, in addition, are often either unemployed or find themselves in occupations with irregular employment patterns or with low wages and poor fringe benefits.

These issues were especially evident during the 1950s and 1960s when voluntary health insurance was covering a constantly increasing percentage of the population. Opposition to major federal programs to deal with these two groups was based on the persuasive argument that the voluntary system could do the job. Consequently, two titles were added to the Social Security Act in 1965. The first, Title XVIII, was the Medicare program for those age 65 and older; the second was Title XIX, the Medicaid program, which substantially expanded the financial assistance provided to states and counties to pay for medical services for the poor.

Hospital insurance is provided to the elderly, and more recently to the permanently and totally disabled, beginning in the thirtieth month after disability, as well as to victims of end-stage renal disease, through Part A of Medicare. Part A also offers coverage in extended care facilities for posthospital convalescence and home health services. Part B of Medicare, supplementary medical insurance, resembles major medical insurance for other than hospital services. Part B includes inpatient and outpatient physician services, ancillary services, and a wide range of other related medical services.

Part A is available without cost to the enrollee for virtually the entire elderly population. All other elderly persons may enroll at any time through the payment of a premium. Ninety-five percent of all persons age 65 and over are enrolled. This hospital coverage includes a deductible that is roughly equivalent to the cost of 1 day of care in the hospital. The amount increases from time to time and in 1982 was

$260. Coverage is provided for 90 days of hospital care for each illness episode, with a copayment for the last 30 of these days equal to one-fourth of the deductible, and 100 days of coverage per illness episode for extended care, with a copayment equal to one-eighth of the hospital deductible for the last 80 days. Additional coverage for hospital days is available in the forms of a "lifetime reserve," each day of which involves a copayment. The lifetime reserve of 60 hospital days may be applied to any episode of care up to the reserve limit. These days are subject to a copayment equal to one-half of the hospital deductible.

Part B of Medicare also includes a deductible, but on an annual basis. In 1982, this amount was $75. A coinsurance of 20% of the reasonable charge is also applied. Often, the beneficiary must also make up the difference between reasonable and actual physician charges. Although it varies by region, overall approximately 50% of claims payments are accepted by physicians as payment-in-full (assignment). There are further limitations for mental and nervous conditions. A very high proportion of the elderly population (96%) is covered by Part B in addition to Part A. Unlike Part A, Part B is available on a voluntary basis, with the requirement that the elderly person pay a monthly premium that is intended to be half the actual rate, based on loss experience. The other half is to be financed by the Health Care Financing Administration (which in reality finances more than two-thirds of the premium). The portion of the premium charged to the individual in 1982 was $12.20 per month.

The effects of deductibles, coinsurance, limitations in coverage, such as for psychiatric benefits, and service exclusions, such as routine dental and vision care, hearing aids, and particularly custodial skilled nursing home services, result in a Medicare program for the elderly that covers somewhat less than half of the expenditures for health services paid by this population. Thus, the inadequacies are similar to those of private health insurance, with the important exception that the governmental programs provide coverage for a very high-risk segment of the population that would ordinarily not be eligible for coverage under the voluntary system.

Medicare Part A is financed almost entirely by a portion, slightly over 1%, of the Social Security payroll tax through contributions by employees and employers. These funds are deposited in a separate trust fund and account for 91% of the fund. Premiums paid directly by a relatively small number of individuals who have not been participants in the Social Security or Railroad Retirement systems also contribute to the trust fund. Another trust fund receives monies from the voluntary premium payments of enrollees under Part B and premium payments from Medicaid on behalf of welfare recipients. The Part B trust fund also receives general revenues to make up the remainder of the funds required. Because of the rising costs of medical care, the amounts paid into the Medicare system from all sources have been substantially increased over the years.

Payments from these trust funds for both the administration of claims processing and reimbursement of providers are made through fiscal intermediaries, who are voluntary underwriters, largely Blue Cross/Blue Shield and commercial carriers, rather than directly by the government. As the program was developing in the late 1960s, the use of existing underwriters that had established administrative systems and relationships with both consumers and providers offered many advantages. More recently, the use of fiscal intermediaries has had the further advantage of requiring responsiveness to changes in federal policy under threat of changes in the designation of fiscal intermediaries, a process that could not be used if administration were directly by the federal government. A major disadvantage of using fiscal intermediaries for claims processing and provider relations is the inevitable variations in practices that develop over time across the country; even with Blue Cross, the federal program is using scores of local plans, although they are tied together through a national association.

The Medicaid program for low income families is quite different in concept from the Medicare program. The Medicaid program developed out of the welfare system, which was originally local in both its administration and its financing. During the Great Depression, local and state funds for welfare were quickly exhausted and the need for federal assistance became evident. The system that developed was one of federal matching funds to the states in support of welfare payments to various categories of the poor. Over the years, new categories were added, such as the totally and permanently disabled. An obvious need of the poor was assistance in paying for medical expenses. There developed a mechanism, *vendor payments*, which simply meant that medical care provided to welfare recipients would be reimbursed by the county or state welfare authorities. A system of matching grants to the states from the federal government to offset partially the states' cost for vendor payments was formalized and expanded in the early 1960s. Medicaid built upon this welfare-oriented system of federal grants to the states by matching state expenditures.

As originally envisioned, Medicaid included matching funds to states that met a set of requirements or standards, including payment for five basic services, inpatient and outpatient hospital care, physician services, laboratory and x-ray services, and nursing home care, and reimbursed providers on a basis consistent with federally established Medicare policies, including retrospective cost reimbursement for hospitals and fee-for-service payments to physicians. Thus, states were obliged to reimburse hospitals on a reasonable cost basis, for example. These services had to be financed by the states for categorical welfare recipients such as families with dependent children, the elderly, the blind, and the totally and permanently disabled.

The original 1965 Medicaid law mandated certain minimum state standards in order for the states to receive matching funds, the amount of the match, ranging from 50 to 83%, being inversely related to the relative affluence of the residents of the state. States were also permitted to offer a much wider range of services than the minimum requirement, with partial federal reimbursement. Further, the states were permitted to establish their own income cutoff levels for determining eligibility. It was originally envisioned that by 1975, all states would be obliged to offer a full range of services to all residents in the state falling below a state-determined income level, without regard to whether or not they were categorical welfare recipients.

The cost to the federal government of the Medicaid program in its first year of operation and in subsequent years was substantially higher than had originally been forecast. Some states set income levels that were quite high by the standards then prevailing and offered a wide range of services. In the following years, amendments to the Medicaid law passed by the Congress reduced the freedom of the states to set high income cutoff levels, removed the requirements for expansion of services and eligibility originally envisioned, and tightened standards along a number of dimensions.

At the same time, state Medicaid budgets were stretched to the breaking point as a result of the rapid increase in costs of care due to the development and use of new services, upgraded services such as in nursing homes, and other factors. The original objective of eliminating second-class medical care for the poor was gradually eroded, in part because of the financial constraints that were placed on the programs, but also because of the great difficulty state governments had in administering such a complex third-party payment program.

There was, and continues to be, considerable hostility toward state Medicaid programs by providers, but at the same time this source of funding remains crucial for the poor and is dominant in certain sectors such as long term care. Because Medicaid is not a program fully financed and administered by the federal government, there is tremendous variation among states with respect to benefits, eligibility, and administration. As a result, a truly national plan for health services has been seriously debated by federal policymakers.

PUBLIC POLICY ISSUES

It is evident from the preceding description of health services financing that a number of pressing issues are facing our society in this area. This concluding section summarizes the more important issues and considers general outlines of various proposed solutions, including strategies along the fundamental continuum that underlies the current debate, ranging from substantial government underwriting and direct regulation to a competitive market approach.

The major issues fall in the general categories of equity, effectiveness, and economy. With respect to equity, there are problems of risk sharing across the population and income redistribution. The primary concerns with regard to effectiveness are access to primary care and future technological development. The broad issue of economy encompasses concerns about total health services costs, cost effectiveness, and the visibility of expenditures.

Spreading the risk of substantial family expense due to medical care was a very early and very compelling motive in the development of voluntary health insurance. Further, the inability of private health insurance effectively to cover the high risk associated with the elderly and the poor led to the passage of Medicare and Medicaid legislation. After the passage of these two programs, it was widely believed that the problem of risk-sharing in our society had been largely resolved with voluntary insurance providing adequate protection to the majority of the population (generally those employed), and governmental programs (Medicare, Medicaid, and other programs designed for specific segments of the population) providing protection for the remainder.

Ironically, the reduction in the effective price of services at the time of delivery attributable to third-party coverage, coupled with cost reimbursement, have led to an elaboration of technological medical care to the point where, even with health insurance coverage, the population currently runs the risk of catastrophic loss. So-called halfway technologies, or those that are very expensive relative to the measurable benefits because they do not definitively deal with the problem, seem to have further aggravated the problem of adequate risk sharing through third-party coverage. Further, even with the federal and voluntary programs now in effect, there is still a segment of the population, as noted earlier in the chapter, that falls between the eligibility cracks. A potential solution to these problems would be federally legislated universal entitlement with a mechanism to ensure that every resident has access to some form of third-party coverage in practice as well as in theory. Universal entitlement might be coupled with a program of catastrophic health insurance coverage that is federally underwritten or, alternatively, federally mandated but underwritten on a voluntary or mixed governmental and voluntary basis.

Another facet of the equity issue is the effect of income redistribution as a result of policies followed in the financing of health services. Three basic sources of revenue have been described in this chapter: out-of-pocket payment for health services, premium payments by employers or employees, and tax revenues (primarily federal Social Security contributions and income taxes). The passage of a national health plan, and its implementation, would result in changes in the relative money costs of health care to families at various income levels. The various proposals that have been put forth over the years differ substantially in their impact on families, with the regressive or progressive nature of a particular plan related not only to the use of a payroll tax versus the income tax (or general revenues) but also to the nature of mandated employer/employee paid premiums when this is part of the proposal and the design of the benefit structure (yielding varying out-of-pocket burdens). It should be sufficient to note here that with expenditures for health services accounting for almost one-tenth of the GNP, and assuming universal entitlement, the redistributive effects of any national health plan will be given serious consideration.

The broad issue of effectiveness includes the impact of third-party coverage and reimbursement policies on the nature of the services that are encouraged or discouraged. Under the present system, the breadth and depth of coverage for inpatient care, coupled with cost reimbursement, have resulted in an increasing proportion of all health care expenditures being devoted to hospital care. It is interesting to note that in those parts of the country, particularly the West Coast, where third-party coverage of out-of-hospital services and favorable reimbursement arrangements for physicians' care developed very early (in some cases before the establishment of Blue Cross), there is a markedly lower proportion of expenditures for hospital care and a lower rate of growth in per capita hospital costs.

Third-party coverage is an important factor in the issue of access to primary care. Beyond this, however, there is evidence to suggest that in large organized systems with enrolled populations, such as prepaid group practice, there appears to be a shift in resources from expensive and elaborate inpatient care to greater amounts of primary care, particularly for enrollees who are younger and healthier. In most parts of the country, however, the pattern is one of little or no coverage for preventive services and relatively poor coverage for routine ambulatory care in general.

At the other extreme, it is common to find substantial coverage for high-cost diagnostic and therapeutic technologies. Further, federally underwritten or mandated catastrophic coverage to address the problem of risk sharing, cited earlier in this section, would further encourage this disparity. Major efforts are just now getting underway to deal with the question of technology assessment in a manner that would give some guidance on the effectiveness of various clinical strategies and therefore the merits of providing third-party coverage in greater or lesser depth for particular types of services (as discussed in Chap. 9).

Under the general rubric of economy, an important factor is the cost effectiveness of medical care. The present financing system removes much of the incentive for consideration of cost effectiveness at the doctor-patient level, as well as at the broader community or regional level. On the other hand, it is becoming clear that increases in total costs that exceed the growth rate of the economy as a whole are stirring the interest of a broad political coalition involving not only organized labor but industry as well. At the same time, the public has been less conscious of rising personal health expenditures since ever-expanding third-party coverage has kept out-of-pocket costs at a fairly stable level measured on a constant dollar basis. In other words, and as noted earlier in this chapter, costs have not been very visible to the consumer in comparison to the obvious increases in complexity, quality, and the amenity level of most health services. With respect to the last, the public has rather high expectations that generally seem to be met.

Discussions of national health insurance up to the late 1960s were almost exclusively concerned with improving risk sharing across the community and providing better and more equitable access to care. In the last 15 years, however, greater attention has focused on the potential for cost containment and the correction of many of the market defects described in this chapter. As the debate has progressed, some have argued that it would be inflationary to implement a national health plan without first having firmly established a strong regulatory strategy designed to constrain both entry of capital into the health field and increases in hospital expenditures and, more generally, to promote cost effectiveness in the delivery of care. Others have argued that the only way to implement such regulation effectively is to incorporate it into a comprehensive national health insurance plan that both concentrates the dollars flowing into the system (through the federal government in order to provide more force to the regulatory effort) and makes the costs of the system more visible by such concentration.

More recently, the fundamental policy differences that have emerged address the relative merits of heavy regulation and/or limitations on reimbursement of the health care industry to contain costs, perhaps coupled with national health insurance, versus a restructuring of the system so as to rely on competition between voluntary health plans to provide a self-correcting market. Such plans would include both underwriting and delivery of care as exemplified by the HMO.

In reality, there is currently substantial regulation of the industry, as discussed in other chapters, and no plausible system has been proposed that does not require a continuation of governmental regulation of some aspects of the field, including the framework within which market competition would take place. Similarly, even proposals that rely heavily on direct governmental financing and/or regulation must recognize that the forces of competition in the market will be at work, undoubtedly distorting the intended outcomes of any regulatory strategy.

To conclude this chapter, some of the problems with governmental underwriting and direct regulation on the one hand, and with the competitive market approach on the other, are described. A good summary of the key weaknesses of the governmental approach is presented by Enthoven (14). In describing the weaknesses of the extreme case of a government monopoly on health insurance, and therefore direct government involvement in the regulation of the delivery system, Enthoven points out the following: 1) Government differs from private enterprise in that it responds to well-focused producer interests whereas competitive markets respond to broad consumer interests, thus weighing decisions in the direction of the former rather than the latter. 2) Political decisions tend to be made on the basis of doing no direct harm but paying much less attention to indirect shortcomings. For this reason, government-regulated systems are designed rigidly, with bureaucrats having very limited discretion. 3) "When every dollar in the system is a federal dollar, what every dollar is spent on becomes a federal case" (14). 4) Government tends to encourage uniformity, which often means a bargained compromise that is satisfactory to no one. 5) If government were involved in direct provision of care, it would face the weakness that it generally does a poor job of delivering direct services to individuals. 6) The government is not a cost-effective purchaser, partially because governmental employees are limited in exercising their judgment. 7) Government is disinclined to take chances and is intolerant of individuals' mistakes. This attitude makes innovations within a governmental system difficult.

An alternate strategy would be to provide enough regulation to structure competitive markets in which comprehensive systems would be competing against one another (e.g., HMOs), and individuals would be responsible for enough of the premium payment to encourage prudent selection among competing plans. To deal with some of the difficulties that have been described throughout this chapter, the regulatory framework for a competitive market model would need to include at least requirements regarding: 1) the information provided to consumers; 2) open enrollment and premium rationing; and 3) minimum benefit packages. In addition, subsidies could be provided to assist those with lower incomes. This subsidization might be accomplished through vouchers to be used only for the purchase of health insurance. The remainder of the population might be provided with partial payment for health insurance premiums either through tax credits or mandated employer payments, but would bear a substantial cost of the premium so as to encourage shopping for the most economical plan, given the family's quality preferences. It would be important to let premiums and/or health plan benefits vary so that the advantages of more efficient plans would accrue to the individuals making the choice.

The principal difficulties with the market competition approach to improving current financing of health services are twofold: uncertainties with respect to provider response, and the degree to which there would be substantial competition (as opposed to a tendency toward ever-increasing industry norms for standards of operation and professional practice). Up to this point, providers have understandably been generally satisfied with the financial arrangements for health services. Certain organized comprehensive systems of care such as prepaid group practice have developed and grown in selected geographic areas, although the growth has not been as impressive as many would have liked. It has been argued that prepaid group practices are substantially more efficient than the rest of the medical care market, because they must be in order to finance the more comprehensive benefits that attract those who choose this approach. If competing systems offered equally comprehensive care but at higher premium levels, one could imagine the prepaid group practice or other HMO-type system having little incentive to do other than ease the pressures toward efficiency, allowing premiums to approach but not quite equal those of its competitors.

With respect to the impact of professional standards, even existing HMOs find it difficult to encourage the practice of substantially different styles of medicine from those that are found generally in the society. In a less highly organized system such as the IPA, group norms would be weaker and greater reliance would have to be placed on financial incentives to providers. However, as was noted in an earlier section, it is not clear to what degree moderating financial incentives can offset the drive for more scientific, technological, and expensive patterns of diagnosis and treatment.

The coming years portend continued debate regarding the many issues raised in this chapter and broader recognition of some of the underlying problems. The solutions to a number of the issues are incompatible, and all are politically sensitive. If it were otherwise, the country would probably have already come to grips with them, and would have adopted a coherent national policy on the financing of health services. These financing issues are also among the central uncertainties in the continuing evolution of approaches to health planning and regulation, as discussed in detail in the following chapters.

REFERENCES

1. Waldo DR: National health expenditures. *Health Care Financing Rev*, 1982; 4(1):1.
2. Waldo DR: Information through March 1982 on: Health Care Prices. *Health Care Financing Trends, Health Care Financing Adm* 1982; 2(5):13.
3. Birnbaum H: *The Cost of Catastrophic Illness.* Lexington, Mass, Lexington Books, 1978, pp 1, 2.
4. Scitovsky A, McCall N: *Changes in the Costs of Treatment of Selected Illnesses: 1951–1964–1971.* Research Digest Series, National Center for Health Statistics, US Dept of Health, Education and Welfare, 1976.
5. Somers AR: The high cost of health care for the elderly: Diagnosis, prognosis, and some suggestions for therapy. *J Health Polit Policy Law* 1978; 3(2):163–180.
6. Fisher G: National health expenditures, fiscal year 1977. *Soc Secur Bull* 1978; 41(7):9.
7. O'Tousa M: Management rounds. *Hospitals* 1982; 56(13):31–32.
8. Jacobs P, Bauerschmidt AD, Furst RW: Hospital cost inflation and health insurance: A complex market model. *Inquiry* 1978; 15:217–224.
9. Carroll MS, Arnett RH: Private health insurance plans in 1978 and 1979: A review of coverage, enrollment, and financial experience. *Health Care Financing Rev* 1981; 3(1):55–87.
10. Mueller MS: Private health insurance in 1975: Coverage, enrollment, and financial experience. *Soc Secur Bull* 1977; 40(6):5.
11. Robert Wood Johnson Foundation: *America's Health Care System: A Comprehensive Portrait.* Special Report, no 1. Princeton, NJ, Robert Wood Johnson Foundation, 1978.
12. Richardson WC: Group payment since the CCMC: Policy implications of the ignored and the unforeseen, mimeo. Seattle, Wash, University of Washington, 1978.
13. Carroll MS, Arnett RH: Private health insurance plans in 1978 and 1979: A review of coverage, enrollment, and financial experience. *Health Care Financing Rev* 1981; 3(1):58.
14. Enthoven AC: Consumer-choice health plan (part one): Inflation and inequity in health care today—Alternatives for cost control and an analysis of proposals for national health insurance. *N Engl J Med* 1978; 298:650–658.

PART FIVE

Assessing and Regulating
System Performance

CHAPTER 12

Health Services Planning and Regulation

Thomas W. Bice

In the post-World War II era, modern nations of all political and economic colorations have turned increasingly to planning and regulation to guide economic and social development (1). Expanding conceptions of the welfare state, imperatives of technologic complexity and change, and unwanted consequences of industrialization and urbanization have given rise to new forms of collective rationality and control that extend over enlarging segments of economic and social life (2). Nowhere is this trend more evident than in modern nations' health services industry. While the basic forms of their organization and financing vary considerably among countries, all are being subjected to direction by mixtures of the market and of state planning and regulation (3).

In the United States, where health care is provided and financed through private institutions, governments' roles in planning and regulation have developed only recently and have evoked considerable debate. This chapter reviews the historic origins and growth of health planning and regulation in the United States. The discussion begins by defining planning and regulation and laying out the rationales underlying their use as instruments of social and economic control. Then major milestones in the development of planning and regulation aimed at improving the health care industry's performance are described. In the concluding section, lessons and issues drawn from this nation's experiences with planning and regulation are discussed.

PLANNING AND REGULATION

Definitions

Rational action by individuals or collectivities involves four fundamental steps: 1) delineation of objectives; 2) formulation and valuation of alternative means of attaining them; 3) implementation of chosen means; and 4) evaluation of program processes and impacts (4,5). This chapter makes a somewhat arbitrary distinction between the'steps involving the delineation of objectives and selection of strategies for attaining them, which are regarded as planning, and the implementation of programs, which may involve regulation.

Accordingly, *planning* is viewed as an essentially symbolic process, the results of which are statements of alternative ends and means and choices among them. *Regulation,* by contrast, refers to a diverse set of means by which individuals or organizations are either induced or compelled to behave in specified ways (6).

Rationales for Planning and Regulation

The rationales for planning and regulation derive from several features of modern industrialized nations. Among these are the complexity and interrelationships among specialized institutions, the expansion of the concept of the *general welfare,* and a variety of circumstances referred to as *market failures.*

Modern industrialized nations comprise highly specialized institutions that, to accomplish their objectives, must coordinate their activities. In countries whose political and economic institutions are based on the principles of political pluralism and free enterprise, such coordination is accomplished primarily through the market mechanisms of mutual adjustment and contractual agreements. Such arrangements minimize the need for government-sponsored planning, particularly when society collectively has no particular interest in what is produced and consumed and when other assumptions of the market are met.

Because no society is totally indifferent to the living conditions of its members or to the types of goods and services that are produced and consumed, governments assume powers and functions aimed at protecting individual rights and promoting the general welfare (7). These powers and functions grow in proportion to the number and variety of rights, entitlement, and other claims that citizens can legitimately make upon government. Faced with increasing claims, governments have two broad alternatives: to provide goods and services directly through publicly owned and operated facilities or to induce or compel private actors to provide them. Socialist countries are inclined toward the former solution, and capitalist nations favor the latter. In either case, the amount and extent of government-sponsored planning and control expand.

Another impetus for planning and regulation is a variety of *market failures.* The presumption that market mechanisms will achieve a socially optimum allocation of goods and services rests on several assumptions about the structures of markets that may be untenable in some situations (8). These assumptions include the following:

1. Individuals know what they want and are able to make informed choices among alternative products.
2. Individuals pay the full costs of the products they consume and enjoy their full benefit.
3. People can select from among products offered by a large number of independent suppliers.
4. Suppliers bear the full costs of producing their products.

The first two assumptions pertain to consumers' ability to make informed choices and to the consequences of their decisions for others. Instances of departures from these conditions abound in highly industrialized and urbanized nations, where consumers have only limited knowledge about many of the products they consume and where opportunities for "neighborhood effects" multiply. The lack of consumers' knowledge about pharmaceutical products, for instance, combined with the potential risks of learning by experimentation, leads government to plan and regulate the production and distribution of drugs. The harmful and bothersome pollutants emitted by automobiles lead government to require drivers to equip their vehicles with emission control devices.

The second pair of assumptions deals with the characteristics of a market's structure and so-called externalities of production. The former assumes that industries are composed of large numbers of competitive suppliers who freely enter and leave markets and who independently decide what to produce and what price to charge for their products. The several circumstances that violate these assumptions call for planning and regulation. In situations where it is economically efficient for particular goods or services to be supplied by a single producer (e.g., natural monopolies), government applies public utility regulation to protect the public against monopolistic practices. In other situations, high costs of entry and other barriers limit the number of suppliers, or collusive decision making among suppliers limits the ranges of products and prices available to consumers. Finally, as in the case of the polluting driver, government intervention is evoked by producers who pass along to the public costs such as those associated with environmental pollution.

The combination of these conditions in the health services industry makes it particularly subject to government planning and regulation (9). The composition of the industry and the nature of the demands made upon it cause it to be one of the more complex sectors of the economy, and trends of the past few decades have greatly increased the need for coordination. Advances in medical knowledge and technology have created high degrees of specialization and segmentation within the medical profession and vast increases in the number and variety of ancillary medical personnel and services. Concomitantly, the types and relative prevalence of health problems have changed from a preponderance of acute and infectious diseases to chronic, emotional, and social problems that require long term management by other helping professionals and agencies, as well as by traditional health care providers. Yet, the prevailing modes of organization and financing within the industry continue to reflect their roots in earlier periods and discourage voluntary coordination of the various levels and types of services that might better meet the needs of patients. Because the industry is dominated by private entrepreneurs, each being reimbursed independently for services provided, few incentives exist to encourage coordination and change. The industry is thus prone to continue oversupplying the highly sophisticated and expensive services of medical specialists and acute care hospitals, and undersupplying less technologically complex primary medical care and life support services.

The intimate relationships between health services and modern nations' notions of the general welfare also invite planning and regulation. Because health care is prominent among the necessities of life, all nations have established means to ensure their citizens access to health services. In the United States, the federal and state governments subsidize consumers and suppliers of health services and those who train health care personnel and conduct research, and directly provide services to particular population groups. Because health services are cloaked in the public interest and because governments are paying growing shares of their costs, public pressure is brought to bear on governments to ensure that services are equitably and efficiently allocated. In the recent past, governments have responded by instituting various regulatory controls.

Finally, virtually all of the market failures that often evoke planning and regulation apply to the health services industry. Given the complexity of medical knowledge and technology, few people are equipped to select among alternative modalities of treatment. Hence, patients essentially abdicate to physicians the responsibility for choosing the goods and services they consume. Even if consumers were able to make such decisions, extensive insurance coverage renders them virtually indifferent to the relative prices of alternative modes of treatment. On the suppliers' side, the industry is dominated by professions that limit entry into their ranks and discourage competitive pricing, and by hospitals that enjoy the status of nonprofit community institutions. Neither physicians nor hospitals bear the full costs of producing their services. Physicians are typically free to employ the facilities and personnel of hospitals in treating their patients without regard for the costs imposed on the hospitals. In turn, the now common practice of reimbursing hospitals retrospectively on the basis of their costs allows hospitals to pass these costs on to the insurers and, through them, to the public. In consequence, neither physicians nor hospitals would be expected to economize voluntarily.

Many of the features of the health services industry that invite planning and regulation were visible nearly a half century ago. Others have developed only rather recently. Despite changing circumstances, however, the appeals for comprehensive planning and greater coordination voiced in the opening decades of this century are strikingly similar to those advanced today by proponents of planning and regulation.

ORIGINS AND DEVELOPMENT OF HEALTH SERVICES PLANNING

Health services planning began in the United States in the 1930s as voluntary efforts and subsequently developed primarily under the auspices of the federal and state governments. Since the beginning of the federal government's involvement in the 1940s, the objectives, scope, and organization of planning have been largely determined by federal policy as expressed in five programs: the Hill-Burton Program, the Hospital Survey and Construction Act of 1946 (PL 79-725); the Regional Medical Programs, the Heart Disease, Cancer, and Stroke Act of 1965 (PL 89-239); the Comprehensive Health Planning Program, the Partnership for Health Act of 1967 (PL 90-174); the Experimental Health Services Delivery Program; and the National Health Planning and Resources Development Act of 1974. The provisions of these programs and the processes they established are milestones in the transformation of health planning from its origins in elite-dominated, categorical planning to the present participatory, comprehensive planning, and from planning in the absence of regulation to the partial joining of these functions (10).

Origins of Health Planning

Health services planning emerged in the United Staes in the 1930s, joining two elements that continue to shape the organization and objectives of planning. One established the organizational foundations of health planning in local voluntaristic groups. The other developed the idea of a regionalized health services system that remains to this day the ideal to which comprehensive health planning is directed.

Before the 1940s, health planning was limited to localized efforts aimed primarily at coordinating activities of municipal public health and welfare departments and hospitals. The attention of the health and welfare councils established to accomplish these ends focused on problems of providing services for the indigent rather than on fundamental reforms of the health services industry (11). The first organized attempt to deal specifically with such matters was made in the 1930s in New York City with the founding of the Hospital Council of Greater New York (12). The Great Depression had produced severe overcrowding of municipal facilities, which provided free services and depleted patient censuses in the voluntary hospitals. These and other conditions were documented in an extensive survey of hospitals, leading the group of prominent citizens that sponsored the study to recommend the establishment of a permanent planning body. A few other cities followed New York's example, urged by philanthropists interested in seeing that their contributions to hospitals were being wisely used (13).

Supported largely by philanthropic donations, these early planning agencies functioned outside the ambit of government. Their governing boards typically were composed of influential citizens who oversaw the activities of their small staffs. Initially, planning concentrated almost exclusively on estimating the number of hospital beds needed in communities.

The concept of health services planning achieved national prominence in the early 1930s with the publication of findings and recommendations of the prestigious Committee on the Costs of Medical Care. This committee had been established in 1927 after a national conference on health care attended by leading physicians, social scientists, public health practitioners, and the lay public (14). With funds provided by several philanthropic foundations, the committee undertook extensive studies of the use, organization, and financing of health services that culminated in 28 published reports and numerous staff papers. Among the committee's principal conclusions was a recommendation calling for the establishment of local and state agencies for the purposes of conducting research and devising plans for coordinating health services. Further, the committee presented a plan for organizing health services institutions and personnel in accordance with the principles of regionalization detailed in the Dawson Report, issued 12 years earlier in the United Kingdom (14).

The notion of regionalization outlined in the Dawson Report and in the recommendations of the Committee on the Costs of Medical Care envisioned a division of functions among hospitals, clinics, and medical personnel based on vertically integrated levels of specialization and intensity of services. Choices of sites of care and the placement of patients would be dictated by the level of services required. Such arrangements were already being initiated in Sweden and Denmark by the beginning of this century, and the idea has been adopted as a guiding principle for health planning in the United Kingdom and elsewhere.

The rationales offered for health services planning in the 1930s and early 1940s combined several notions that appealed to deeply rooted social values. As practiced in New York City and later in Rochester (New York), Detroit, and Pittsburgh, planning was a voluntary endeavor in which leading citizens and health care providers applied the tools of business management to attain greater efficiency and improved health care. Moreover, the concept of regionalization embodied ultimate designs of rationality and offered possibilities for resolving the then pressing problem of providing health services to the nation's small towns and rural areas.

The Hill-Burton Program

World War II and its aftermath placed health services planning on the public agenda as the Great Depression had done the decade before. Concerns about the educational and physical fitness of the population raised by findings from examinations of military inductees led to a Senate inquiry into the adequacy of the nation's health services and their bearing upon the health of the population. Pursuant to its charge, the Senate Subcommittee on Wartime Health and Education conducted hearings at which the then Surgeon General of the U.S. Public Health Service proposed establishing planning agencies throughout the country to guide the development of "coordinated hospital systems" (14). His testimony and subsequent discussions with members of the subcommittee clearly showed the influence of the Dawson Report, and although his proposal referred specifically to "coordinated hospitals," the plan itself extended to virtually all aspects of contemporary comprehensive health planning.

After the war, hospital conditions prompted the federal government to establish the nation's first major health services planning and construction subsidy program. Given 2 decades of neglect imposed first by the Depression and then by the war, the country's stock of hospital facilities was obsolete and unevenly distributed; and wartime migrations of people from rural areas to cities, rapid population growth, and rising construction costs strained the private sector's ability to make needed improvements. In response, Congress enacted the Hospital Survey and Construction Act of 1946, as discussed in Chapter 6, a two-part law that provided funds for states to:

> (1) inventory their existing hospitals, to survey the need for construction of hospitals, and to develop programs for construction of such public and other non-profit hospitals as well, in conjunction with existing facilities, afford the necessary physical facilities for furnishing adequate hospitals, clinics, and similar services to all people, and (2) construct public and other non-profit hospitals in accordance with such programs (15).

The avowed purpose of the program was to eliminate shortages of hospitals, particularly in the nation's rural and economically depressed regions. This objective was incorporated in the formula devised to allocate funds among the states and, within the states, in the fixed bed/population ratios used to identify underserved areas. Over its more than 20 years of operation, the program was successful in distributing construction funds to hospitals, and as the shortage of hospital beds diminished, the act was repeatedly amended to extend its benefits to hospital modernization and replacement, and later to neighborhood health centers and emergency rooms. Additionally, the idea that increasing the number of hospitals in rural areas would entice physicians to locate there appears in retrospect to have had at least some validity (16).

The record of the Hill-Burton program in planning and inducing coordination among hospitals is less favorable, however. The program was administered in each state by an agency of state government assisted by an advisory Hospital Planning Council typically composed of hospital administrators and representatives of trade associations and local government agencies. These councils reviewed applications for grants and provided other assistance. In view of their members' ties to the industry, one would not have expected them to be vigorous proponents of major changes and, even if they had been so, Hill-Burton agencies faced other problems that limited their ability to plan and coordinate. Initially, they were given few resources with which to plan. Consequently, their decisions on whether to award grants to particular applicant hospitals were often made without the benefit of well-formulated guidelines (17). Furthermore, agencies' purviews encompassed only a minority of the nation's hospitals, and their authority to enforce compliance with plans was strictly circumscribed. An applicant whose request for assistance was denied was free to engage in construction projects using funds from other sources, and those who were either ineligible for subsidies or chose not to apply for them were outside the agency's control altogether.

Despite these limitations, the program provided states with at least some experience in planning hospital facilities and dealing with the difficult problems of defining and estimating the population's need for hospital beds. The replacement of the bed/population formula by a more sensitive indicator of need represented an important advance in the techniques of planning, and the grants for research and demonstration programs authorized in 1964 stimulated investigation into a variety of issues pertaining to the structure and dynamics of hospitals.

By the early 1970s, however, history had reversed itself: The problem of shortages of hospital beds had been eclipsed by concerns about their oversupply. Hence, Hill-Burton's *raison d'être* evaporated, as had its focal role of planning with the establishment of the Regional Medical Programs and Comprehensive Health Planning Program in the mid-1960s. In 1974, the Hill-Burton authority was allowed to expire, and its few remaining functions were incorporated in the National Health Planning and Resources Development Act.

Regional Medical Programs

Among the enduring problems of the American health services industry has been the variation in the quality of health services rendered in medical research and teaching centers versus that provided by community-based practitioners. Once licensed upon completion of their training, physicians find it difficult and have few incentives to stay abreast of new discoveries and improved techniques. Medical schools, in turn, have had little contact with community-based providers. Throughout this century, the gap has widened as specialization has accelerated the growth of medical knowledge (18).

To remedy this situation, Congress enacted in 1965 an amendment to the Public Health Service Act intended, among other purposes, to "encourage and assist in the establishment of regional cooperative arrangements among medical schools, research institutions, and hospitals, for research and training (including continuing education) and related demonstrations of patient care" (19). The law was an outgrowth of a report by the President's Commission on Heart Disease, Cancer, and Stroke, which had been empaneled to make recommendations regarding the control and treatment of these three dreaded diseases (20). Upon completion of its task, the commission envisioned the establishment of regional centers through which advanced technology would be channeled to communities from research and training institutions, and where services would be delivered and community-based physicians informed of new techniques through continuing education.

The amendment, however, authorized considerably less than the commission had recommended. The program was essentially stripped of its services-providing authority and was thereby transformed primarily into a grants-in-aid program (21). Powerful interest groups, particularly the American Medical Association, opposed the federal government's sponsoring centers, which would compete with local practitioners in the practice of medicine. Hence, the compromises required to attain passage led to a program that was to coordinate services without interfering with existing patterns of health services delivery.

The Regional Medical Programs Act was implemented by Regional Advisory Groups (RAGs) established in 56 regions. Composed of representatives of medical schools, teaching hospitals, state and local health departments, private practitioners, and the general public, RAGs were charged with devising plans and authorizing expenditures of federal grant monies for innovative programs. Thus, the Regional Medical Programs were to enhance coordination and integration of health services through a voluntary, pluralistic mechanism that transferred decision making from the federal government to the 56 RAGs, which were dominated by the interests of providers, particularly those of the medical schools and teaching hospitals. Although most of the regions included portions of various states, state governments were given no role in the program's implementation or funding.

Because the substance of Regional Medical Programs was left within broad limits to local determination, considerable variation occurred in their structures and activities. In consequence, as Glaser notes (22), it became increasingly difficult over time to characterize the program's national purposes (23). The RAGs stimulated federally funded demonstrations of a variety of innovations, including continuing education for physicians and training for ancillary personnel. However, no overlapping plans appeared in any of the 56 regions. When other local planning agencies began to be established pursuant to the Partnership for Health Amendments of 1967, the Regional Medical Programs' stated goals shifted from concern with specific diseases to the promotion of comprehensive health services. Federal monies were then made available through the programs for several types of system-oriented demonstrations, prominent among which were efforts to develop and improve emergency medical services (24). In Glaser's words, "the Regional Medical Programs became an effort to obtain federal money for worthy projects rather than a disciplined system for framing and implementing plans" (22).

Because the Regional Medical Programs Act was popular among the nation's medical schools and teaching hospitals, it was able to withstand the Nixon administration's attempts to abolish it. However, in 1974 the program was swept with Hill-Burton and other planning efforts under the umbrella National Health Planning and Resources Development Act, and shortly thereafter the Regional Medical Programs became extinct.

The Comprehensive Health Planning Program

Although the federal government had attempted to promote planning and coordination of health services through Hill-Burton and the Regional Medical Programs, it had used categorical approaches. Hill-Burton dealt only with construction of and planning for facilities; the Regional Medical Programs ostensibly concentrated, at least at the outset, on particular diseases. No agency had responsibility for overall, comprehensive health planning. Only 1 year after enactment of the Regional Medical Programs legislation, Congress moved to fill this void. The instrument was to be a network of voluntary comprehensive health planning agencies with mandates to develop long-range, statewide, and local plans for environmental as well as personal health services.

As with the Regional Medical Programs, Comprehensive Health Planning (CHP) legislation was preceded by a report of a national commission that called for more sweeping roles and powers than were ultimately incorporated in the authorizing statute (25). *Planning* was defined as an "action process" in which councils would not only devise blueprints but would also take steps to implement their plans. Based on a careful and extensive study of health service needs and through the exercise of their pluralistic influence, councils were to effect major and permanent changes in health services delivery (25).

However, legislation authorizing the CHP program, as with the Regional Medical Programs before it, specified that planning was to be accomplished without interfering with the prevailing patterns of medical practice. This constraint and the absence of any regulatory authority over health services institutions left CHP agencies created under the act devoid of official powers to pursue "active planning" as defined by the National Commission on Community Health Services. In effect, these agencies were given the mandate to develop plans but were prevented from implementing them.

CHP was organized in two layers. Each participating state established a statewide—CHP(a)—agency to oversee planning throughout the state. At the local level, areawide—CHP(b)—agencies were responsible for planning within designated regions. Plans developed by these so-called *b* agencies were to be reviewed by the umbrella *a* agency and incorporated in its statewide plan.

Unlike the Regional Medical Programs, CHP was structured as a cooperative effort of the federal and state governments and local areas rather than as a direct federal-to-local decentralization. Moreover, the Partnership for Health Amendments reflected the policy of encouraging maximum feasible participation that was incorporated in much of the social legislation of the 1960s. CHP(a) agencies were to be advised by councils with a membership of at least 51% consumers. Similarly, CHP(b) agencies were to be voluntary corporations with equivalently constituted boards. To preserve local autonomy, CHP agencies were funded by formula grants in which federal monies were to be augmented by contributions from states and localities, which were divided about evenly (26).

It is generally agreed that CHP agencies were unable to accomplish all of their intended aims. Although empirical data on improvements in health levels, health care costs, and the like attributable to CHP planning are virtually nonexistent (27), observations accumulated since 1967 on the organization and process of planning at various sites suggest that CHP was structurally, fiscally, and politically unable to bring about the kinds of changes that are required to affect significantly major trends in the costs, quality, and accessibility of health services (28). Few statewide or areawide agencies were able to develop long-range plans; most lacked the resources to gather information to develop them, and few had the power to enforce compliance with their recommendations. As a result, CHP agencies existed on the fringes of the major forces that shape the nation's health services industry. They attempted to plan in a turbulent and recalcitrant environment, while the power to act remained in the hands of institutions and associations that comprised their memberships and provided local funds.

During the late 1960s and early 1970s, CHP agencies began to acquire advisory roles in federal and state regulatory processes. In keeping with its New Federalism policy, the Nixon administration delegated to CHP agencies the function of review-ing and commenting on requests for federal Public Health Service grants by institu-tions within their jurisdictions. Also, several states assigned advisory roles to CHP agencies in their implementation of certificate of need controls (29). However, for the most part, CHP agencies continued to practice consensus planning, lacking the clout to move forcefully to the implementation stage. Moreover, by the early 1970s, it had become apparent to officials in the Nixon administration that federal agencies engaged in planning had become as confused as the health services industry itself. On that point, the then Secretary of the Department of Health, Education, and Welfare remarked:

> . . . six years ago, the federal government attempted to systematize and bolster planning efforts by creating and funding state and local comprehensive health agen-cies [sic]. Today, all states and territories have comprehensive health planning agen-cies. And more than 170 local and areawide agencies now serve about 70 percent of the nation's population.
>
> But from their inception, these agencies have been underfunded and under-staffed. Even more pertinent, they haven't had any real authority to coordinate planning. They have served principally as advisory groups and, while some can claim successes here and there, for the most part, their advice has been ignored.
>
> Thus we see a planning system in which, as with its operational counterpart, interrelationships among functions are very poorly thought out—if any real thought has even been given to the possibility of interrelationships—and which is thus hopelessly confusing and sometimes duplicative and overlapping.
>
> It is, again, a "non-system" incapable of either rationally identifying shortfalls or gaps in performance or of rationally addressing needs (30).

Dedicated to the elimination of programs that did not work and to streamlining of the federal bureaucracy (31), the Nixon administration had sought to combine the Regional Medical Programs and the CHP program under a single authority. Its proposal, submitted to Congress as the National Health Care Improvement Act of 1970, had failed, leaving these programs intact as separate entities. The consolida-tion was ultimately accomplished with the enactment of the National Health Plan-ning and Resources Development Act of 1974, when CHP gave way to a more vigorous form of planning linked to regulatory controls.

The Experimental Health Services Delivery Program

The federally sponsored health services planning programs previously described shared an important feature: The principal impetus behind each was the federal government's recognition of deficiencies within the health services industry. By the late 1960s, however, other elements were becoming sources of concern to the fed-eral government, namely, the "bureaucracy problem" (32) and the rapidly escalat-ing health care costs stemming from the Medicare and Medicaid programs. Hence, several problems within the health services industry were increasingly being attrib-uted to the federal government's involvement. Such recognitions gave rise to yet another planning effort, the Experimental Health Services Delivery System (EHSDS) program.

The EHSDS program grew out of attempts to reorganize the internal affairs of the federal bureaucracy and its dealings with local communities. Beginning with the Johnson administration's War on Poverty in the early 1960s and continuing throughout the decade, Congress enacted a landslide of health legislation that vastly increased the federal government's administrative responsibilities (33). Characteristically, programs bypassed the states, going directly to targeted areas in which local groups dealt directly with federal agencies (34,35). A variety of demonstration authorities had established health centers for the impoverished—first under the Office of Economic Opportunity and, later, others under the Partnership for Health Programs—migrant workers' health centers, maternal and infant care centers, mental health centers, and Model Cities health clinics. All were supported with federal funds administered by newly created or expanded federal agencies (18).

Several of these agencies were brought together in 1968 under the administration of the newly created Health Services and Mental Health Administration (HSMHA). Established as part of a general reorganization of the health activities of the Department of Health, Education, and Welfare (36), HSMHA's nine agencies and fiscal year 1970 budget of $1.3 billion made it one of the three largest federal organizations concerned exclusively with health and health services (37–39).

Impressive as the scope of activities subsumed under HSMHA was, the creation of the agency by no means solved all the problems of disorganization among the federal government's health programs. Most of the government's health effort, as measured by budgets, remained with other agencies (e.g., Medicare and Medicaid), and each of HSMHA's programs operated under congressional authorizations that defined at least in general terms how their appropriations were to be allocated. HSMHA was not an integrated agency with a set of well-ordered priorities or the ability to combine the budgets and personnel of its member programs. It was, rather, a confederation of programs, each with its own purposes, procedures, constituencies, and interests (40).

The need to transform HSMHA's disparate functions and programs into a coherent whole gave impetus to ideas that ultimately led to the EHSDS program. A solution that emerged was the notion of *conjoint funding*: HSMHA programs were to increase their efficiency by working together and, more importantly, by pooling their resources and delegating allocative decisions to local groups.

Within HSMHA, the National Center for Health Services Research and Development (NCHSR&D) was designated as the lead agency to develop the EHSDS program. NCHSR&D was a newly established agency whose principal mission was to provide grants and contracts for research into and development of health services (41). The agency came to view EHSDS as the ultimate embodiment of rationality and as a mechanism for bringing together various innovations being developed and tested under its grants and contracts (42). In selected states and communities, systemwide planning based on research and development was to combine with the rational allocation of funds by local management agencies, that is, EHSDS corporations. These funds were to be channeled from various federal agencies directly to the management corporations, thus eliminating federal agencies' direct administrative involvement in determining the uses of federal monies in local communities.

To accomplish these aims, in 1971 NCHSR&D established 12 EHSDS corporations scattered throughout the United States, and six others were added the following year. Like CHP (b) agencies, EHSDS corporations were voluntary, nonprofit corporations. Unlike the *b* agencies, however, boards of EHSDS corporations were mandated to include representatives of four interest groups (the "four Ps")—public, providers, payors (i.e., insurance companies and government agencies), and politicians—in proportions such that no group constituted a majority.

While EHSDS members could also participate on CHP and Regional Medical Program boards, the EHSDS corporations were to remain distinct from these and other agencies. NCHSR&D developed a triangular model of the division of labor among Regional Medical Programs, CHP, and EHSDS bodies. Regional Medical Programs were seen as instruments of providers to develop and test innovations in the delivery of health services. CHP agencies would, in turn, incorporate these ideas in their long range plans and communicate to the Regional Medical Programs the issues that planners deemed important for research and development. EHSDS bodies would then incorporate these priorities in their shorter term investment decisions. In sum, NCHSR&D envisioned a network of cooperative and mutually facilitating exchanges among the three planning and coordinating bodies.

As the EHSDS experiment proceeded, none of the prerequisites required for its full implementation materialized. Each EHSDS site was given 2 years to charter a conforming corporate body and to conduct community surveys and other studies with which to establish priorities. Meanwhile, NCHSR&D and HSMHA endeavored to conjoin funds of HSMHA and other federal agencies and to deliver these to EHSDS corporations. No such conjoining occurred, however. As might have been expected, other HSMHA agencies resisted NCHSR&D's urgings to delegate funding decisions to EHSDS bodies and declined even to give EHSDS communities priority claims upon their funds. In consequence, the principal functions of the EHSDS corporations were vitiated, and their activities became increasingly indistinguishable locally from those of CHP and Regional Medical Programs. Instead of mutual cooperation and coordination, conflict and duplication characterized the triangle of agencies. On this point, in 1974 the acting associate director for health resources planning of the Bureau of Health Resources Development observed that the EHSDS experiment demonstrated that communities will accept federal funds when they are offered and will engage in conflict when competing programs are established (43).

While the EHSDS experiment failed to attain its principal objectives, it introduced a new element into the evolving debate about health planning that had reemerged in the early 1970s, and it contributed valuable experience to the body of planning methods. The experiment's focus on implementation and systemwide management of conjoined federal funds—although none were forthcoming—was in marked contrast to the long range perspectives of CHP and the narrower categorical interests of the Regional Medical Programs. Also, EHSDS's emphasis upon linking decisions to thorough empirical research on communities' health services needs and use patterns and their flows of health services monies was notably different from the paucity of such information in most CHP agencies. Indeed, the vision of regional health authorities not unlike those in the United Kingdom, which underlay the EHSDS ideology, anticipated by several years the contemporary debate about the roles of current planning agencies in gathering and analyzing data and in implementing regulatory controls.

The experiment never gained the support of officials in the Nixon administration, who in 1973 ordered its termination. Lacking explicit legislative authorization, the EHSDS program thus died within the bureaucracy, causing little comment. With Hill-Burton and the two other sides of the planning/innovation-management triangle, EHSDS corporations closed their doors shortly after the enactment of PL 93-641.

The National Health Planning and Resources Development Act of 1974

By the close of the 1960s, it had become apparent that the collection of planning activities scattered among the several existing programs was unable to deal with the mounting costs of health care and other problems of the health services industry. Congress responded by enacting the National Health Planning and Resources Development Act of 1974 (PL 93-641), which consolidated most of the functions and powers of the existing programs in a single planning structure. The new program preserved the basic participatory logic of the CHP program while greatly enlarging the responsibilities of the federal and state governments. It also, for the first time, assigned a variety of regulatory functions to health planning agencies, the most prominent being capital expenditures and services review authority. In this section, we describe the organization of the planning structure and discuss some of the issues it has raised.

The organizational structure mandated by PL 93-641 builds upon and modifies that of the CHP program that it succeeded (44). Like CHP, the current program is built upon a local agency, the Health Systems Agency (HSA). These HSAs are chartered as nonprofit corporations or local government agencies with boards composed of representatives of several interest groups, including consumers, health services providers, local government officials, and others. To ensure representation of minority groups, the law explicitly requires HSA boards to include minority group members in proportion to their numbers in their regions. At the state level, PL 93-641 created State Health Planning and Development Agencies (SHPDAs). These units are agencies of state governments, as were the CHP(a) agencies they replaced.

Two new groups were added to the planning structure. Within the states, State Health Coordinating Committees (SHCCs) were created to advise SHPDAs. These SHCCs are composed of representatives of the states' HSAs and other persons appointed by state governors. At the federal level, the law established a National Health Planning Council to advise the Secretary of Health and Human Services on the national health planning goals, guidelines, and standards that the secretary is directed to formulate and disseminate.

Each of the agencies and advisory groups established by PL 93-641 is charged with specific functions and authorities within the overall planning network (45). HSAs produce Health Systems Plans and Annual Implementation Plans for their respective Health Services Areas. The former incorporate HSAs' long range recommendations regarding numbers and types of health care facilities, services, and manpower. The latter are formulations of shorter range strategies for implementing components of Health Systems Plans. In addition, HSAs review and make recommendations regarding the issuance of certificates of need and proposed uses of federal grant funds in their areas, and they are directed to review periodically the appropriateness of the facilities that serve the populations within their jurisdictions. At the state level, the SHPDA develops State Health Plans and State Medical Facilities Plans and exercises final decision-making authority for the granting of certificates of need. The preliminary statewide plans produced by SHPDAs are supposed to reflect the recommendations embodied in HSAs' plans. With advice from the SHCC, the SHPDA then produces its own plans. Finally, the entire planning network is overseen by the Secretary of Health and Human Services. Day-to-day direction is provided by the department's Bureau of Health Planning and Resources Development, and the National Health Planning Council is consulted on larger policy issues pertaining to national health planning goals and guidelines.

The program is funded by federal formula grants that allow for additional federal matching of funds contributed by state and local governments and other permissible donors. The latter excludes named groups and organizations whose contributions might be construed as constituting conflicts of interest (e.g., individual hospitals).

The planning and regulatory program mandated by PL 93-641 is considerably more explicit with respect to goals and functions and immeasurably more complex structurally than earlier planning programs. Experience has proved that it is more controversial as well. Since its inception, the program has been the subject of debate, often leading to litigation. Many of the controversies have centered on the program's regulatory authorities, which will be discussed later in this chapter. Others have stemmed from structural issues, particularly those dealing with intergovernmental relations and the participatory structure mandated for HSAs.

Because PL 93-641 promised to exercise greater authority over the organization and financing of health care than had earlier planning efforts, it attracted greater interest among federal and state officials regarding the issue of who would control planning agencies and functions. These considerations led to extensive debate during initial congressional hearings (46) and subsequently surfaced during the program's implementation and reauthorization amendments. State and local officials were concerned about the extensive powers granted to the Secretary of Health and Human Services. These included such responsibilities as approving governors' designations of Health Services Areas, reviewing and approving the composition of HSA boards, defining the formats and contents of state and areawide plans, and formulating national planning goals and guidelines. These provisions led several states to test the program's constitutionality. Several governors who found portions of their states being joined in HSAs with parts of other states challenged the secretary's authority to define Health Service Areas. Some joined the American Medical Association and other parties in suits alleging that the law's regulatory provisions violated constitutional guarantees of states' rights. Still others brought suit to enjoin the secretary from interfering in the determination of the composition of HSA and SCHCC boards. In these early challenges the courts ruled consistently in favor of the provisions of PL 93-641, both on constitutional matters and on specific authorities granted to the Secretary of Health and Human Services (47). However, the flood of dissenting comments evoked by the secretary's issuance of the first set of planning guidelines in 1978 (48) was a clear indication of the extent of dissatisfaction with what many regarded as an overly centralized planning structure. This mood was, in turn, reflected in the 1979 amendments to PL 93-641, which placed greater control over health planning in the hands of state governors (49).

A second major organizational issue stems from the compositional requirements of PL 93-641 and the theory of interest group participation that underlies them. As noted earlier, PL 93-641 preserved the notion of participatory health planning that was embodied in CHP. Moreover, PL 93-641 took elaborate precautions to ensure that consumer representatives would control the planning process. HSAs were required by law not only to be governed by consumer majorities but also to include particular categories of consumers on their boards, namely, the poor and ethnic, racial, and linguistic minorities. These requirements greatly complicated the task of developing organizations and, in the opinion of several critics, perpetuated the erroneous conception of the consumer as a proponent of cost control (50,51). Several observers have noted that consumer members of HSA boards, especially representatives of minority groups, are likely to join providers in supporting the growth of new services and facilities, thereby diverting health planning from its cost-controlling mission (52).

Differences in states' orientations and the composition of agencies, along with the broad and ambiguous purposes of the planning program, have given rise to the great diversity of emphases and procedures among the programs. Some are aimed primarily at developing the various plans required by PL 93-641, while others emphasize their regulatory responsibilities (53,54). The resulting heterogeneity precludes the possibility of making generalizations about either the activities or the effects of health planning per se. It would appear, however, that the program is in jeopardy due to changes in the larger national political mood. By the late 1970s, health care cost containment had become the nation's most visible health issue. Accordingly, efforts such as PL 93-641 increasingly came to be evaluated in terms of their ability to control increases in health care expenditures. The 1980 elections brought to power a presidential administration firmly convinced that planning and regulation could not effectively deter rising costs and dedicated to repealing PL 93-641. As of the early 1980s, the program remains in force, albeit with fewer resources and less political support than it enjoyed at its inception (55).

ORIGINS AND DEVELOPMENT
OF HEALTH SERVICES REGULATION

It was noted at the outset of this chapter that regulation includes a variety of instruments by which government induces or compels persons to engage in (or refrain from) behaviors that promote (or are injurious to) some aspect of the public interest or general welfare. The objectives pursued through regulation embrace a large and growing set of socially desirable ends, including directing the development of entire industries and sectors of the economy and protecting persons from a host of hazards accompanying modern life (56,2). The means available to government to pursue such ends are nearly limitless, ranging from subsidies provided either indirectly through tax policies or directly through cash transfers to direct command and control mechanisms enforced by a variety of legal and economic sanctions (56). Further, the types of agencies involved in the implementation of regulatory programs defy simple enumeration. All branches of government—legislative, executive, and judicial—are directly implicated (57), and in many instances basically private bodies are enlisted in governments' regulatory efforts.

In view of this complexity, one cannot hope to comprehend all forms of regulation in the United States or even in a single sector of the economy (58). Accordingly, the discussion that follows is selective, highlighting the general features of and trends in regulation rather than attempting to describe comprehensively the highly fluid and uncertain regulatory environment surrounding the health services industry.

Specifically, the origins and development of three types of regulation that have recently been imposed upon the health services industry are examined: 1) capital expenditures and services (CES) controls, 2) use review as practiced by the Professional Standards Review Organizations (PSROs), and 3) prospective rate setting applied to hospitals and nursing homes. Each of these programs is intended, *inter alia*, to contain health care cost inflation, and each contributes an ingredient to a whole that approximates public utility regulation as applied in other industries.

Objects of Regulation

	Individuals	Institutions

Subsidies	Supply
	    Training grants
	
	Demand
	    Medicare / Medicaid
	    Tax exemptions
		Supply
		    Construction grants, loans,
		    loan guarantees
		    Tax exemptions
		Demand
		    Tax exemptions to
		    employers

Entry Restrictions	Personnel licensure	Facilities licensure Capital expenditures controls

Rate
Controls
	Fee schedules under
	    Medicaid & the Economic
	    Stabilization Program
		Rate setting commissions
		Medicare and Medicaid
		reimbursement limits

Quality Controls	Professional Standards Review Organization	Certification for Medicare and Medicaid

(Regulatory Instruments — row axis label)

Figure 12-1. A typology of regulatory instruments and examples from the health services industry.

Before proceeding to these particular forms of regulation, the principal types of regulation are briefly described and illustrated.

Types of Regulation

In the interest of simplicity, Figure 12–1 is presented to categorize roughly and illustrate the types of regulatory instruments that are operative in the health services industry. The four fundamental instruments in the rows of the figure are 1) subsidies, 2) entry controls, 3) rate or price setting, and 4) quality controls. The columns classify objects of regulation as natural and corporate persons.

Subsidies are generally the oldest and most widespread means employed by governments to regulate the supply of and demand for health services. These subsidies take many forms. On the supply side, governments have conferred a tax exempt status upon voluntary, nonprofit hospitals and nursing homes and have provided them with direct grants, loans, and loan guarantees for construction, renovation, and modernization. Likewise, governments support the training of health services professionals and the conduct of health-related research and development, and have made available construction subsidies to institutions that engage in training and research. On the demand side, tax credits offered to employees and employers defray the costs of health insurance; also, above specified limits, individuals' health care expenditures are exempt from the personal income tax. Governments also act as third parties for the aged under Medicare, for the impoverished under Medicaid, and increasingly for persons receiving treatment for chronic, catastrophic diseases (e.g., end-stage renal disease).

Ordinarily, subsidy programs are accompanied by administrative regulations that define eligibility criteria, specify the legitimate uses of subsidies, and increasingly define terms of trade. Examples of the last are provisions of the Hill-Burton program requiring hospitals to provide specified volumes of free care in return for government grants, and sections of personnel training legislation that establish for medical schools target mixes of types of physicians to be educated and trainees' forgiveness clauses. Furthermore, it should be noted that the principle that there is no free lunch applies to all subsidy programs and, under current fiscal constraints, increasingly so. That is, eligibility requirements and definitions of the scope of goods and services covered by subsidy programs often entail for both givers and receivers considerable administrative costs in the forms of paperwork and red tape (59).

Entry controls apply to producers, generally seeking to limit their ability to offer particular goods or services to those who have satisfied at least minimal tests of competence or character or to those whose products are needed in their communities. In the case of health personnel and facilities, these controls take the familiar forms of licensure and certification. More pertinent to the discussion below, capital expenditures and services controls are applied to health care institutions to assure the public that offerings of health services are in balance with communities' needs.

Rate- or price-setting powers are usually assumed by governments as a quid pro quo for protection afforded producers in markets that are subject to mandated entry restrictions or in industries where government is the dominant (i.e., monopsonistic) purchaser of their outputs. The former rationale is applied most purely in so-called natural monopolistic markets, such as the production and distribution of electrical power and local telephone services. In these and similar situations, where a sole producer is optimally efficient, governments protect monopolies from competition by restricting entry and, in turn, protect the public from the monopolies by controlling their rates and the quality of their products. The latter rationale—that of the government monopsony—appears to underlie the imposition of price controls in the health services industry, even where governments are not the principal purchasers of its services. In the inpatient sector of the industry, such controls are universally applied by states to nursing homes, and various combinations of voluntary and state-mandated rate-setting efforts are imposed on hospitals in about a dozen states.

The category of quality controls includes various regulatory mechanisms aimed at reducing dangerous risks and other socially undesirable practices associated with the product or consumption of goods and services. This class is frequently labeled *social regulation,* as opposed to *economic regulation,* which embraces the other types of controls described above (60,2). Especially important in social regulation are efforts to eliminate hazards in workplaces, environmental pollution, and other so-called external costs of production, and to ensure the safety and efficacy of consumer goods and services. These controls differ from entry restrictions, some of which attempt to assure quality, in that they apply to all designated suppliers whether or not they exist in markets with entry controls. In the health services industry, for instance, hospitals, like all other firms, must comply with construction and fire codes, fair employment rules, and environmental pollution standards. Further, the Food and Drug Administration's reviews of the safety of drug products and PSROs' scrutiny of physicians' practices are intended, respectively, to assure consumers that the drugs they ingest and the medical services they receive are not injurious to their health or proffered fraudulently.

Having covered a great deal of the regulatory apparatus that affects portions of the health services industry, we can now focus on features of the structure and financing of hospital services that have prompted the imposition of entry restrictions and quality and price controls.

The Bases of Controls on Hospitals

Hospitals are the principal targets of regulatory programs, as discussed in Chapter 6, aimed at controlling health care cost inflation (61). This situation may be due to the hospital industry's large and growing share of the nation's health care expenditures. It accounts for about 40% of the total and has been increasing annually at a rate of approximately 15%. It may also reflect tradition and political forces. As discussed previously, it follows that controls on hospitals would be the first to appear. It is also the case, as noted in Chapter 6, that hospitals have historically been a less potent political force than physicians and, therefore, are correspondingly more vulnerable to government intervention. Alternatively, if one takes the view that regulatory controls—particularly entry restrictions—are sought by industries to thwart competition, it might be argued that physicians' greater power was exercised earlier in this century in the establishment of their cartel and that hospitals have only recently been able to accomplish this feat (28). Regardless of one's conception of the origins of regulation, the fact remains that the newest forms of regulation concentrate on hospitals.

The principal problem that has stimulated regulation of hospitals is cost inflation attributable to inefficiencies in the industry. Basically, two related arguments are advanced: 1) hospitals overinvest in sophisticated and expensive services, and 2) such services are overused by the population (62). The overinvestment and overuse, in turn, result in unnecessary expenditures for health services that contribute wastefully to cost inflation.

Recalling the earlier comments on the structure and financing of the health services industry, several features of the market for inpatient hospital services appear to warrant regulation. Specifically, assuming consumer ignorance, four features combine to justify regulation: 1) the nonprofit status of most hospitals, 2) their relationships with community-based physicians, 3) the so-called Roemer Law (more generally, the availability effect), and 4) insurance.

The hospital industry is dominated by multiproduct, nonprofit firms whose investment and output decisions are amalgams of interests of their communities, lay boards of trustees, management, and medical staffs. Because hospitals must be responsive to the demands of these various constituencies, their investment decisions reflect considerations other than profit maximization. Among the various objectives attributed to hospitals by economists are prestige and status (63), the quality and quantity of services produced (64), and social welfare (65). While all such specifications are conceived as being subject to the constraint that revenues must cover costs, all of them imply that nonprofit hospitals' investment and output decisions do not conform to the model of a pure profit maximizer.

Related to these observations is the argument that hospitals' investment and output decisions are strongly influenced by physicians' preferences (66,67). Because physicians select both the hospitals for their patients and the mix of services patients receive, they exert pressures on hospitals to provide the types of amounts of facilities, services, and support personnel that they desire. These pressures join with competition among hospitals for prestige to encourage investment in expansion and, more importantly, in upgrading styles of care (68). Moreover, the role of the physician as both an advocate for the patient and an entrepreneur invites con-flicts of interest that apparently are frequently resolved in favor of the entrepre-neurial segment (69). As physicians' incomes are enhanced by their use of hospital services, whose costs are paid by insurance, one would expect them to give little attention to hospital cost inflation (70).

The availability effect observed in the hospital industry protects the hospital from losses due to investment in facilities and services for which demand is low (68). In effect, this phenomenon implies that the availability of health services stimulates their use. Hence, within limits, hospitals can expand their capacity and services with the assurance that additional beds will be filled and services will be used.

Insurance for hospital services affects hospital investment in two ways. First, the coverage of inpatient services, which typically is more extensive than the ser-vices rendered in ambulatory care settings, shifts patients into hospitals, where, due to low deductibles and coinsurance rates, patients pay out-of-pocket only a small portion of their charges. Patients are therefore relatively indifferent to the costs incurred at the time of treatment. Second, retrospective cost-based reimbursement schemes protect hospitals from losses that might otherwise occur from poor invest-ment decisions. Together, the assurances of high cash flows due to the availability effect and insurance and the guaranteed retroactive payment of costs (including debt service) place hospitals in favored positions in the capital market (71,72). This situation, in turn, facilitates more investment. The three types of regulation dis-cussed next are intended to rectify the consequences of these structural and financial characteristics.

Capital Expenditures and Services Controls

Capital expenditures and services (CES) controls attempt to eliminate unnecessary investment in expansion of capacity and to halt offerings of new services that are deemed to duplicate existing ones (73,74). To the extent that this situation occurs, needless expenditures for health services will be averted by preventing initial outlays for construction, renovation, and new equipment and avoiding future oper-ating costs. Proponents of CES regulation point to two indicators of unnecessary expenditures: excess capacity and inappropriate use. Excess capacity, as evidenced by empty hospital beds and idle equipment and services, is taken to be an obvious sign of overinvestment and a portion of the hospital's fixed costs as an indication of unnecessary expenditures. Also, expenditures for inpatient services are considered to be unnecessarily high when patients' problems are viewed as amenable to treat-ment in less expensive ambulatory care settings and, for patients who require hospi-talization, when less expensive combinations of diagnostic and therapeutic services could be substituted for more costly ones.

These controls are mandated by state certificate of need (CON) and the feder-ally sponsored Section 1122 program. Both attempt to attain equilibrium between supplies of and needs for services by requiring hospital plans for major capital investments and offerings of new services to be certified by regulatory agencies as needed in their communities. State CON statutes typically levy legal sanctions against institutions that either fail to seek certificates or proceed with their plans after certificates have been denied. The Section 1122 program employs only financial sanctions: Institutions that implement plans that have not received prior authorization are denied reimbursement for costs associated with their investments (e.g., interest payments) by the Medicare, Medicaid, and Maternal and Infant Care programs. Because PL 93-641 initially required states to adopt CON laws by 1980 in order to qualify for various grants-in-aid from the U.S. Public Health Service, it is likely that this more stringent form of CES regulation will soon blanket the nation.

CES programs are administered by agencies created by the National Health Planning and Resources Development Act of 1974. The review process is initiated when a hospital submits a proposal for a major capital investment or a significant change in its services to its local HSA. This body determines whether there is a need for the proposed project and transmits its recommendation to the SHCC and the SHPDA. Based on its review and the recommendations from the HSA and SHCC, the SHPDA decides whether to issue or deny a certificate (75,76).

Research on the impact of CES controls has shown that they have not had significant effects on the costs of health care, although they may have limited the growth of some types of expensive technologies. One study of CON programs in force before 1974 found that these programs had no effect on overall investment by hospitals but may have altered its composition (77,78). Specifically, findings indicated that rates of increase in the number of hospital beds were lower in states with CON programs, while increases in other forms of investment (e.g., new equipment, modernization) were higher. Studies of experience after the enactment of PL 93-641 have not revealed any appreciable effects of CES regulation on the growth of hospital beds, total investment, or expenditures for hospital services (79,80). Some evidence suggests, however, the CES controls may have prevented hospitals from acquiring particular types of technology such as cobalt and radium therapy (81), open heart surgery and renal dialysis (82), and computed tomography scanners (83).

Professional Standards Review Organizations

The soaring costs of Medicare and Medicaid prompted Congress to enact in 1972 sweeping reforms in these programs' reimbursement procedures. Among the amendments attached to the Social Security Act by PL 92-603 were provisions establishing PSROs, discussed also in Chapter 13. These organizations were

> to promote the effective, efficient, and economical delivery of health care services of proper quality for which payment may be made (in whole or in part) under this Act and in recognition of the interests of patients, the public, practitioners, and providers in improved health care services, it is the purpose of this part to assure, through the application of suitable procedures of professional standards review, that the Social Security Act will conform to appropriate professional standards for the provision of health care (84).

The clear intent of the statute was to curtail overuse and excessive costs of inpatient hospital services by subjecting physicians' admitting and treatment decisions to reviews by colleagues. For this purpose, PSROs composed of local physicians were created throughout the nation. These bodies were to establish standards of medical care for categories of health problems, develop profiles of individual physicians' practices, and monitor the inpatient services they provide or order for beneficiaries of the Medicare, Medicaid, and Maternal and Infant Care programs (85). Failing this test, the federal government withholds payment to the offending physician for the unnecessary services and levies more severe financial penalties on repeating and fraudulent offenders.

At the federal level, a National PSRO Council was empaneled to review local PSROs' standards and to advise the Secretary of Health and Human Services on the program's structure and operation.

From its inception, the PSRO program has been beset by controversy. During the legislative process, the American Medical Association mounted a ferocious, albeit belated and unsuccessful, campaign to defeat the bill. While the association endorsed the bill's delegation of responsibility and authority to its members, it was appalled by what it regarded as an unwarranted and ominous gambit that allowed the federal government to intrude directly in individual physicians' practices. Associations representing other health professions viewed the program as a government endorsement of the dominance of physicians, and spokesmen for consumers' interests saw it as a sellout akin to appointing the fox to guard the henhouse (86). Moreover, as the program has developed, its principal mission has become clouded. Physicians are inclined to view it primarily as aimed at improving the quality of health services, while advocates of the PSRO in Congress and the federal bureaucracy see it as a cost containment effort (87).

Research on the effects of the PSRO program and its predecessor prototype programs have shown that peer review may affect uses of particular types of medical services (88). However, it is unclear whether PSRO review has produced lower overall use or reduced the cost of hospital care. Studies conducted by the Department of Health and Human Services indicated that savings attributable to PSRO review more than offset the program's administrative costs (89). However, analyses produced by the Congressional Budget Office disputed these findings (55). Thus, as of the close of the 1970s, it was not clear whether the PSRO program has materially lowered hospital cost inflation.

Because PSRO has not proved its worth as a cost-containment program, it has received dwindling support. In 1979, the Carter administration threatened to withhold further federal funding; more recently, the Reagan administration has cut PSRO's budget.

Prospective Rate Setting

By the late 1960s, the impact of health care cost inflation from the Medicaid program was being felt in state legislatures. Among the several factors identified as causing the problem was the prevailing mode of paying hospitals for their services. The reimbursement scheme for the Medicare and Medicaid programs had initially been modeled after the Blue Cross procedure of retroactively paying hospitals for their costs plus a fixed percentage (90). As noted earlier, this approach to financing in combination with other features of the hospital industry reinforced its tendency toward inefficiency. To remedy this situation, regulatory programs have been established in several states that either set prospectively the rates that hospitals may charge for particular units of service or fix their overall budgets (91). The assumption behind this approach is that fixed rates or budgets will encourage hospitals to be more efficient (92). In principle, such programs reward efficient institutions by permitting them to retain revenues in excess of their costs and penalize inefficiency by placing institutions at risk for costs that exceed allowable rates or budgets.

By the late 1970s, some form of rate setting or rate review was in force in more than half of the states (93). In 1977, Congress failed to enact the Carter administration's hospital cost containment bill that would have established a national rate-setting program, thus leaving this form of regulation to the states (94). Nine states have statutorily mandated programs; those of other states are sponsored by private organizations, principally state hospital associations and Blue Cross plans.

Although the procedures by which prospective rates or budgets are set vary among programs, most of them employ comparisons among similar hospitals. Hospitals are categorized according to factors that influence costs, and the average experience of a particular group is taken as the standard for all hospitals categorized in that group. Comparisons, and units upon which prospective rates are based, include costs per diem and per stay. One state (New Jersey) has adopted average costs for the treatment of particular conditions as its unit for calculating prospective rates (see Chapter 11).

Programs mandated by state laws are generally regarded as being more stringent than those operated under private auspices. State-sponsored programs typically cover more sources of hospital revenues. They also employ more thorough and systematic procedures in setting rates and use stricter means of enforcing prospectively determined rates (95).

Evidence from evaluations of rate-setting programs indicates that they are lowering the rates of increase of per diem and per capita expenditures for hospital services (95,79). Moreover, studies have shown that prospective rate setting has lowered the rates at which hospitals acquire expensive technologies (83,96).

The apparent effectiveness of rate-setting programs prompted Congress in 1982 to adopt amendments to the Social Security Act mandating prospective payment for hospital services rendered to Medicare beneficiaries. The same legislation that allows states to experiment with novel reimbursement schemes for Medicaid beneficiaries led California to implement a prospective payment program for its MediCal recipients. It would appear that, unlike the other forms of regulation discussed in this chapter, prospective rate setting is likely to become a more significant and widespread reform.

AN ASSESSMENT OF PLANNING AND REGULATION

The comprehensive health planning and regulatory movements began in this nation in an era in which philanthropic and, later, government subsidies sought to develop health care resources and to assure their equitable and efficient deployment. Over the years, the nation took sometimes halting but compassionate steps toward the fulfillment of deeply rooted political and social values by expanding government's role as the guarantor of an elusive right to health care. It did so, however, in the characteristically American fashion of muddling through, attempting to enlarge government's functions without at the same time extending its authority. Gradually but inevitably, the country reached an impasse that became in the 1970s a rush to regulation to contain the costs of our beneficence. While our society has not abandoned the values that spawned the planning movement nearly a half century ago, the economic meanings of these ideals are painfully in view and perhaps on a collision course with the growing mood of fiscal conservatism.

Equally apparent is the conflict between this nation's devotion to free enterprise as the bedrock of its economy and the widespread reliance on increasingly stringent regulatory controls (97). The federal government first embraced this politicoeconomic instrument to protect free enterprise from the abuses of monopolies (98,99). The government continues to employ controls for that purpose, but increasingly they are imposed to remedy the problems of existence and, in health care, to rectify the behavior of an industry that has enjoyed a half century of virtually unfettered subsidies. Regulation has not yet reached its intended goals in the health services industry, and the regulatory movement is now evoking its antithesis in the form of a deregulation movement.

Faced with pervasive and significant strains, people voice extreme and all-encompassing proposals for their resolution. Ideas abound in the debate about health services planning and regulation. One view holds that planning and regulation have been ineffective because we have pursued the strategy only halfheartedly with fragmented responsibilities and partial authorities. The solution, from this perspective, lies in the welding of the fragments and extending the resulting super-structure more broadly over and more deeply into the health services industry (100). At the opposite pole is the belief that planning and regulation are inherently clumsy—in Lindblom's words, "thumbs without fingers" (1)—and that they should therefore be abandoned in favor of other incentives that would unleash latent market forces (101,102).

By the beginning of the 1980s, the latter view had gained considerable political currency. The election of Ronald Reagan brought to the federal government an administration with a deeply rooted ideological animus toward regulation and an abiding faith in free enterprise. Devoted to trimming the federal government's budget, the Reagan administration reduced federal funds for the health planning and PSRO programs to levels that threatened their survival (55). At the same time, the administration promised to devise a health care policy that would replace current regulatory controls with market-oriented incentives.

As the specific features of market-oriented reforms have been slowly revealed, their planning and regulatory implications are unknown. It is unlikely, however, that planning and regulation will disappear altogether. Rather, responsibilities for controlling and performance of health care institutions appear to be passing back to the states and private organizations from which they originally sprang.

REFERENCES

1. Lindblom CE: *Politics and Markets: The World's Political-Economic Systems.* New York, Basic Books, 1977.

2. Weidenbaum ML: *Business, Government, and the Public.* Englewood Cliffs, NJ, Prentice-Hall Inc, 1977.

3. Blanpain J, Delesie L, Nys H: *National Health Insurance and Health Resources: The European Experience.* Cambridge, Mass, Harvard University Press, 1978.

4. Dahl RA, Lindblom CE: *Politics, Economics, and Welfare.* New York, Harper & Row Publishers Inc, 1953.

5. Bice TW, Eichhorn RL: Evaluation of public health programs, in Guttentag M, Struening EL (eds): *Handbook of Evaluation Research.* Beverly Hills, Calif, Sage Publications, 1975, vol 2, pp 605–620.

6. Breyer S: *Regulation and Its Reform.* Cambridge, Mass, Harvard University Press, 1982.

7. Okun AM: *Equality and Efficiency: The Big Tradeoff.* Washington, DC, The Brookings Institution, 1975.

8. Cohodes DR: Where you stand depends on where you sit: Musing on the regulation/competition dialogue. *J Health Polit Policy Law* 1982; 7 (Spring):54–79.

9. Fuchs VR: Health care and the United States economics system—An essay in abnormal physiology, in McKinlay JB (ed): *Economic Aspects of Health Care*. New York, Prodist, 1973, pp 57–94.

10. Bice TW, Kerwin C: Governance of regional health systems, in Saward EW (ed): *The Regionalization of Personal Health Services*. New York, Prodist, 1976, pp 61–105.

11. Palmiere D: Community health planning, in Corey L, Saltman SE, Epstein MF (eds): *Medicine in a Changing Society*. St Louis, CV Mosby Co, 1972, pp 59–82.

12. Klarman HE: Planning for facilities, in Ginzberg E (ed): *Regionalization and Health Policy*. Government Printing Office, 1977, pp 25–36.

13. Thompson P: Voluntary regional planning, in Ginzberg E (ed): *Regionalization and Health Policy*. Government Printing Office, 1977, pp 123–128.

14. Pearson DA: The concept of regionalized personal health services in the United States, 1920–1975, in Saward EW (ed): *The Regionalization of Personal Health Services*. New York, Prodist, 1976, pp 10–14, 5–10, 14–19.

15. Cited by May JJ: *Health Planning: Its Past and Potential*. Chicago, Center for Health Administration Studies, Perspectives No. A5, University of Chicago, 1967, p 25.

16. Lave JR, Lave LB: *The Hospital Construction Act: An Evaluation of the Hill-Burton Program, 1948–1973*. Washington, DC, American Enterprise Institute for Public Policy Research, 1974, pp 41–43.

17. Gottlieb SR: A brief history of health planning in the United States, in Havighurst CC (ed): *Regulating Health Facilities Construction*. Washington, DC, American Enterprise Institute for Public Policy Research, 1974, pp 7–26.

18. Stevens R: *American Medicine and the Public Interest*. New Haven, Conn, Yale University Press, 1971, pp 496–527.

19. Cited by Hilleboe HE, Barkhuus A: Health planning in the United States: Some categorical and general approaches. *Int J Health Serv* 1971; 1:37.

20. President's Commission on Heart Disease, Cancer and Stroke: *A National Program to Conquer Heart Disease, Cancer and Stroke*. Government Printing Office, 1964, vol 1.

21. For a comparison of the commission's recommendations and the actual provisions of the amendment, see Pollack J: Health services and the role of medical school, *Milbank Mem Fund Q/Health Society* 1968; 46(pt 2):151–152.

22. Glaser WA: Experience in health planning in the United States, mimeo. Paper prepared for the Conference on Health Planning in the United States: Past Experiences and Future Imperatives. New York, Columbia University, June 1973.

23. Bodenheimer TS: Regional medical programs: No road to regionalization. *Medical Care Review* 1969; 26:1125–1166.

24. Regional Medical Programs Service: *Selected Vignettes on Activities of Regional Medical Programs*. Health Services and Mental Health Administration, US Dept of Health, Education, and Welfare, 1971.

25. National Commission on Community Health Services: *Health Is a Community Affair*. Cambridge, Mass, Harvard University Press, 1966.

26. Comptroller General of the United States: *Comprehensive Health Planning as Carried Out by State and Areawide Agencies in Three States*. US General Accounting Office, US Congress, April 1974, p 8.

27. May's studies are a notable exception. See May JJ: *Health Planning: Its Past and Potential*. Chicago, Center of Health Administration Studies, Perspective No. A5, University of Chicago, 1967, pp 25–36.

28. Havighurst CC: Regulation of health facilities and services by "certificate of need." *Virginia Law Rev* 1973; 59:1143–1232.

29. These and other regulatory controls are discussed below.

30. Richardson EL: Address before the Institute of Medicine. Washington, DC, National Academy of Sciences, May 10, 1972.

31. Iglehart JK, Lilley W III, Clark TB: New federalism report/HEW department advances sweeping proposal to overhaul its programs. *Nat J* 1973; 6:1–10.

32. Wilson JQ: The bureaucracy problem. *Public Interest* 1967 (Winter):3–9.

33. US Congress, Senate Committee on Government Operations, Subcommittee on Executive Reorganization and Government Research: *Federal Role in Health: Report Pursuant to S Res 390.* 91st Congress, 2nd Session, S Report 91-801, 1970.

34. Sundquist JL, Davis DW: *Making Federalism Work.* Washington, DC, The Brookings Institution, 1969.

35. Liebman L: Social intervention in a democracy. *Public Interest,* 1974; 34 (Winter):14–29.

36. US Congress, House of Representatives: *Hearings Before the Subcommittee on Department of Labor and Health, Education, and Welfare and Related Agencies of the Committee on Appropriations.* 91st Congress, 1st Session, 1969, pp 426–431.

37. English JT: Mission of the Health Services and Mental Health Administration. *Public Health Rep* 1970; 85:95–99.

38. All of the planning programs discussed in this chapter were within MSMHA.

39. The Health Services and Mental Health Administration was abolished in 1973, and its agencies were divided between the present Health Services Administration and the Health Resources Administration.

40. For a more complete enumeration of such programs, see US Congress, Senate Committee on Government Operations, Subcommittee on Executive Reorganization and Government Research: *Federal Role in Health: Report Pursuant to S Res 390.* 91st Congress, 2nd Session, S Report 91-801, 1970.

41. The National Center for Health Services Research and Development is now the National Center for Health Services Research. For a description of this agency's history and current functions, see The Institute of Medicine: *Health Services Research.* Washington, DC, Institute of Medicine, National Academy of Sciences, 1979, chap 5.

42. Sanazaro PJ: Federal Health Services research and R and D under the auspices of the National Center for Health Services Research and Development, in Flook EE, Sanazaro PJ (eds): *Health Services Research and R and D in Perspective.* Ann Arbor, Mich, Health Administration Press, 1973, pp 150–183.

43. Rubel EJ: Testimony before the US Congress, House of Representatives, Committee on Interstate and Foreign Commerce, Subcommittee on Public Health and Environment. *Hearings on the National Health Policy and Health Resources Development Bill and Related Bills.* 93rd Congress, 2nd Session, March 15, April 30, May 1, 6–9, and 14, 1974, p 408.

44. Klarman HE: Health planning: Progress, prospects, and issues. *Milbank Mem Fund Q/ Health Society* 1978; 56 (Winter):78–112.

45. Atkisson AA, Grimes RM: Health planning in the United States: An old idea with a new significance. *J Health Polit Policy Law* 1976; 1 (fall):295–318.

46. Raab GG: National/state/local relationships in health planning: Interest group reaction and lobbying, in *Health Planning in the United States: Selected Policy Issues.* Washington, DC, National Academy Press, 1981, vol 2, pp 105–130.

47. Glantz LH: Legal aspects of health facilities regulation, in Hyman HH (ed): *Health Regulation: Certificate of Need and Section 1122.* Germantown, Md, Aspen Systems Corp, 1977, pp 75–104.

48. Public Health Service, US Department of Health, Education, and Welfare: National guidelines for health planning. *Federal Register* 1978; 43:13,040–13,050.

49. Budetti PP: Congressional perspectives on health planning and cost containment: Les-

sons from the 1979 debate and amendments. *J Health Human Resources Adm* 1981; 4 (Summer):10–19.

50. Vladeck BC: Interest-group representation and the HSAs: Health planning and political theory. *Am J Public Health* 1977; 67:23–29.

51. Brown LD: Some structural issues in the health planning program, in *Health Planning in the United States: Selected Policy Issues*. Washington, DC, National Academy Press, 1982, vol 2, pp 1–46.

52. Morone JA: The real world of representation: Consumers and the HSAs, in *Health Planning in the United States: Selected Policy Issues*. Washington, DC, National Academy Press, 1981, vol 2, pp 1–46.

53. Cohodes DR: Interstate variation in certificate-of-need programs—a review and prospectus, in *Health Planning in the United States: Selected Policy Issues*. Washington, DC, National Academy Press, 1981, vol 2, pp 47–80.

54. Altman D, Greene R, Sapolsky HM: *Health Planning and Regulation: The Decision-Making Process*. Washington, DC, AUPHA Press, 1981, pp 52–73.

55. Davis K: Reagan Administration health policy. *J Public Health Policy* 1981; 2:312–332.

56. Stone A: Planning, public policy and capitalism, in Lowi TJ, Stone A (eds): *Nationalizing Government: Public Policies in America*. Beverly Hills, Calif, Sage Publications, 1978, pp 427–442.

57. Woll P: *American Bureaucracy*, ed 2. New York, WW Norton and Co, 1977.

58. For a personalized attempt to do so for a single state's health services regulatory structure, see Kinzer DM, *Health Controls Out of Control: Warnings to the Nation from Massachusetts*. Chicago, Teach'Em Inc, 1977.

59. Weidenbaum ML: The costs of government regulation of business. A study prepared for the use of the Subcommittee on Economic Growth and Stabilization of the Joint Economic Committee, US Congress. Government Printing Office, 1978.

60. Green M, Nader R: Economic regulation vs. competition: Uncle Sam the monopoly man. *Yale Law J* 1973; 82:871–889.

61. Zubkoff M (ed): *Health: A Victim or Cause of Inflation*. New York, Prodist, 1976.

62. Throughout this section, terms are used such as *need, overinvest, unnecessary costs*, and the like, with the recognition that these are elusive concepts. For a critique of the practice of basing health planning on notions of need, see Klarman HE: Planning for facilities, in Ginzberg E (ed): *Regionalization and Health Policy*. Government Printing Office, 1977, pp 25–36. For a more general critique of the language of health planners, see Kessel R: Commentary on the papers, and Posner RA: Certificates of need for health care facilities: A dissenting view, in Havighurst CC (ed): *Regulating Health Facilities Construction*. Washington, DC, American Enterprise Institute for Public Policy Research, 1974, pp 33–35, 113–118.

63. Lee ML: A conspicuous production theory of hospital behavior. *South Economic J* 1971; 38:45–58.

64. Newhouse JP: Toward a theory of nonprofit institutions: An economic model of a hospital. *Am Economic Rev* 1970; 60:64–74.

65. Feldstein PJ: *An Empirical Investigation of the Marginal Cost of Hospital Services*. Chicago, Graduate Program in Hospital Administration, University of Chicago, 1961. For a review of economics literature on hospitals' objective functions, see Berki SE: *Hospital Economics*. Lexington, Mass, Lexington Books, 1972, pp 19–30.

66. Fuchs VR: *Who Shall Live: Health Economics and Social Choice*. New York, Basic Books, 1974.

67. Redisch MA: Physician involvement in hospital decision making, in Zubkoff M, Raskin IE, Hanft RS (eds): *Hospital Cost Containment*. New York, Prodist, 1978.

68. Feldstein MS: Hospital cost inflation: A study of nonprofit price dynamics. *Am Eco-*

nomic Rev 1970; 60:853–872. Pauly MV, Redisch M: The not-for-profit hospital as a physicians' cooperative. *Am Economic Rev* 1973; 63:87–99.

69. Monsma GN Jr: Marginal revenue and the demand for physicians' services, in Klarman HE (ed): *Empirical Studies in Health Economics*. Baltimore, Johns Hopkins University Press, 1970, pp 145–160.

70. Pauly MV, Redisch M: The not-for-profit hospital as a physicians' cooperative. *Am Economics Rev* 1973; 63:87–99.

71. Clapp DC, Spector AB: A study of the American capital market and its relationship to the capital needs of the health care field, in MacLeod GK, Perlman M (eds): *Health Care Capital: Competition and Control*. Cambridge, Mass, Ballinger Publishing Co, 1978, pp 275–304.

72. Kelling RS Jr, Williams PC: The projected response of the capital markets to health facilities expenditures, in MacLeod GK, Perlman M (eds): *Health Care Capital: Competition and Control*. Cambridge, Mass, Ballinger Publishing Co, 1978, pp 319–348.

73. Salkever DS, Bice TW: *Hospital Certificate of Need Controls: Impact on Investment, Costs, and Use*. Washington, DC, American Enterprise Institute for Public Policy Research, 1979.

74. Urban Systems Research and Engineering and Policy Analysis, Inc: *Certificate of Need Programs: A Review, Analysis, and Annotated Bibliography*. Government Printing Office, November 1978.

75. Of course, the process rarely proceeds so simply. See Kinzer DM: *Health Controls Out of Control: Warning to the Nation from Massachusetts*. Chicago, Teach'Em, Inc, 1977. See also Lewin and Associates, Inc: *Evaluation of the Efficiency Effectiveness of the Section 1122 Review Process, Part I*. US Dept of Commerce, National Technical Information Services, 1975.

76. Public Health Service, US Dept of Health, Education, and Welfare: Health planning: Capital expenditure review, certificate of need and review of new institutional health services. *Federal Register* 1977; 42:4,002–4,032.

77. Salkever DS, Bice TW: The impact of certificate-of-need controls on hospital investment. *Milbank Mem Fund Q/Health Society* 1976; 54:185–214.

78. Salkever DS, Bice TW: *Hospital Certificate of Need Controls: Impact on Investment, Costs, and Use*. Washington, DC, American Enterprise Institute for Public Policy Research, 1979, pp 53–73.

79. Sloan FA, Steinwald B: Effects of regulation on hospital costs and input use. *J Law and Economics* 1980; 23:81–109.

80. Policy Analysis, Inc and Urban Systems Research and Engineering, Inc: *Evaluation of the Effects of Certificate-of-Need Programs*. Final report of Contract No. 231-77-0114, Bureau of Health Planning and Resources Development, US Dept of Health and Human Services, 1980.

81. Cromwell J: *Incentives and Decisions Underlying Hospital Adoption and Utilization of Major Capital Equipment*. Cambridge, Mass, Abt Associates, Inc, 1975.

82. Russell LB: *Technology and Hospitals: Medical Advances and their Diffusion*. Washington, DC, The Brookings Institution, 1979.

83. Bice TW, Urban N: *Effects of Regulation on the Diffusion of Computed Tomography Scanners*. Final report of Grant No. HS 03750, National Center for Health Services Research, US Dept of Health and Human Services, 1982.

84. 42 United States Code 1301, Sec. 1151.

85. Blumstein FJ: The role of PSROs in hospital cost containment, in Zubkoff M, Raskin IE, Hanft RS (eds): *Hospital Cost Containment*, New York, Prodist, 1978, pp 461–488.

86. Bellin LE: PSRO: Quality control? or gimmickry? *Med Care* 1974; 12:1012–1018.

87. Havighurst CC, Blumstein FJ: Coping with quality/cost tradeoffs in medical care: The role of PSROs. *Northwestern Law Rev* 1975; 70:6–68.

88. Brook RH, Williams KN, Rolph JE: *Controlling the Use and Cost of Medical Services: The New Mexico Experimental Medical Care Review Organization—A Four-Year Case Study*. Santa Monica, Calif, Rand Corporation, November 1978.

89. *Professional Standards Review Organization 1978, Program Evaluation*, publication No. HCFA-03000. Health Care Financing Administration, US Dept of Health and Human Services, 1979.

90. The plus portion of this formula was subsequently deleted. For a detailed analysis of the original Medicare reimbursement procedures, see Somers HM, Somers AR: *Medicare and the Hospitals: Issues and Prospects*. Washington, DC, The Brookings Institution, 1967, pp 154–196.

91. Dowling WL: Prospective reimbursement of hospitals. *Inquiry* 1974; 11:163–180.

92. Bauer KG: Hospital rate setting—this way to salvation? in Zubkoff M, Raskin IE, Hanft RS (eds): *Hospital Cost Containment*. New York, Prodist, 1978, pp 324–369.

93. Editorial: State rate controls: Documentation of the bureaucracy's imperfect plan. *Fed Am Hosp Rev* December 1978, pp 11–13.

94. Abernethy DS, Pearson DA: *Regulation Hospital Costs: The Development of Public Policy*. Washington, DC, AUPHA Press, 1979.

95. Coelen C, Sullivan D: An analysis of the effects of prospective reimbursement on hospital expenditures. *Health Care Financing Rev* 1981; 2 (Winter):1–40.

96. Joskow PL: *Controlling Hospital Costs: The Role of Government Regulation*. Cambridge, Mass, MIT Press, 1981, pp 162–168.

97. Schultze CL: *The Public Use of Private Interest*. Washington, DC, The Brookings Institution, 1977.

98. Hofstadter R: *The Age of Reform*. New York, Vintage Books, 1960.

99. Lowi TJ: *The End of Liberalism: Ideology, Policy, and the Crisis of Public Authority*. New York, WW Norton and Co, 1969.

100. For broad outlines of extensive regulatory strategies, see Blum HL: *Expanding Health Care Horizons: From a General Systems Concept of Health to a National Health Policy*. Oakland, Calif, Third Party Associates, 1976, pp 161–196; Joe T, Neddleman J, Lewin LS: Health care capital financing: Regulation, the market, and public policy, in McLeod GK, Perlman M (eds): *Health Care Capital: Competition and Control*. Cambridge, Mass, Ballinger Publishing Co, 1978, pp 63–80; and Krause EA: *Power and Illness: The Political Sociology of Health and Medical Care*. New York, Elsevier, 1977, pp 324–350.

101. Enthoven A: Consumer choice health plan. Parts I and II. *N Engl J of Med* 1978; 298:650–658, 709–730.

102. McClure W: The medical care system under national health insurance: Four models, *J Health Polit Policy Law*, 1976; (Spring):22–68.

CHAPTER 13

The Quality of Health Care

James P. LoGerfo

Robert H. Brook

The purpose of this chapter is to create an understanding of major issues relevant to the assessment of the quality of health care and to provide an overview of existing mechanisms that have been established to ensure that patients receive good personal medical care. The first portion of the chapter will discuss the relationship between health and medical care; potential sources and selection of data on provider performance; issues of measurement including reliability of data, sensitivity, and specificity concerning judgments about the quality of care; specific methods of measuring quality of care and each method's strengths and limitations; and the implications of imperfect knowledge concerning the true effectiveness of many medical services. Illustrative studies of the quality of care are presented. The last portion of the chapter deals with those mechanisms and programs that have been established to assure that medical care is of appropriate quality. While the chapter addresses most of the major issues in the above areas, it is not an exhaustive review; the reader may wish to consult other reviews and bibliographies on the assessment and assurance of the quality of medical care (1–5).

Assessment of the quality of care is inextricably intertwined with societal, professional, and patient expectations concerning the role of health care in society. Quality—the degree of excellence or confirmation to standards—cannot be definitively assessed without a clear understanding about the expected standards of excellence. Unfortunately, many of society's expectations concerning health and medical care have not been explicitly delineated. However, improvement in the health of society at large, or of some persons within that society, is an expectation of the medical care system. With this fact in mind, the quality of health care could be asessed by the extent to which the society's or the person's health is improved by a specified level of resources, provided in a manner that is most consonant with the cultural and social mores of the society. If there are good methods for measuring health, the quality of a system could be measured by the relationship between actual health and the expected level for the amount of resources used. Unfortunately, the relationship between medical care and the improvement of health is not as well defined as one would like, and this ambiguity raises significant problems for the assessment of the quality of medical care. The following section deals with some of these important implications.

THE RELATIONSHIP BETWEEN HEALTH AND MEDICAL CARE

The improvement and maintenance of health are nearly universally accepted as objectives of medical care. These objectives would ideally be achieved by the sequence of events, represented in Figure 13-1 and discussed in more detail in Chapter 3. As has been known for more than 20 centuries, however, many factors other than medical care have a profound effect on health, including personal behavior, environmental factors, and genetic endowment. In addition, as reflected in various ancient codes of law dealing with the adverse outcomes of care, such as removing the hand of a surgeon for a poor-quality operation, not all care is efficacious; that is, not all care contributes to a positive outcome. Indeed some care has the potential to be harmful, leading to iatrogenic illness caused by the care itself (e.g., infections after surgery). Accordingly, a more extensive model is presented in Figure 13-2.

The final outcome of care for any patient is a function of the likelihood that the patient actually needs care, that a correct diagnosis is made, that the correct treatment is given, that the treatment is efficacious, and that the treatment was adhered to by the patient. The probability of all of these events occurring represents the positive contribution of medical care to health. Most of these probabilities are not precisely known. Even if the probabilities are known for specific medical care interventions, it is critical to recognize the contributions of the nonmedical factors (such as environment) to the production of health. This recognition is important because lack of an understanding of the multifactorial determinants of outcomes of disease process can lead to major errors in evaluation of health services. For example, critics of the U.S. health care system often cite this country's higher infant death rate and lower life expectancy compared to those of selected European nations as evidence that the health care system in this country is inferior. Infant death rates, however, are influenced by demographic and social factors that are difficult to adjust for when performing these comparisons. Similarly, life expectancy is influenced by personal behaviors such as smoking, drinking, and involvement in violence. Thus, criticism of a health care system based on mortality statistics is less

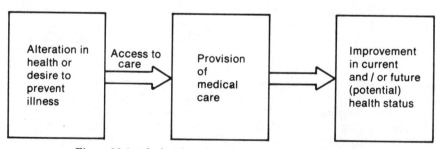

Figure 13-1. Idealized model of an episode of medical care.

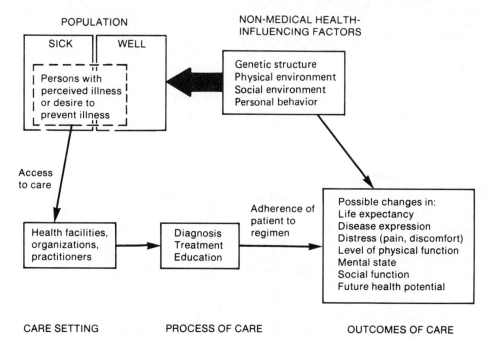

POPULATION   NON-MEDICAL HEALTH-
                                INFLUENCING FACTORS

SICK   WELL

Persons with   Genetic structure
perceived illness   Physical environment
or desire to   Social environment
prevent illness   Personal behavior

Access
to care

Health facilities,   Diagnosis   Adherence of   Possible changes in:
organizations,   Treatment   patient to   Life expectancy
practitioners   Education   regimen   Disease expression
                                                           Distress (pain, discomfort)
                                                           Level of physical function
                                                           Mental state
                                                           Social function
                                                           Future health potential

CARE SETTING   PROCESS OF CARE   OUTCOMES OF CARE

Figure 13-2. Model of a single episode of medical care.

a condemnation of that system than might be thought at first glance. This statement is not meant to imply that medical care has no influence on health as measured by mortality rates, but rather that the rates are imperfect measures for the evaluation of medical care. Accordingly, planners, policymakers, and providers should be cautious in the use of such global measures as the sole basis for criticizing a health care system or recommending changes in it. This argument also applies to other measures of health that are affected by nonmedical factors.

While the above discussion sounds a cautionary note about the use of broad measures of health in assessing medical care, it is also important to note that a focus on very narrow, professionally defined technical measures of health might also cause distortion if they are used as the sole basis of evaluation. For example, triumphs in the treatment of congenital heart disease by surgery and the prevention of strokes through the treatment of high blood pressure are often cited as unequivocal examples of effective medical care. Even in these two areas of undisputed efficacy, however, there could be harmful effects if, for instance, people who do not have the disease were erroneously labeled.

The negative effect of medical care on the health of nondiseased persons was demonstrated in a study of 93 junior high school children in Seattle, Washington, who had notations in school records indicating the presence of a heart condition (6). On detailed examination of these students, only 18 had evidence of heart disease; the other 75 were probably misdiagnosed. In the latter group, 30 were significantly restricted either psychologically or physically. The result was that screening for cardiac disease that is potentially curable by surgery may have produced more disability among those with no disease than it cured in those with heart disease.

In another study, the effects of labeling were noted in a hypertensive screening program. Absenteeism significantly increased when persons were identified as hypertensive even though many had had documented but unlabeled elevated blood pressure before screening (7). If the program had used narrowly defined measures of program outcome, such as number of cases identified, this important effect would have been missed. After the demonstration of the labeling effect, another study has shown that special attention can partially offset the effect of labeling. These examples illustrate the importance of knowing the effects of medical care on the health of populations and being careful to select appropriate measures to assess health programs.

Use of Population-Based Rates for Assessing Quality

An important and often neglected concern in assessing the quality of care by a system or institution is the use of measures that are directed at the entire population at risk rather than simply the users of services. The latter approach commonly implies assessment of care only for patients definitively diagnosed as having a specific disease (case rate analysis). The importance of using population-based rates (occurrence of diseases in populations) rather than case rates has always been accepted by epidemiologists concerned with "denominators." The point is vividly illustrated in assessing the effect of various organizations or hospitals on the disease appendicitis, which is frequently included in evaluations of care.

In cases of appendicitis, the dilemma confronting physicians is a choice between operating on patients who have abdominal pain at a time when the signs and symptoms are such that some of the patients may have a less serious, nonsurgical illness mimicking appendicitis versus waiting until the signs and symptoms are more definite and clearly indicate that an inflamed appendix is the cause of the pain. Unfortunately, if one waits too long, the inflamed appendix may perforate and produce peritonitis (a general inflammation and infection of the abdomen). The choice is between operating too early on some people with abdominal pain and removing some normal appendices versus operating too late and having a few patients with appendicitis progress to peritonitis. Recognition of this trade-off has led to acceptance of the fact that even the best surgeons will sometimes operate at a time when the diagnosis is not certain so as to decrease the number of perforations. This means that some people who have undergone surgery will be found to have a normal appendix. The optimum rate of such removals per 100 cases of true appendicitis has not been rigorously defined, but the implications of the trade-off have been discussed in detail (8).

In view of the above considerations, the logical inference is that the evaluator could assess the results described in the operative and pathology reports to classify the proportion of a facility's cases that are either normal (unnecessary), or abnormal but not perforated (best result), or perforated—possibly reflecting unnecessary delay before surgery. The case rate for these outcomes has been used to judge the extent to which a hospital or provider organization acts to reduce unnecessary surgery without significantly increasing the risk of perforation. Interestingly, the natural course of appendicitis is such that not all abnormal appendices will perforate; rather, some will improve without specific therapy or surgical intervention. The possible fate of patients who have abdominal pain are represented in Figure 13-3. Surgical intervention is beneficial only to groups III and IV, in the former case to prevent perforation and in the latter to prevent continued leakage of bacteria into the abdomen by removing the source of the bacteria and draining any abscess that

Patient group	State of appendix when first seen for abdominal pain		State of appendix at removal

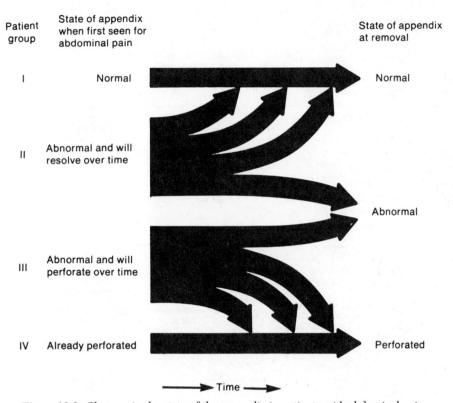

Figure 13-3. Changes in the state of the appendix in patients with abdominal pain.

might be present. Note that in an absolutely biologic sense, all operations on patients in groups I and II are unnecessary. In assessing the performance of a provider, a crucial question is the extent to which physicians can differentiate between groups II and III. If they can, and if case rates are used, the relative sizes of those groups in any population will have a dramatic impact on the results of an assessment of care (Fig. 13–4).

Assume that two different medical organizations provide care to biologically similar populations of 100,000 people each. The staff in organization A cannot distinguish patients with abdominal pain who have abnormal appendices that are likely to perforate, either initially or after careful observation, from those patients whose abnormal appendices are not likely to perforate. Thus, they admit all such patients to the hospital and operate on them. The physicians in organization B can make this distinction and do not admit or operate on patients in group II. In addition, they are able to distinguish correctly all patients with normal appendices from those with abnormal ones and thus do not hospitalize or operate on anyone in group I. Analysis of operative case rates using only hospitalized patients would suggest that organization B is trading off lives (more than 50% higher death rate) for efficiency. On a population basis, however, organization B has exactly the same number of deaths as organization A and, in addition, performed less than one-half as many operations. A practical demonstration of this problem in evaluating health care has been described (9).

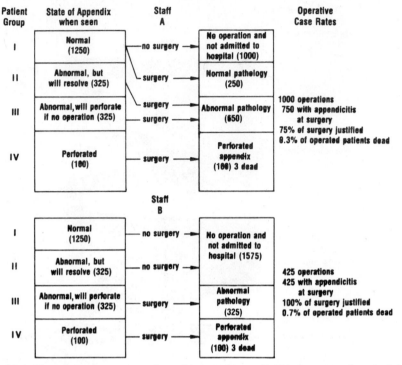

Figure 13-4. Hypothetical outcomes of care for two cohorts of 2,000 patients each with abdominal pain managed under two different systems of care.

This illustration has implications for both quality assurance and cost containment programs that are aimed at hospitals. For example, a hospital might respond to a cost containment program by reducing admissions. An evaluation of the effect of that program on the quality of care may require a population-based assessment. Unfortunately, the identification of a hospital's denominator population is difficult, especially in large cities. Thus, one might need to identify areawide variations for all hospitals in a small area. The task is much easier when dealing with well-defined geographic areas served by only one hospital.

QUALITY ASSESSMENT IN HEALTH CARE

The following discussion shifts from health care for a population to the assessment of care at the level of the individual provider and patient. As noted in previous chapters, there are annually more than 1 billion visits to physicians in the United States. While some care might be for trivial reasons, most of it has potential for either enhancing or harming the health of patients. It is essential, therefore, to use knowledge of the assessment and assurance of the quality of care to help achieve improved health. Most of the knowledge acquired thus far has been based on care given by physicians, but the general principles apply to care given by other health professionals, especially nurses (10–12).

Before discussing specific methods of assessing quality of care, it is important to note that certain general issues of sampling and measurement have major relevance for the conclusions that might be drawn from any assessment of the quality of care.

Focus of Assessment

Before embarking upon any assessment of the quality of care, it is important to state specifically why the assessment is being performed and what is its target, or focus. At the extreme, studies are undertaken either because of substantive concern about problems in quality that may exist or because of a requirement of a regulatory group to demonstrate ongoing analysis of the quality of care. This issue may seem trite, but numerous professional groups have found that studies undertaken because of a perceived problem in quality are far more likely to yield important results than assessments that are done simply to satisfy the requirements of external agencies. Also, studies performed because of a substantive concern about quality will more likely have a clear focal point, which is important in considering what sample of care will be reviewed. In general, the focal point of studies will be either specific providers, care for specific conditions, or care received by selected groups of patients.

Provider-based studies (e.g., physicians or hospitals) involve either sampling selected aspects of care given by all providers rendering that care or sampling all the care given for a large number of conditions by only a few providers. The specific sample chosen will depend on whether one assumes that deficiencies in care are likely to be randomly distributed across all providers, or whether poor care is more likely to be associated with only a few providers. If the latter is assumed to be true, then one might attempt to identify providers whose practice pattern with respect to the use of such items as laboratory tests, drugs, or number of visits characterizes them as "outliers" in comparison to their peers.

An alternative assessment strategy is to select random persons, independent of the nature of their diagnosed medical problems or their usual provider, and determine whether they have received appropriate care. This approach is particularly helpful in evaluating case finding for an asymptomatic disease that may benefit from early treatment. It has been incorporated into a population-based quality assessment strategy known as the *tracer method* (13).

Finally, the focus of a study may be a specific medical topic (e.g., a particular disease, a specific treatment, or provision of preventive care). The sampling unit for such studies is either all patients receiving care or all patients at risk. The former is more appropriate for assessment of errors of commission; the latter two are appropriate for detecting errors of omission.

Sources of Data for Quality Assessment

Data sources that can be used to study the quality of care are numerous and include direct observation, video or audio recordings of patient-provider contacts, direct interviews and examinations of patients, review of medical records; review of insurance claims forms, and review of public documents such as birth or death certificates.

MEASUREMENT ISSUES

After specifying the subject or sample frame, topic, and data source, there are measurement problems that must be considered. Included are issues of validity, reliability, sensitivity, and specificity.

Validity and Reliability

The validity of a measure is the extent to which it actually assesses what it purports to measure. For instance, if a measure is supposed to reflect the quality of care, one would expect improvements in quality to affect the measure positively. In this regard, it has already been noted that death rates may not be valid measures of care for a variety of disease processes. For instance, deaths due to cancer of the pancreas are, at the present time, not a good indicator of quality of care for that disease because it tends to be generally incurable. In general, the most valid measures of the quality of medical care will be defined quite narrowly (e.g., the proportion of patients in a given practice who have uncontrolled blood pressure).

Reliability reflects the extent to which the same result occurs from repeated application of a measure to the same subject. Reliability has been of considerable interest at two levels: the reliability of clinical observations by professionals and the reliability of the judgments of quality as assessed by certain methods. The reliability of a clinical observation can be determined by having the same observer repeat the same examination on the same subject (e.g., a repeat physical examination or a rereading of x-ray films) to determine if the same results (e.g., normal versus abnormal, getting better versus getting worse, need for a treatment versus no need for treatment) are obtained. This phenomenon is termed *intraobserver reliability*.

A second method involves having different observers review the same subject and compare the results of the observations made. This phenomenon is termed *interobserver reliability* and is similar to what occurs in second-opinion surgery programs in which more than one surgeon determines whether surgery is indicated. The results of observer-reliability testing have generally demonstrated poor levels of reliability of clinician-based data and judgments (14). For example, substantial lack of reliability has been shown for such information as whether or not patients have a heart murmur, or a diagnosis of coronary artery disease, or whether they should have a certain elective surgical procedure. The order of magnitude of such disagreements varies from 5 to 40% using conventional reliability tests. When more sophisticated (kappa statistic) tests are performed, the results are even more disquieting. The advanced method adjusts for the expected distribution of agreement based on chance alone (14). The implications of these problems in the reliability of clinical observations have not been adequately explored, and most methods of assessing quality assume that clinical observations are correct.

Reliability of Secondary Data Sources

Assuming that clinical observations are reliable, the next level of concern is the recording of data and its incorporation into data systems useful for quality assessment purposes. This process includes entering data into the medical record by providers, followed by abstracting or synthesis of that information by medical rec-

ords personnel. Abstracts include discharge diagnoses listed on the cover or summary sheets of medical records, summary abstracts such as those prepared for the
Commission on Professional and Hospital Activities, insurance claims forms, and
hospital discharge summaries; these abstracted sources are termed *secondary* data.
There have been very few studies of what bias occurs when the events occurring in
a patient-provider encounter are recorded in the medical record. Studies have compared tape recordings of medical encounters to determine the extent to which the
physician's notes of these encounters reflected the verbal content (15). Significant
underrecording occurred and was most pronounced for information relating to patient education and number of pills prescribed. A study of patients undergoing
tonsillectomy and/or adenoidectomy indicated that phrases in hospital records such
as "frequent" and "numerous" episodes of tonsillitis were open to considerable
variation in intrepretation when compared to the actual disease experiences of the
patients (16).

It is assumed that there is greater discordance between actual care provided
and that recorded in office settings as compared to such discordance in inpatient
settings. Indeed, one large study of office care provided for children documented
numerous deficiencies in recording and found that more than half of the physicians
felt that their records did not adequately reflect the care they provided (17).

Finally, with respect to data reliability, there is concern over information that is
routinely abstracted from medical records and recorded on magnetic computer
tapes. Studies conducted by the Institute of Medicine of the National Academy of
Sciences assessed the reliability of hospital discharge diagnostic data and showed
major disagreements on such critical information as principal diagnosis (18). As a
result, concern has been raised regarding the utility of such data for many quality
assessment programs. These studies do not negate the utility of such data systems
for identifying possible areas for more intensive review at the individual case level.
Reliable judgments of the quality of care at the individual level (either patient or
physician) may require the use of the medical record, however, except for those few
providers whose practice patterns are so deviant from the norm that problems such
as those discussed above are inconsequential.

Evaluating Methods Used to Assess Quality of Care

The sensitivity, specificity, and predictive value of methods of quality assessment
have major implications for the efficiency of quality of review procedures. To illustrate these concepts, assume the presence of an omniscient quality assessor who
knows whether or not people are sick, what happens to them, and what the relative
contribution of medical care is to improving their illness. Such an assessor would
provide a "gold standard" for true judgments against which other methods of assessing quality could be compared. If a new method of identifying cases of bad-quality
care were proposed, a comparison of the new and true methods would result in a
distribution of cases into four categories (Fig. 13-5). The sensitivity of the new
method represents the extent to which it identifies all truly bad cases of quality; in
this case, sensitivity $= a/(a + c)$. Specificity reflects the extent to which cases that
are classified as good by the test actually are good; specificity $= d/(b + d)$. At the
operational level, methods that have high sensitivity and specificity are desirable.
In general, increases in the sensitivity of a method achieved by loosening the
criteria for bad versus good care, without changing the method itself, will tend to
decrease the specificity of the method.

Results by "New" Method	Results by "True" Method	
	Bad care	Good care
Bad care	**a**	**b**
Good care	**c**	**d**

Figure 13-5. Testing a new method of assessing the quality of care.

The concepts of positive or negative predictive value of a method are also of interest. In Figure 13-5 the new method attempts to identify bad care as indicated by a positive test result. The positive predictive value of the test is the probability that a positive result by the new method reflects a positive result by the true method; the positive predictive value $= a/(a + b)$. The accurate reflection of a negative result yields a negative predictive value $= d/(c + d)$.

Knowledge of these characteristics of a method for assessing quality of care helps one to use such methods. If the primary goal of an assessment of quality is to identify all episodes of bad care, then highest priority should be given to increasing the sensitivity of the method used. If a primary goal is to lower the cost of identifying a case of bad care, then the specificity or positive predictive value of the method is emphasized.

QUALITY ASSESSMENT METHODS

The preceding discussion sets the stage for presenting the categories of measures of quality that can be monitored. The selection and design criteria outlined above are generic and apply to all measures of the quality of care. Quality of care measures generally fall into one of three categories: 1) outcome measures that reflect the results or impact of care (e.g., changes in health status); 2) process measures that reflect what was done (e.g., number and types of laboratory tests performed); and 3) structural measures that reflect the setting in which care is provided (e.g., licensure of personnel or facilities).

Outcome Measures of Quality

Outcomes of care reflect the net changes that occur in health status as a result of health care and are appealing because of their face validity; their use in assessing care has been extensively reviewed elsewhere (19,20). As discussed previously, many factors affect health. Therefore, if outcomes are to be used as an indicator of the quality of care, they must be sensitive to different levels in the quality of the process or content of care; that is, outcomes should change when the process changes.

The two major groups of outcome measures are general health status indicators and disease-specific indicators. A general health status measure is multidimensional and may include physical, emotional, and social aspects of health. The measures can be based on a person's own perception of his or her health or on independent assessments that do not rely on the patient's own perceptions (21–24). An example of a health status measure that relies on self-reported perceptions and covers several dimensions of health is the Sickness Impact Profile (25). This profile is an index based on patients' responses to a series of statements such as: 1) I am going out less to visit people; 2) I do not walk at all; 3) I often act irritable toward my work associates, for example, snap at them, give sharp answers, criticize easily; 4) I am doing less of the regular daily work around the house than I usually do; and 5) I stop often when traveling because of health problems. Changes in these aspects of an individual's function can be produced by a variety of diseases.

General health status indicators have the advantage of reflecting changes in several dimensions of health that might not be detected by technically derived, disease-specific measures (e.g., changes in blood pressure level). They have the disadvantage of possibly being too sensitive to nonmedical factors. For instance, in assessing outcomes of care for an operation to fuse a spine because of back pain, a general health status instrument might detect deficiencies in work productivity and in the emotional state of the patient, but there are many factors other than the surgery that could affect a patient's productivity and propensity to depression.

Disease-specific outcome indicators include death rates due to a given disease, the presence of symptoms known to occur with a disease, or behavioral disabilities commonly associated with a specified disease. For example, in patients with coronary artery disease, assessments could be based on deaths from heart attacks, on the number of people with symptomatic chest pain on exertion, or on the avoidance of specific work or social activities by patients with heart disease due to fears of incurring a heart attack.

Data on many outcome measures must be obtained directly from patients because such data may not be recorded in the medical record. Obtaining reliable outcome information by either a self-administered or interviewer-administered questionnaire may be expensive, and the cost may limit the usefulness of the outcome methods on a routine basis.

Outcome measures can be used in operational settings to assess quality of care. At the very least, adverse outcomes related to treatment can be monitored as indicators of suboptimal quality (e.g., infections after surgery). Similarly, while 5 years may have to elapse before one can determine if survivors of a surgical procedure have better or worse than expected death rates, immediate (within a short time period) surgical mortality can be used as an indicator of poor technical quality for such procedures as gastrectomies for patients with stomach cancer or replacement of heart valves in patients with rheumatic heart disease. Before passing judgment on such mortality data, however, the severity of illness in the patients treated must be considered, as was done in a recent study of the variation by hospitalization in surgical death rates (26). In this study, unadjusted death rates for various operations varied fivefold across study hospitals, but the differences were generally less than twofold after adjustments for case severity were made.

In addition to the use of treatment-related adverse outcome measures, quality of care can be reflected in intermediate outcomes that are known to relate to a final outcome that is a goal of care. For example, the treatment for high blood pressure seeks to avoid the future occurrence of stroke, heart attack, or heart failure by lowering blood pressure. Rather than waiting 10 to 14 years to determine if the incidence of stroke or heart failure has been altered by a treatment program, an intermediate outcome can be measured. In this case, one could assess the extent to which blood pressure has been reduced to levels that are known to be associated with a lower long term probability of stroke or heart failure.

The use of intermediate outcomes is inherent in the staging approach to assessing quality of ambulatory care (27). This technique is very useful in the diagnosis of cancer, since death rates from certain cancers are related to how advanced the disease is at the time of detection. Many cancers should be detectable at an early stage if the quality of ambulatory care is high. The stage of a cancer is reflected in pathology, laboratory, and x-ray reports, and presumably a good-quality ambulatory care program will identify tumors at an early stage (i.e., the intermediate outcome) and improve long term survival.

Process Measures of Quality

The process of care, as defined by Donabedian, refers to what is done to patients (28). DeGeyndt has elaborated this concept into the notion of the content of care (i.e., activities performed) and uses the word *process* to denote the sequence and coordination of these activities (29). A further refinement of the concept separates the technical aspects of care from the affective and interpersonal skills (how the patient was treated) implied in the art of care (30).

The use of process measures has considerable attraction because they are operationally much easier to collect than outcome measures. Specifically, they are less time dependent and less dependent on expensive patient follow-up studies because the medical record, despite its imperfections, does reflect certain processes of care reasonably well. Most of the process approaches to assessing care depend on the establishment of agreed-upon criteria for good care and the application of these criteria to individual cases.

The most common process method used is based on the development of a list of elements of good care and on whether or not these elements are documented in the medical record. Physicians frequently argue that they do not think in checklist fashion or, more perjoratively, in a "laundry list" format. Instead, they argue correctly that in making decisions they use a contingency-based format that considers case severity, test results, and the presence or absence of certain signs and symptoms. Accordingly, simple checklists may not be the optimal or most relevant means of assessing the process of care.

An approach to assessing the process of care that more closely mirrors clinical decision making is the criteria-mapping approach (31). In this approach, criteria for good care can be met in a variety of ways depending on the presence or absence of certain signs, symptoms, laboratory test results, or more general reflections of case severity. The criteria-mapping approach should be as sensitive in detecting poor care as the list, but should also be more specific. Additionally, it may afford the possibility of identifying excess use of certain tests or procedures that should be done only in very selected circumstances. A comparison of criteria that might be used by these two approaches is shown in Table 13-1.

While assessment of the process of care is inherently attractive, several criticisms have been voiced about the use of process measures. The most common

TABLE 13-1. Comparison of Lists and Mapping Approaches for Assessing the Process of Care: Hypothetical Criteria for Diagnostic Tests in Patients with Newly Discovered Hypertension.

Checklist Approach	Illustrative Criteria-Mapping Approach
Abdominal examination for bruits	Abdominal examination for bruits
Serum potassium level	Serum potassium level
Serum bicarbonate level	Serum bicarbonate level
Fasting glucose level	Fasting glucose level
Test of catecholamine or vanillylmandelic acid excretion for pheochromocytoma	Test for pheochromocytoma only if there is a history of palpitations, weight loss, elevated fasting glucose level, orthostatic drop in blood pressure without treatment, or a family history of this tumor
Plasma renin or intravenous pyelogram to rule out renal artery stenosis	Test for renal artery stenosis only if there is one of the following: abdominal or flank bruit, serum potassium less than 3.6 mEq/L or bicarbonate level greater than 28 mEq/L

criticism is that outcomes should be of most concern, and few studies have demonstrated a strong relationship between the process and the outcome of care. While this contention is often correct, there are several biologic and methodologic reasons for this failure. The biologic explanation is that not all health care is necessarily efficacious. Accordingly, variations in the process of care will not alter outcomes. For example, in past years, many surgeons might have listed radical mastectomy as an element of good process for treating breast cancer. But this procedure is not clearly superior to a simple mastectomy, and no difference in outcomes may be measured for patients who had either a good or suboptimal process. Examples of process criteria for good care that have not been validated are numerous, including time-honored exhortations such as requiring all patients with sore throats to have a throat culture before antibiotic therapy is started (32).

There are also conceptual and methodologic deficiencies in those studies that demonstrate low (or even negative) correlations between process and outcome. The choice of the strategy used to assess the quality of care is critical; a strategy that emphasizes diagnosis rather than treatment ignores those aspects of process that are most proximate to determining a good outcome. For example, hypertension is a treatable condition, and therapy for it is efficacious. In more than 90% of treated cases, hypertension is *not* due to a readily identifiable etiology, yet it will respond to therapy. Process-oriented studies of the quality of care given to hypertensive patients frequently focus on the degree to which physicians establish the level of end-organ damage when a hypertensive patient is identified, and the extent to which a differential diagnostic strategy is pursued to identify those few patients with a specific etiology for their hypertension. A more critical factor in changing outcomes, however, is whether an antihypertensive drug is prescribed. For the vast majority of patients, an antihypertensive drug is more important in determining whether blood pressure is lowered than a laboratory test to detect rare causes of hypertension. Accordingly, unless much greater weight is attached to initiation of therapy than to ruling out a rare diagnosis, there will be very little positive correlation between process and outcome assessments of quality care.

The use of criteria for good care that are process oriented but not of proven efficacy in operational quality assurance programs may result in the increased use of unnecessary tests and drugs without any improvement in outcome. Much of the concern about using a process-oriented approach can be alleviated if it is employed primarily to identify a lack of optimal process in cases with known poor outcomes, (e.g., use of antihypertensive drugs in patients with uncontrolled hypertension) or to discourage the use of practices that are known to be harmful (e.g., most applications of chloramphenicol in ambulatory care).

The lack of definitive studies on efficacy of some clinical strategies does not require that they be excluded from a quality of care study. Practicing physicians should not be expected to conduct basic research to demonstrate conclusively the efficacy of a procedure that overwhelming professional opinion already believes is appropriate to use; that should be the role of academic research centers. This reiterates the fundamentals of good care developed 50 years ago by Lee and Jones (33):

> Good medical care is the kind of medicine practiced and taught by recognized leaders of the medical profession at a given time and period of social, cultural, and professional development in a community or population group . . .
> The concept of good medical care . . . is based upon certain "articles of faith" which can be briefly stated:
>
> 1. Good medical care is limited to the practice of rational medicine based on the medical sciences . . .
> 2. Good medical care emphasizes prevention . . .
> 3. Good medical care requires intelligent cooperation between the lay public and the practitioners of scientific medicine . . .
> 4. Good medical care treats the individual as a whole. . . . Good practice requires that the patient be considered as a person, a member of a family living in a certain environment. All factors which concern his [her] health—mental and emotional, as well as physiological—must be weighed in diagnosis, prevention, and treatment. It is the sick or injured person and not merely the pathologic condition which must be treated . . .
> 5. Good medical care maintains a close and continuing personal relationship between physician and patient . . .
> 6. Good medical care is coordinated with social welfare, work . . . love of [people] must be clarified by an understanding of [people] and must take note of his [her] social environment and economic needs . . .
> 7. Good medical care coordinates all types of medical services . . .
> 8. Good medical care implies application of all the necessary services of modern scientific medicine to the needs of all the people. Judged from the viewpoints of society as a whole, the qualitative aspects of medical care cannot be dissociated from the quantitative. No matter what the perfection of technique of one individual case, medicine does not fulfill its functions adequately until the same perfection is within reach of all individuals.

Structural Measures of Quality

Measures of the structure of care relate to the personnel and facilities used to provide services and the manner in which they are organized. Examples of structural measures of care are presented in Table 13-2.

TABLE 13-2. Examples of Structural Measure of Quality

Resource	Illustrative Criteria
Facility	Does it meet fire and safety codes? Is it clean?
Personnel	Are the physicians licensed? Are the physicians board certified? Is the ratio of registered nurses to practical nurses over 0.3? Is the ratio of nurses to patients over 0.2?
Organization	Is there an organizational structure with clearly defined responsibility? Is there a mechanism for peer review?

From an administrative viewpoint, structural assessments are attractive because much of the information they require can be readily obtained from existing documents or a simple inspection of a facility. Assessments based solely on the structure of care assume that if the structure is optimal, then the appropriate processes will necessarily follow and outcomes will be maximized. The assumptions underlying many structural criteria, however, have not been validated. For example, consider the criterion of whether or not the physicians in a hospital are board certified. Presumably physicians with longer training programs who become board certified in their specialty will treat diseases related to that specialty better than noncertified physicians. Much medical training, however, is oriented toward teaching the process of care as best known at the time of training. Because the presumed best process of care 10 years ago may not now result in the best outcome, board-certified status may not be a powerful prediction of quality of care.

There is also some evidence that better-qualified physicians do not necessarily perform at a substantially higher level, that is, have higher process scores, than similarly trained physicians who are not board certified. A large study in Hawaii showed that self-declared specialists tended to treat diseases related to their specialty better than nonspecialists, but it also found little difference in the quality of care provided by physicians with formal board certification in a specialty versus those who were self-identified specialists, but not board certified (34). This example is especially pertinent in view of recent trends stressing board certification as an indicator of quality in consumer's guides to choosing a physician, and as a mechanism to control the number of unnecessary surgical procedures. The objective of making all physicians board certified could increase the total costs of care for society substantially, with only a marginal affect on the quality of care, and perhaps no positive effect on outcomes. Similar concerns can be raised in regard to many other structural criteria for good care, including an increased interest in having only nurses with baccalaureate training be eligible for licensure as registered nurses.

Do limitations of structural measures mean that they should not be included as an element of a quality assessment or assurance program? While reliance on structural criteria does not guarantee that good processes and outcomes will follow, some level of structure must be obtained in areas such as professional responsibility, peer review, and life safety if good processes are to occur. Good structure is a necessary but not sufficient correlate of good care.

Efficiency and Quality

Efficiency of care reflects how much care of a given quality is provided for a specified cost, and can be expressed as net outcomes achieved per unit of cost. With concern over the rising costs of health care in relation to the gross national product (Chap. 11), increasing attention has been directed toward inefficient use of resources as reflected by such terms as *inappropriate hospitalization, unnecessary surgery,* and *defensive medicine.* A hypothesized relationship between costs and outcomes is presented in Figure 13-6. Initial investments in care produce rapid increases in positive outcomes (zone A). When only difficult and costly problems are left to be overcome, there is little and eventually no increase in positive outcomes from further investments (zone B). Finally, a negative slope could even occur in one of two ways (zone C). First, direct application of increased medical care at very intensive levels might produce more iatrogenic injury than benefit. Second, costs of care could become so high that resources that might be used to produce health through means other than medical care are diverted to medical care. Thus, auto safety devices may not be produced in favor of investments in medical care that produce less impact on health. Note, however, that Figure 13-6 is very simplistic. A more complex figure would have a series of curves that takes account of the multidimensional nature of the outcome of care, (e.g., disability days, symptoms status, mortality) and relates each of these outcomes to costs of care.

Because outcomes are multidimensional, even a simple disease process produces a family of efficiency curves rather than a single curve; the trade-offs of favoring one efficiency curve over another must be understood. For example, two outcomes of interest in the management of high blood pressure might be work status and age-specific death rate. There is no question that investing more resources in the identification and adequate treatment of all hypertensives would reduce overall cardiovascular age-specific death rates. There may be, however, high rates of work loss in treated patients secondary to the psychologic effects of being labeled hypertensive, or because of complications of therapy such as depression. These latter effects occur when treated patients are in their third or fourth decade of life, while reduction in death rate might not occur until the fifth decade of life. The net effect might be substantially more disability days in a treated as compared to an untreated population in order to achieve a reduction in strokes and heart failure in later life. Many people who would never have had a stroke or heart failure are

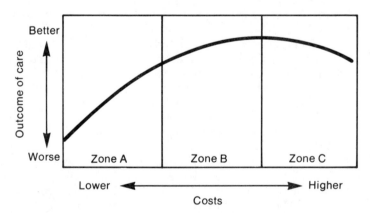

Figure 13-6. Hypothetical relationship between the outcomes and costs of care.

treated to prevent these events that will occur in some hypertensives. For those individuals who would never have developed a stroke or congestive heart failure, the treatment may have a negative effect on physical health. Unfortunately, trade-offs such as these are common in current medical practice and will need to be considered in efforts to improve the quality of care. Donabedian and colleagues have presented an integrated framework relating quality, costs, and health outcomes (35).

Efficiency and Provider-Patient Relationship

There has been considerable interest in increasing efficiency in recent years. When efficiency is stressed, providers must play a larger role of social policeman vis-à-vis their role of patient advocate. This shift in emphasis has substantial implications for patient-provider relationships, especially under prepayment arrangements.

For example, a physician may know that fewer than one out of 100 patients with adult-onset seizures have a treatable form of brain tumor. The physician may also know that certain associated signs and symptoms make that possibility more or less likely. The physician cannot determine with absolute certainty, however, whether a given patient is, or is not, that one in 100. It is unethical for the physician to tell the patient that there is a 100% likelihood that there is no serious and treatable problem. How many tests and what expense should be incurred to determine if the patient is the rare one with a treatable disease? What should be the provider's response to a patient who says, "Look, Doc, I'm fully covered by insurance, and I'd like you to order a computerized axial tomography scan for me because I just want to be sure?" These and similar questions have no simple answer, and they pose major ethical dilemmas for professionals entrusted with the dual functions of advocate and policeman. These dilemmas may prove to be too uncomfortable to place major emphasis on cost cutting in the individual patient-physician encounter. Rather, the emphasis might be placed at the institutional or payer level (e.g., restriction of benefits), so that patients and physicians do not develop a somewhat adversarial relationship concerning provision of certain services.

Patient Satisfaction and the Quality of Care

Patient satisfaction is a measure that can reflect the outcome, process, and structure of care. Satisfaction has been viewed as a multidimensional concept involving the cost, convenience, technical and interpersonal aspects of care, and outcome of care (36,37). Satisfaction with care can be assessed for a specific illness episode, for a patient's personal care, or for medical care in general. From a technical medical perspective, satisfaction is important because it is positively correlated with patient adherence to prescribed therapeutic regimens. It may positively affect subsequent care-seeking behavior, and probably has some impact on the propensity to file a malpractice claim.

At any point in time, using existing measures, the overwhelming majority (usually more than 85%) of people are satisfied with their own health care. The level of satisfaction may appear to be high because most patients finally find a provider who meets their needs after a long odyssey, or because existing measures are not sensitive to all components of satisfaction. However, despite the generally high rate of satisfaction with most aspects of personal medical care, there is room for improvement, especially in the areas of interpersonal aspects of care and costs of care.

Access to Care

Access to care, which has been discussed in earlier chapters, is an important element of quality assessment at the programmatic and social levels. Access to care as a dimension of quality at the individual provider level is more difficult to conceptualize and measure. A provider who agrees to be a regular source of primary care for a panel (those patients who identify that provider as their regular source of care) should be responsible for assuring access to services for those patients. Poor access may be reflected in delayed care seeking, absence of preventive care, and low patient satisfaction. Whether equity of access for all members of society is a measure of quality at the individual provider level is an unresolved issue. This issue includes questions about the extent to which individual providers should be accountable for assuring access to care by working longer hours, treating more patients, working more efficiently, or encouraging or actively seeking out potential patients with limited access to care, as reflected in the types of measures presented in Chapter 3.

A provider's patterns of practice can markedly affect access to care, and studies of physicians in group practices show large variations in the number of patients per physician and number of visits per patient despite relatively similar populations of patients (38). In the absence of optimal visit schedules for acute and chronic illnesses by which such data could be judged, it is difficult to determine which physicians are practicing better medicine or are requiring too many or too few follow-up visits. If providers who treat widely varying numbers of patients have similar outcomes, there should be considerable concern about the relationships among efficiency, quality, and access to care.

ILLUSTRATIVE STUDIES OF THE QUALITY OF CARE

The quality of care assessment literature has expanded rapidly in the past 3 decades. Selected major studies performed since 1950 are highlighted here for illustration purposes.

Outcome-Oriented Studies

Outcome-oriented studies have been based on death certificates, face-to-face and telephone interviews with patients, medical records, and secondarily abstracted medical records. Shapiro and associates studied the quality of care under two different organizational systems in New York by analyzing the perinatal mortality of infants born to low income women (39). Their findings indicated a lower death rate for those infants whose mothers were enrolled in a prepaid practice plan. The study highlights the importance of defining a denominator population and raises several issues concerning epidemiologic and statistical adjusting procedures when dealing with problems of selection bias in quality of care studies based on outcome measures.

Forrest and associates studied the outcome of surgical care in 17 hospitals by making direct assessments of the status of patients during a 40-day postoperative period (26). They found significant variations across hospitals, with death rates that were nearly twice as high in the worst as compared to the best hospital in the sample. This study is important because it illustrates the need to adjust for case severity. Forrest and associates also found that the use of data from a medical abstracting service as opposed to a direct assessment produced results with similar trends but not similar magnitudes. This means that with proper adjustments for such factors as case mix, hospitals with unusually adverse outcome rates can potentially be identified for further investigation by means of analysis of data collected by a medical abstracting service. Additionally, the study identified some organizational features of hospitals that might be associated with better care (40). For example, both stringent control over membership on the surgical staff and the ratio of registered nurses to other nurses were positively related to better outcomes of care. Interestingly, teaching status, size of medical staff, and board certification of surgeons were not significantly correlated with quality of care. Because of the nature of the study, a causal relationship between these structural features and outcomes of care could not be inferred, but prospective studies using this information are clearly in order.

An analysis of death rates for selected surgical procedures was carried out by Luft using Medicare data. He demonstrated a significant association between better outcomes with higher volumes of procedures for some operations, but not for others (41,42). While the analyses were hindered by limited measures of case severity, and inadequate sample size for procedures with very low expectations of death, the data for several major surgical procedures do support the notion of better outcomes in institutions that have greater experience with selected procedures.

Kessner and associates conducted a population-based study of the quality of ambulatory care for children using the outcome-oriented tracer method (43). They assessed outcomes for iron deficiency, ear infection, and vision correction. The study sample consisted of 1,436 families with 2,780 children aged 6 months to 11 years in Washington, D.C. More than 25% of the children aged 6 months to 3 years had anemia, 20% had ear disease, and nearly 25% of those aged 4 to 11 failed a vision screening test. After controlling for the social class of the patients, no significant correlation between outcome and type of provider organization was found. Inappropriate or ineffective treatment was provided to a large proportion of children in the sample. Subsequent analyses of the same data did suggest different outcomes among different providers using a finer categorization of providers (44). In particular, it was suggested that outcomes were poorest among patients of solo practitioners.

Schroeder and Donaldson applied the outcome-oriented method known as *health accounting* to a Health Maintenance Organization (45). This method was developed by Williamson and requires a consensus estimate of what outcomes are achievable with specific interventions. The extent to which the outcomes achieved deviate from expected outcomes is then determined. The outcome assessment can usually be performed by telephone survey or mailed questionnaire. Applied to the diagnoses of depression, high blood pressure, and contraception, the method revealed major problems of underdiagnosis for all the conditions (44–74%) and unacceptable therapeutic outcomes for depression and high blood pressure. The operational difficulties for using this outcome-based method in ambulatory facilities delivering care to large numbers of disadvantaged people were also emphasized.

Intermediate outcomes have been assessed from medical records in several studies. Gonnella and colleagues applied the staging approach to hospitalized patients as an outcome measure of the quality of their ambulatory medical care (27).

They studied 5,000 patients admitted to hospitals in two cities in California. For six of the 18 conditions studied, they showed significant differences in the stages of disease present at the time of hospitalization in patients from various population groups. Disease was generally more severe in patients with government sponsorship other than Medicare.

Process-Oriented Studies

Process-oriented studies can be conducted by direct observation of medical encounters, by review of medical records, and by review of insurance claims. Observational studies provide a wealth of information not otherwise obtainable, but suffer from high cost and potential alteration of behavior resulting from the presence of an observer. These problems notwithstanding, a few observational studies of process have been completed, the most noteworthy of which in the United States was a study of 88 general practitioners in North Carolina by Peterson and associates in 1953 (46). They developed a semistructured review protocol that included observable elements of history taking, physical diagnosis, use of laboratory services, preventive care, and clinical record keeping. In addition to an index score based on these observations, the authors developed a 5-point qualitative ranking system. With the ranking system, 8% of the physicians were in rank 5 (essentially outstanding) and 18% in rank 1. The physicians in rank 1 had a very superficial, disorganized approach to clinical medicine. Overall, 39 of the 88 physicians were in rank 1 or 2. This study was of considerable importance because it showed the feasibility of carrying out direct observations of practicing physicians in their offices and demonstrated major deficiencies in the level of care in office settings. The study also highlighted the need to assess the quality of care in an organized manner.

There have been numerous large scale process-oriented studies of hospital and ambulatory care using medical records. In his pioneering work in Monroe County, New York, Lembcke identified numerous deficiencies in care given to patients undergoing hysterectomies (47). Similar findings were noted by Doyle in a study of more than 6,000 hysterectomies in the Los Angeles area (48). More recently, major problems in surgery judged to be unnecessary by process criteria were noted in a population-based study of hysterectomies in Saskatchewan (49). McCarthy and Widmer have identified potentially unnecessary surgery in nearly one-third of patients recommended for a variety of elective procedures in a second surgical opinion program (50). They and others have found reductions in surgery after starting such programs, but the significance of the results is not yet clear.

In one of the largest studies of the process of care, Payne and Lyons found numerous deficiencies in care provided to patients admitted to hospitals in Hawaii. This study was based on a random sample of all hospital patients in the state who had selected discharge diagnoses in 1968 (34). A group of practicing physicians established criteria for good care that were then applied to the hospital records. For each disease, a physician's performance index (PPI) was developed that represented the percentage of process criteria (e.g., performance of certain laboratory tests) for which evidence of compliance could be found in the medical records. Overall, they found a PPI of 0.71 for hospitalized patients. In a companion study of office-based care in 1970, they found an average PPI of only 0.40 (34). These studies are important demonstrations of the feasibility of carrying out large-scale quality assessments. They have identified several organizational and structural features that tend to be associated with good care, even though the correlations were relatively low.

In addition to studies using direct observation or medical record review, the process of care has been studied through the use of claims forms. In Tennessee, Ray and associates established criteria for the appropriate use of certain drugs and applied them to claims data (51). Their first analysis was concerned with chloramphenicol, a broad-spectrum antibiotic that can cause death due to agranulocytosis (absence of white cells necessary to fight infection). The use of this drug has been recommended only for serious, well-defined infections for which there are no reasonable therapeutic alternatives. The analysis indicated that nearly 6% of all antibiotic prescriptions filled by pharmacies were for this drug, and it was prescribed by 6% of the physicians participating in the Tennessee Medicaid program. About half of the prescriptions were for upper respiratory tract infections, for which the drug is never indicated. Most of the remaining prescriptions were also appropriate. This study is important because it documented the ability to identify inappropriate practice patterns by analysis of claims data. In a similar study, Brook and colleagues analyzed the use of injectable antibiotics in Medicaid patients in New Mexico and showed that claims data could identify physicians whose practice patterns were both atypical and inappropriate (52). They further showed that practice patterns could be altered by the use of an ongoing monitoring system with feedback to physicians whose practice patterns were at variance with established and accepted standards.

QUALITY ASSURANCE IN MEDICAL CARE

The application of quality assessment methods in assuring acceptable care to patients is of considerable concern to providers. *Quality assurance* refers to those activities that are designed to guarantee, in part, that the care received meets reasonable professional standards. In general, there are two major mechanisms that serve this purpose: structure-oriented systems, or systems that actively monitor the events and outcomes of the care actually provided. The notion of assurance implies that when deficiencies occur, they will be corrected in some way, ultimately by changing physician behavior. As will be discussed below, our understanding of how to alter physician behavior is fragmentary, but there is accumulating evidence that some strategies are effective.

Structure-Oriented Approaches to Quality Assurance:Licensure

The most pervasive, oldest, and most fundamental assurance mechanism is licensure. With rare but highly publicized exceptions, licensure assures a patient that a physician or nurse has a specified level of educational achievement relevant to the profession. For physician licensure, states require graduation in good standing from a recognized medical school, passing of a state-required examination or its equivalent (e.g., examinations offered by the National Board of Medical Examiners), no record of conviction for any major crime (such as a felony), and letters of recommendation from other licensed physicians. In addition, virtually all states require the applicant to have completed an accredited internship program. Persons not meeting these requirements are denied the right to practice their profession legally in a defined geographic area. In essence, the licensing mechanism sets a floor on the quality of the personnel available to provide care.

It is interesting to note that in professional licensure, the licensing body represents public interests, but the determination of whether certain schools are acceptable often lies (to a great extent) in the hands of nonpublic groups. In this instance, the accreditation of a given medical school is determined by a mixture of academic and professional organizations. This arrangement has raised the question of whether an organization representing professional interests, such as the American Medical Association, should have any direct or indirect influence in determining whether certain training programs are accredited because potential conflicts of interest might exist.

Licensure mechanisms are very general in relation to actual professional practice. For example, most physicians' licenses state only that they are physicians and surgeons; in theory, they are allowed to perform any act within the scope of medical practice. Accordingly, they could attempt procedures that they had not been specifically trained to do. For instance, there is great concern about the use of potentially toxic chemotherapeutic drugs in cancer patients by physicians not trained in this area. In view of such concern, the general nature of licensing laws may represent a substantial weakness. Because of this weakness, one could argue for the passage of limited licensure laws that would restrict surgery to those with surgical training in accredited programs, or the use of cancer drugs to oncologists. Obviously, such laws would be complex to administer and might reduce some of the highly beneficial flexibility given to practicing physicians. They presumably would, however, also prevent uncommon but egregious abuse of the medical license. Whether they would produce more good than harm is an open question.

A further weakness of licensure has been its static nature, although this situation appears to be changing in many states. Once licensed, individuals need only send in a fee on a regular basis, indicate that they had not been convicted of a felony in the past year, and provide other minimal information about themselves to be relicensed. Given the rapid changes in medical knowledge and practice, it has been proposed that professionals should demonstrate evidence of up-to-date knowledge to be licensed. This concern has led to the development of relicensure requirements by which the individual must show proof of a certain amount of continuing medical education (CME). For instance, in several states, physicians must be able to document 150 hours of CME every 3 years to be relicensed. These CME credits can be obtained through attendance at special courses, teaching, independent study, and similar activities.

While mandatory CME resolves some of the problems inherent in what amounts to lifetime licensure, it does not resolve those related to the general nature of the license itself and, more seriously, does not address the failure of structural mechanisms to guarantee the appropriateness of care.

A few states (e.g., Washington) have strengthened their licensure systems through the establishment of medical disciplinary boards that have the power to revoke or severely restrict the licenses of physicians who are found to be impaired due to alcoholism or drug abuse, or who are involved in several malpractice cases or in professional misconduct.

Licensure has also been applied to hospitals and long term care institutions. In general, such licenses heavily emphasize physical structure with a modicum of required organization structure. To the extent that medical care is provided in organized settings, institutional licensure represents a pervasive mechanism that can contribute to assuring the quality of care; however, given the present form of most licensing mechanisms, this potential might not be realized.

Certification and Accreditation

The second most pervasive structural assurance mechanism has been voluntary professional certification and accreditation. For physicians, this procedure consists of certification by specialty boards that require completion of at least 3 years of postgraduate training and the passage of a special examination. Several specialty boards also require 1 or more years of practice after completion of residency training and/or submission of a series of records of actual cases for review by members of the board.

Specialty certification goes one step beyond licensure in setting minimal standards of quality for the provider's training and knowledge; however, it has limitations similar to those of licensure. As in the case of relicensure, there has been a trend toward mandatory periodic recertification of many specialty boards to assure updating of knowledge. While recertification tends to be structure oriented and based on tests of knowledge, at least one board, the Academy of Family Practice, requires that records of selected cases be submitted for review.

Accreditation through the Joint Commission on Accreditation of Hospitals (JCAH) is the most pervasive and influential accreditation mechanism (see also Chapter 6). The JCAH functions as an independent accrediting body, with representation from the American Hospital Association, the American Medical Association, the American College of Surgery, and the American College of Physicians.

For many years, the JCAH emphasized a structural approach to quality assurance, with formal requirements for such matters as the organizational framework of hospitals, adequacy of medical records, safety standards, a requirement for periodic review of tissue removed at surgery, hospital infections, and mortality reviews. In more recent years, the actual accreditation process has required demonstration of ongoing performance-based assessments of quality, including documentation that any deficiencies found were specifically corrected.

At the present time, the JCAH reviews the extent to which hospitals meet its quality assurance standard, which states: "There shall be evidence of a well-defined, organized program designed to enhance patient care through the ongoing objective assessment of important aspects of patient care and the correction of identified problems" (53). Given the interpretation of this standard and other required activities of the JCAH, there are several dimensions of quality assurance that are expected of an accredited institution. These include an organized system for the granting of clinical privileges, with requirements for periodic review based on demonstrated performance; a system of evaluation studies of perceived problems in patient care; and a series of monitoring activities that may indicate when problems arise in selected areas such as tissue review, blood use, antibiotic use, or deviation in performance from other hospitals as reported by local peer review organizations.

As part of its standard, the JCAH requires coordination of quality assurance efforts throughout the hospital, and involves administrative, nursing, and other professional groups in addition to the medical staff.

Overall, the JCAH reviews about 75% of all hospitals for accreditation. Accreditation can be given for 3 years on an unconditional basis, or contingencies can be established for interim hospital reports and/or additional on-site review. About one-half of hospitals receive the full 3-year unconditional approval, and only about 1% are not approved for accreditation.

The historical impact of the JCAH and its current standards on quality of care are difficult to evaluate because this organization has had major direct and indirect effects on virtually all hospitals, even those it does not review. However, the emphasis on the coordination, delineation of accountability, and visibility of quality assurance efforts is consistent with existing research on organizational features that are positively associated with better quality of care using performance-based measures (54).

Performance-Based Assurance Approaches

Structural mechanisms focus on the providers of care rather than care for selected patients or groups of patients, and generally do not rely on assessments of how the system is actually performing. In view of this deficiency, there is considerable interest in performance-based assurance programs that include use review and review of both processes and outcomes of care.

Use Review.   Use review represents one of the earliest forms of process assurance to be instituted on a large scale. In essence, it assures that care is actually required and that the facility is not inappropriately costly for the level of care provided. Not surprisingly, use review developed out of a desire to control the costs of hospital care, and was developed through cooperation between insurers and professional groups. It grew slowly in the private sector in the late 1950s and 1960s and gained considerable attention in the public sector with the establishment of Medicare and Medicaid. Use review was also subsequently embodied in the Professional Standards Review Organization (PSRO) program.

There are three forms of use review: review of the necessity of care before the provision of a service, review during the care process, and review after the care has been provided. These are known as *prospective, concurrent,* and *retrospective* review, respectively. In general, use review has been directed at costly institutionally based care, but it can also be applied in ambulatory care, dental care, and elsewhere.

How does use review relate to the quality of care? While it is true that efforts aimed at controlling inappropriate hospital admissions or lengths of stay in hospitals were begun because of interests in cost containment, they definitely represent a form of quality assurance. Patients spared admission to a hospital for surgical removal of a gallbladder because they do not require surgery as determined by a peer review group forego the pain, distress, and potential life-threatening hazards of major surgery; this is certainly a quality assurance function. Similarly, patients who might otherwise be kept in a hospital despite the availability of equally appropriate care at home, or in other less intense settings, are spared exposure to a host of nosocomial infections and other risks that can produce injury in the hospital. Because of their orientation toward cost control, use review programs are generally designed to avoid unnecessary care and do not specifically promote increased use where underprovision of services could occur (i.e., increased access).

The mechanism of review used by use review groups and PSROs include establishment of explicit criteria for both appropriate indications for hospitalization and length of stay. Cases not meeting these criteria might not be reimbursed by the insurance program. In practice, the review body (e.g., Foundation for Medical Care or PSRO) usually sets explicit criteria that can be applied by review coordinators, who most commonly are specially trained nurses or medical records personnel. Cases are reviewed shortly after admission (concurrent review) and periodically during the hospital stay. Cases that do not appear to meet the indications for hospitalization are then formally reviewed by a physician or panel of physicians. Most systems also include an appeal mechanism. Cases that are not found to meet indications for continued stay are then denied payment (after a small grace period) by the insurer for any further durations of stay.

Some use review programs have a mechanism for prehospital admission review that is applied to elective hospitalization. Second-surgical opinion programs represent such a review mechanism and require approval by an independent physician of the need for the planned surgery.

The extent to which use review programs have reduced inappropriate use or saved money spent for hospital care is unclear at present, and various studies suggest mixed results (55–59). It may be that there is a sentinel effect such that simple awareness of being watched has altered provider behavior substantially from what might have occurred had use review programs not been implemented. However, even if hospital costs are reduced, it does not necessarily follow that total medical care costs to individual persons or society are reduced because some substitution may occur.

Peer Review Assurance Programs. While most use review programs represent forms of peer review, they are not designed to monitor patient-specific aspects of care once it has been decided that a certain procedure or level of care is appropriate. For example, once a decision has been made that a diseased gallbladder can be removed, use review systems are not designed to assess the technical adequacy of the procedure performed, or whether there were preventable operative complications. This latter question can be addressed only by peer review systems that focus on specific aspects of quality of care. Examples of peer review programs are provided elsewhere; this discussion will focus primarily on an approach originally known as *medical audits,* but now also termed *patient care evaluation studies* (59).

The medical audit concept has been embellished in recent years, but essentially consists of the following six steps: 1) selection of a topic for study, such as care for a specific disease or use of a certain procedure or drug; 2) selection of explicit criteria for good care using both process and outcome criteria, which might include whether specific diagnostic tests and treatments were performed, whether the status at discharge compared favorably with the expected status, and whether there were avoidable complications or unnecessary lengths of stay; 3) review of medical records to determine if the criteria for good care are met, usually by a medical records analyst; 4) review by professional peers of all cases that do not meet the criteria for good care; 5) development of specific recommendations for assuring that any deficiencies found will be avoided in the future (e.g., education programs, changes in administrative procedures, requirements for consultations); and 6) restudy of the topic at a future date to ascertain if deficiencies have actually been reduced or eliminated. These elements of quality assurance have been incorporated into two complementary programs—the PSRO and the guidelines suggested by the JCAH.

Professional Standards Review Organization. The PSRO program, also discussed in Chapter 12, represents the most ambitious publicly mandated performance-based quality assurance program in existence (60,61). The program incorporates the features of use review and medical care evaluation studies carried out at the hospital and nursing home levels, as well as an overall analysis of patterns of care by different providers carried on at the agency (i.e., PSRO) level.

The PSRO program was established in 1972 and, administered at the federal level through the U.S. Department of Health and Human Services, as discussed in previous chapters. It is currently under the Health Care Financing Administration, which is also responsible for administering the Medicare and Medicaid programs. The law (PL 92-603) establishing PSROs provided that care under the Medicare, Medicaid, and Title V (Maternal and Child Health) programs will be paid for if it meets the criteria for medical necessity and is provided in the appropriate level of facility. Thus, hospital care may not be covered if appropriate care could be given on an outpatient basis or in a less costly facility such as a nursing home.

The implementation of the PSRO program was federally mandated, but the actual establishment of the 195 state- or areawide PSROs was left in the hands of practicing physicians. The individual PSRO must assure that the review activities are carried out in its area. It can delegate the review process to hospitals that meet certain requirements, or it can elect to perform all of the review activities itself. Under these arrangements, criteria for review of care can vary at the local level, so that considerable flexibility exists.

The primary activities of use review and quality assurance employ the strategies described above. The medical audits tend to be process oriented but usually include criteria covering avoidance of complications and the expected state of the patient at discharge. Reports of the audit and use review activities are monitored by the PSRO staff, who in turn are responsible to the physician board of the PSRO.

In general, PSRO activities are oriented to hospital care, but the legislation provided for review of ambulatory and long term care as well, and one-third of the PSROs have begun efforts in the long term care area.

What has been the effect of the PSRO program? An evaluation of such a broadly mandated program is difficult because of the absence of ideal control versus experimental groups and the long time required to organize and implement such an ambitious departure from the status quo. Despite these problems, evaluations suggest a positive net benefit/cost ratio in terms of the effects of the impact of use review on hospital costs. Additionally, a number of PSROs were able to document improvements in quality of care above and beyond their use function.

In 1982, the nature of the PSRO program was substantially revised by federal legislation. The basic requirements of use review and quality assurance for Medicare and Medicaid were left intact. However, the contracts for the review can now be awarded to groups other than the 195 existing organizations representing a majority of physicians in each PSRO area. As of 1983, other physician-based review groups can compete for the review contracts. In 1984, the competition will be expanded to other groups that have access to a substantial number of physicians to assist in review. It is likely that various insurance companies will actively seek such arrangements. Additionally, there will be significant consolidation of existing PSRO areas to represent more closely statewide areas.

While the notion of opening PSRO review contracts to competitive bidding may have some benefits, it is possible the entire thrust of awards will be based on cost/benefit ratios. Thus, emphasis may be placed on reducing hospital costs, and programs may have difficulty maintaining major forms of quality assurance other than a reduction in unnecessary hospital days.

Malpractice Litigation and Quality Assurance

The legal system plays a role in quality assurance because of patients' ability to sue for malpractice, which is to some extent a quality assurance mechanism (62). Despite possible abuses by a minority of patients and lawyers, most malpractice awards do relate to less than optimal care, and all physicians are aware that they are in jeopardy of suit for egregious deficiencies in the quality of care. Interestingly, until recently there was almost no linkage between the malpractice system and licensure. Thus, a physician could have been involved in several cases of malpractice, settled them out of court, and continued to maintain his or her license without having it reviewed with extra scrutiny. However, some states now require insurance companies to report a physician to a state discipline board if a few malpractice cases involving the physician occur in a limited time period. The board may then make an independent judgment about this person's future suitability for practice.

Another trend in malpractice insurance that may have an effect on quality assurance is self-insurance by state medical societies and hospitals. As the size of the self-insurance unit becomes smaller than it was under usual insurance programs, it is highly likely that these units will be forced to exercise increasing self or peer vigilance. The net impact on quality of care of these newer aspects of the malpractice litigation and insurance systems cannot yet be ascertained. However, at this point, a positive impact is quite likely.

Assessment of Quality of Care

This chapter has reviewed salient issues with regard to quality assessment strategies and described basic quality assurance mechanisms. The uncertainty concerning the impact of various medical strategies on the health of persons limits our ability to assess and assure the quality of medical care. However, there is sufficient medical knowledge to provide a solid foundation for systems of quality assessment and assurance that, as a minimum, could help us to avoid harmful strategies, promote known helpful strategies, and allow identification of practice patterns that deviate significantly from reasonable professional practice. While the chapter has dealt primarily with examples of physician and hospital behavior, the concepts presented are analogous for assessing care by other professionals or institutions.

A final note concerns the importance of personal motivation in improving the quality of health care. No matter how systems are structured, the final common pathway of assessment will rely on the best professional judgment of a variety of persons. The development, quality, and acceptance of those judgments will be a function of the professional's personal commitment to promoting good care in the context of a supportive organizational framework. Without strong positive commitments by practicing professionals, all of the structure will prove to be of no avail. Conversely, without appropriate structural support, the best professional commitments and energy expenditure will be as efficacious as Cervantes' sorrowful figure of the lone would-be knight tilting at windmills.

REFERENCES

1. Donabedian A: *Exploration in Quality Assessment and Monitoring*, vol 1: *The Definition of Quality and Approaches to Its Assessment.* Ann Arbor, Mich, Health Administration Press, 1980.
2. Donabedian A: *Exploration in Quality Assessment and Monitoring*, vol 2: *The Criteria and Standards of Quality.* Ann Arbor, Mich, Health Administration Press, 1981.

3. Williamson JW: *Improving Medical Practice and Health Care: A Bibliographic Guide to Information Management in Quality Assurance and Continuing Education.* Cambridge, Mass, Ballinger, 1977.

4. Barro AR: Survey and evaluation of approaches to physician performance measurement. *J Med Ed* 1973; 48(suppl):1047–1093.

5. Williams KN, Brook RH: Quality measurement and assurance. *Health Med Care Serv Rev* 1978; 1:3–15.

6. Bergman AB, Staemm SJ: The morbidity of cardiac non-disease in school children. *N Engl J Med* 1967; 276:1008–1013.

7. Sackett DL, Taylor DW, Haynes RB, et al: The short term disadvantage of being labeled hypertensive. *Clin Res* 1977; 25:266.

8. Neutra R: Indications for the surgical treatment of suspected acute appendicitis: A cost-effectiveness approach, in Bunker JP, Barnes BA, Mosteller F (eds): *Costs, Risks and Benefits of Surgery.* New York, Oxford University Press, 1977, pp 277–307.

9. Watkins RN, Howell L: A population based quality assessment of the treatment of appendicitis. Presented at the 105th Annual Meeting of the American Public Health Association, Washington, DC, November, 1977.

10. Bloch D: Evaluation of nursing care in terms of process and outcome: Issues in research and quality assurance. *Nurs Res* 1975; 24:256–263.

11. Lang N: *Quality Assurance in Nursing. A Selected Bibliography,* publication No. 12, HHR-80-30. US Dept of Health, Education and Welfare, 1980.

12. Lang N (ed): *Nursing Quality Assurance Management/Leasing System.* Northridge, Calif, American Nurses Association and Sutherland Leasing Association Inc, 1982.

13. Kessner DN, Kalk CE: *Contrasts in Health Status,* vol 2: *A Strategy for Evaluating Health Services.* Washington, DC, National Academy of Science, 1973.

14. Koran LM: The reliability of clinical methods, data and judgments (parts 1 and 2). *N Engl J Med* 1975; 293:642–646, 695–701.

15. Zuckerman AE, Starfield B, Hochreiter C, et al: Validating the content of pediatric outpatient medical records by means of tape-recording doctor-patient encounters. *Pediatrics* 1975; 56:407–411.

16. LoGerfo JP, Dynes IN, Frost F, et al: Tonsillectomies, adenoidectomies, audits: Have surgical indications been met? *Med Care* 1978; 16:950–955.

17. Osborne CE, Thompson NH: Criteria for evaluation of ambulatory child health care by chart audit—development and testing of a methodology. *Pediatrics* 1975; 56(suppl pt 2):625–692.

18. Demlo LK, Campbell PN, Spaght S: Reliability of information abstracted from patients' medical records. *Med Care* 1978; 16:995–1004.

19. Shapiro S: End-result measurements of quality of medical care. *Milbank Mem Fund Q* 1967; 45:7–30.

20. Brook RH, Davies-Avery A, Greenfield S, et al: *Quality of Medical Care Assessment Using Outcome Measures: An Overview of the Method.* Santa Monica, Calif, Rand Corp, 1976.

21. Stewart AL, Ware JE, Brook RH: *Conceptualization and Measurement of Health for Adults in the Health Insurance Study,* vol 2: *Physical Health in Terms of Functioning.* Santa Monica, Calif, Rand Corp, 1978.

22. Ware JE, Johnston SA, Davies-Avery A, et al: *Conceptualization and Measurement of Health for Adults in the Health Insurance Study,* vol 3: *Mental Health.* Santa Monica, Calif, Rand Corp, 1978.

23. Donald CA, Ware JE, Brook RH, et al: *Conceptualization and Measurement of Health for Adults in the Health Insurance Study,* vol 4: *Social Health.* Santa Monica, Calif, Rand Corp, 1978.

24. Ware JE, Davies-Avery A, Donald CA: *Conceptualization and Measurement of Health for Adults in the Health Insurance Study*, vol 5: *General Health Perception*. Santa Monica, Calif, Rand Corp, 1978.

25. Bergner M, Bobbitt RA, Krenel A, et al: The Sickness Impact Profile: Conceptual formulation and methodological development of a health status index. *Int J Health Serv* 1976; 6:393–415.

26. Forrest WH, Scott WR, Brown BW: *Study of the Institutional Differences in Postoperative Mortality*, Project report (PB 250-940). National Center for Health Services Research, Hyattsville, Md, 1974.

27. Gonnella J, Louis DZ, McCord JJ: The staging concept—an approach to the assessment of outcome of ambulatory care. *Med Care* 1976; 14:13–21.

28. Donabedian A: Promoting quality through evaluating the process of patient care. *Med Care* 1968; 6:181–202.

29. DeGeyndt W: Five approaches for assessing the quality of care. *Hosp Adm* 1970; 15:21–42.

30. Brook RH, Williams KN, Davies-Avery A: Quality assurance today and tomorrow: Forecast for the future. *Ann Intern Med* 1976; 85:809–817.

31. Greenfield S, Lewis CE, Kaplan SH, et al: Peer review by criteria mapping: Criteria for diabetes mellitus. The use of decision-making in chart audit. *Ann Intern Med* 1975; 83:761–770.

32. Tompkins RK, Burnes DC, Cable WE: An analysis of the cost-effectiveness of pharyngitis management and acute rheumatic fever prevention. *Ann Intern Med* 1977; 86:481–492.

33. Lee RI, Jones LW: *The Fundamentals of Good Medical Care*. Chicago, University of Chicago Press, 1933.

34. Payne BC, Lyons TF, Dwarshius L, et al: *The Quality of Medical Care: Evaluation and Improvement*. Chicago, Hospital Research and Educational Trust, 1976, pp 7–19.

35. Donabedian A, Wheeler JR, Wyszewianski L: Quality, cost, and health: An integrative model. *Med Care* 1982; 20:975–992.

36. Zyzanski SJ, Hulka BS, Cassel JC: Scale for the measurement of "satisfaction" with medical care: Modifications in content, format, and scoring. *Med Care* 1974; 12:611–620.

37. Ware JE, Davies-Avery A, Stewart PE: The measurement and meaning of patient satisfaction. *Health Med Care Serv Rev* 1978; 1:1–15.

38. Lyle CB, Applegate WB, Citron DF, et al: Practice habits in a group of eight internists. *Ann Intern Med* 1976; 84:594–601.

39. Shapiro S, Jacobziner H, Densen PM, et al: Further observation on prematurity and perinatal mortality in a general population and in the population of a prepaid group practice medical plan. *Am J Public Health* 1960; 50:1304–1317.

40. Scott WR, Forrest WH Jr, Brown BW Jr: Hospital structure and postoperative mortality and morbidity, in Shortell S (ed.), *Organizational Research in Hospitals—An Inquiry Book*, Chicago, Ill, Blue Cross Association, 1976.

41. Luft HS, Bunker JP, Enthoven AC: Should operations be regionalized? An empirical study of the relation between surgical volume and mortality. *N Engl J Med* 1979; 301:1364.

42. Luft HS: The relation between surgical volume and mortality: An exploration of causal factors and alternatives models. *Med Care* 1980; 18:940–959.

43. Kessner DM, Snow CK, Singer J: *Contrasts in Health Status*, vol 3: *Assessment of Medical Care for Children*. Washington, DC, National Academy of Sciences, 1974.

44. Dutton DB, Silber R: Children's health outcomes in six different ambulatory care delivery systems. *Med Care* 1980; 18:693–714.

45. Schroeder SA, Donaldson MS: The feasibility of an outcome approach to quality assurance—a report from one HMO. *Med Care* 1976; 14:49–56.

46. Peterson OL, Andrews LP, Spain RS, et al: An analytic study of North Carolina general practice 1953–1954. *J Med Ed* 1956:31(12, pt 2):1–165.

47. Lembcke PA: Medical auditing by scientific methods: Illustrated by major female pelvic surgery. *JAMA* 1956; 162:646–655.

48. Doyle JC: Unnecessary hysterectomies—study of 6,248 operations in 75 hospitals during 1948. *JAMA* 1953; 151:360–365.

49. Dyck FJ, Murphy FA, Murphy JK, et al: Effect of surveillance on the number of hysterectomies in the province of Saskatchewan. *N Engl J Med* 1977; 296:1326–1328.

50. McCarthy E, Widmer G: Effects of screening by consultants on recommended elective surgical procedures. *N Engl J Med* 1974; 291:1331–1335.

51. Ray W, Federspiel CP, Schaffner W: Prescribing of chloramphenicol in ambulatory practice. An epidemiologic study among Tennessee Medicaid recipients. *An Intern Med* 1976; 84:266–270.

52. Brook RH, Williams KN, Rolph JE: Controlling the use and cost of medical services. The New Mexico experimental medical care review organization—a four year case study. *Med Care* 1978; 16(suppl 9):1–76.

53. *Accreditation Manual for Hospitals*, 1983 ed. Chicago, Illinois, Joint Commission on Accreditation of Hospitals, 1982, p. 151.

54. Shortell SM, LoGerfo JP: Hospital medical staff organization and quality of care: Results from myocardial infarction and appendectomy. *Med Care* 1981; 19:1041–1056.

55. Chassin M: The containment of hospital costs: A strategic assessment. *Med Care* 1978; 16(suppl 10):1–55.

56. Ruchlin HS, Finkel ML, McCarthy EG: The efficacy of second-opinion consultation programs: A cost-benefit perspective. *Med Care* 1982; 20:3–20.

57. Martin SG, Shwartz M, Whalen BJ, et al: Impact of a mandatory second-opinion program on Medicaid surgery rates. *Med Care* 1982; 20:21–45.

58. Brook RH, Lohr KN: Second-opinion programs: Beyond cost-benefit analyses. *Med Care* 1982; 20:1–2.

59. Ertel PY, Aldredge MG (eds): *Medical Peer Review: Theory and Practice*. St Louis, CV Mosby Co, 1977.

60. Jessee WF, Munier WB, Fielding JE, et al: PSRO: An educational force for improving quality of care. *N Engl J Med* 1975; 292:668–675.

61. Goran MJ, Roberts JS, Kellogg MA, et al: The PSRO hospital review system. *Med Care* 1975; 13(suppl 4):1–33.

62. Brook RH, Brutoco RL, Williams KN: The relationship between medical malpractice and quality of care. *Duke Law J* 1976; 75:1197–1231.

CHAPTER 14

Evaluating Health Care Programs and Services

Arnold D. Kaluzny

James E. Veney

While the previous two chapters have discussed the structuring of the health services system, including the regulation of its performance and the assessment of the quality of services provided, this chapter focuses on the *evaluation* of those services and the programs under which they are provided. Evaluation represents an important component of the overall process of assessing and regulating the performance of the health services system. While a great deal has been written about the techniques and methods appropriate to evaluation in various kinds of program and research activities, this chapter presents an overview of evaluation in the health services field. Specifically, it defines evaluation, discusses the uses and abuses of evaluation, presents a historical perspective on evaluation efforts, and illustrates various evaluation strategies. The chapter concludes with some speculation about the future of evaluation in health services.

WHAT IS EVALUATION?

As with many terms used in health services, the definition of *evaluation* should be intuitively obvious. Yet even the casual reader encounters a number of alternative and often conflicting definitions. The following are definitions that vary by the emphasis given to focus and method. For example, the Shortell and Richardson definition (1) focuses primarily on program objectives and suggests that evaluation be conducted through the use of scientific and explicit methodologies. Definitions of evaluation follow:

- The use of the scientific method or approximation in assessing the degree to which an organized set of activities has reached intended objectives. The primary purpose is to inform the decisions of program operators (1).

- The process of making reasonable judgments about program effort, efficiency, and effectiveness, based on systematic data collection and analysis. Information generated by this process is used in program management. The focus is especially on issues of assessibility, acceptability, awareness, availability, comprehensiveness, continuity, integration, and cost of service (2).
- The determination (whether based on opinions, records, subjective or objective data) of the results (whether desirable or undesirable, transient or permanent, immediate or delayed) attained by some activity (whether a program or part of a program, a drug or a therapy, an ongoing or one-shot approach) designed to accomplish some valued goal or objective (whether ultimate, intermediate, or immediate effort or performance, longer or short range) (3).

While Attkisson and Broskowski (2) retain the emphasis on explicit methodology, they broaden the focus to include evaluation of process activities. Another perspective appears in the definition presented by Suchman (3), which focuses on program objectives but includes more subjective methodologies.

These are important distinctions, but they do not represent conflicting definitions of evaluation. As described by Weiss: "Evaluation is an elastic word that stretches to cover judgments of many kinds—what all uses of the word have in common is a notion of judging merit. Someone is examining and weighing a phenomenon—against some explicit or implicit yardsticks" (4).

With this in mind, the range of variation can be simply indicated by defining health services evaluation as follows: "The collection and analysis of information by various methodological strategies to determine the relevance, progress, efficiency, effectiveness and impact of health service program activities" (5). This definition includes the use of implicit and explicit methodology, as long as evaluation is conducted in a systematic manner and focuses on the achievement of project objectives as well as program process. The various evaluation functions, and illustrations of issues addressed by each function, in the evaluation of health care programs and services are as follows (6):

Relevance concerns the question of need for the program—the basic rationale for having a program or set of activities to meet the health needs or service demands of a community. The development of relevance as a legitimate evaluation topic in health services is a recent phenomenon. Historically, health services have been considered relevant a priori, and the critical questions have focused on the delivery of services. In more recent years, the concern for delivery and extent of use have been supplemented by concern regarding the underlying rationale for the program. The very basis of a program in terms of objectives, scope, depth, and coverage becomes the primary issue. Questions central to this type of evaluation include the following:

What problem does the program address?
Does that problem need attention?
How accurate is the information about the problem?
How adequate is the definition of the problem?
How adequate is the definition of the program?
Is the program appropriate to the defined problem?

Progress evaluation refers to the tracking of program activities. Here attention is focused on the degree to which program implementation complies with the predetermined plan. Traditionally, progress evaluation has been considered an integral part of the management process. Illustrative questions concerning progress include the following:

Are appropriate personnel, equipment, and financial resources available in the right quantity, in the right place, and at the right time to meet program needs?

Are expected products of the program actually being produced? Are these products of expected quality and quantity? Are these outputs produced at the expected time?

Efficiency evaluation concerns the relationship between the results obtained from a specific program and the resources expended for its operation. This form of evaluation is gaining increasing attention as programs compete for limited resources. It plays an important role in determining whether or not new programs are funded, continued or terminated, and expanded or contracted. Questions addressed by evaluations of efficiency include the following:

Are program benefits sufficient for the cost incurred?

Are program benefits more or less expensive per unit of outcome than benefits derived from other programs designed to achieve the same goal?

Effectiveness evaluation emphasizes program outputs and the immediate results of program efforts, and considers their success in meeting predetermined objectives. Evaluations of effectiveness are aimed at improving program formulation and thus have a relatively short term time perspective. The questions central to this type of evaluation include the following:

Did the program meet its stated objectives?

Were program providers satisfied with the effects of program activities?

Were program beneficiaries satisfied with the effects of program activities?

Are things better as a result of the program's existence?

Impact evaluation concerns the long term implications of the program—the changes observed over time in characteristics that the program is designed to influence. While evaluation of effectiveness focuses on program outputs, impact evaluation considers whether program outputs have the desired effects on the fundamental problems the program is designed to solve. It is possible that a program may prove to be both efficient and effective in producing short run outputs, yet have minimal long term impact. Illustrative questions for this type of evaluation include the following:

Did a particular program produce the observed effects?

Could the observed effects occur in the absence of the program or in the presence of some alternative program?

Evaluation and the Managerial Process

Health service managers are forced daily to make judgments and plan actions on the basis of program evaluations. Evaluations may deal with such apparently mundane affairs as determining whether program resources and personnel are in the right places at the right time (progress) or with more glamorous issues, such as whether a program has made any difference. However, any activity aimed at making decisions about whether a program should be implemented, how the program should be carried out, whether program activities are being pursued in a timely manner, if the program is producing expected outcomes, or whether the outcomes are as desirable as anticipated is essentially evaluation.

Two views of evaluation and the role of each in the managerial process need to be considered: linear and nonlinear.

Linear Process.   One approach to evaluation and its role in the management process is consideration of a sequence of events in which program planning comes first, followed by implementation and finally by evaluation (7). This logical sequence of steps is often perceived as including feedback from evaluation to both planning and implementation, so that program modification occurs, allowing the program to proceed·at a new level of effectiveness. Figure 14-1 presents this sequence of activities.

There is nothing basically wrong with this formulation; still, it is somewhat limited as far as the role of evaluation in program planning and implementation is concerned. The difficulty with the linear model is its assumption that evaluation takes place after program planning and implementation.

Nonlinear Process.   An alternative view of evaluation, and the view taken here, is to consider evaluation as an integral part of the management cycle. Figure 14-2 shows a nonlinear model of planning, implementation, and control as three interconnected activities. From this perspective, evaluation occurs during all phases of the management cycle. For example, program evaluation may accompany the planning and design stage of a program, focusing on such issues as the current state of the system to be affected by the program, the specific nature of problems to be addressed, and alternative approaches to solving those problems.

Once a program is in operation, a number of evaluation issues arise. A general question concerns whether the process works as intended. Do resources, funds, doses of vaccine, students to be trained, medical supplies, or other types of inputs arrive at the proper place, on time, and in sufficient quantity? Are activities undertaken in a timely manner and in proper order? Are various components of the program coordinated? These and many other questions are addressed as aspects of program progress.

Once the program has been implemented, is it effective and efficient? Are the costs of the program reasonable? Do the results expected from the program appear in the projected time frame? Are there other less expensive or more timely ways of producing the same results? Are the results of the program meeting predetermined objectives?

Finally, have the desired results been achieved? Has the problem the program was designed to solve been solved, or is it being solved on a continuing basis? Would the problem have been solved in the absence of the program? Could any other program have solved the problem?

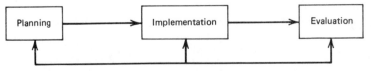

Figure 14-1. Linear model of program planning management and evaluation cycle.
Source: From Veney JE, Kaluzny AD: *Evaluation and Decision Making in Health Service Programs.* Reprinted by permission of Prentice-Hall, Inc., Englewood Cliffs, N.J. © 1983.

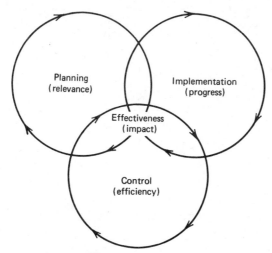

Figure 14-2. Nonlinear model of program planning, implementation, and evaluation.
SOURCE: From Veney JE, Kaluzny AD: *Evaluation and Decision Making in Health Service Programs.*
Reprinted by permission of Prentice-Hall, Englewood Cliffs, N.J. © 1983.

Who Does Evaluation?

All health service managers need evaluation for various purposes. Many social scientists and persons involved in health services research have the skills necessary to conduct evaluation studies. The involvement of both groups depends on the degree to which formal evaluation research techniques are used and the extent to which the manager collaborates with persons skilled in their use.

Figure 14-3 presents a continuum showing the various levels of involvement by managers and evaluation research personnel. At one end of the continuum, the manager has the most influence. Here, emphasis is on evaluation focusing on relevance and program progress. At the other end of the continuum, where researchers have the most influence, emphasis is on assessing impact and effectiveness. These evaluations involve more sophisticated methodologic approaches and techniques.

This continuum also illustrates an often made distinction between formative and summative evaluation (8). *Formative evaluation* concerns the activities associated with the ongoing operations of a program. Emphasis is placed on improving the management of the program through data gathering and analysis. *Summative evaluation,* on the other hand, refers to activities associated with more long term effects of a program—whether the program, in fact, has had an impact on critical indicators or performance and/or meets specific previously determined program objectives.

In reality, evaluation along the continuum requires collaboration between program administrators and persons trained in research and evaluation methodologies. The relationship of health services research and management activities resembles the interface between program evaluation and management. Joel May suggests the following:

> Important opportunities for innovation, improvement and refinement of health services delivery systems are lost because of the administrators' lack of awareness of research (evaluation) findings or their inability to use them. At the same time much

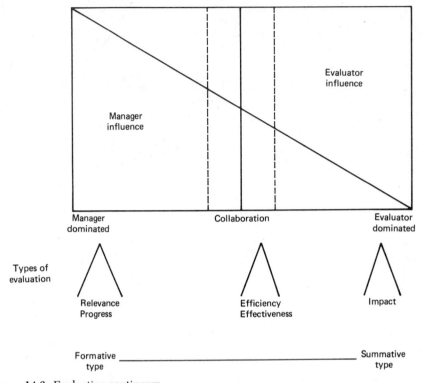

Figure 14-3. Evaluation continuum.
SOURCE: From Veney JE, Kaluzny AD: *Evaluation and Decision Making in Health Service Programs.* Reprinted by permission of Prentice-Hall, Englewood Cliffs, N.J. © 1983.

time and money is being invested in research (evaluation) that addresses questions not relevant to current needs of decision-makers or is too abstract or narrowly oriented to be useful to them. Research and development (program evaluation) are too important to leave the research design and executive responsibility solely to the researchers. And it is too important to leave the choice questions and formulation to administrators. The focus, content, quality, pertinence, and timeliness of health services research (program evaluation) efforts represent areas for which all interested parties share responsibility (9).

Collaboration requires considerable change in the way managers and evaluators function. For managers, collaboration requires recognition that they do not really know whether program X will be effective or is even relevant to the many problems faced by their organization. Instead of advocating a particular solution, the manager needs to present solutions as a series of options and develop ways to address them, at the same time considering effects on the community and organization. In essence, this approach requires a:

shift from the advocacy of a specific reform to the advocacy of the seriousness of the problem, and hence to the advocacy of persistence in alternative reform efforts should the first one fail. The political stance would become: "This is a serious problem. We propose to initiate Policy A on an experimental basis. If after five years there has been no significant improvement, we would shift to Policy B." By making explicit that a given problem solution was only one of several that the administrator or party could in good conscience advocate, and by having ready a plausible alternative, the administrator could afford honest evaluation of outcomes. Negative results, a failure of the first program, would not jeopardize his job, for his job would be to keep after the problem until something was found that worked (10:410).

For individuals involved in research and formal evaluation, an equally important shift must occur. Currently, many staff members view the research/evaluation community as the center of knowledge and its primary function as disseminator of information about program operations to the manager or community. A more realistic view for achieving collaboration is to recognize that much of the knowledge generated by social science represents only one approach to resolving important social problems (11). This perspective focuses on management as the center, with the various social sciences, including program evaluation, contributing to the main activity. To use evaluation studies for effective decision making, managers must be trained to understand research and evaluation skills as part of their overall arsenal in program management. In essence, given this approach, managers must be as knowledgeable about various evaluation methodologies as they are in other managerial skills, such as cost accounting and personnel management.

Uses of Evaluation

While general agreement exists that evaluation is an integral part of the decision-making process, the critical issue concerns actual use of information generated by evaluation methods. Recent investigations of the extent of use of evaluation and other research studies indicate that decision makers use information in a variety of ways and at different levels, but not necessarily as a direct guide for decision making. For example, Weiss and Buculavas (12), in a survey of evaluation studies in the health field, found that these studies served primarily to provide background information to managers. Energy and commitment on the part of the manager are important preconditions for the use of evaluation studies. Review of studies indicates that decision makers were receptive to research findings that challenged preconceived notions, at least in the area of mental health.

Despite some indications of use, expectations far exceed reality. Several factors contribute to the discrepancy.

Timeliness.   Timeliness, or rather lack of it, is often cited as an important factor in the nonuse of evaluation studies. Evaluations of large health service programs may require years of study, but policymakers and project managers want to know study results within a few weeks or, at most, months. Since managers and policymakers have a propensity for action (13), evaluations, to be useful, must fit within management's limited time frame.

A good example of the lag between the need for information and completion of a program to satisfy that need is the Rand Corporation's experiment assessing the effect of various types of health insurance coverage on the use of services (14,15). The project began in 1972, is still underway, and has yet to produce final results. While the project is well designed, the results, when they are available, may have little influence on policymaking in regard to any national health insurance scheme. The issue of national health insurance, important in the 1970s, has become more or less irrelevant to federal decision making in the early 1980s. Perhaps in the next decade, new concerns with health insurance may emerge; however, a study conducted in the 1970s may be considered too dated to be of value.

Relevance.   A second factor contributing to the failure of program evaluation to affect decision making is that evaluation has developed a dynamic of its own. That is, evaluation activities have become increasingly professional, based on an expanding esoteric body of knowledge almost independent of basic service delivery activities. In essence, evaluation activities tend to be self-limiting and self-controlling, organized around their own technical requirements and processes. Administrators do not see the work of evaluators as relevant to their decision-making needs.

Resolution of this problem does *not* require that program evaluation redefine its task as purely a technical function or abandon methodologic rigor. Instead, evaluation must focus on questions of interest to program managers involved in decision-making processes necessary to direct a program. Often these questions have counterparts in theory: issues derived from theory can be translated into practical policy and administrative issues (16,17).

Alternative Decision Making.   A third factor contributing to the apparent discrepancy between expectations and actual use is that information and analysis derived from program evaluation represent only one approach to the resolution of problems confronting decision makers. As described by Lindblom and Cohen:

> Information and analysis provides only one route because . . . a great deal of the world's problem-solving is acomplished through the various forms of social interaction that substitute action for thought, understanding or analysis. Information and analysis are not a universal or categorical prescription for problem-solving (11:10).

Lindblom and Cohen's challenging analysis indicates that a significant portion of decision making depends upon ordinary knowledge, social learning, and interaction. *Ordinary knowledge* does not owe its origin, testing of degree of verification, truth status, or currency to distinctive evaluation or research methodologies and techniques. Instead, ordinary knowledge requires common sense, causal empiricism, and thoughtful speculation and analysis. Decision making regarding health programs will always depend heavily on ordinary knowledge.

Social learning results from actual participation and ongoing social phenomena through which persons learn new behavior. Information generated from evaluation is likely to be of little use until social learning occurs. In a sense, social learning must occur before researchers can raise the significant questions appropriate for evaluation.

Finally, decision making based on *interactive problem solving* is considered to be an important alternative to program evaluation and occurs through resolution of problems with actions substituting for thought. This method introduces solutions to alleviate a problem or improve a situation without any understanding of the dilemma or systematic assessment of remedies or preferred outcomes. This approach to problems in health services is particularly pervasive because of the dominant role of physicians with their propensity of action (18).

LONG AND SHORT HISTORY
OF PROGRAM EVALUATION

From one perspective, evaluation may be considered a well-established activity in the health services field (19). This perspective stems from the tradition of research and development (R & D) characteristic of the medical field. As described by Freeman and Rossi:

> The R & D perspective is part of the vast medical research enterprise, dedicated to the detection, diagnosis, prevention, treatment, and management of disease. The evaluation of R & D efforts takes place at various levels within the medical enterprise. At one extreme, individuals and households are the targets of programs that seek to find efficacious ways to control or lessen harmful individual or household practices. Examples of such programs are those that seek to lower the incidence and prevalence of substance abuses—alcoholism, drug addiction or smoking—or to instill health practices such as weight control or the use of dental floss, or to maximize participation in mass preventive efforts such as vaccinations, chest x-rays, or routine examinations for breast cancer.
>
> At the other extreme, the R & D efforts are directed at larger aggregates that include communities and the nation as a whole. Such programs are directed at improving public sanitation, abating noise, or controlling polluting substances (19:342).

The R & D approach has been used in health services research. While the term *health services research* commonly refers to broad, heterogeneous activities, a fairly extensive review of the field defines it as inquiry to produce knowledge about the structure, processes, or effects of personal health services (20). The definition incorporates a number of program evaluation activities such as technology assessment, quality assessment, comparative use studies, and overall evaluation of the effects and impact of various types of health service programs.

To facilitate this type of evaluation, Congress in 1971 empowered the Secretary of Health, Education, and Welfare (HEW) to spend up to 1% of appropriations under the Public Health Service Act for evaluation of programs carried out under that act. The primary concern in Congress was on problems of equal access to health care and controlling the spiraling cost of medical services—basic issues of public policy and accountability of public funds.

Specific projects focused on basic questions of effectiveness of health services in accordance with the requirement that all ongoing activities within the federal government have an evaluation component. Examples of substantive evaluation are presented below:

Illustration A (21): The purpose of this project is to develop, implement, and evaluate the newly proposed health care cost containment strategy entitled *physician-based group insurance (PBGI)*. PBGI is a plan combining the concepts of prepayment and containment of health care costs. Under this scheme, the patient selects his or her own primary care physician. The primary care physician, in turn, must render and coordinate the total care of the patient in return for a yearly capitation payment. Consequently, premiums vary across physicians because of the relative efficiency with which a practice and patients make selections. Premiums are therefore the prime allocator of patients and resources to physicians. PBGI will be implemented in rural Baldwin County, Georgia, and a systematic effort will be made to evaluate the administrative feasibility of the strategy as well as health care cost, quality, and access. To meet these objectives, the demonstration and subsequent evaluation will involve five different population groups:

Group A—Medicare patients enrolled in PBGI who go to PBGI participating physicians (treatment group) in Baldwin County

Group B—Medicare patients not enrolled in PBGI who go to PBGI primary care physicians in Baldwin County

Group C-1—Baldwin County Medicare patients not enrolled in PBGI who go to primary care physicians not participating in PBGI

Group C-2—Residents in counties immediately surrounding Baldwin who are Medicare patients not enrolled in PBGI who go to primary care physicians not participating in PBGI

Group C-3—Medicare patients in the control counties who are not enrolled in PBGI and go to primary care physicians not participating in PBGI

Group D—Non-Medicare patients who go to primary care physicians participating in PBGI in Baldwin County

Group E—Non-Medicare patients who go to primary care physicians not participating in PBGI in Baldwin County

The study applies an elaborate set of measures to gather data on access to care, quality of care, physician adoption of preventive medicine approaches, physician satisfaction, cost, use, enrollment, and referral patterns among physicians. Data collection and analysis will cover a 5-year period beginning in 1981.

Illustration B (22): This project evaluates the impact of the National Institutes of Health consensus development program on the knowledge and practice of medical practitioners, and public awareness of and behavior regarding subjects of consensus conferences. Specifically, the project attempts 1) to analyze the impact of conducting and distributing the results of consensus conferences, particularly the contribution of these programs to professional decisions to modify practice, and 2) to develop recommendations for future activities to strengthen the dissemination process, enhance the diffusion, and increase the impact of the consensus development programs. The project gives special attention to evaluating the incremental benefit of the consensus program, over and above traditional modes of analysis and dissemination. Moreover, the project attempts to disclose, to the fullest extent possible, the factors facilitating or impeding changes in knowledge and behavior among health care providers and recipients. The analysis will provide the basis for developing a monitoring system to assess continuously the effectiveness of the consensus development program.

While evaluation may be considered part of a long tradition, it may also be viewed as a more recent phenomenon, as demonstrated in the requirement that Department of Health and Human Services (DHHS) projects incorporate an evaluation component to enhance their management. For example, the National Cancer Institute has attempted to develop evaluation guidelines for its centers' outreach program (23). Under these guidelines, 1) activities performed by the program should have defined and designated measures of performance, including use of staff and their resources; 2) each activity intended to have impact should be defined and measured to provide an indication of how the activity affects cancer incidence, morbidity, and mortality; 3) proposals should define the characteristics and capability of the evaluation system to handle various experimental designs and analyses; and 4) proposals should indicate how the project staff will use evaluation information to improve operations.

As a result of both types of evaluation activities, evaluation units and staff have developed at various levels of the federal health establishment. Consulting firms and universities have also developed a particular interest in evaluation to help meet the federally mandated demand.

A second implication was a recognition of the need for personnel to conduct evaluations. To satisfy this need, funds were allocated at the federal level to prepare persons with expertise in various evaluation methodologies.

Given this increased attention, evaluation as a set of activities developed its own dynamic, creating problems of timeliness and relevance vis-à-vis program decision makers. More recently, evaluation activities have been the target of federal budget cuts since they often focus on basic changes to achieve socially defined ends (1).

METHODS OF EVALUATION

Evaluation incorporates a range of methodologic strategies and procedures borrowed from social and management sciences. In general, five different types of evaluation strategies are relevant to health services programs: monitoring, case studies, survey research, trend analysis, and experimental design (5).

Below is a definition with selected illustrations for each of these methodologies. While the strategies are presented individually, use of one generally does not exclude use of the others. In fact, any well-designed evaluation requires multiple strategies to reveal different aspects of empirical reality, reduce threats to internal and external validity, and improve the ability to view the phenomena in a dynamic rather than a static fashion (24).

Monitoring

Monitoring systematically compares expectations with reality as the plan is implemented. Comparisons involve a range of activities including:

- Whether financing meets budgetary expectations
- Whether the personnel of the program meet personnel needs of the plan
- Whether the materials and other resources available meet the plan's specifications
- Whether the timing of activities follows the timetable of the plan
- Whether the quality of care provided meets established (explicit) criteria

When the plan and reality do not coincide, the plan, as reflected in the established criteria, can be modified or action can be initiated to change reality. In either case, the data generated by monitoring are critical to the decision.

The particular form monitoring takes depends upon the primary focus of activity and may vary in complexity. Below is a fairly simple scheme developed to monitor the operations of a number of community-based drug treatment programs. (For a more elaborate system as applied to public health programs see Ref. 25.)

Illustration: Monitoring Community Drug Treatment Programs (26).   Given a set of program goals, it is possible to identify relevant activities and targets associated with the respective goals. These targets represent the plan against which comparisons can be made.

For example, consider the following goal: the establishment of a crisis intervention service for the delivery of an immediate help service for a variety of drug, drug-related, and other crises.

Suggest that activities addressed to this goal include:

- Providing intervention services
- Providing a rap house or walk-in center
- Providing a hotline

Once a program has established a set of activities for a given reporting period, it must establish a corresponding set of targets and target levels for the same period. For example, prototype targets for the first activity, providing intervention services, are:

Hours per week of services provided

Referrals sent to other agencies per quarter

Staffing sessions per quarter involving staff members

Helping service agencies

Hours per week of telephone counseling/information

Hours per week of face-to-face counseling

Target levels are established for each target at the beginning of every reporting period. For example, the target levels for the first target (hours per week of services provided) might be 10 hours. At the end of each reporting period, the program manager reports the actual accomplishment vis-à-vis each target. For instance, in the above example, the target level measurement might be 8 hours for the same first target.

The program director is also required to assign a relative importance weight to each target (relative importance within an activity), for each activity (relative importance within a goal), and to each goal (relative importance vis-à-vis respective goals). For simplicity, the rating scale is from 1 to 5, representing levels of increasing importance. Just as activities, targets, and target levels may change between reporting periods, so may the relative importance weights assigned by the program director.

The five items—goals, activities, targets, target levels, and relative importance weights—comprise the management profile. In essence, the management profile describes what the program director plans for the program and the relative importance placed on each goal, activity, or target for that program.

A scoring system provides a numerical measure of how well a program is doing against its own targets based on the achievements it reports in each target area. For example, on a 0–1 scale, target fulfillment or success is arbitrarily assigned the value 0.6. Thus, if intervention services were provided for 10 hours per week, a score of 0.6 would be assigned. A target nonfulfillment or failure level is also set and arbitrarily assigned a value of 0.4. For example, 6 hours per week of services provided might be selected as failure of target level; that is, less than 6 hours would be considered unsatisfactory. On a given actual achievement level for the reporting period, for example, 8 hours per week, a score is found between 0 and 1. In this case, 8 hours per week would be assigned a score of 0.5.

Uses and Limitations.   Monitoring as an approach to evaluation is perhaps no more than good management. In fact, the decisions that can and should be made as a result of a well-designed monitoring effort are the day-to-day management decisions required in any organization. While monitoring is an important aspect of evaluation, its application in health services programs is subject to several limitations, in part generic to the monitoring process and in part a function of the unique characteristics of health services (19).

- *Informal versus formal activity.*   Monitoring may often be carried out in a highly informal manner. However, as programs become larger and more diverse, systematic and explicit monitoring efforts tend to underestimate the complexity of the process.
- *Measurement difficulties.*   As programs become more complex, difficulties develop with accurate measurement of resources, time, frequency of events, and finances. The problem becomes particularly critical to health services in which programs require health care professionals to compromise. Thus, goals often set at a level to achieve consensus are far too general to be used for developing specific indicators of performance.
- *Substitution of monitoring for program performance.*   A problem arises if monitoring begins to replace actual products desired from the program. One illustration comes from the area of family planning, where monitoring the number of contraceptive devices dispensed does not ensure the expected outcomes of a program. This difficulty makes essential the need for a clear relationship between monitoring and the desired program outcome.
- *Propensity to gather too much data.*   Monitoring may gather a great deal of data that is never used. Monitoring should deal with those aspects of the program directly relevant to decision making. It should not be conceived as a general data collection activity to cover all aspects of program operations.
- *High level of cynicism among organizational personnel.*   Organizational personnel are veterans of many monitoring programs, such as management by objectives (MBO) and program budgeting systems (PBS), as well as a host of other techniques. From previous experience, many personnel are skeptical, if not cynical, about the usefulness of such approaches to health services programs. Thus, while it may be possible to impose a monitoring scheme within a health services program organization, the critical factor in its success is the manager's effort to promote adoption of the program by organizational personnel.

Case Studies

Case studies concern the observation and analysis of a single unique activity, organization, or entity as representative of a general category. Case studies may use either qualitative or quantitative data, and are particularly appropriate where the boundaries of the program and its context are not clearly evident (27). The approach provides a great deal of information and depth of understanding about the particular phenomena under study.

In addition to providing a single focus and depth of understanding, the case study technique uses a number of different approaches in obtaining, analyzing, and using information. Case studies may involve a fairly unstructured set of historical and participant observations, more structured and systematic efforts such as probability samples, or specific techniques such as content analysis, nominal group process, and delphi procedures. An example of a case study using a combination of historical and participant observations is presented.

Illustration: Implementation of Health Center Concepts in a Rural Community: A Case Study (28).   The development of a comprehensive health center integrating inpatient and outpatient treatment in public health services within the same medical and administrative structure is a significant event worthy of documentation. Using a combination of historical records and participant observation, the authors document the successful implementation of a health center concept in a sparsely populated area of northwestern New Mexico. The case study describes the environmental and population characteristics of the catchment area within which the center operates, using information derived from secondary sources as well as surveys specifically designed to assess the service needs and demands of the area. Based on this background material, the case study proceeds to document the growth and development of the center over a period of time. Three stages are identified: initial implementation, transitional stage, and stabilization. In each stage the major actors are described, and significant events during each phase are analyzed. Special emphasis is given to identifying critical events, as well as to describing programmatic developments either facilitating or impeding the implementation of the program. The case study concludes with the implications of these findings for implementation of similar centers throughout the United States.

Uses and Limitations.   Case studies are important because they are a relatively inexpensive way to acquire information about how a particular program works. Specifically, the technique provides information about relevance (i.e., the nature and extent of the problem) and progress (i.e., how well the program is doing). Case studies also provide supplemental information that is useful in assessing efficiency, effectiveness, and impact.

Case studies, however, have limitations. First, particularly when data are collected in an unstructured manner, the evaluator is inundated with information. Lacking clear categories, it is difficult, if not impossible, to use the data to affect managerial decisions. Second, the approach is particularly vulnerable to selective perceptions, not only in how questions are perceived and recorded but also in how they are formulated.

A third limitation is the reactiveness of the strategy, that is, the extent to which the evaluation methodology (i.e., observation or other data collection effort) affects the operations of the program. While this problem is also prevalent in other evaluation methodologies, a major difficulty in case studies lies in the actual measurement of its effect on study results.

Case studies are perhaps appropriate when other types of evaluations are not, particularly when initial planning failed to include any systematic evaluation effort. When no comparison groups or criteria were established, case studies offer the only strategy available for evaluating the program.

Survey Research

Survey research uses information collected through questionnaires or interviews involving a sample of persons drawn from a population of interest. For instance, a survey may be directed to any or all of the following groups: the recipients or potential recipients of health services and the providers of services, including planners and managers as well as health professionals. Information about the perceptions and feelings of the recipients or providers of services on such issues as adequacy, effectiveness, and continuity of program services is typically obtained through interviews or questionnaires.

Survey research and evaluation methodology fall into two primary categories: descriptive or analytic. *Descriptive surveys* give an accurate picture of the situation. In the context of evaluation, a survey might describe a problem requiring some type of program activity, characterizing the program itself from the perspective of providers or service recipients, or simply describing results of the program or project. Below is an illustration of a descriptive survey.

Illustration: Using Survey Data to Plan Geriatric Mental Health Services (29). Within a given community:

- What is the rate and distribution of mental and physical disorders for persons aged 65 years or older?
- What is the perceived need for services of the mentally impaired elderly?
- How are existing services used, and what factors affect their use?

To answer these as well as other questions, a university medical center and a community mental health center undertook a descriptive survey of elderly patients and used the data to plan a geriatric mental health program. Using a random sample of 1,173 county residents 65 years or older, interviews were conducted to attempt to measure five areas of functioning: social resources, economic resources, mental health, physical health, and activities of daily living. Analysis indicated that 13% of the sample had mental impairment, and that mental impairment was highly correlated with other measures of functioning (e.g., 0.42 with social and economic resources, 0.55 with physical health, and 0.61 with activities of daily living). The analysis indicated that mentally impaired persons were likely to be impaired in other areas of functioning as well. These findings led to the development of new programs to accommodate multiple problems among patients.

Analytic surveys concern primarily relationships between various aspects of the phenomena under study. For example, an analytic evaluation survey might deal with whether program recipients with different characteristics view the program more or less favorably, or whether there is some differential effect of the program on recipients with certain characteristics. Consider the following example involving the productivity of nurse practitioners and physician assistants.

Illustration: Productivity of Nurse Practitioners and Physician Assistants (30).

Is productivity higher in practices employing nurse practitioners and physician assistants than other practices?

Do nurse practitioners and physician assistants make greater contributions to practice productivity when working independently of physicians (indirect supervision) or when working under the close supervision of physicians?

Do practices employing nurse practitioners and physician assistants deliver more services than other practices?

Does the use of nurse practitioners and physician assistants result in a shift of the location where services are delivered (e.g., more home visits)?

To evaluate the effect of nurse practitioners and physician assistants on practice activity and productivity, a national survey of 455 ambulatory care practices employing nurse practitioners and physician assistants was conducted. A matched sample of primary care physicians not employing nurse practitioners and physician assistants was also surveyed. Participants (physicians, nurse practitioners and physician assistants) in the survey were requested to complete a self-administered log diary for collecting detailed data on all patient encounters and professional activities recorded for a randomly selected 3-day period. Productivity data were measured by seven basic variables relating to patient volume, time, patient care, and revenue generated; number of minutes spent in direct patient care per day, number of, and minutes spent in, each direct patient encounter, number of, and minutes spent in, telephone patient encounter per day, and gross dollar income per day and per patient encounter. Data were subject to extensive reliability and validity checks.

Analysis revealed that physician assistants are considerably more productive than nurse practitioners, although the latter spent more time with individual patients. To provide a better understanding of the differences, productivity was assessed by rural-urban setting of the practice, availability of community resources, practice arrangement, complexity of services provided, severity of problems, and level and type of supervision. Nurse practitioners were shown to be equally productive in rural and urban settings; however, those in resource-poor areas tended to be slightly more productive. Nurse practitioner productivity in resource-rich areas can be measured by the number of patients seen and the amount of time spent in direct patient care; however, the opposite is not true. Finally, productivity was greatly modified by practice arrangement. For example, nurse practitioners were more productive in single-specialty groups and partnerships, while physician assistants were more productive in solo practice.

Uses and Limitations.   Survey research is a valuable methodology for gaining insight into program relevance, progress, efficiency, effectiveness, and impact. However, although it is an important approach, survey research has a number of limitations. First, it is an extremely costly process in terms of time and resources. Often, decisions have already been made by the time survey data are gathered and analyzed. Second, survey research focuses on subjective data. While this fact is often cited as a disadvantage, in reality it may be a major advantage since what persons perceive as real is real in its consequences.

Trend Analysis

Trend analysis involves the examination of trends in program outputs over a period of time. It provides an opportunity to ascertain 1) whether observed changes occurred before or after the initiation of a particular health service activity; 2) whether these changes are outside the normal expected range of variation; and 3) in certain instances, whether other possible explanations of the changes can be eliminated.

Trend analysis depends on information collected at more than one point in time. In a sense, it is similar to monitoring. Trend analysis, however, generally involves somewhat more sophisticated data analysis techniques than monitoring and is concerned primarily with program effects or impacts. Consider the following illustration.

Illustration: *Effect of the Mandated Highway Speed Limit Reduction of 1974 (31).*   This study was an attempt to determine whether it was possible to assess the effect, if any, of the change in speed limit laws that was implemented nationally in 1974. The data used in this study were highway deaths in the state of North Carolina from January 1975 to June 1980. The question addressed by the study was this: Was the lowered speed limit of 55 miles an hour, introduced in January 1974, associated with a concomitant reduction in the total number of highway or accident deaths?

The technique used to examine this question was ordinary least squares regression, in which the number of automobile deaths in each month was treated as the dependent variable. The independent variables consisted of time as a predictor, a dummy variable for each month of the year (to eliminate the differential effect of various months), and a dummy variable that was coded as 0 before the introduction of the speed limit law and 1 after the speed limit law went into effect. On the basis of this analysis, it was found that there was an average decrease of approximately 36 deaths per month after the introduction of the reduced speed limit. This decrease represented approximately a 25% reduction and was statistically significant.

Uses and Limitations.   Trend analysis provides important information for decision makers. In terms of relevance, it supplies background information about the situation that health services are designed to affect. An existing data system forms the base for the analyses and provides a continuous source for defining the nature of the problem.

Trend analysis also provides information about program progress. Because data are available over a period of time, it is possible to assess changes outside the normal expected range of variation. This characteristic is critical for initiating corrective action during the life of a program.

Trend analysis gives managers the opportunity to assess effectiveness and impact. Since data are collected over time, it is possible for the manager to 1) observe changes before and after the implementation of program and 2) suggest other explanations of change and thereby clearly decide whether the specific program has had a desired effect.

Like other methodologies, trend analysis has limitations. First, the costs of maintaining data over time are very high. Second, even when data are maintained, there may be various changes in categories or coding procedures, making longitudinal comparisons difficult. Finally, it is often difficult to account for other changes that may have occurred at the time the study program was introduced.

Experimental Design

Experimental design makes a structured and systematic comparison of output or output measures between a setting in which a program is provided and one in which the program is not provided. (For a detailed presentation of these and experimental and quasi-experimental designs, see Refs. 32 and 33.) This simple formulation includes a number of different strategies directly applicable to health service settings. Presented next are descriptions of basic experimental designs appropriate to health services.

Experimental Design Type:
Pretest/Posttest Design

	t (1)		t (2)
E	O (1)	X	O (2)

In the pretest/posttest design, the only group considered is the experimental group. At time one [t(1)], a first observation is made [O(1)]. Between t(1) and time two [t(2)], an experimental effect (E) is introduced (X). Finally, at t(2), a second observation is made [O(2)], and the effect of the program is the difference between the measure of the state at t(2) and at t(1).

An illustration of this type of evaluation in the health services setting is presented.

Illustration: Evaluating the Health Insurance Plan (HIP) Peer Review Program (34).   The HIP Peer Review Program involves a systematic application of explicit process criteria to medical care for selected types of conditions recorded in patient records. Under this program, findings are reported to 26 physician groups participating in the HIP program. Each group is required to respond with a plan for resolving identified problems.

To evaluate the effectiveness of the Peer Review Program, a total of 6,788 records were reviewed in terms of clinical management of acute otitis media, hypertension, and breast lesions. Evaluation involved a comparison of compliance with the explicit initial criteria with findings reporting compliance with these criteria on a reaudit.

Analysis revealed a statistically significant improvement in the quality of clinical practice as measured by assessment parameters. For example, in the area of hypertension, comparison of audit and reaudit compliance showed a statistically significant improvement on criteria associated with diagnostic processes such as history taking, physical examination, and laboratory tests, as well as therapeutic process criteria, including regimen specification and referral. Similar results are reported for otitis media and breast lesions.

Experimental Design Type:
Pretest/Posttest with a Control Design

	t (1)		t (2)
E	O (E1)	X	O (E2)
C	O (C1)		O (C2)

This design involves an experimental group (E) as well as a control group (C). At [t(1)], an observation is made on the experimental group [O(E1)] and on the control group [O(C1)]. Between t(1) and t(2), an experimental variable (X) is introduced in E. At t(2), another set of observations is made on both the experimental [O(E2) and control group [O(C2)]. The effect is determined by comparing the observation on an experimental group at t(2) minus the observation taken on the group at t(1), subtracted from the observation of the control group taken at t(2) minus that at t(1). The following illustration involves the evaluation of a psychologic intervention on medical care utilization.

Illustration: Impact of Psychologic Intervention on Medical Care Utilization (35).   Can utilization of medical services be reduced without reducing the quality of care by providing psychologic interventions? To answer this question, an experiment was designed to determine how the use of medical services would be affected by applying rational-emotive therapy principles and behavioral principles emphasizing stimulus control.

To evaluate the intervention, the number of outpatient visits of matched treatment ($N = 17$) and control groups ($N = 17$) were compared 6 months before and 6 months after the intervention. Subjects were matched on age, sex, marital status, and general medical symptoms.

TABLE 14-1. Mean Number of Outpatient Visits During the 6 Months Before and 6 Months After Treatment Initiation or Abstention

Group	Before	After
Treatment	7.47	2.71
Comparison	6.94	7.12

The results of the study, summarized in Table 14-1, demonstrate a significant reduction in the use of medical services after the intervention. The study suggests that for certain patients utilization of medical services can be decreased by the use of psychologic counseling.

Experimental Design Type: Multishot Pretest-Posttest (with Control Group) Design

The multishot pretest-posttest design, represented in Table 14-2, involves multiple experimental groups [E(n)] with an observation each at time one [O(En1)], an experimental variable introduced between time one and time two, [x(n)] and observation on each of the experimental groups at time two [O(En2)]. Control groups [c(m)] may or may not be used in this design; however, when control groups are used, they act as control against any experimental effects. The major interest in this design is to compare the various experimental effects against each other, as opposed to comparing a program input with no program interventions. For this design to have maximum effect, allocation to the various groups should be on a random basis. Presented next is an example of this design in a health services setting.

Illustration: Psychosocial Treatment of the Cancer Patient: A Multiple Experiment (36). Providing various types of psychosocial support services to cancer patients nd their families is increasingly recognized as an important part of the management of the cancer patient. A study was designed to consider the impact of psychosocial services on the cancer patient. Hospitalized cancer patients were

TABLE 14-2. Multiple Treatment Pretest-Posttest (with Control Group) Design

	t (1)		t (2)	
E (1)	O (E11)	X (1)	O (E12)	
E (2)	O (E21)	X (2)	O (E22)	
E (3)	O (E31)	X (3)	O (E32)	
—				
—				
—				
E (n)	O (En1)	X (n)	O (En2)	
C (1)	O (C11)		O (C12)	⎤
—				
—				⎬ Optional
—				
C (m)	O (Cm1)		O (Cm2)	⎦

randomly assigned to one of three treatment groups. Patients assigned to group A received no special psychosocial support services. These patients served as the control group for the study.

Patients in group B received the services of the Psychosocial Intervention Program (PIP). A basic premise of PIP is that the needs of a cancer patient are best met by a single health care provider who follows the patient from initial diagnosis through hospital discharge and continues long term contact with the patient. This role was filled by a psychologist or social worker (psychosocial worker). An advisory board consisting of other health care professionals worked with the psychosocial worker in developing specific interventions, which varied according to a number of factors, including site of the cancer, severity, type of medical treatment, frequency and nature of psychosocial problems, and scores on psychometric tests. In group B, as in group A, the individual patient was the focus of psychosocial interventions.

Patients assigned to group C received PIP, as described for group B. However, the families of group C patients were also treated. Treatment was oriented toward the needs of patients and family members as individuals and as interacting members in a social network.

Psychometric tests and problem-oriented interviews were administered to all patients and the major significant other person in the patients' lives at hospital admission, before discharge, and 3, 6, and 12 months after discharge. Demographic and medical data were also collected. Results are pending analysis.

Experimental Design Type:
Posttest Design (with Randomization)

R	t (1)		t (2)
E	—	X	O (E1)
C	—		O (C1)

As this design indicates, no observation is made at time 1. An experimental variable (X), such as a program, is introduced, and observations on both the experimental and control group are made at t(2). Consider the following illustration.

Illustration: Controlled Clinical Trial Family Care Coupled with Child Care Only in Comprehensive Primary Care (37).   Is there a difference between the effectiveness of providing primary care to children as opposed to providing care to both children and their parents? To evaluate these alternative patterns of care, the Morrisama Comprehensive Health Center randomly assigned new registrants at the center to either family care or child care only. Persons in the family care group were offered comprehensive care for both parents and children, while only children in the child care group were offered comprehensive care.

Results indicate few measurable differences between the two groups of children in terms of utilization or outcome. Where there were differences, most tended to favor the family pattern of care. Older children continued to use the center, immunizations were somewhat more timely, and children over time appeared to make fewer visits to sources of ambulatory care other than the health care center.

Uses and Limitations.   When properly planned and executed, the experimental design approach is the most powerful evaluation technique available for assessing the effectiveness or impact of a given health service program. No other evaluation approach, with the possible exception of time series methodology, can give such a

TABLE 14-3. Limitations of Various Types of Experimental Designs

Problem	Pretest/ Posttest	Pretest/Posttest with Control Group	Randomized Posttest	Multiple Group Pretest/Posttest with Control Group
Extraneous variable	−	+	+	+
Regression to the mean	−	+	+	+
Sensitization	−	−	+	+
Reactiveness	−	−	−	+

+ indicates that the design is able to resolve or control the problem.

− indicates that the design is not able to resolve or control the problem.

clear and definitive assessment of the true value of the efficiency, effectiveness, and impact of a program.

The application of various experimental methodologies requires a firm understanding of the problems associated with each design. Table 14-3 presents the limitations of the various experimental designs as related to four formative problems associated with experimentation. The first problem with experimental design is that of extraneous variables, that is, the extent to which the design is able to determine the real effects of the programs (i.e., the experimental variable) from other simultaneous factors. For example, in the course of a major program such as primary care, family planning, or other major activities, a number of factors other than the program itself are likely to influence the desired effects. The design must be able to control or at least identify these factors.

A second problem concerns regression to the mean. Over a period of time, a general shift may occur back toward the basic trend line, either higher or lower, without regard to any effect of the program introduced to influence the phenomena.

A third problem is that of sensitization, in which participation in the experiment has an effect on performance. Again, the concern is the extent to which the design is able to control or at least identify this factor. Finally, reactiveness is a problem that affects various designs and concerns the effect of knowledge about a situation upon the situation itself.

As seen in Table 14-3, the effects of these problems vary by type of design. For example, a pretest/posttest design is strongly affected by all four types of problems. This design is unable to control for extraneous variables, or to assess whether the effects are derived from the program or simply represent a general regression to the trend line. Similarly, because the design lacks any control, it is impossible to deal with the problems of sensitization or reactiveness.

The pretest/posttest with the control group, while unable to resolve the problems of sensitization or reactiveness, can resolve the problems of extraneous variables and regression to the mean. The use of a control group provides a basis for determining whether observed changes are a function of program effect or extraneous variables. Similarly, use of the control group provides a basis for determining whether observed changes over time are the result of program effects or simply regression effects.

Randomized posttest designs provide a mechanism for dealing with effects of extraneous variables, regression, and sensitization. The critical factor is randomization. Unfortunately, this design does not control the effects of reactiveness.

The multiple treatment pretest/posttest with the control group is obviously the most effective means of dealing with these problems. Random assignment among various interventions as well as use of a control group permits an adequate solution to the problems of extraneous variables, regressions to the mean, sensitization, and reactiveness.

THE FUTURE OF EVALUATION

As with many activities, the potential of evaluation far exceeds its accomplishments to date. Projections of the future need to be set in terms of long range versus short range expectations. In the long term, the role of evaluation will undoubtedly expand, focusing on various programmatic as well as technologic aspects of health services. The increasing cost of services will expand the need for evaluation and provide more sophisticated approaches to the evaluation process.

The major policy changes initiated by the Reagan administration will shape the short term future of evaluation. While President Reagan and his colleagues have proven that program survival does not depend upon evaluation findings, a more optimistic view suggests that the new policies provide an opportunity to refocus evaluation efforts and redefine the process in a manner that increases overall impact and in the end produces stronger health services programs. Discussed next are some specific issues that will guide the role of evaluation in the foreseeable future.

- It must be explicitly recognized that evaluation is only one method of resolving health services problems. Evaluation must not be considered a substitute for other types of problem solving. It merely supplements or complements other methods. Failure to recognize this fact reduces the overall effect of evaluation. As described by Lindblom and Cohen: "[Evaluators] will indiscriminately attempt too many tasks rather than selectively choosing critical supplements or complementarities to the other inputs; will spend their energies on tasks that they cannot do well, as well as those they need not do; and will fail to focus on tasks they can do" (11:54).

  To the extent that expectations can be reduced, and that evaluation can adapt to the realities of the problem-solving process, it will play an important role. Health services managers, for example, require information to help improve decision making. Managers face problems of expanding or contracting services and recruiting, retaining, and allocating personnel, as well as deciding what types of services and personnel are required. To solve these problems, information generated by various evaluation methodologies is critical. Industrial managers spend a great deal of time and money to make these decisions more effectively. A similar investment is likely to be worthwhile for health services managers.

- It must be recognized that evaluation resources, like program resources, are limited and should be allocated to activities likely to benefit from the process. Thus, while all programs can be evaluated, there is often merit in delaying any substantive evaluation until preliminary assessment of the program's basic design is made. Increased emphasis will be given to what Wholey (38) defines as *evaluability assessment*, that is, the process of determining whether objectives are well defined, whether program assumptions are plausible, and whether intended uses of evaluation information are clearly stated.

TABLE 14-4. Decision-making Factors Affecting the Choice of Future Program Evaluations

Beliefs About Cause/Effect Relationships	Preferences Regarding Desirability of Possible Outcomes	
	Certain	Uncertain
Certain	Progress evaluation No need for formal program evaluation efforts, although ongoing monitoring is important	Effectiveness evaluation Rigorous program evaluation efforts useful in selling and defending the program in political battles, particularly if program effects are small
Uncertain	Impact evaluation Impact, summative program evaluation most appropriate	Relevance evaluation Process-oriented formative evaluation most appropriate

(efficiency) (efficiency)

SOURCE: Adapted from Shortell SM, Richardson WC: *Health Program Evaluation*. St Louis: CV Mosby Co, 1978.

- More selective identification of evaluation issues provides an opportunity to match types of evaluation with basic characteristics of the program within its political context. This approach is illustrated nicely by Shortell and Richardson's formulation of program evaluation using Thompson's (39) typology of organizational decision-making strategies. Table 14-4 presents the basic decision-making factors affecting the choice of future program evaluation activities, as well as the types of evaluation appropriate for these basic conditions.

As presented in Table 14-4, the type of evaluation that is appropriate is a function of 1) whether there is certainty or uncertainty about the cause-and-effect relationship and 2) whether there is certainty or uncertainty about the desirability of program outcomes. Where there is certainty regarding both of these factors, a *progress* type of evaluation is considered the most appropriate. The purpose is simply to ensure that the program is following the expected plan.

Where there is certainty about cause-and-effect relationships but uncertainty about the desirability of possible outcomes, a far more elaborate evaluation effort is required. Here attention needs to be given to *effectiveness*, to determine whether the program is meeting stated objectives. Evaluation information becomes critical in providing a justification and/or defense for continuation of the program.

Where there is uncertainty about the cause-and-effect relationship but certainty about the desirability of possible outcomes, an *impact* type of evaluation is most appropriate. This approach determines whether observed effects occurred in the absence of the program or in the presence of some alternative activity.

Finally, where there is uncertainty about both the cause-and-effect relationship and the desirability of possible outcomes, the basic issue is *relevance*, that is, whether the program is actually needed. As noted in the table, *efficiency* evaluations are critical under these conditions.

Failure to diagnose the basic problems accurately and to initiate the appropriate type of evaluation activity undermines the ability to respond to critical health services needs. Unfortunately, there is often a preoccupation with issues of relevance when, in fact, there is certainty about cause and effect as well as about the desirability of outcomes. Similarly, there is often concern with progress when, in fact, there is uncertainty about cause and effect, as well as about the desirability of outcomes.

REFERENCES

1. Shortell SM, Richardson WC: *Health Program Evaluation.* St Louis, CV Mosby Co, 1978.
2. Attkisson CC, Broskowski A: Evaluation and the emerging human service concept, in Attkisson CC, Hargreaves WA, Horowitz MJ, et al (eds): *Evaluation of Human Service Programs.* New York, Academic Press, 1978.
3. Suchman EA: *Evaluative Research.* New York, Russell Sage Foundation, 1967.
4. Weiss CH: *Evaluation Research.* Englewood Cliffs, NJ, Prentice-Hall Inc, 1972.
5. Veney JE, Kaluzny AD: *Evaluation and Decision Making in Health Service Programs.* Englewood Cliffs, NJ, Prentice-Hall Inc, 1983.
6. Second draft: Provisional guidelines for health program evaluation, HPC/DPE/78.1. Geneva, World Health Organization.
7. Borus ME, Buntz CG, Tash WR: *Evaluating the Impact of Health Programs: A Primer.* Cambridge, Mass, MIT Press, 1982.
8. Scriven M: The methodology of evaluation, in Tyler RW, Gagne RM, Scriven M (eds): *Perspectives of Curriculum Evaluation.* Chicago, Rand McNally, 1967.
9. May JJ: Symposium: The policy uses of research. *Inquiry* 1975; 12:228–230.
10. Campbell DT: Reforms as experiments. *Am Psychol* 1969; 24(4):409–429.
11. Lindblom CE, Cohen DK: *Usable Knowledge: Social Science and Social Problem Solving.* New Haven, Conn, Yale University Press, 1979.
12. Weiss CH, Buculavas MJ: The challenge of social research to decision making, in Weiss CH (ed): *Using Social Research in Public Policy Making.* Lexington, Mass, Lexington Books, 1977.
13. Mintzberg H: *The Nature of Managerial Work.* New York, Harper & Row Publishers Inc, 1973.
14. Newhouse JP: A design for a health insurance experiment. *Inquiry* 1974; 11:5–27.
15. Newhouse JP, Manning WG, Morris CN, et al: Some interim results from a controlled trial of cost sharing in health insurance. *N Engl J Med* 1981; 305:1501–1507.
16. Shortell SM: Organizational theory and health service delivery, in Shortell SM, Brown M (eds): *Organizational Research in Hospitals,* Chicago, Blue Cross Association, 1976.
17. Kaluzny AD, Veney JE: *Health Service Organizations: A Guide to Research and Assessment.* Berkeley, McCutchan Publishing Co, 1980.
18. Freidson E: *Profession of Medicine: A Study of the Sociology of Applied Medicine.* New York, Dodd, Mead & Co, 1970.
19. Freeman H, Rossi P: Social experiments. *Health Society: Milbank Mem Fund Q* 1981; 59(3):340–373.
20. National Academy of Sciences: *Report of a Study, Health Services Research.* Washington, DC, National Academy of Sciences, 1979.
21. Freund D: Implementation and evaluation of physician based group insurance. Proposal submitted to the Health Care Financing Administration, Chapel Hill, North Carolina, University of North Carolina, 1980.
22. US Dept of Health and Human Services: Assess the impact of the NIH Consensus Development Program, RFP No. NIH-00-82-06. U.S. Department of Health and Human Services, 1982.

23. Caban CE, Fink DJ: A structural model for cancer control programs, discussion paper 1. Bethesda, Md, Division of Cancer Control and Rehabilitation, National Cancer Institute, 1979.

24. Denzin NK: *The Research Act: A Theoretical Introduction to Sociological Methods.* New York, McGraw-Hill Book Co, 1978.

25. Hauver JH, Goodman JA: The evaluation of performance and cost in a hypertension control program. *Med Care* 1980; 18(5):485–502.

26. Zalkind DL, Zelon HS, Moore MD, Kaluzny AD: *North Carolina Drug Abuse Program Evaluation Report.* Chapel Hill, Department of Health Administration, University of North Carolina, 1976.

27. Yin RK: The case study crisis: some answers. *Adm Sci Q* 1981; 26:58–65.

28. Reid RA, Bartlett EE, Kozoll R: Implementation of the health center concept in a rural community: A case study. *J Community Health* 1981; 7(1):57–66.

29. Blazer DB, Maddox G: Using epidemiologic survey data to plan geriatric mental health services. *Hosp Community Psychiatry* 1982; 33(1):42–45.

30. Mendanhall RC, Repicky PA, Neville RE: Assessing the utilization and productivity of nurse practitioners and physician's assistants: Methodology and findings on productivity. *Med Care* 1980; 18(6):609–623.

31. Veney JE, Luckey JW: Effect of the mandated highway speed limit reduction of 1974. *Soc Indicators Res,* in press.

32. Campbell DT, Stanley JC: *Experimental and Quasi-Experimental Design for Research.* Chicago, Rand McNally, 1966.

33. Cook T, Campbell D: *Quasi-Experimentation: Design and Analysis Issues for Field Settings.* Chicago, Rand McNally, 1979.

34. Deuschle JM, Alvarez B, Logsdon DN, et al: Physician performance in a prepaid health plan: Results of the peer review program of the Health Insurance Plan of Greater New York. *Med Care* 1982; 20(2):127–142.

35. Longobardi PG: The impact of a brief psychological intervention on medical care utilization in an Army health care setting. *Med Care* 1981; 19(6):665–671.

36. Gordon WA, Freidenberg I, Diller L, et al: Efficacy of psychosocial intervention with cancer patients. *J Consulting and Clin Psychology* 1980; 48(6):743–759.

37. Agustin MS, Sidel VW, Drosness DL, et al: A controlled clinical trial of "family care" compared with "child-only care" in the comprehensive primary care of children. *Med Care* 1981; 19(2):202–213.

38. Wholey JS: *Evaluation: Promise and Performance.* Washington, DC, Urban Institute, 1979.

39. Thompson J: *Organizations in Action.* New York, McGraw-Hill Book Co, 1967.

PART SIX

Health Care Policies and Politics

CHAPTER 15

Health Policy and the Politics of Health Care

Philip R. Lee

A. E. Benjamin

Political considerations have significantly affected nearly all of the developments discussed in this book. However, the importance and central role of health care policy analysis and politics can best be highlighted by directly discussing these issues. That is the purpose of this chapter. While many of the topics mentioned here have been discussed from a variety of perspectives in other chapters, the policy and politics of changes in health care in the nation is the focus here, and examples of developments in health care serve as illustrations of the central role of political forces in shaping our health services system. The philosophies and processes discussed in other chapters, and especially in Chapters 4 and 12, are further analyzed here.

Government plays a major role in planning, directing, and financing health services in the United States. The significance of the public sector is apparent as one considers the following: Public programs account for approximately 40% of the nation's personal health care expenditures; most physicians and other health care personnel are trained at public expense; almost 65% of all health research and development funds are provided by the government; and most nonprofit community and university hospitals have been built or modernized with government subsidies. The bulk of governmental expenditures are federal, with state and local governments contributing significant, but much smaller, amounts.

The health policies and programs of the U.S. government have evolved piecemeal, usually in response to needs that were not being met by the private sector or by state and local governments. The result has been a proliferation of federal categorical programs administered by more than a dozen government departments. Over the years, new programs have been added, old ones redirected, and numerous efforts made to integrate and coordinate services. Functions of the public and private sectors have become increasingly interrelated, and roles are often blurred. There can be little argument that the primary function of most government programs in health has been to support or strengthen the private sector (e.g., hospital construction, subsidy of medical student training, Medicare) rather than to develop a strong system of publicly provided health care.

Although U.S. government policies have evolved over a 200-year period, most of those affecting health services have developed since the enactment of the Social Security Act in 1935. Many federal health programs evolved because of failures in the private sector to provide necessary support, for example biomedical research; others arose because results of the free market were grossly inequitable, for example hospital construction; and some programs, such as Medicare and Medicaid, developed because health care was so costly that many could not afford to pay for necessary health services. Some federal health programs, such as biomedical research, potentially benefit everyone, while others, such as the Indian Health Service, reach only a small but needy segment of the population. Some programs, such as poliomyelitis immunization and health personnel development, have been effective in achieving their goals; others, such as health planning, have probably failed to realize even limited objectives; still others, such as Medicare, have reached some goals, although at a much higher cost than originally anticipated.

The process by which health policy is made in this country can best be understood by considering a fundamental paradox in American health care: Government spends more and more money to support a wide range of health programs, services, and agencies, yet the role of government in the reform of our health care system remains limited and halting. Government is faced with a crisis in health care, defined primarily in terms of rising costs to public treasuries, while proposed solutions are framed in terms that do not address in any comprehensive fashion the sources of demand on the public purse. Indeed, solutions to the cost crisis commonly are limited to withdrawing benefits from those very recipient populations whose health care needs justify government intervention. To understand this paradox, it is necessary to consider several characteristics of public policymaking and thus to explore the sources of the paradox and the nature of policy processes in health.

DIMENSIONS OF POLICYMAKING IN HEALTH

The making of health policy across several levels of government and hundreds of programs is complex, and no single analytical scheme can do it sufficient justice. Still, students of public policy have identified five characteristics of the policy process: 1) the relationship of government to the private sector; 2) the distribution of authority within a federal system of government; 3) pluralistic ideology as the basis of politics; 4) the relationship between policy formulation and administrative implementation; and 5) incrementalism as a strategy of reform. Each will be considered in detail.

Public and Private Sector Politics

Although in recent years the role of government in health care has grown considerably, that role remains relatively limited. The U.S. government is less involved in health care than are those of many other industrialized countries (1). This circumstance derives primarily from a persistent ideology that identifies the market system as the most appropriate setting for the exchange of health services, and from a related belief that private sector support for public sector initiatives can be acquired only through accommodation to the interests of health care providers. The significance of the market ideology has been elaborated in analyses of the passage of Medicare and Medicaid in 1965 (2,3). The persistence of doubts about the appropriate role of government is certainly apparent in the renewed vitality of neoconservatism, in which it is argued that the market can better respond to the economic and social problems of our time if it is unfettered by government intervention (4).

Uncertainty about the role of government in health care has numerous consequences. Primary among them is the absence of any design or blueprint for governmental reform (5). Instead, the public sector (with its relatively immense capacity to raise revenues) is called upon periodically to open and close its funding spigots to stimulate the health care market. Hospital construction and physician education are prominent examples of public activity. Not only is there no blueprint for public sector action, but governments in America harbor grave doubts about the appropriateness of regulation as a public sector activity. Dependence at the federal level upon "voluntary approaches," such as the reduction of hospital costs in the late 1970s, delayed serious consideration of more stringent measures even as the costs to government of hospital care continued to rise dramatically (6).

A Federal System

The concept of *federalism* has evolved dramatically in meaning and practice since the founding of the republic more than 200 years ago. Originally, federalism was a legal concept that defined the constitutional division of authority between the federal government and the states. Federalism initially stressed the independence of each level of government to the other, while incorporating the idea that some functions, such as foreign policy, were the exclusive province of the central government, whereas other functions, such as education, police protection, and health care, were the responsibility of regional units—state and local governments. Federalism represents a form of governance that differs both from a unitary state, where regional and local authority derive legally from the central government, and from a confederation, in which the national government has limited authority and does not reach individual citizens directly (7,8).

Shifts in responsibilities assigned to various levels of government do not pose a serious problem for health policy if at least two conditions are met: 1) administrative or regulatory responsibilities and financial accountability are consonant and 2) the various levels of government possess the appropriate capacities to assume those responsibilities assigned to them. Important questions can be raised regarding whether either of these conditions has been met in the development of health policy during the last 2 decades.

Analysis of federal-state relationships in programs as divergent as Medicaid, provider licensure, and health planning under PL 93-641 have suggested that the structure of these relationships produces outcomes widely held to be dysfunctional (e.g., Medicaid cutbacks) because one level of government (e.g., the states) can do nothing else under the conditions established by another (e.g., the federal government). The disjuncture between administrative responsibilities and financial accountability (i.e., the terms of federalistic arrangements) in these cases yielded results for which governments and the recipients of health care ultimately paid. What seems to matter most in the structure of relationships within federalism is not so much the distribution of activities as it is the relationships among levels of governments (9).

For allocations of authority among levels of government to work, it is important that governments possess those capacities appropriate to the responsibilities they confront. Governments must possess the revenue capacity, the capability to plan and manage policies and programs, and the political will necessary for responsiveness and reform. State and local governments have been found wanting in each of these respects. Because state governments do not tax as heavily as the federal government (10), their capacity for generating new revenues is limited. Many states, moreover, are viewed as having inadequate administrative infrastructures, being short on sophisticated management techniques, and having limited capabilities in the conduct of policy analysis and planning.

Finally, there is evidence that state and local governments may have less political will to make decisions in the public interest than the federal government. Wide variations among states in program outputs (e.g., Medicaid) suggest significant inequities. The argument is not that every state, if freed from federal constraints, would establish standards for health programs that are certain to fall below former federal standards. Rather, it is that some states will surely exceed some federal standards, and others will fall far below what is generally considered adequate. At the heart of this problem, many argue, is the reputedly greater susceptibility of state governments to interest group pressures and narrow conceptions of the public good.

For at least two of these sets of arguments, there is some countervailing evidence that the capacity and will to govern is becoming more widely diffused within the federal system. States (taken as a group) spent a higher percentage of their budgets on health care than did the federal government in 1978, even though absolute federal expenditures for health grew to more than double the state and local health expenditures combined (11). A considerable increase at the state level in the conduct of policy analysis and its use in policy deliberations is one indication that the capacity of states to plan and manage is improving (12). Regarding inequities and political will, on the other hand, little counterevidence has emerged to challenge the argument that the states are more vulnerable to interest groups (e.g., provider groups in health) and that the result is wide program variation among states in response to provider—not consumer—interests. The structure of federalism enables provider groups to maximize their power at the expense of consumer interests (9,13).

Pluralistic Politics

Pluralism is a term used by political theorists to describe a set of values about the effective functioning of democratic governments. Pluralists argue that democratic societies are organized into many diverse interest groups, which pervade all socioeconomic strata, and that this network of pressure groups prevents any one elite group from overreaching its legitimate bounds. As a theoretical framework for explaining the political context of policymaking, this perspective has been criticized relentlessly and appropriately (14,15). As an ideology that continues to influence the way elites and masses think about government, pluralism becomes a basis for considering some essential elements of the process of public decision making in this country.

Interest groups play a powerful role in the health policy process. Most federal and state laws designed to address the health care needs of the population are shaped by the interaction among interest groups, key legislators, and agency representatives. Ginsberg (16) has identified four power centers in the health care industry that influence the nature of health care and the role of government: 1) physicians, 2) large insurance organizations, 3) hospitals, and 4) a highly diversified group of participants in profit-making activities within the health care arena.

The growing influence of these power centers is evident in policies at all levels of government. The development of Medicare and Medicaid policies reflects the powerful influence of physicians, hospitals, and nursing homes as well as their allies in the health insurance industry. For example, in enacting Medicare, Congress ensured that the law did not affect the physician-patient relationship, including the physician's method of billing the patient. The system of physician reimbursement adopted by Medicare is highly inflationary, because it provides incentives to physicians to raise prices and to provide ancillary services, such as laboratory tests, electrocardiograms, and x-ray films. Hospital reimbursement is based on costs incurred in providing care, creating strong incentives to provide more and more services. Despite the impact of rapidly rising Medicare costs on the Social Security trust fund, on Social Security taxes (paid by employers and employees), and on the elderly, Congress has steadfastly refused to alter Medicare's methods of payment to physicians and hospitals. Many features of the program, patterned on principles developed by the medical industry, have had remarkable staying power.

As the case of Medicare suggests, health policy in the United States has been largely a product of medical politics (17). Health policy reform has been characterized as a series of new opportunities for the medical system to expand its influence, scale, and control (18). Marmor et al. (19) describe the political "market" in health (i.e., institutional arrangements among actors in the political system) as imbalanced. In an imbalanced market, participants have unequal power, and those with concentrated rather than diffuse interests have a greater stake in the effects of policy. At least until recently, provider interest groups have had a far greater stake in shaping health policy than have consumer interests.

Some observers argue that the rising costs of health care may change the configuration of interest groups seeking to influence health policy. In recent years, steadily escalating costs have stimulated other interests, especially labor, business, and governments themselves, to giving greater attention to health policy and its implications. In other words, their interests may be shifting from diffuse to concentrated. The result may be that increased competition in the political marketplace from a more diverse set of participants will lessen the dominance of medical provider groups (20). The pluralist dream of effective interest groups that prevent any one group from overreaching its legitimate bounds continues to influence our thinking about health care.

Policy Implementation

The nature of the health policy process is determined not only by the balance between provider and consumer interests but also by the relationships of these interests to government actors. Students of public policy have observed that policymaking moves through at least three stages: 1) agenda setting, the continuous process by which issues come to public attention and are placed on the agenda for government action; 2) policy adoption, the legislative process by which elected officials decide the broad outlines of policy; and 3) policy implementation, the process by which administrators develop policy by addressing the numerous issues unaddressed by legislation (13,21). An important element of the health policy process involves the relative roles of elected officials and professional administrators. As one moves from agenda setting to policy adoption and implementation, it can be argued that the role of elected officials becomes more remote and that of administrators more crucial.

No policy theorist has pressed this argument with more conviction than Lowi (22). A central theme in what he calls *interest-group liberalism* is the growing role of administrators in politics. According to Lowi, in a period of resource richness and government expansion, such as the 1960s, government responded to a range of major organized interests, underwrote programs sought by those interests, and assigned program responsibility to administrative agencies. Through this process, the programs became captives of the interest groups because the administrative agencies themselves were captured. Interest groups dominate the policy process, he argues, not only through their influence on the legislative process (policy adoption) but also through control of administration. In effect, governments in the United States make policies without laws and leave the lawmaking to administrators.

The study of policy implementation in health has received increased attention in recent years (23). Not surprisingly, the landmark legislation creating Medicare and Medicaid in 1965 has been the subject of much of this analysis. A study of Medicare by Feder is especially enlightening. She describes a number of crucial decisions related to the nature of the federal role that were not addressed by the legislation, and she discusses the process by which the Social Security Administration subsequently addressed these decisions. Feder argues that the agency could have pursued two fundamentally different strategies. Using a cost-effectiveness strategy, the agency could assess the impact of alternative approaches to a problem (e.g., hospital payment) on cost and quality and select a course that would achieve maximum health care value per dollar spent. Alternatively, with a balancing strategy, the agency could seek to identify relevant political actors (e.g., the American Hospital Association), weigh their capacity to aid or threaten program survival, and select those policies that minimize political conflict (24).

Feder makes a persuasive argument that the Social Security Administration selected a balancing strategy. She traces the various consequences for the public interest of an approach that administratively transfers policy discretion to those provider groups with the greatest stake in the content of that policy. For those who are directly involved in the implementation of the Medicare program, the primary motivation was not to minimize political conflict but to assure access for elderly Social Security beneficiaries to hospital and physician services. At one point, this access was jeopardized because of the vigorous enforcement of the Civil Rights Act by the U.S. Public Health Service and the Social Security Administration on instructions from the Secretary of Health, Education, and Welfare. When compliance with the Civil Rights Act was assured in hospitals, particularly in the South and Southwest, access barriers disappeared. Reimbursement policies followed the intentions of Congress and achieved the initial objective of assuring high levels of hospital and physician participation in Medicare.

Incremental Reform

The powerful role of administrators in the implementation of policy is derived in part from the broad and ambiguous nature of much federal and state health legislation. Despite dramatic improvements in the capacity of congressional staffs to conduct policy analysis, the constraints of politics are such that ambiguity frequently is employed to assure the passage of legislation.

The public policy process in American government can best be described in terms of an incremental model of decision making (25,26). Simply stated, this model posits that policy is made in small steps (increments) and is rarely modified in dramatic ways. Major actors in the political bargaining process, whether legislators, interest groups, or administrators, operate on the basis of certain rules, and these rules are based on adherence to prior policy patterns. Because the consequences of policy change are difficult to predict and because unpredictability is risky in the political market, policymakers prefer reform in small steps to more radical change.

The incremental model was elaborated by decision theorists concerned with understanding how policymakers managed a large information load and the uncertainty of their political environment. Quite a different view, but one that is compatible with this perspective, has been developed by Alford (27). Alford addresses the nature of reform in health care and its ideological basis. He identifies three approaches to reform, including market reformers, who call for an end to government interference in health care delivery and the restoration of market competition in health care institutions, and bureaucratic reformers, who blame market competition for defects in the system and call for increased administrative regulation of health care. What these perspectives share, notes Alford, is that each leads to incremental reform, and the extent to which they challenge fundamental patterns of policy is limited. A third approach, the structural interest perspective, begins with an analysis of the ways in which the other two accept and benefit from current arrangements in health care. This perspective is formulated to challenge the effective institutional control exercised by dominant structural interests that benefit from continuance of the system in its present form. As Alford makes clear, the market and bureaucratic approaches describe the limits of health care reform, and they underlie resistance to change in the health system.

Relatively little research in the United States has examined the institutional and class basis of public policy, including health policy (28). Those who hold that defects in health care are rooted in the structure of a class society would radically alter the present health care system, creating a national health service, with decentralization of administration and community control over health care institutions and health professionals. Those who view defects in health care as having a class basis believe that tinkering with the health care system itself cannot achieve the desired outcomes, but that these outcomes will follow major structural changes in society.

Policy developments of the coming decades will depend on which of these views of health care politics—pluralist, bureaucratic, or class—predominates. To date, the pluralists have played the most influential role in health care politics and policies.

A HISTORICAL FRAMEWORK: THE DEVELOPMENT OF HEALTH POLICY FROM 1798 TO 1982

After a long initial period in which the federal government played virtually no role, the concepts of federalism, pluralistic politics, and incremental reform began to appear, particularly with respect to the role of government, intergovernmental relations within federalism, and the role of the private sector. The private sector in the United States has always maintained a larger role in health care than it has in most other industrial nations, figuring largely in both the financing and delivery of services. While it is not possible in a short space to do full justice to the rich history of health care policy, an effort is made here to present highlights in the development of health policy that reflect the manner in which much has changed and much has stayed the same.

The Evolution of Health Policy: Dual Federalism and the Role of the Private Sector

The slow emergence of public policies and programs related to health and health care in the United States has generally followed the pattern of other industrial countries, particularly those in Western Europe (29). At least three stages in the process have been identified:

1. Private charity, including contracts between users and providers, and public apathy or indifference
2. Public provision of necessary health services that are not provided by voluntary effort and private contract
3. Substitution of public services and financing for private, voluntary, and charitable efforts

Although these three stages have been identified in many nations, different patterns have been observed among industrial countries. Political parties in the United States have been more reluctant than those in European countries or Canada to challenge the medical profession, hospitals, and the health insurance industry to promote health care reform.

The role of government at the federal, state, and local levels in public health and health care evolved in response to changes occurring in the health care system (30). With the major changes in health care that have occurred over the past 200 years, and particularly in the past 50 years, has come a transformation in the role of government.

During the early years of the republic, the federal government played a limited role in public health and health care, which were largely within the jurisdiction of the states and the private sector. Private charity shouldered the responsibility of care for the poor. The federal role in providing health care began in 1798, when Congress passed the Act for the Relief of Sick and Disabled Seamen, which imposed a 20-cent per month tax on seamen's wages for their medical care. The federal government later provided direct medical care for merchant seamen through clinics and hospitals in port cities, a policy that continues to this day. The federal government also played a limited role in imposing quarantines on ships entering U.S. ports in order to prevent epidemics (29). It did little or nothing, however, about the spread of communicable diseases within the nation, a problem that was thought to lie within the jurisdiction of the individual states.

Throughout the eighteenth, nineteenth, and early twentieth centuries, the major diseases in the United States, as in Europe, were infectious diseases, as discussed in Chapter 1. Tuberculosis, pneumonia, bronchitis, and gastrointestinal infections were the major killers. As the sanitary revolution progressed in the nineteenth century, social and economic conditions advanced, nutrition improved, and reproductive behavior was modified, the burden of acute infection declined. National health policies during the nineteenth century were limited to the imposition of quarantines to stop epidemics and the provision of medical care to merchant seamen and members of the armed forces. In laws beginning with the Port Quarantine Act, Congress preempted state and local authority and put an end to long-standing federal-state disagreements over the authority to prevent and control epidemics of yellow fever and cholera, as well as recurring outbreaks of plague and smallpox (31).

States have always played a role in protecting the health of the public, as discussed in detail in Chapter 4. Indeed, state constitutions invariably protect the health of every citizen under the authority of state law (32). States first exercised their public health authority through special committees or commissions. Most active concern with health matters was at the local level. Local boards of health or health departments were organized to tackle problems of sanitation, poor housing, and quarantine. Later, local health departments were set up in rural areas, particularly in the South, to counteract hookworm, malaria, and other infectious diseases that were widespread in the nineteenth and early twentieth centuries. Originally, the emphasis of local health departments in the cities was on environmental sanitation and epidemic diseases (33).

The first state health department was established by Louisiana in 1855, and Massachusetts followed in 1869. Gradually, other states followed suit. By 1915, public health agencies were established in all states. Because of advances in bacteriology, the role of state health departments moved beyond the early concerns with quarantine and sanitation to the scientific control of communicable disease.

The most significant role played by state governments in personal health care was in the establishment of state mental hospitals (Chap. 8). These hospitals first developed as a result of a reform movement in the mid-nineteenth century led by Dorothea Dix. Over the next century, state mental institutions evolved into isolated facilities for custodial care of the chronically mentally ill. The development of these asylums reinforced the stigma attached to mental illness and placed the care of the severely mentally ill outside the mainstream of medicine for more than a century (34).

Hospitals began to evolve in the nineteenth century from almshouses that provided shelter for the poor. Hospital sponsorship at the local level was either public (local government) or through a variety of religious, fraternal, or other community groups. Thus, the nonprofit community hospital was born; this institution, rather than the local public hospital, was gradually to become the primary locus of medical care. Physicians provided voluntary services to the sick poor in order to earn the privilege of caring for their paying patients in the hospital (35). Hospital appointments became important for physicians in order to conduct their practices. Hospitals increased in the late nineteenth century and began to incorporate new medical technologies, such as anesthesia, aseptic surgery, and later radiology. Although charity was the major source of care for the poor, public services also began to grow in the nineteenth century. Gradually, the public sector assumed responsibility for indigent care. The development of the hospital is discussed further in Chapter 6.

The Civil War brought about a dramatic change in the role of the federal government. Not only did the federal government engage in a war to preserve the Union, but it began to expand its role in other ways that significantly altered the nature of federalism in the United States. This changing federal role was reflected in congressional passage of the first program of federal aid to the states—the Morrill Act of 1862, which granted federal lands to each state. Profits from the sale of these lands supported public institutions of higher education, known as *land grant colleges* (36). Toward the end of the nineteenth century, the federal government began to provide cash grants to states for the establishment of agricultural experiment stations. While the federal role generally was expanding, this change had little impact on health care. An important exception occurred in the late 1870s when the Surgeon General of the Marine Hospital Service was given congressional authorization to impose quarantines within the United States. This marked the first time that the federal government assumed public health responsibility in an area where the states had previously held jurisdiction.

The next major change in the role of the federal government was in the regulation of food and drugs. After 20 years of debate and much public pressure, Congress enacted the Federal Food and Drug Act in 1906 to regulate the adulteration and misbranding of food and drugs. The law was designed primarily to protect the pocketbook of consumers, not their health. It represented a major change in the role of the federal government, which assumed a responsibility previously exercised exclusively by the states. The legislation provided some measure of control over impure foods, but it had little impact on impure or unsafe drugs (37).

It was not until 1938, after the death of a number of children due to the use of elixir of sulfonamide, that health protection became a real issue. The result of this disaster was the Food, Drug and Cosmetic Act of 1938, which required manufacturers to demonstrate the safety of drugs before marketing them. This law was a further extension of the federal role, and was consistent with major changes in that role that occurred during the Depression of the 1930s. After the passage of this act, little change was made in drug regulation law until the thalidomide disaster in the early 1960s. Amendments to the Food, Drug and Cosmetic Act in 1962, which were enacted in response to that disaster, specified that drugs must be demonstrated to be effective, as well as safe, before they could be approved for marketing. Advertising was also strictly regulated, and more effective provisions included the removal of unsafe drugs from the market (37).

A number of other important developments in the early decades of the twentieth century had a strong impact on health care and health policy. Among the most significant were reforms in medical education that transformed not only education but professional licensing and, eventually, health care itself. The American Medical Association and the large private foundations (e.g., Carnegie and Rockefeller) played a major role in this process. Voluntary hospitals also grew in number, size, and importance. Medical research discovered new treatments. Infant mortality declined as nutrition, sanitation, living conditions, and maternal and infant care improved. Health care changed in significant ways, but it was little affected by public policy.

The Great Depression had brought action by the federal government to save banks, support small business, provide direct public employment, stimulate public works, regulate financial institutions and business, restore consumer confidence, and provide Social Security in old age. The role of the federal government was transformed within a few years. Federalism evolved from a dual pattern, with a limited role in domestic affairs for the federal government, to a cooperative one, with a strong federal role.

The Evolution of Health Policy: From Dual Federalism to Cooperative Federalism

The Social Security Act of 1935 was the most significant domestic social legislation ever enacted by Congress. It marked the real beginning of what has been termed *cooperative federalism*. The act established the principle of federal aid to the states for public health and welfare assistance. It provided federal grants to states for maternal and child health and crippled children's services (Title V) and for public health (Title VI). It also provided for cash assistance grants to the aged, the blind, and destitute families with dependent children. This cash assistance program provided the basis for the current federal-state programs of medical care for the poor, first as Medical Assistance for the Aged in 1960 and then as Medicaid (Title XIX of the Social Security Act) in 1965. Both later programs linked eligibility for medical care to eligibility for cash assistance. More importantly, however, the Social Security Act of 1935 established the Old Age, Survivors' and Disability Insurance (OASDI) programs that were to provide the philosophical and fiscal basis for Medicare, a program of federal health insurance for the aged, also enacted in 1965 (Title XVIII of the Social Security Act). While passage of the Social Security Act was significant, providing the basis for direct federal income assistance to retired persons and for federal aid to the states in health and welfare, it did not include a program of national health insurance. This omission was due principally to the opposition of the medical profession to any form of health insurance, particularly publicly funded insurance.

Growing attention to maternal and child health, particularly for the poor, was reflected in a temporary program instituted during World War II to pay for the maternity care of wives of Army and Navy enlisted men. This means-tested program successfully demonstrated the capacity of the federal government to administer a national health insurance program. With rapid demobilization after the war and opposition by organized medicine, the program was terminated; but it was often cited by advocates of national health insurance, particularly those who accorded first priority to mothers and infants.

Introduction of the scientific method into medical research at the turn of the century and its gradual acceptance had a profound effect on national health policy and health care. The first clear impact of the growing importance of research was the transformation of the U.S. Public Health Service Hygienic Laboratory, established in 1901 to conduct bacteriologic research and public health studies, into the National Institutes of Health (NIH) in 1930, with broad authority to conduct basic research. This change was followed by enactment of the National Cancer Act of 1937 and the establishment of the National Cancer Institute within the framework of NIH (Chap. 9). There followed multiple legislative enactments during and after World War II that created the present institutes, primarily focused on broad classes of disease such as heart disease, cancer, arthritis, neurologic diseases, and blindness. In the 15 years immediately after World War II, NIH grew from a small government laboratory to the most significant biomedical research institute in the world. NIH became the principal supporter of biomedical research, quickly surpassing industry and private foundations. Indeed, in the period after World War II and until the 1960s, federal support for biomedical research represented one of the few areas of health policy in which the federal government was active. The influence of organized medicine was a critical factor in limiting the federal role in other areas during this period.

In addition to federal support for biomedical research, largely through medical schools and universities, and a limited program of grants to states for public health and maternal and child health programs, federal policy related to hospital planning and construction became of primary importance, as mentioned in Chapter 12. After World War II, it was evident that many of America's hospitals were woefully inadequate; in response, the Hill-Burton federal-state program of hospital planning and construction was launched. Its initial purpose was to provide funds to states to survey the hospital bed supply and develop plans to overcome the hospital shortage, particularly in rural areas. The Hill-Burton Act was amended numerous times as its initial goals were met. This legislation provided the stimulus for a massive hospital construction program, with federal and state subsidies primarily for community, nonprofit, voluntary hospitals. Public hospitals, supported largely by local tax funds to provide care for the poor, received little or no federal support until the needs of private institutions were met. The program became a model of federal-state-private sector cooperation in the distribution of substantial federal resources. It was a prime example of cooperative federalism and the major force—until the enactment of Medicare and Medicaid—behind modernization of the voluntary community hospital system.

After World War II, President Harry S Truman urged Congress to enact a program of national health insurance funded through federal taxes. President Truman's efforts and those of his supporters in Congress and organized labor were thwarted, again largely by the American Medical Association. No progress was made in extending the federal role in financing medical care because of the opposition of the medical profession. It was argued that voluntary health insurance, such as Blue Cross, and commercial insurance could do the job.

By 1953, when the Department of Health, Education, and Welfare (now the Department of Health and Human Services) was created, the federal government's role in the nation's health care system, although limited, was firmly established. This role was designed primarily to support programs and services in the private sector. Biomedical research, research training, and hospital construction were the major pathways for federal support. Traditional public health programs, such as those for venereal disease control, tuberculosis control, and maternal and child health, were supported at minimal levels through categorical grants to the states. Federal support for medical care was restricted to military personnel, veterans, merchant seamen, and native Americans until 1960, when enactment of the Kerr-Mills Law authorized limited federal grants to states for medical assistance for the aged. This program proved short-lived, but it highlighted the need for a far broader federal effort in medical care for the poor and the aged.

The Transformation of Health Policies: The New Frontier, the Great Society, and Creative Federalism (1961–1969)

A number of major federal health policy developments took place between 1961 and 1969, during the presidencies of John F. Kennedy and Lyndon B. Johnson. Although federal support was extended directly to universities, hospitals, and nonprofit institutes conducting research, most federal aid in health was channeled through the states. The term *creative federalism* was applied to policies developed during the Johnson presidency that extended the traditional federal-state relationship to include direct federal support for local governments (cities and counties), nonprofit organizations, and private businesses and corporations to carry out health, education, training, social services, and community development programs (7). The primary means used to forward the goals of creative federalism were grants-in-aid. More than 200 grant programs were enacted during the 5 years of the Johnson presidency.

The categorical programs that developed during the period of creative federalism were numerous and varied. Some programs were based on disease (heart disease, cancer, stroke, and mental illness); some on public assistance eligibility (Medicaid); some on age (Medicare, crippled children); some on institutions (hospitals, nursing homes, neighborhood health centers); some on political jurisdiction (state or local departments of public health); some on geographic areas that did not follow traditional political boundaries (community mental health centers, catchment areas, the Appalachian Regional Commission); and some on activity (research, facility construction, personnel training, and health care financing) (31).

Among the more important new laws enacted during the Johnson presidency were the Health Professions Educational Assistance Act of 1963, which authorized direct federal aid to medical, dental, pharmacy, and other professional schools, as well as to students in these schools; the Maternal and Child Health and Mental Retardation Planning Amendments of 1963, which initiated comprehensive maternal and infant care projects and centers serving the mentally retarded; the Civil Rights Act of 1964, which barred racial discrimination, including segregated schools and hospitals; the Economic Opportunity Act of 1964, which provided authority and funds to establish neighborhood health centers serving low income populations; the Social Security Amendments of 1965, particularly Medicare and Medicaid, which financed medical care for the aged and the poor receiving cash assistance; the Heart Disease, Cancer and Stroke Act of 1965, which launched a national attack on these major killers through regional medical programs; and the Comprehensive Health Planning and Public Health Service Amendments of 1966 and the Partnership for Health Act of 1967, which reestablished the principle of block grants for state public health services (reversing a 30-year trend of categorical federal grants in health). This legislation also created the first nationwide health planning system, which was dramatically changed in the 1970s to focus on regulation of health care as well as health planning (38) (Chap. 12). Of the many new health programs initiated during the Johnson presidency, only Medicare was administered directly by the federal government.

The programs of the Johnson presidency had a profound effect on intergovernmental relationships, the concept of federalism, and federal expenditures for domestic social programs. Grant-in-aid programs alone (excluding Social Security and Medicare) grew from $7 billion at the beginning of the Kennedy-Johnson presidencies in 1961 to $24 billion in 1970, at the end of that era. In the next decade, the impact was to be even more dramatic as federal grant-in-aid expenditures for these programs grew to $82.9 billion in 1980. "Grants-in-aid," note Reagan and Sanzone (7), "constitute a major social invention of our time and are the prototypical, although not statistically dominant (they now constitute over 20 percent of domestic federal outlays), form of federal domestic involvement."

Not only did the programs of the Johnson presidency have a significant effect on the nature and scope of the federal role in domestic social programs; they also had important consequences for health care. Federal funds for biomedical research and training, health personnel development, hospital construction, health care financing, and a variety of categorical programs were designed primarily to improve access to health care and secondarily to improve its quality. Increased attention during this period was given to the notion of health care as a right, a concept similar to the principle of the "earned right" that underlies the Social Security system (39,40).

Although there was a profound change in the role of the federal government, many policies adopted during this time reflected the interests of the medical profession, the hospitals, and the health insurance industry. Medicare and Medicaid hospital reimbursement policies were designed to assure hospital participation. Adoption of the cost-based method of reimbursement proved a boon for hospitals but was very costly for taxpayers. Policies designed to meet the physician shortage of the 1960s eventually developed the full support of organized medicine. Designed to strengthen the capacity of the nation's medical schools to respond to a nationally perceived need, these policies also provided direct benefit to an interest group of growing power—medical schools.

Health Policy in an Era of Limited Resources: From Creative Federalism to New Federalism and Increasing Dependence on Market Forces and the Private Sector

During the 1970s, President Richard M. Nixon coined the term *new federalism* to describe his efforts to move away from the categorical programs of the Johnson years toward general revenue sharing, through which federal revenues are transferred to state and local governments with as few federal strings as possible, and toward block grants, which are allocated to state and local governments for broad general purposes. During the Nixon and Ford presidencies (1969–1977), considerable conflict developed between the executive branch and the Congress with respect to domestic social policy, including the new federalism strategy originally advocated by President Nixon. Congress strongly favored categorical grants, with their detailed provisions, and was opposed to both revenue sharing and block grants. This period also witnessed an erosion of trust between federal middle management and congressional committees and subcommittees (41).

President Nixon also differed sharply from President Johnson in his explicit support for private rather than public efforts to solve the nation's health problems. On this fundamental issue the Nixon administration made its position clear:

> Preference for action in the private sector is based on the fundamentals of our political economy—capitalistic, pluralistic and competitive—as well as upon the desire to strengthen the capability of our private institutions in their effort to provide health services, to finance such services, and to produce the resources that will be needed in the years ahead (42).

Although the Nixon administration attempted to implement its new federalism policies across a broad front, progress was made primarily in the fields of community development, personnel training, and social services. Categorical grant programs in health continued to expand despite attempts by both the Nixon and Ford administrations to transfer program authority and responsibility to the states and to reduce the federal role in domestic social programs. During the period 1965–1975, more than 75 major pieces of health legislation were enacted by Congress, indicating continued support for the categorical approach by the federal government (38).

Although categorical health programs proliferated in the 1960s and 1970s, the expansion of two programs—Medicare and Medicaid—dwarfed the others. While these programs contributed to medical inflation, their growth was due largely to the rising costs of medical care in the 1970s. The federal and state governments became third parties that underwrote the costs of a system that had few cost-constraining elements, and the staggering expenditures had profound effects on health policy.

The federal government's response to skyrocketing medical care costs (and thus governmental expenditures) took a variety of forms. Federal subsidies for the construction of hospitals and other health facilities were replaced by planning and regulatory mechanisms designed to limit their growth. In the mid-1970s, health personnel policies focused on specialty and geographic maldistribution of physicians rather than on physician shortage, and by the late 1970s, concern was expressed about an oversupply of physicians and other health professionals (43). Direct subsidies to expand enrollment in health professions schools were cut back and then eliminated. Funding for biomedical research began to decline in real dollar terms when an abortive "war on cancer" launched by President Nixon appeared to produce few concrete results and when Medicare and Medicaid preempted most federal health dollars.

More important than the constraints placed on resources allocated for health care were regulations instituted to slow the growth of medical care costs (Chap. 12). Two direct actions were taken by the federal government: first, a limit on federal and state payments to hospitals and physicians under Medicare and Medicaid (included in the 1972 Social Security Amendments); second, a period of wage and price control applied to the general economy when the Economic Stabilization Program was introduced to dampen increasing inflation. Wage and price controls on hospitals and physicians were continued after the general restrictions were removed. When controls were lifted in 1974, health care costs again began to climb.

Another regulatory initiative was designed to control costs by limiting the use of hospital care by Medicare and Medicaid beneficiaries. Although the original Medicare and Medicaid legislation required hospital use review committees, these groups appeared to have little effect on hospital use or costs. In 1972, amendments to the Social Security Act (PL 92-103) required the establishment of Professional Standards Review Organizations (PSROs) to review the quality and appropriateness of hospital services provided to beneficiaries of Medicare, Medicaid, and maternal and child health and crippled children programs (paid for under the authority of Title V of the Social Security Act). PSROs are composed of groups of physicians who review hospital records in order to determine if the length of stay and the services provided are appropriate. Results of these efforts have been mixed. In only a few areas where PSROs are in operation is there evidence that cost increases have been restrained, and in these areas it is not clear that the PSRO has been a critical factor.

An attempt was also made to control costs through major changes in the organization of medical care. Efforts were made to stimulate the growth of group practice prepayment plans, which provide comprehensive services for a fixed annual fee. These capitation-based prepayment organizations were defined in federal legislation enacted in 1973 as Health Maintenance Organizations (HMOs). Studies have demonstrated that HMOs provide comprehensive care at significantly less cost than fee-for-service providers, primarily because of lower rates of hospitalization (Chaps. 5 and 11) (44). Predictably, the federal stimulus for development of HMOs encountered strong resistance from organized medicine. Nevertheless, the program enhanced professional and public awareness of HMOs and assisted in the development of a number of small prepaid group practices. The impact on costs at the national level, however, remained minimal.

An additional regulatory initiative enacted during President Nixon's second term was the National Health Planning and Resource Development Act of 1974 (PL 93-641), also discussed in Chapters 6 and 12. This law incorporated some of the planning principles from the Partnership for Health Act of 1967 and the Heart Disease, Cancer and Stroke Act of 1965, both of which were terminated with the enactment of PL 93-641. In addition to the health planning responsibility assigned to State Health Planning and Development Agencies (SHPDAs) and to local Health Systems Agencies (HSAs), the law required that health care facilities obtain prior approval from the state for any expansion, in the form of a certificate of need (CON).

The National Health Planning and Development Act was enacted when decentralization of government authority and the new federalism were primary strategies for achieving national objectives and when the role of special interests, such as organized medicine, was expanding at both federal and state levels. State and local health planning agencies created by the law resisted efforts to impose what they considered to be too much federal direction and regulation. With few exceptions, HSAs were not part of local government, but rather nonprofit private agencies strongly influenced by health care providers, particularly physicians and hospitals represented on their boards of directors. Although health planning agencies were concentrating their efforts on health care costs, particularly those generated by additional hospital beds and technology, these efforts appeared to have little effect in the face of inflationary pressures from the hospital reimbursement policies of Blue Cross, Medicare, Medicaid, and commercial health insurance carriers. The regulatory role that they were required to play, particularly the approval (or disapproval) of the certificate of need required for new hospital and nursing home construction, created growing resistance among providers. Although this regulatory role apparently has had little impact on total investments by hospitals (45), provider opposition to it has led to efforts to limit the authority of health planning agencies.

Although the new federalism advocated by President Ronald Reagan was a dramatic departure from past policies and trends because of the scope of his proposals, these policies were rooted in the comprehensive Health Planning and Public Health Service amendments enacted in 1966 during the presidency of Lyndon Johnson. They were increasingly evident in both the policy initiatives and the budgetary decisions of Presidents Nixon and Ford. Not only were the Nixon and Ford new federalism policies similar to those later advocated by President Reagan, but their fiscal and monetary policies were also designed to reduce the growth of federal spending and program responsibility.

During the presidency of Jimmy Carter (1977–1981), there were few new health policy initiatives. The Carter administration tried without success to push Congress to enact hospital cost containment legislation. Special interests, particularly hospitals and physicians, again prevailed. They were able to convince Congress that a voluntary effort would be more effective. Escalating health care costs did moderate during the debate in Congress, but when mandatory controls were discontinued, costs rose at a record rate. The picture in the late 1970s was one of frustration with efforts to control costs. Concern about access to care became a secondary consideration.

In 1979, when legislative authority for health planning was renewed, two conflicting congressional attitudes emerged: 1) an antiregulatory, procompetitive sentiment that was to grow in the 1980s (46), and 2) a continuing movement toward decentralization of existing planning and regulatory programs, which provided state and local authorities with increasing responsibility. Congress was not anxious to spend more money on medical care, and the procompetitive approach was promoted as a more effective means of cost containment than continued expansion of regulatory cost controls.

Since it is inherently difficult to make specific changes in health planning and regulatory processes that increase beneficial competition, these new provisions simply added impossible goals to the already lofty purposes identified for health planning—improving access and assuring quality of care while controlling costs. These procompetitive, antiregulatory, and prodecentralization forces found full expression 2 years later with the enactment of the Omnibus Budget Reconciliation Act of 1981 and in efforts in 1982 to eliminate federal support for local health planning efforts.

The Reagan administration accelerated the degree and pace of change in policy that had been developing since the early years of the Nixon presidency. The most prominent shifts in federal policy advanced by the Reagan administration that have directly affected health care are 1) a significant reduction in federal expenditures for domestic social programs; 2) decentralization of program authority and responsibility to the states, particularly through block grants; and 3) deregulation and greater emphasis on market forces and competition to address the problem of continuing increases in the costs of medical care. A fourth policy development of major importance, the Economic Recovery Tax Act, will have direct and indirect effects on health care—first, by reducing the fiscal capacity of the federal government to fund programs, and second, by providing possible incentives for private philanthropy. These effects will be mediated largely through philanthropic contributions to independent (nonprofit) institutions, but they cannot begin to compensate for federal revenue losses. The effects of the policy shifts are difficult to gauge, in part because of severe problems in the economy.

An important consequence of the block grants enacted by Congress at the urging of the Reagan administration is that the wide discretion they provide to the states fosters inequities in programs among the states. These inequities, in turn, make it impossible to assure uniform benefits for target populations, such as the poor and the aged, across jurisdictions or to maintain accountability with so many varying state approaches (13). Because the most disadvantaged persons are heavily dependent on state-determined benefits, they are especially vulnerable in this period of economic flux. These policies have also increased pressure on state and local governments to underwrite program costs at the same time that many states, cities, and counties are under great pressure to curb expenditures.

Although the Reagan administration strongly favors deregulation and stimulation of procompetition market forces, this movement has had little impact on federal health care policies except in the health planning area. Indeed, in the Medicare program, the use of regulations to limit hospital reimbursement and physicians' fees has increased. At the state level, however, major changes are underway in response to the growing influence of the free market ideology. In California, major reforms were enacted in 1982 in an attempt to increase competition among hospitals and reduce the costs of Medicaid in that state. Private insurance companies were also authorized to contract directly with hospitals through preferred provider contracts in an attempt to stimulate price competition among hospitals.

Congress has considered a number of procompetition proposals related to Medicare, Medicaid, and private health insurance. Although these proposals differ in detail, several elements characterize the procompetitive approach. These are 1) changes in tax treatment for employers, employees, or both regarding employer contributions to health insurance plans; 2) establishment of incentives or requirements for employers to offer employees multiple choices of health insurance plans, subject to certain limitations with respect to coverage of services and cost sharing, including catastrophic benefits and preventive care; and 3) establishment of Medicare and Medicaid voucher systems under which elderly, disabled, and blind persons would receive a fixed value voucher that could be used toward the purchase of a qualified health insurance plan.

Although President Reagan's new federalism and procompetition-deregulation policies have attracted the greatest attention, it is the dramatic reduction in federal fiscal capacity due to tax cuts and high interest rates that have had the most significant effect on health services. While the federal government is debating cost containment strategies, a number of states have moved to restrict expenditures for Medicaid beneficiaries because of the continued impact of high costs on Medicaid expenditures at the state and federal levels. Several states, including California, have enacted dramatic policy changes, restricting patients' freedom to choose providers, reducing levels of hospital and physician reimbursement, and shifting the burden of large numbers of the poor back to local government. The fiscal crisis—recession, reduced government revenue growth, and record high interest rates—is certain to have a profound effect on health policy at all levels of government.

The politics of limited resources began to dominate the U.S. political scene in the 1970s, and are continuing into the 1980s with little prospect of change. Controlling the costs of health care has become a critical need at the federal and state levels. To date, policy efforts have focused more on limiting federal and state expenditures for Medicare and Medicaid than they have on dealing with the root causes of the problem—reimbursement incentives in Medicare, Medicaid, and private insurance mediated through the fee-for-service health care system that have led to enormous inflation in health care costs.

Given a policy process characterized by limited government roles, federalism, pluralism, administrative bargaining, and incrementalism, prospects are dim for controlling expenditures in ways that protect vulnerable groups such as the poor and the elderly. There is reason to fear that those groups whose needs originally inspired special programs will be asked to relinquish the gains achieved in access to care. Because in terms of potential for political action the interests of these groups remain diffuse, it is unlikely that they can compete effectively in the policy process with the interest groups that have long influenced the shape of public policy in health.

REFERENCES

1. Jonas S, Banta D: Government in the health care delivery system, in Jonas S (ed): *Health Care Delivery in the United States.* New York, Springer Publishing Co, 1981.
2. Marmor TR: *The Politics of Medicare.* Chicago, Eldine Publishing Co, 1973.
3. Vladeck BC: *Unloving Care: The Nursing Home Tragedy.* New York, Basic Books, 1980.
4. Wade RC: The suburban roots of new federlism. *The New York Times Magazine,* August 1, 1982:20, 21, 39, 46.
5. Ginzberg D: Health reform: the outlook for the 1980's. *Inquiry* 1978; 15:311–326.

6. Pechman JA (ed): *Setting National Priorities: The 1980 Budget*. Washington, DC, The Brookings Institution, 1979.

7. Reagan MD, Sanzone JG: *The New Federalism*, ed 2. New York, Oxford University Press, 1981, 7.

8. Hale GE, Palley ML: *The Politics of Federal Grants*. Washington, DC, Congressional Quarterly Press, 1981.

9. Vladeck BC: The design of failure: Health policy and the structure of federalism. *J Health Polit Policy Law* 1979; 4:522–535.

10. Reagan MD: *The New Federalism*. New York, Oxford University Press, 1972.

11. Clarke GJ: The role of the states in the delivery of health services, in Jain SC (ed): *Role of State and Local Governments in Relation to Personal Health Services*. Chapel Hill, University of North Carolina, 1981.

12. Lee RD, Staffeldt RJ: Executive and legislative use of policy analysis in the state budgetary process. *Policy Analysis* 1977; 3:395–405.

13. Estes CL: *The Aging Enterprise*. San Francisco, Jossey-Bass Publishers, 1980.

14. Schattschneider EE: *The Semisovereign People*. New York, Holt, Rinehart & Winston Inc, 1960.

15. Bachrach P: *The Theory of Democratic Elitism: A Critique*. Boston, Little, Brown and Co, 1967.

16. Ginsberg E (ed): *Regionalization and Health Policy*. Government Printing Office, 1977.

17. Silver GA: Medical politics, health policy, party health platforms, promise and performance. *Int J Health Serv* 1976; 6:331–343.

18. McKnight J: The medicalization of politics. Unpublished paper, May 1975.

19. Marmor TR, Wittman DA, Heagy TC: The politics of medical inflation. *J Health Polit Policy Law* 1976; 1:69–84.

20. Feldstein PJ: The politics of health, in Lee PR, Brown N, Red IVSW (eds): *The Nation's Health: Article Booklet*. San Francisco, Boyd and Fraser Publishing Co, 1981, pp 40–42.

21. Sabatier B, Mazmania D: Conditions of effective implementation. *Policy Analysis* 1979; 5:481–504.

22. Lowi TJ: *The End of Liberalism: The Second Republic of the United States*. New York, WW Norton and Co, 1979.

23. Silver GA: Preface: *Uncertainties of Federal Child Health Policies*. Hyattsville, Md, National Center for Health Services Research, 1978.

24. Feder JM: *Medicare: The Politics of Federal Hospital Insurance*. Lexington, Mass, Lexington Books, 1977.

25. Lindblom CE: The science of "muddling through." *Public Adm Rev* 1959; 10:79–88.

26. Wildavsky A: *The Politics of the Budgetary Process*. Boston, Little, Brown and Co, 1964.

27. Alford RR: *Health Care Politics: Ideological and Interest Group Barriers to Reform*. Chicago, University of Chicago Press, 1975.

28. Estes CL: Austerity and aging in the United States: 1980 and beyond. *Int J Health Serv* 1982; 12:573.

29. Lee PR, Silver GA: Health planning—a view from the top with specific reference to the USA, in Fry J, Farndale WAJ (eds): *International Medical Care*. Oxford, Medical and Technical Publishing Co, Ltd, 1972.

30. Torrens PR: Overview of the health services system, in Williams SJ, Torrens PR (eds): *Introduction to Health Services*. New York, John Wiley & Sons Inc, 1980.

31. Lewis I, Sheps C: *The Sick Citadel: The American Academic Medical Center and the Public Interest*. Cambridge, Oelgeschlager, Gunn and Hain, Publishers, Inc, 1983.

32. Miller CA, Gilbert B, Warren DG, et al: Statutory authorizations for the work of local health departments. *Am J Public Health* 1977; 67:940–946.

33. Miller CA, Moos MK, Kotch JB, et al: Role of local health departments in the delivery of ambulatory care, in Jain SC (ed): *Role of State and Local Governments in Relation to Personal Health Services.* Chapel Hill, University of North Carolina, 1981.

34. Foley HA: *Community Mental Health Legislation.* Lexington, Mass, Lexington Books, 1975.

35. Silver GA: *A Spy in the House of Medicine.* Germantown, Md, Aspen Systems Corp, 1976.

36. Hale GE, Palley ML: *The Politics of Federal Grants.* Washington, DC, Congressional Quarterly Press, 1981.

37. Silverman M, Lee P: *Pills, Profits, and Politics.* Berkeley, University of California Press, 1974.

38. US Dept of Health, Education, and Welfare: *Health in America 1776–1976,* publication No. (HRA) 76-616. Government Printing Office, 1976.

39. Lee PR, Jonsen AR: The right to health care. *Am Rev Respir Dis* 1974; 109:591–593.

40. Callahan D: Health and society: Some ethical imperatives. *Daedalus* 1977; 106:1.

41. Walker D: *Toward a Functioning Federalism.* Cambridge, Mass, Winthrop Publishers Inc, 1981.

42. Richardson EL: *Towards a Comprehensive Health Policy in the 1970s.* Dept of Health, Education, and Welfare, 1971.

43. Lee PR, LeRoy L, Stalcup J: *Primary Care in a Specialized World.* Cambridge, Mass, Ballinger Publishing Co, 1976.

44. Luft HS: *Health Maintenance Organizations: Dimensions of Performance.* New York, Wiley Interscience, 1980.

45. Salkever DS, Bice TW: The impact of certificate-of-need controls on hospital investment. *Milbank Mem Fund Q* 54:185–214, 1976.

46. Budetti P: Congressional perspectives on health planning and cost containment: lessons from the 1979 debate and amendments. *J Health Human Resources Adm* 1981; 4:10–19.

EPILOGUE

Issues for the Future

What is the future of the American health care system? What are the issues about which health professionals and others who are interested in health care must be concerned over the next 20 years? What are the pressures and trends that will shape the American health care system in the future?

There seem to be a number of key issues and forces that are becoming increasingly influential in shaping and molding the future. This epilogue briefly identifies these issues and describes why they will be important.

The Real Purpose of Health Care

At the present time, the United States really has a "sickness care" system, not a "health" system. Tremendous amounts of money, energy, and personal resources are presently being spent on the treatment of illnesses after they have started, sometimes (apparently) *long* after they have started. While this country probably has the most sophisticated and elaborate technologic establishment in the world for the treatment of illness, it must be admitted that this is the wrong area of the disease spectrum in which to excel. If, excellence in health is what we want, we should be trying to attack disease earlier, when it may be amenable to simpler treatment or even when it may still be preventable.

The challenge for the future will be one of remaking and reshaping a health care system so that it emphasizes *first* methods of preventing illness from happening, rather than treating illness after it is already present. This process will involve a change in values and attitudes, a change in reimbursement patterns, a change in the provider system, and, most important of all, a change in the power structure of health care. None of these changes will happen easily, and perhaps none of them will happen at all. One thing is certain: The next health care "revolution" in this country, the next major advance, will certainly have to be the establishment of a system that actively promotes healthier life styles and works to prevent or limit the occurrence of chronic disease in all its aspects.

The Establishment of Priorities for Health Care

In 1980, the people of the United States spent $247.2 billion, or 9.4% of the Gross National Product (GNP), on health care. This amounted to $1,067 for every person in our country.

While the amount is staggering, and while the percentage of the GNP spent on health care seems to be increasing each year, these two items by themselves are not of major concern. What should really worry all interested people is that we have no idea whether these funds were spent according to any sort of priority ranking. There is no indication that the money was intentionally and purposefully channeled toward those problems that have the most direct relationship to the *real* health needs of our people. We have no means of identifying the major health problems and translating that information into priorities for organized and concerted action to alleviate them.

For the future, one of the greatest challenges facing our health care system, particularly as it begins to experience the economic realities of budget limitations and reductions, is to establish a means whereby we as a nation can focus our combined resources and energies on those health problems that are most critical for us to solve (or at least soothe). Although it will certainly take a Herculean effort and test the good will and good spirits of everyone involved, we can no longer afford the rather scattered and random approach of spreading our national resources over as wide an array of situations and conditions as possible, with the hope that by using enough money and resources, we will somehow impact everything. There simply will not be enough money available. As a result, we have to establish a more rational system of identifying and attacking the most important conditions.

The Control and Direction of the American Health Care System

A parallel to the issue of better social priorities for health care is the question of control and direction of the American health care system, when (and if) those priorities are ever established. The issue here is the ability of any person to be able to insist that social priorities for health are carried out.

At the present time, the American health care system is a far-flung, eclectic, and internally unrelated collection of separate institutions, programs, and personnel—a genuine nonsystem, to use a much overused term. There is no central organizing or controlling force, either nationally or locally, that can ensure that any portion of the health care system will respond to the highest social priorities, if those priorities are ever set.

Instead, by default, power in the health care system has been exercised by indirection and almost by accident. For a while, power rested in the hands of physicians and the medical professions. Later, it moved to physicians and hospitals, acting in concert. Then power began to move into governmental regulatory and planning agencies. Most recently, it has moved to the major health insurance plans, such as Medicare and Medicaid, Blue Cross, and the employer purchasers of health insurance, where it seems destined to reside for some time. We have not developed a means whereby the parties involved can cooperatively and voluntarily come together to create a set of priorities and a plan under which everyone can move forward in a coordinated and cooperative manner.

This is not to say that there need be a rigid, single, governmentally operated national health care system, as exists in other countries. Rather, the point needs to be made that unless we develop a more acceptable means of establishing social control and direction of our health care system and its parts, that type of national health care system may become inevitable.

The Control of Health Care Costs and the Development of New Financing Mechanisms for Health Care

Little added commentary is needed to emphasize the central importance of controlling the rise in health care costs in the future. It should be noted that health care costs have been rising rapidly again in the last few years (an increase of almost 1% in the proportion of GNP spent on health care—8.9% to 9.8%—from 1980 to 1981) after having been stable for a while (8.6% of the GNP in 1975, 8.7% in 1976, 8.8% in 1977, 8.8% in 1978, and 8.9% in 1979) (Chap. 11). There is an urgent need to stabilize this rather sudden and uncontrolled surge in health care costs, and perhaps even reverse it.

At the same time (and probably in connection with the need to control health care costs), we will certainly have to decide how health care should be financed in the future. This issue will involve a review of both parts of the health care financing equation: how money is gathered to fuel the health care system, and how that money is paid out to providers for doing the work.

In terms of gathering money, one of the key issues will certainly be the individual, out-of-pocket contribution that people will make in the future. Over the past 20 years, this portion of the health care income has shrunk considerably, dropping from 54.9% of the health care dollar in 1960 to 32.4% in 1980 (1). With regard to high cost items such as hospital care, the percentage of personal, out-of-pocket payment is considerably less. The result of this trend has been to shelter the public from the impact of health care costs to such a degree that they no longer are directly involved in or really concerned with these costs; they certainly are no longer an active force in keeping health care costs down. One of the key questions in the future will be how to reinvolve people in the management of their own health care costs, either by reducing their benefits, by increasing their out-of-pocket expenses, or by somehow increasing their own stake in controlling those costs.

In terms of paying out to providers, one of the key issues will be to develop new payment mechanisms that reverse the incentives in such a way as to make the providers more cost conscious and to involve them more directly in the control of health care costs. Health Maintenance Organizations (HMOs), preferred provider organizations, diagnosis-related groups, capitation payments—all these will become increasingly important, as will any number of presently unknown and untried new mechanisms of finance.

Probably the most important single issue in health care financing in the future will be the development of a mechanism that draws physicians into a joint effort with hospitals for the control of health care costs. At the present time, physicians are not at risk in any way for their use of hospital services for their patients and, as a result, are virtually untouched by most cost control efforts aimed at hospitals. The challenge for the future will be to develop a new mechanism (perhaps a single payment to hospitals for all services, medical as well as hospital) that joins the physician's ability to order and use health services to some form of financial and economic accountability and control.

New Mechanisms for Providing Health Care

While all of the other major issues are being debated and deliberated, the usual process of improving the organizational capacity of the health care system will have to continue. In particular, new organizational forms and new programs of service must be continuously designed, tested, and if more effective than those we have now, implemented.

Some of these developments are already taking place with the creation of such diverse new entities as hospice programs, preferred provider organizations, and social HMOs (organizations that attempt to coordinate and provide both social and health services to an enrolled elderly population for a capitation reimbursement). Hopefully, these will be only the first of a wave of new arrangements that will transform the present health care system into one that is more effective and more economical.

Special Areas of Interest or Need

In addition to the new organizational forms that will be required, there are a number of disease states or life situations that will still require special emphasis in the future. These are the subject of health care activity rather than new organizational forms.

What are some of these high priority areas? Certain disease states or conditions such as alcoholism, depression, and emotional disability in general will need increasing attention in the future. Programs of life style change and health promotion that aim at influencing those precursors to chronic disease will also be needed. Programs to promote safety at the work site and the whole subject of using the work environment for general health education and promotion must be explored. Care for the elderly, primarily at home and then in first-stage care facilities, will have to be expanded, and the skilled nursing facilities and nursing homes that already exist must be improved. Problems related to the environment and to hazards that are breathed in, ingested, or otherwise absorbed without our knowledge must be handled more directly and adequately in the future. The list could go on and on, and probably will as one new problem is solved and we move on to the next.

Technology and Health Care

Finally, the whole issue of technology—its development, distribution, and use—will have to be carefully reviewed in the future. The explosion of health care technology that has taken place since World War II shows no sign of abating; indeed, it gives every indication of expanding. Expansion by itself is neither bad nor good, but if it is not controlled by thoughtful people, technology will continue to be the master rather than the servant, and an expensive, sometimes inhuman, master at that.

In contrast to the usual view of technology as a potential monster that needs to be curbed is the belief that while there may be a gross overproduction and over-availability of health care technology, its actual distribution to the population is spotty and frequently inequitable. There are significant subgroups in our population who do not have adequate access to technology because we do not have a universal system of health care delivery; the issue for these subgroups may not be less technology but more.

Maintenance of Pride, Confidence, and Hope

Finally, perhaps the most difficult challenge for the future will be for health care workers to maintain their sense of equilibrium in the midst of the vigorous challenges they face, and their sense of pride in the face of all the criticism and bad publicity they sometimes receive. One of the saddest commentaries on the state of our health care system is the frequent expression of frustration and occasionally hopelessness that one hears from health care workers throughout the country.

There is, in fact, no need for sadness, frustration, or hopelessness about health care in the United States, either now or in the future. Indeed, although the challenges are perhaps stronger and more immediate than they have ever been, the status of health care in the United States has never been better. The health care system is better supported, both financially and emotionally, by the people of this country than it has ever been. What health care workers are able to offer their patients and what can be accomplished by health care is more impressive than ever before. Results are obtainable now for patients in this country that were formerly unheard of and that still cannot be obtained in most other countries. The challenges will certainly remain and perhaps even grow, but it is important for health care professionals to maintain a sense of pride in what they are able to achieve and confidence that good health care will continue to be available to the people of this great country.

REFERENCES

1. Gibson RM, Waldo DR: *Health Care Financing Review*, HCFA publication No. 03123. Health Care Financing Administration, September 1981.

Index

Access to care, 420
Accreditation, 424–425
Act for the Relief of Sick and Disabled
    Seamen, 468
Action for Mental Health Report, 259
Active medical staff, 194
Activities of daily living (ADL), 221
Alcohol Abuse, Drug Abuse, and Mental
    Health Block Grant, 128
Alcohol Abuse and Drug Abuse Act, 132
Almshouses and pesthouses, 173, 174
Alternative decision making, evaluation and,
    440
Ambulatory health care services, 135–171
    design criteria, 166
    governmental programs, 161–163
    historical perspective, 136–139
    institutionally based, 156–161
        emergency room, 160
        outpatient clinics, 157–160
        surgery centers, 160
    list of providers, 138
    middle income America, 17–18
    military system, 24
    noninstitutional, 163–165
    office-based practice, 139–153
        diagnostic and therapeutic services, 142
        distribution by type of service, 140
        drugs prescribed, 143
        group, 145–153
        physicial visits, 139
        reasons and diagnosis, 141
        solo practitioners, 144–145, 150
    organization, 165–169
    poor family, 20
    prepaid group and HMOs, 153–156
    primary, 137
    regionalization, 136–137
    secondary and tertiary, 137–139
    use of, 56
American Cancer Society, 279
American College of Physicians, 205
American College of Surgeons, 205
American Heart Association, 279
American Hospital Association (AHA), 178,
    203, 205
American Medical Association (AMA), 42,
    106, 147, 177, 205, 472
American Psychiatric Association, 252, 258,
    260, 261
American Psychological Association, Vail
    Conference of 1973, 261
American Public Health Association (APHA),
    104, 105, 106, 107, 109, 110–111, 113,
    114
American Rheumatism Association, 37
Antibiotics, 6, 177
APHA, see American Public Health
    Association (APHA)
Appalachian Regional Commission, 473
Area Health Education Centers (AHEC), 319
Arthritis, 300–301
Artificial heart, 42
Asbestos, 41
Associate medical staff, 194–195
Association of State and Territorial Health
    Officials (ASTHO), 114–118
Atherosclerosis, 39–41, 280, 299

Behavioral model, health services use, 66–70
    effect of medical variables, 69–70
    enabling variables, 68
    overview, 67
    predisposing variables, 68
Bellevue Hospital, 3, 8, 176
Blood pressure test, 58

Blue Cross/Blue Shield, 4, 12–13, 16, 74, 178, 204, 206, 395, 476, 482
  common rate approach, 357
  financing health services and, 349, 350, 351, 354, 357–358, 361, 363–364
  operating expenses, 358–360
Breast examination, 57
Bronchitis, 38, 468
Bubonic plague, 4, 91
Bureau of Health Professions, 329

Cancer, 38, 103, 177, 475
Capital expenditures and services (CES), 389, 393–394
Cardiopulmonary resuscitation (CPR), 297
Care for the walking patient, see Ambulatory health care services
Carnegie Foundation, 470
Case management, 233, 363
Categorical grants, 103–104
CDC, see Centers for Disease Control (CDC)
Center for Disease Investigation and Diagnosis, 126
Center for Environmental Health, 126
Center for Epidemiologic Studies, 254
Center for Health Promotion and Education, 126
Center for Prevention Services, 126
Center for Professional Development and Training, 126
Centers for Disease Control (CDC), 125, 126
Cerebrovascular accident (stroke), 37
Certificate of need (CON), 393–394
Certification, 424–425
Chamberlain-Kahn Act of 1918, 100, 101
Charity Organization Societies, 261
Child health care, 80–81
Cholera, 4, 41, 91, 299
Cholesterol, 7
CHP, see Comprehensive Health Planning (CHP)
Chromatography, 286
Chronic illnesses, 6–7
Cigarette smoking, 7, 38
Civilian Health and Medical Program of the Uniformed Services (CHAMPUS), 26
Clean Air Act of 1965, 122
Coinsurance, 360
Commission on Professional and Hospital Activities, 411
Committee on the Costs of Medical Care, 137, 146, 355, 379
Community hospitals, 184–185
  administration, 192–194
  facilities and services, 186–187

governing board, 190–192
  medical staff, 194–196
Community Hypertension Evaluation Clinic Program, 58
Community Mental Health Act, 132
Community Mental Health Centers, 162, 260, 263, 268, 270
Community Mental Health Services, 259, 260
Community rating, 357
Comprehensive Alcohol Abuse and Alcoholism Prevention, Treatment, and Rehabilitation Act of 1970, 128
Comprehensive Health Assessment and Treatment for Poor Children (CHAP), 125
Comprehensive Health Planning (CHP), 206, 378, 381, 382–384, 386, 387, 388
Comprehensive Health Planning and Public Health Service Amendments of 1966, 121, 473
Computerized axial tomography (CAT) scanners, 289
Conjoint funding, 385
Consulting medical staff, 195
Continuing medical education (CME), 424
Cooperative federalism, 471
Coronary bypass surgery, 299, 300
Cost controls, hospital, 206–207
Cost shifting, 354
Council on Scientific Affairs, 42
Courtesy medical staff, 195
Creative federalism, 472–473
Credentials committee, community hospital, 195
Cultural influences, disease and, 43–47
Curandero, 257

Dawson Report, 137, 379, 380
Death, leading causes of (1900–1978), 5
Deductible insurance, 360
Degeneration, disease, 38
Demand, health service, 50–51
Dementia praecox, 250
Dental examinations, 59–60
Dentistry and dentists, 323–328
  auxiliary personnel, 326–328
  geographic distribution, 325–326
  number of, 324
  solo practice, 325
Descriptive trends, use of health services, 51–63
  ambulatory care, 56
  dental examination, 59–60
  hospital use, 60–61
  nursing home, 62

physician use, 52–55
prescription use, 62
selective preventive services, 56–59
summary, 62–63
Diabetes, 36
Diagnosis-related groups (DRGs), 207,
    352–353
Diagnostic and Statistical Manual (DSM), 252
Diagnostic technologies, 282–293
    basic medical research, 285–286
    CAT scanners, 289
    conversion of basic research, 286
    detection of asymptomatic disease, 294–295
    drugs, 295–296
    effects of energy probes on costs, 291–292
    electronics industry, 292–293
    expenditures, 283, 284
    external energy probes, 287–289
    intrinsic energy sources, 286–287
    medical uncertainty principle, 293–294
    radioisotopes, 291
    thermography, 291
    ultrasound, 289–290
Dietary habits, disease and, 43
Digitalis, 38
Diphtheria, 41, 91
Disease, 35–47
    definining, 35–37
    physiologic bases, 37–41
        patterns, 41–43
        symptom production, 39–41
    social and cultural influences, 43–47
    see also names of diseases
Division of Maternal and Infant Hygiene, 100
Donaldson v. O'Conner, 271
DRG, *see* Diagnosis-related groups (DRGs)
Drugs, dangers of, 295–296

Economic Opportunity Act of 1964, 473
Economic Recovery Tax Act, 477
Economic regulation, 391
Economic Stabilization Program (ESP), 206,
    343
Effectiveness evaluation, 435
Efficiency evaluation, 435
EHSOS, *see* Experimental Health Services
    Delivery System (EHSDS)
Electrocardiogram (EKG), 40, 176, 343
Electroencephalogram (EEG), 176
Electronics industry, diagnostic equipment,
    292–293
Elizabethan Poor Laws of 1601, 250
Emergency Medical Services Systems Act of
    1972, 297
Emergency room, 20, 160–161, 297

Emerson Report, 105–106, 109, 110
Emphysema, 38
Employment trends, 305–308
    by decade (1910–1980), 306
    selected occupations (1950–1980), 308
Endometrial carcinoma, 41
Energy probes, effects (on health care costs),
    291–292
Environmental Protection Act of 1970,
    116–117
Epidemiologic Catchment Area (ECA)
    program, 254
Evaluation, 433–457
    definitions, 433–440
    future, 454–456
    managerial process, 435–436
    methods, 443–454
        case studies, 445–446
        experimental design, 449–454
        monitoring, 443–445
        survey research, 446–448
        trend analysis, 448–449
    program, 440–443
    uses of, 439–440
Executive committee, community hospital,
    195
Experience rating, 357
Experimental design, evaluation, 449–454
Experimental Health Services Delivery
    Program, 378
Experimental Health Services Delivery
    System (EHSOS), 384–386
External energy probes, 287–289

Federal Employees Health Benefits Program,
    74
Federal Employees Health Insurance Plan,
    266
Federal health grants, 104
Federalism, 463–464
Federal Mediation and Conciliation Service
    (FMCS), 203–204
Ferrell Study, 98
Financing, health services, 340–371
    arrangements and economic relationships,
        344–355
        hospital, 347–355
        patient-physician, 345–346
        physician reimbursement, 346–347
    expenditures, 340–344
        distribution and sources, 340–342
        trends, 342–344
    insurance coverage, 355–367
        benefit structure, 360–361
        development of, 355–358

Financing, insurance coverage (*Continued*)
  government-financed, 364–367
  HMOs, 361–364
  premiums, 358–360
  public policy issues, 367–371
  mental health, 265–266
  public policy issues, 367–371
Flame photometry, 286
Flexner Report, 177, 278
Food, Drug and Cosmetic Act of 1938, 470
Food, Drug and Cosmetic Act of 1962, 470
Food and Drug Act of 1906, 470
Food and Drug Administration, 132, 391
Foreign medical graduates (FMGs), 309, 312
Formative evaluation, 437
For-profit, investor-owned, or proprietary
    hospitals, 182–184
Frontier Nursing Service (Kentucky), 163

Gastrointestinal infections, 468
"Gay bowel" syndrome, 42
General purpose(block grants), 103
General welfare, concept of, 376
Geriatric assessment units, 233–236
Gonorrhea, 299
Governing board, community hospitals,
    190–192
Government Accounting Office (GAO), 220,
    232
Governmental ambulatory care programs,
    161–163
Graduate Medical Education National
    Advisory Committee (GMENAC), 311,
    312, 323, 334, 335
Gravely disabled, 271
Great Depression, 12, 101, 178, 179, 188,
    355, 366, 379, 380, 470
Group Health Cooperative of Puget Sound,
    146
Group practice, 145–153
  advantages and disadvantages, 151
  assessment, 150–153
  history, 146–147
  number and distribution, 148, 149
  organization, 147–149
  physicians, 149–150
  prepaid, 153–156

Head Start, 123
Health accounting, 421
Health behavior, defined, 71
Health belief model, research findings, 70–73
Health Care Financing Administration
    (HCFA), 30
Health Care personnel, *see* Personnel

Health education, 97
Health insurance, growth of, 177–178. *See
    also* Insurance coverage
Health Insurance Plan of New York, 146
Health Maintenance Organization (HMOs), 7,
    50, 74–75, 153–156, 158–159, 199, 236,
    266, 333, 354, 361–364, 369, 370, 475,
    483
Health officers, 93
Health Planning and Resource Development
    Act of 1974, 117
"Health planning" approach, 30
Health Professions Education Assistance Acts
    (HPEA), 309, 321, 322, 473
Health Services and Mental Health
    Administration (HSMHA), 385, 386
Health services system:
  causes and characteristics, 33–38
    factors associated with services, 49–88
    physiologic and psychologic bases, 35–48
  historical evolution, 3–14
    problems of American people, 4–8
    technology, 8–14
  issues for the future, 481–485
    control and direction, 482–483
    new mechanisms, 483–484
    pride, confidence, and hope, 484–485
    priorities, 481–482
    purpose, 481
    special areas, 484
    technologies, 484
  overview, 14–28
    local government care, 19–23
    military care, 23–28
    private practice, fee-for-service system,
        17–19
    summary of perspectives, 28–31
    trends (1850-present), 15
  policies and politics, 459–480
    dimensions, 462–467
    historical framework, 467–478
  providers, 89–273
    ambulatory care, 135–171
    hospital, 172–215
    LTC versus tender loving care, 216–248
    mental health, 249–273
    public health services, 91–134
  resources, 275–371
    financing services, 340–371
    personnel, 305–339
    technologies, 277–304
  system performance, 373–457
    evaluation, 433–457
    planning and regulation, 375–402
    quality of care, 403–432

use of services, 49–88
  categories and conceptual distinctions,
    50–63
  models and findings, 63–83
Health Systems Agency (HSA), 387, 388
Health to Underserved Rural Areas (HURA),
  69
Heart attack, 40
Heart disease, 5, 177
Heart Disease, Cancer, and Stroke Act of
  1965, 378, 473, 476
Heart failure, 41
Hepatitis, 299
Hill-Burton Act (Hospital Survey and
  Construction Act), 4, 179, 205, 378,
  380–381, 386, 391, 472
Historical development, 3–14
  hospitals, 173–179
  predominant problems of American people,
    4–8
  summary, 14
  technology and, 8–14
    availability, 8–11
    social organization, 11–14
Home health services, 163
Hospital Council of Greater New York,
  379
Hospitals, 6, 172–215, 469
  characteristics, 179–180
    community, 184–185
    financing and ownership, 188–189
    for-profit, 182–184
    multihospital, 185–188
    nonprofit, 184
    public hospitals, 180–182
  development, 3–4
  forces affecting development, 175–179
    health insurance, 177–178
    medical education, 177
    medical science, 175–176
    professional nursing, 176–177
    role of government, 178–179
    specialized technology, 176
  historical development, 173–179
  inpatient services for the poor, 20–21
  internal organization, community hospitals,
    189–196
    administration, 192–194
    governing board, 190–192
    medical staff, 194–196
  nongovernmental insurance relationships,
    353–355
  outpatient clinics, 27
  prospective reimbursement, 351–353
  regulation, 392–393

reimbursement, equity, and growth,
  350–351
reimbursement mechanisms, 347–350
short-stay by geographic area, 62
trends and issues, 196–208
  controls on facilities and services,
    205–206
  control of utilization, 207–208
  cost controls, 206–207
  inflation, 197–200
  regulation, 204
  small and rural hospitals, 200–203
  unionization of personnel, 203–204
use of, 60–61
VA, 26, 28, 162, 258
wards, 21
Hospital Survey and Construction Act of
  1946, see Hill-Burton Act (Hospital
  Survey and Construction Act)
House staff, 195
Human Population Laboratory Longitudinal
  Study, 221
Hypertension, 36–37
Hyperglycemia, 36, 44

"Iatrongenic diseases of institutional life," 240
Ileojejunal bypass, 42
Illness:
  attempts to link with disease, 36
  defining, 35
Illness behavior, 71
Impact evaluation, 435
Independent practice associations (IPAs), 74,
  363, 364
Independent Practice Plan (IPPs), 154
Indian Health Service, 28, 163
Individualism, philosophy of, 12
Inflammation, 38
Inflation, hospital cost, 197–200
Influenza, 4, 299
Informal support, 216
Innovations in Ambulatory Primary Care
  program, 319
Inpatient care:
  ambulatory services, 136–137
  mental disorders, 253
Institutionalization, 3–4
Institutionally based ambulatory services,
  156–161
  emergency room, 160
  outpatient clinics, 157–160
  surgery centers, 160
Insurance coverage, 355–367
  benefit structure, 360–361
  development, 355–358

Insurance coverage (*Continued*)
  government-financed, 364–367
  HMOs, 361, 364
  premiums, 358–360
  public policy issues, 367–371
Interactive problem solving, 440
Interest-group liberalism, 466
Intraobserver reliability, 410
Intrinsic energy sources, diagnostic
    technologies, 286–287
Investor-owned hospital corporations, 183

Johns Hopkins University, 4, 6
Joint Commission on Accreditation of
    Hospitals (JCAH), 184, 204, 205,
    425–426
Joint conference committees, 195
Journal of the American Medical Association,
    278

Kaiser Foundation, 75, 319
Kaiser Foundation Health Plans, 146, 154
Kaiser Permanente, 362
Kaposi's sarcoma, 41
Kear-Mills Law, 472

Laissez-faire approach, 30, 31
Land grant colleges, 470
Learned helplessness, 240
Licensure, 423–424
Linear process, approach to evaluation, 436
Local government health care (poor, inner
    city, minority America), 19–23
Local health department growth (after 1935),
    104–112
  Emerson Report, 105–106
  federal role, 119–120
  period 1946–165, 107–110
  public policy implications, 110–112
Local public health services (before 1935),
    92–97
Long term care (LTC), 80, 216–248
  alternate programs, 234–235
  case management, 232
  definition, 216
  federal programs, 228–232
  in-home services, 231
  as an issue, 217–218
  medical versus social models, 241–244
  nursing home, 216, 218, 219–232
    admission versus resident statistics, 225
    characteristics, 223–224
    discharges, 226
    funding, 226–232
    homes and patients, 222–224

    number of residents, 220
    risk factors, 219–222
    role, 222–226
  quality of care, 237–239
  quality of life, 239–241
  resources, 231
Los Angeles County General Hospital, 259
LTC, *see* Long term care (LTC)

Malaria, 5, 91, 299
Malpractice litigation, 428–429
Managerial process, evaluation and, 435–436
Manhattan Project, 279
Marine Hospital Service, 99–100, 470
Market failures, 376
Market shortage, notion of, 51
Massachusetts General Hospital, 3, 174, 176
Massachusetts Sanitary Commission, 98
Maternal and Child Health (MCH), 116
Maternal and Child Health and Mental
    Retardation Planning Amendments of
    1963, 473
Maternal and Child Health Services Block
    Grant, 120, 124, 127, 128, 129
Mayo Clinic, 146
Measles, 41, 91
Mechanical heart, 301–302
Medical audits, 427
Medical education, 320–321
  advances in, 177
Medical science, advances in, 175–176
Medical staff, community hospital, 194–196
Medical uncertainty principle, 293–294
Medicare and medicaid, 4, 16, 21, 30, 63, 68,
    75, 119, 122, 125, 178, 179, 182, 184,
    188, 191, 199, 200, 204, 206, 207, 217,
    227, 231, 237, 266, 384, 390, 394, 396,
    421, 428, 441–442, 463, 465, 466, 472,
    473, 474, 475, 476, 477–478, 482
  effects of, 13
  expenditures, 13
  financing health services and, 342, 344,
    349, 350, 355, 357, 364, 365–367
  physician visits, 54, 55
  poor family care, 22–23
Medicine man, 257
Mental health services, 249–273
  definitions, 251–252
  development, 257–260
    early system, 257–258
    outpatient services, 258–260
  extent of disorders, 252–257
    admissions to facilities, 255, 256
    inpatient and outpatient care, 253
    prevalence and incidence, 252–254

use of services, 254–257
historical perspectives, 249–252
issues and trends, 268–271
  barriers to service, 269–270
  coordinating services, 269
  mental health law, 270
organization, 265–268
  financing care, 265–266
  insurance coverage, 266–267
  private sector services, 267
  public sector services, 267–268
personnel, 260–265
  miscellaneous providers, 263–265
  psychiatrists, 260
  psychologists, 260–261
Mental Retardation Facilities and Community
  Mental Health Centers Construction
  Act of 1964, 259
Mesothelioma, 42
Metabolic diseases, 38
Middle class, system of health care, 17–19
Military medical care system, 23–28
  VA system, 26–28
Model Cities (Housing and Urban
  Development), 123
Monitoring methods:
  diagnostic technologies, 296–297
  evaluation, 443–445
Morrill Act of 1862, 470
Mountin Report, 105
Multihospital systems, 185–188
Mumps, 41, 91
Municipal health departments, 105
Myocardial infarction, 40

National Academy of Sciences, 279
National Aeronautics and Space
  Administration (NASA), 279
National Ambulatory Medical Care Survey
  (NAMCS), 140, 144
National Association of Social Workers, 261
National Board of Health, 99
National Board of Medical Examiners, 423
National Cancer Act of 1937, 471
National Cancer Institute, 471
National Center for Health Care Technology,
  10
National Center for Health Services Research
  and Development (NCHSR&D), 385,
  386
National Center for Health Statistics, 243
National Center for Prevention and Control of
  Rape, 259
National Channeling Demonstration project,
  233

National Commission on Community Health
  Services, 383
National Health Care Improvement Act of
  1970, 384
National Health Planning and Resources
  Development Act of 1974, 13, 30, 179,
  204, 206, 378, 381, 382, 384, 387–389,
  394, 476
National Health Planning Council, 387
National Health Service (Great Britain), 30,
  137, 347
National Health Services Corps (NHSC), 162,
  319
National High Blood Pressure Education
  program, 58
National Institute for Occupational Safety and
  Health, 126
National Institute of Mental Health (NIMH),
  254, 258
National Institutes of Health (NIH), 4, 9, 279,
  280, 281, 282, 471
National Mental Health Act of 1946, 258, 259
National Public Health Program Reporting
  System (NPHPRS), 114–118
Need, health service, 50
Neighborhood Health Centers, 13, 123
Neoplastic disease, 38
Nephritis, 5
New Haven Hospital, 174, 176
New Jersey State Nurses Association, 262
New York City Health Department, 96
New York Hospital, 174
New York State Nursing Association
  (NYSNA), 333
NIH, see National Institutes of Health (NIH)
NIMH, see National Institute of Mental
  Health (NIMH)
Nonlinear process, alternative evaluation,
  436
Nonprofit hospitals, 184
Nurse practitioners (NPs), 307, 333–336
Nurses and nursing, 328–333
  education and role changes, 331–333
  number of, 330
  supply and shortages, 328–331
  training, 8, 10
Nursing homes, 21–22
  long term care (LTC), 216, 218, 219–232
    admission versus resident statistics, 225
    characteristics, 223–224
    discharges, 226
    funding, 226–232
    homes and patients, 222–224
    number of residents, 220
    risk factors, 219–222

Nursing homes, *(Continued)*
    role, 222–226
    use of, 62
Nursing schools, development of, 176–77

Obesity, 43
Occupational Safety and Health Act, 132
Office-based practice, ambulatory care,
        139–153
    diagnostic and therapeutic services, 142
    distribution by type of service, 140
    drugs prescribed, 143
    group, 145–153
        advantages and disadvantages, 151
        assessment, 150–153
        history, 146–147
        number and distribution, 148, 149
        organization, 147–149
        physicians, 149–150
        prepaid, 153–156
    physician visits, 139
    reasons and principal diagnosis, 141
    solo practitioners, 144–145, 150
Office of Economic Opportunity (OEO), 13,
        123
Office of Technology Assessment (OTA), 11
Ohio River Valley Sanitation Compact, 122
Old Age, Survivors' and Disability Insurance
        (OASDI), 471
Older Americans Act, 227, 230–232
Omnibus Budget Reconciliation Act of 1981,
        120, 127
Ordinary knowledge, evaluation and, 440
Outcome measures of quality, 412–414
Outcome-oriented studies, 420–422
Outpatient care, mental disorders, 253
Outpatient clinics, 157–160
Outpatient services, mental health, 258–250

Pacemakers, 42, 300
Papanicolaou smear, 44, 57
Pancreatic cancer, 41–42
Partnership for Health Act of 1967, 378, 473,
        476
Partnership for Health Amendments of 1967,
        121
Peer Review Assurance Programs, 427
Penicillin, 6
Pennsylvania Hospital, 174
Peptic ulcer, 39
Personnel, 305–339
    dentistry, 323–328
    employment trends, 305–308
    future issues, 336–337
    mental health, 260–265

nurse practitioners (NPs), 333–336
    nursing, 328–333
    physician assistants, 333–336
    physicians, 309–323
Pertussis, 41
PHs, *see* U.S. Public Health Service
Physician-based group insurance (PBGI),
        441–442
Physician draft, 25–26
Physicians, 309–323
    geographic distribution, 316–320
    in group practice, 145–153
    medical education, 320–323
    number of, 310, 311, 313
    patient relationships, 345–346
    ratio of supply to estimated requirements,
        315
    reimbursement, 346–347
    shortage and surplus, 309–311
    solo practitioners, 144–145, 150
    training, 8, 10
    trends in specialty distribution, 311–316
Physicians' assistants (PAs), 307, 333–336
Physician use, 52–55
Physiologic bases, care-seeking behavior,
        35–48
    changing patterns, 41–43
    defining illness and disease, 35–47
    processes involved in, 37–39
    social and cultural influences, 43–47
    symptom production and pathologic
        process, 39–41
Placebos, 45
Plague, *see* Bubonic plague
Planning and regulation, 375–402
    assessment, 396–397
    definitions, 375–376
    origins and development, 378–396
        planning, 378–389
        regulation, 376–378
    rationales, 376–378
Pluralistic politics, 464–9465
Pneumocystis carinii pneumonia, 42
Pneumonia, 5, 468
Policies and politics, 459–480
    dimensions, 462–467
        federalism, 463–464
        incremental reform, 466–467
        pluralism, 464–465
        policy implementation, 465–466
        public and private sector, 462–463
    historical framework, 467–478
        evolution, 468–472
        limited resources, 474–478
        transformation (1961–1969), 472–474

Polio, 41
Pollock v. *Farmer's Loan and Trust Co.*, 102
Poor, inner city minority system of health
    care, 19–23
Poorhouses or workhouses, 173, 174
Port Quarantine Act, 469
Preferred Provider Organization approach, 19
Prepaid group practice, 153–156
    organizational relationships, 153
President's Commission on Heart Disease,
    Cancer, and Stroke, 381
President's Commission on Mental Health,
    254, 260
Preventive Health and Health Services Block
    Grant, 127–128
Preventive services, use of, 56–59
Primary ambulatory care, 137
Primary care, expansion of, 81
Primary Care Block Grant, 128
Private practice, fee-for-service system
    (middle-class, middle income America),
    17–19
Process measures of quality, 414–416
Process-oriented studies, 422–423
Professional nursing, development of, 176–177
Professional Standards Review Organizations
    (PSROs), 199, 204, 207–208, 389,
    394–395, 426, 427–428, 475
Prognostic adjustment factor (PAF), 239
Progress evaluation, 434–435
Project grants, 104, 121–122
PROs, *see* Utilization and Quality Control
    Peer Review Organizations (PROs)
Providers of health services, 89–273
Pseudosolutions, therapeutic technologies,
    301
PSROs, *see* Professional Standards Review
    Organizations (PSROs)
Psychiatric impairment, 254
Psychiatric nurses, 262–263
Psychiatrists, 260
Psychologists, 260–261
Psychotropic drugs, 258
Public and private sector politics, 462–463
Public health departments, 17
Public Health Service Act, 120, 122, 127,
    381, 441
Public health services, 91–134, 164–165, 394,
    466
    disparity between tax base and
        responsibilities, 101–104
    future, 131–132
    period after 1935, 104–131
        local department growth, 104–112
        state agencies, 112–119

period before 1935, 92–101
    federal role, 98–101
    local organization, 92–97
    state agencies, 97–98
    traditional focus, 91–92
Public hospitals, 180–182

Quality of care, 232–239, 403–432
    assessment, 408–409
        data sources, 409
        evaluation, 411–412
        focus, 409
        use of population-based rates, 406–408
    assurance, 423–429
        assessment, 429
        certification and accreditation, 424–425
        licensure, 423–424
        malpractice and, 428–429
        performance-based, 426–428
    major studies (since 1950), 420–423
    measurement issues, 410–412
        outcome-oriented, 420–422
        process-oriented, 422–423
        secondary sources, 410–411
        validity and reliability, 410
    quality assessment methods, 412–420
        access to care, 426
        efficiency, 418–419
        outcome, 412–414
        patient satisfaction, 419
        process measures, 414–416
        provider-patient relationship, 419
    relationship between health and medical
        care, 404–408
Quality of life, 239–241

Radioisotopes, 291
Red Cross, 161
Regional Advisory Groups (RAGs), 382
Regional medical programs, 378, 381–382,
    383, 384, 386
Regional Medical Programs Act, 382
Registrars, 94
Regulation, 389–396
    CES controls, 389, 393–394
    hospital, 392–393
    prospective rate setting, 395–396
    PSROs, 389, 394–395
    types of, 390–392
Relevance, evaluation, 440
Resources, 275–371
    financing services, 340–371
        arrangements and economic relationships,
            344–355
        expenditures, 340–344

Resources, personnel (*Continued*)
    insurance coverage, 355–367
    public policy issues, 367–371
  personnel, 305–339
    employment trends, 305–308
    future issues, 336–337
    nurse practioners (NPs), 333–336
    nursing, 328–333
    physician assistants, 333–336
    physicians, 309–323
  technologies, 277–304
    assessment, 302
    diagnostic, 283–293
    diagnostic imperative, 293–296
    emergency services, 297
    future forecasts, 302–304
    historical perspectives, 278–282
    monitoring methods, 296–297
    therapeutic, 287–302
  see also Providers of health services;
      Services, use of
Rheumatoid arthritis, 37
Robert Wood Johnson Foundation, 319
Rockefeller Foundation, 470
Rouse v. *Cameron*, 270–271
Rubella, 41
Rural health care, 82, 163
Rural Health Clinic Services Act of 1977, 335
Rural Practice Project, 319

St. Luke's Hospital (New York), 9
St. Mary's Hospital (London), 6
Sanitarians, 94
Scarlet fever, 91
Scientific technology, 8–14
  availability, 8–11
  social organization, 11–14
Schizophrenia, 250–251, 258
Seattle Prepaid Health Care Project, 73, 75
Secondary ambulatory care, 137–139
Self-care, 81–82
Senile dementia, 38
Senility, concept of, 243
Services, use of, 49–88
  categories and conceptual distinctions,
    50–60
    ambulatory care, 56
    dental, 59–60
    hospital, 60–61
    market shortage, 51
    need, wants, and demand, 50–51
    physician, 52–55
    prescriptions, 62
    preventive services, 56–59
    resources, 52

    summary, 62–63
    utilization, 51
  models and key findings, 63–83
    assessment of utilization, 82–83
    behavioral research, 66–70
    child health care, 80–81
    classification, 65
    critique, 76–77
    description, 63–66
    frameworks of study, 77–79
    health belief, 70–73
    impact, 73–76
    long term care, 80
    primary care, 81
    self-care, 81–82
  see also Providers of health services
SHAs, *see* State health agencies (SHAs)
Sheppard-Towner Act of 1921, 100, 101
SHPDA, *see* State Health Planning and
    Development Agency (SHPDA)
Sick role behavior, 71
Sixteenth Amendment, 102
Small and rural hospitals, 200–203
  consolidation of community health
    resources, 201–202
  functional differentiation, 202
  regionalization, 202–203
Smallpox, 4, 41, 91, 299
SMSA, *see* Standard Metropolitan Statistical
    Area (SMSA)
Social Functioning Index (SFI), 222
Social influences, disease and, 43–47
Social learning, 440
Social organization, use of technology, 11–14
Social psychiatry, 260
Social regulation, 391
Social Security Act of 1935, 92, 101, 104, 119,
    204, 227, 230, 342, 368, 396, 466, 471,
    475
Social Security Amendments of 1972,
    205–206, 473
Social Service Amendment, 230
Social workers, 261–262
Solo practitioners, 144–145
Specialization, medical, 9, 10, 18, 311–316
Specialized technology, development of, 176
Spectroscopy, 286
Standard Metropolitan Statistical Area
    (SMSA), 58, 108, 316
State and Local Fiscal Assistance Act of 1972,
    124
State and Provincial Health Authorities of
    North America, 106
State health agencies (SHAs), 115–118, 119,
    122, 128, 129, 132

State Health Coordinating Committees
    (SHCCs), 387
State Health Planning and Development
    Agency (SHPDA), 117, 119, 476
State Health Plans, 387
State Medical Facilities Plans, 387
State Plan for the SHPDA, 117
State public health agencies (after 1935),
    112–119
    federal role, 119–120
    NPHPRS data, 114–118
    period 1946–1968, 120–123
    period 1969–1980, 123–129
    public policy implications, 118–119,
        129–131
    trends in organizations and functions,
        113–114
State public health agencies (before 1935),
    97–98
Structural measures of quality, 416–417
Summative evaluation, 437
Surgeon General, see U.S. Surgeon General
Surgery centers, ambulatory, 160
Survey of Low-Income Aged and Disabled,
    221
Survey research, evaluation, 446–448
Symptom production, pathologic process and,
    39–41
Syphilis, 41, 250
System performance, 373–457
    evaluation, 433–457
    planning and regulation, 375–402
    quality of care, 403–432

Tax Equity and Fiscal Responsibility Act of
    1982, 200, 208
Tax revenue resources, service responsibilities
    and, 101–104
    redistribution of revenues, 103–104
Technological resources, 277–304
    advances in, 298–299
    assessment, 302
    basic medical research, 285–286
    CAT scanners, 289
    conversion of basic research, 286
    detection of asymptomatic disease, 294–295
    diagnostic, 283–293
    diagnostic imperative, 293–296
    drugs, 295–296
    effects of energy probes on costs, 291–292
    electronics industry, 292–293
    emergency services, 297
    expenditures, 283, 284
    external energy probes, 287–289
    future forecasts, 302–304

historical perspectives, 278–282
    intrinsic energy sources, 286–287
    mechanical heart, 301–302
    medical uncertainty principle, 293–294
    pseudosolutions, 301
    radioisotopes, 291
    structural substitutes, 300–301
    therapeutic, 297–302
    thermography, 291
    ultrasound, 289–290
Tertiary ambulatory care, 137–139
Tetanus, 41
Therapeutic technologies, 297–302
    advances in, 298–299
    mechanical heart, 301–302
    pseudosolutions, 301
    structural substitutes, 300–301
Thermography, 291
Timelessness, evaluation, 439
Title III of the Older Americans Act, 227,
    230–232
Tomography, 289
Toxic bases for disease, 38
Transcultural psychiatry, 260
Trend analysis, evaluation, 448–449
Tuberculosis, 5, 91, 128, 468
Typhoid fever, 4, 41, 91, 299

Ultrasound, diagnostic, 289–290
Unionization, hospital personnel, 203–204
United Health Care, 74
U.S. Constitution, 99
U.S. Children's Bureau, 100, 104
U.S. Department of Agriculture, 116
U.S. Department of Health, Education, and
    Welfare (HEW), 122–123, 384
U.S. Department of Health and Human
    Services (HHS), 205, 207
U.S. Department of Labor, 100, 104, 307
U.S. Public Health Regional Medical
    Program, 205
U.S. Public Health Service, 96, 100, 105,
    125, 132, 163, 380
    declining prestige, 122–123
U.S. Public Health Service Hygienic
    Laboratory, 471
U.S. Surgeon General, 96, 120, 122, 380, 470
Use of services, see Services, use of
Use review, 426–427
Utilization, health service, 51
Utilization and Quality Control Peer Review
    Organizations (PROs), 208

Vascular disease, 37–38
Vehicle accidents, 43

Veterans Administration (VA), 25, 26–28, 162, 258
  expenditures, 27
  financial benefits, 26–27
  hospitals, 26, 28, 29
Veterans Administration Psychology Training Program, 261
Voluntary hospitals, nineteenth century, 174–175

WAMI program (Washington, Alaska, Montana, and Idaho), 319
Wants, health service, 50
Welfare, 21, 122

Western Interstate Commission for Higher Education (WICHE), 319
Whooping cough, 91
Women and Infant Care (WIC), 116, 128, 129
World Health Organization (WHO), 295
World War II, 9, 11, 12, 16, 107, 178, 179, 258, 260, 261, 380
Wyatt v. Stickney, 271

X-rays, 24, 281, 343
  energy probes for diagnostic information, 288

Yellow fever, 4, 91